Managing Psychosexual Consequences in Chronic Diseases

Elena Vittoria Longhi

Editor

Managing Psychosexual Consequences in Chronic Diseases

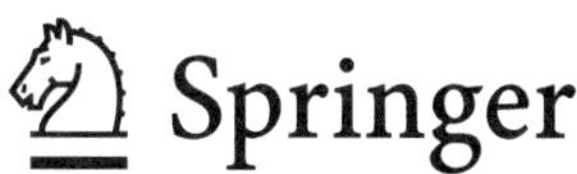 Springer

Editor
Elena Vittoria Longhi
Department of Sexual Medical Center
San Raffaele Hospital
Milano, Italy

ISBN 978-3-031-31309-7   ISBN 978-3-031-31307-3   (eBook)
https://doi.org/10.1007/978-3-031-31307-3

This Springer imprint is published by the registered company Springer Nature Switzerland AG
The registered company address is: Gewerbestrasse 11, 6330 Cham, Switzerland

Foreword

I am very honoured to have the opportunity to write the foreword for the book *Managing Psychosexual Consequences in Chronic Diseases*, a vast field which involved our daily practice in sexual medicine.

Sexual problems in general practice are often hidden from the patient himself or underestimated due to the severity of the chronic disease. The mechanism of interference of chronic illness and its treatments on sexual function may be neurologic, vascular, endocrinologic, musculoskeletal, or psychologic. These issues may have a profound effect on the patient's partner as well as the patient. Doctors need to use and understand colloquial language when describing sexual problems and body parts. Patient education and reassurance are essential. When we are in front of a couple, it is often easier to identify who has the actual problem and work with them individually and establish whether there is a relationship problem.

This is, in many ways, a unique publication because it provides a very comprehensive coverage of difficult psychosexual situations and also an extraordinary collaboration from the top international experts in this challenging field. This book will also prove a valuable reference document for experienced colleagues and for the scientific societies related to Sexual Medicine and Psychosexual Management.

The mission of ESSM is to "promote sexual health and the highest standards of evidence based sexual medicine and clinical care through education, research and the formulation of healthcare". ESSM's scientific and educational partnership with the international societies in this field represents our landmark and points of strength, and these activities are aimed at improving not only our knowledge but above all at the training of doctors who are increasingly able to better manage these problems.

On behalf of the ESSM, I cannot thank enough the Editor, Prof Elena Vittoria Longhi, for having spent a considerable amount of time for motivating and bringing together this amount of information from each author. But at the same time, I also need to thank all the experts in this field for having provided such a high-quality contribution in making this book a reality. Finally, my good wishes to all the readers who would directly benefit from this book.

European Society for Sexual Medicine (ESSM)   Carlo Bettocchi

Foreword

This book, edited by distinguished authors, comprises many in-depth studies on the sexual theme related to chronic illnesses and stands alone as a splendid series of chapters analysing the consequences of chronicity on sexuality. The onset of chronic diseases frequently involves young people and adults, who often share with the partner their illness, their treatment, their deterioration, their improvement, their worries and joys, facing with avoidant or proactive coping the impact on the affective-relational-sexual intimacy.

Several scientific studies correlate the healing of the disease with the recovery of the quality of life, including sexual life.

Sexuality is a complex aspect of human life and is not limited to the sexual act. It is multifactorial and involves biological, psycho-emotional, relational, and socio-cultural factors; it is multi-systemic: from the biological point of view sexual function depends on the integrity and coordination of the nervous, vascular, hormonal, muscular, metabolic, and even immune systems; from the psychological point of view sexual function depends on the relationship with the self and with others.

Sexology requires a multidimensional and multidisciplinary approach and cannot disregard an enriching cultural and methodological "contamination" between professionals in an intra-professional perspective for the "care of the sick person"; this aspect is absolutely central to this volume. The doctor is generally pragmatic and interventionist, operating in a realistic scenario, mainly questioning; the psychologist is expectant and theorizing, dealing with experiences and mental representations, mainly listening; both are potentially victims of an organicistic approach: some address the body, others the mind. The best therapeutic results, however, are obtained with a multidisciplinary approach, and this book, in its treatment of individual illnesses, includes the psychosexual and medical approaches.

The book is a good representation of the interdisciplinary approach that CIS, Centro Italiano di Sessuologia, has been pursuing since it was founded. It is the oldest Italian sexology society and also one of the first in Europe; celebrating its 63rd anniversary this year it was founded in 1959 when Italy was beginning to debate important issues such as voluntary termination of pregnancy and divorce, themes which focus on relationships and sexuality. It is therefore a pleasure to include among our CIS members and trainers at the quadrennial school Dr. Elena Longhi, who by editing this book gives voice to the mission of the CIS: professional integration and the centrality of the patient, taking care or attending to those who ask to be "cured", not simply stopping at the symptom that the person–patient–client brings. To do this it is necessary to know the professional limits and skills of the other professional; we must rethink the pathology of sexual function: symptom or disease? The sick or the sickness?

As Giorgio Rifelli, one of the founders of the CIS and one of the leading exponents of Italian sexology, reminds us: "sexuality is a narrative, a story, a human and social event that cannot be understood solely by analysing its parts without understanding the value of the whole in which its mysterious aspects are revealed. The desire to reduce sexuality to rational knowledge, denying value to emotional knowledge, has created the illusion of being able to access the mystery, revealing it".

Italian Centre of Sexology   Maria Cristina Florini
Bologna, Italy

Foreword

Presently, the world is faced with the most challenging pandemic of the modern era, which is severe acute respiratory syndrome 2 (SARS-CoV-2) infection that causes coronavirus disease (COVID-19). This *book* was developed as a unique and practical means to assist healthcare workers actively engaged in this ongoing pandemic. COVID-19 research has performed incredibly well, although the exceptional speed and quality of the results has often been overshadowed thanks to the publication of insufficiently robust data that was later withdrawn. The initial enthusiasm of politicians and citizens concerning scientific results on SARS-CoV-2 has also faded as a result of public disputes between doctors, scientists, and virologists expressing diverse opinions, and also due to an ill-concealed disappointment that despite all the results obtained the problem still persists. Yet the very fact that unreliable data could be so quickly identified and retracted shows how well science can rigorously evaluate itself, correcting its own path. A plurality of hypotheses and explanations is the heart and lifeblood of scientific research, but these should never be reported as absolute truths, especially if they are not corroborated by robust scientific evidence and validation. The COVID-19 problem is far from solved, but the progress made in its understanding and management seems almost like science fiction to me.

This book is essentially a user's manual to guide the medical practitioner in making adequate clinical judgement quickly with respect to the psychosexual consequences in Chronic Diseases of COVID-19 disease. These aspects are currently little explored and we will see only in the near future the real extent of these consequences.

It is our goal that this book will serve as an effective teaching tool in the recognition and management of the sequelae due to COVID-19 disease.

We hope that you enjoy this book and find it useful.

Dipartimento Scienze Biomediche per La Salute   Fabrizio Ernesto Pregliasco
Università degli Studi di
Milano - IRCCS Galeazzi di Milano
Milan, Italy

Preface

The perception of illness, both acute and chronic, with the resulting clinical complications and impact on quality of life, does not concern the patient alone, but involves all the players in the diagnostic and therapeutic process and the family system to which they belong.

The disease does not only damage the body, but also affects the individual's social, working, emotional, and sexual life. It often compromises compliance, especially in times of pandemic, when the chronic pathology of the patient is compounded by the fear of losing loved ones, the difficulty of locating clinicians (who are involved in intensive care), lifestyle restrictions, and confinement within the home.

Given the context of the volume being written and developed during the first 3 years of the COVID-SARS 19 pandemic, it becomes important to focus on the pathological, social, and individual process involved.

The authors of the various chapters who have shared this project with me have invested their clinical commitment not forgetting their research and drafting of a text that validates the importance of all the systems involved in chronic conditions.

In this sense, the human values inherent in long-term pathology are further reinforced. It does in fact call into question the meaning of existence, self-image, motivation to live, and plans for the future.

In times of pandemic, clinicians, too, often question their own role, as they experience the fragility of their scientific knowledge, and never before, the anguish of death and impotence not only affected doctors but also patients and their relatives.

In all this, it is often forgotten that quality of life also concerns the sexual expression of individuals and their carers. Self-esteem, depression, the chronic pain of certain illnesses, body image, play, the relationship between two people: all this is sexuality.

There is still much to do in terms of the sensitivity of some clinicians in this respect. Asking a diabetic patient, for example, what kind of sexuality they are experiencing is still the prerogative of psychologists and not always of sexologists.

To this end, each chapter of this book presents the clinical part of the chronic disease and the quality of life and sexuality of patients and caregivers. It seeks to offer a systemic description that starts with the pathology and ends with the individual.

The book describes the physiology of chronic pathologies and consequent sexual dynamics, according to the WHO classification. It will be noted that some of these do not show primary sexual dysfunction, such as osteoporosis for example, but indirect intimacy disorders concomitant or consequent to additional disabling pathologies (in the case, fractures or complications of other clinical origin). The treatment thus includes a specialist description of each pathology and the pathophysiology of the resulting male and female sexual dysfunction, primary or secondary.

Clinicians have often wanted to anticipate in their treatment some sexological notes of general indication. Anticipations in this regard show the interest of Clinicians, but not the specific training in this regard, which is therefore deferred to Psychosexologists. The "timidity" in asking patients questions about sexuality is specifically attributable to the specialized training that often defers to an accurate diagnosis and subsequent medical diagnosis and treatment or surgical approach. It follows then that the psychosexologist is often the "facilitator" of a clinical process that safeguards the patient's quality of life in every expression: physical, psychological, relational, sexual, social.

Following the publication of the previous volume *Psychosexual Counseling in Andrological Surgery*, which investigated the quality of life of andrological patients before and after surgery, today *Managing Psychosexual Consequences in Chronic Diseases* enhances clinical research with links to the psychometric questionnaires specific to each of the chronic diseases treated.

Thanks are due to all the co-authors of each individual chapter who have shown faith and invested in this publishing project, the constraints of the pandemic notwithstanding. The Centre for Sexual Medicine, to which I belong, was able to compare its clinical and research experience with other Scientific Institutes and Universities, sharing our interest in a systemic and multidisciplinary clinic.

The prospect of identifying joint strategies to accompany the patient, who has been diagnosed with a chronic pathology, in the path of individualized planning that goes beyond the disease and the restrictive perceptions of daily life is confirmed.

https://novopsych.com.au/assessments/diagnosis/international-trauma-questionnaire-itq/.

Milano, Italy

Elena Vittoria Longhi

Introduction

COVID and the Impact on Individuals and Couples

The COVID-19 pandemic has affected the quality of life of each and every one of us: isolation, restrictions on movement, social distancing, and forced cohabitation have affected people's quality of life and their sexuality. Investigating how the COVID-19 epidemic and its consequences impacted on people's sexuality was the aim of the study by Eleuteri et al. [1] which assessed: variables associated with the improvement or deterioration of the lives of individuals and couples during the pandemic; the use of sex as a coping strategy; the impact of the COVID-19 epidemic on LGBT people.

The results showed that the deterioration of sex life seems to be identical across all genders, men and women, singles, and couples, but also among healthcare workers, whether with or without children.

In addition, a detrimental effect on sexuality was associated with stress, forced cohabitation, routine, anxiety and worry about work and the pandemic, a feeling of distance from one's partner, dissatisfaction with one's partner, and lack of privacy.

During the pandemic, there was an increase in the use of sex toys, passive (often obsessive) viewing of pornographic material, masturbation, and sexual experimentation. Among LGBT people, there was an increase in the number of casual sexual partners, potentially due to the perceived lower likelihood of transmission through sex. In addition, increased sexual activity may have been a strategy to cope with periods of quarantine and the subsequent psychological distress.

This emergency has negatively affected the psychological health of the world's population as a whole, triggering an increase in negative emotions such as anxiety and depression and a decrease in positive emotions and life satisfaction [2]. For example, recent research has shown that this has induced a change in sleep-wake rhythms and a decrease in sleep quality [3], not to mention an increase in anxiety, depression, and harmful alcohol abuse [4]. Other common responses to the pandemic have been fear, anger, guilt, grief and loss, and stress-related post-traumatic symptoms [5].

Mood Disorder

In general, all of the studies that have examined psychological disorders during the COVID-19 pandemic have reported that affected individuals show various symptoms of mental trauma, such as emotional distress, depression, stress, mood swings, irritability, insomnia, attention deficit hyperactivity disorder, post-traumatic stress, and anger [6]. Research has also shown that frequent media exposure can cause distress [7].

Due to the pathogenicity of the virus, the rate of spread, and the resulting high mortality rate, COVID-19 can affect the mental health of individuals in different strata of society, from infected patients and health workers to families, children, students, patients with mental illness, and even workers in other sectors [8].

Luo et al. [9] conducted a systematic review and meta-analysis on the psychological and mental health impact of COVID-19 among healthcare professionals, the general population, and patients at higher risk of COVID-19 published between 1 November 2019 and 25 May 2020.

Sixty-two studies with 162,639 participants from 17 countries were included in the review. The overall prevalence of anxiety and depression was 33% and 28% (23–32%), respectively: especially in patients with COVID-19 (56% [39–73%] and 55% [48–62%]).

The same finding was confirmed among healthcare professionals and the general public. Studies from China, Italy, Turkey, Spain, and Iran reported that common risk factors included being female, being a nurse, having a lower socioeconomic status, having a high risk of contracting COVID-19, and social isolation.

Protective factors included the availability of sufficient medical resources, up-to-date and accurate information, and the adoption of precautionary measures. Policies of social distancing, compulsory lockdowns, periods of isolation, and anxiety about falling ill, together with suspension of manufacturing activity, loss of income and fear of the future, jointly influenced the mental health of both the general population and workers [10].

Mental health problems related to health emergencies, such as anxiety, depression, post-traumatic stress disorder (PTSD), and sleep disorders, are more likely to affect health workers, especially frontline workers, migrant workers, and workers in contact with the public.

Job insecurity, long periods of isolation, and uncertainty about the future worsened the psychological condition, especially in young people and those with a higher education background.

Furthermore, 48 studies were included in a large review.

Between 11 and 73.4% of healthcare workers, including primarily doctors, nurses, and auxiliary staff, reported symptoms of post-traumatic stress during outbreaks, with symptoms lasting 1–3 years in 10–40%. Depressive symptoms were reported in 27.5–50.7%, insomnia symptoms in 34–36.1%, and severe anxiety symptoms in 45%.

General psychiatric symptoms during outbreaks ranged from 17.3% to 75.3%; high levels of work-related stress were reported from 18.1% to 80.1%. Several individual and work-related characteristics could be considered risk or protective factors, such as personality characteristics, level of exposure to affected patients, and organizational support [11].

In contrast, research conducted by Sharif et al. [12] on neurosurgeons after the advent of the first COVID-19 vaccine had a significant impact on the psychological rebalancing of healthcare workers.

Almost half of the 534 neurosurgeons interviewed were from Asia (50.9%), followed by Europe (38.8%). Most of the respondents were under 40 years of age (88%) and almost two thirds were trainees (62.2%). Half of the respondents worked in wards with <40 beds (50.7%) and most practiced in the private sector (72.5%). The majority of the respondents (85.8%) had had COVID-19 positive colleagues in their department and 64% had been exposed to a COVID-19 positive colleague, family member, and/or patient. More than half of the respondents had been exposed to infected patients and/or colleagues and almost half (43.1%) had been tested for COVID-19 when exposed. Almost half of the respondents had been tested for COVID-19 more than twice (52.4%).

Of the respondents, 83% had received at least the first dose of the vaccine. The probability of depression among vaccinated respondents was significantly lower than among their colleagues who had not received the vaccine. Among healthcare workers, neurosurgeons are one of the groups indirectly affected by the pandemic. It is therefore hypothesized that adaptation to the new normal and the advent of vaccines control psychological distress among all groups of health workers, including neurosurgeons.

Sexuality of Individuals and Couples

Let us return to the sexuality of individuals and couples.

In a survey of a sample aged 18 years and over, living in Australia, a qualitative assessment of sex life throughout 2019 and the period after 22 March, coinciding with the lockdown period, was requested [13].

Respondents reported having a sexual partner in both time windows considered, but 89.8% said they did not have a good sexual frequency in 2019 while 60.3% said they had sex during the lockdown. Only 14.3% of participants said they continued to have intimate relationships during the lockdown, compared to the remaining participants (53.5%) who reported no sex at all. The latter were predominantly single (69.1%).

In addition, men who had had sex with men (MSM) reported experiencing less sexual activity during the lockdown compared to 2019, while respondents who lived with their partner were more likely to report the same or increased sexual frequency during the lockdown compared to 2019.

A small proportion of participants (1.2%) reported participating in group sexual encounters, swinging, or troilism since the start of the lockdown compared to 2019.

Further results showed a moderate increase in the number of sexual partners among MSM and an increase in casual sex [14, 15].

Stephenson et al. [16] studied changes in sexual behaviour in a sample of 518 gay, bisexual, and other men who have sex with men (GBMSM). This sample consisted of persons assigned male sex at birth, aged 18–44 years, currently residing in the United States and dependent areas, and reporting sexual experiences in the past 12 months. The authors assessed respondents' experiences of COVID-19 (i.e. employment status, housing stability, food security, drug use, alcohol use, and binge drinking) and perceptions of the prevalence of COVID-19. In addition, changes in sexual behaviour from the start of the COVID-19 epidemic (February 2020 to April/May 2020) compared to 3 months before the pandemic (November 2019 to January 2020) and HIV prevention behaviours were studied.

The results showed that 9% of the sample believed that COVID-19 could be contracted through sexual activities, 94.8% of the respondents believed that the infection could occur through kissing, about half of the participants believed that it could be transmitted through other sexual acts (e.g. oral sex, anal sex, rimming). Men reported that it was not important to reduce the number of sexual partners during COVID-19 and showed willingness to continue their sexual activity during the pandemic. Compared with the previous 3 months, respondents reported a moderate increase in the number of sexual partners and a slight increase in the number of unprotected anal sex partners.

Lack of support and intimacy with family and friends due to COVID-19 restrictions may have worsened LGBT people's vulnerability to depression and negative mental outcomes. A sense of loneliness is typically associated with low levels of well-being and labelled as a risk factor for mental illness (e.g. depression, anxiety, stress, insomnia) [17]. In this sense, it is possible to hypothesize that the individual MSM, who felt more lonely and emotionally distressed, would be more likely to break the rules of restriction and engage in casual sex.

This groundbreaking literature represents the first attempt to understand changes in the sexuality of couples and individuals during a stressful situation such as the COVID-19 pandemic. Its strengths include the investigation of certain factors (e.g. gender, employment, parenting, relationship status) related to changes in the sexual sphere and the transformation of people's sexuality to cope with COVID-related distress, paying attention to different genders and sexual orientations.

Increased substance use was correlated with an increased likelihood of having protected and unprotected sex. Having more free time during quarantine and the disruption of daily routines may have led to more time spent on sexual activities and substance use. In addition, it is possible that increased sexual activity and substance use may represent coping strategies for dealing with quarantine-related distress [18].

Occasional sex during the period of social restrictions due to the pandemic was found to be associated with being younger, being single, having engaged in riskier sexual behaviours prior to the COVID-19 outbreak, and showing lower levels of well-being and higher levels of mental distress. During COVID-19, LGBT people appear to have been at greater risk of social and physical isolation and their condition was worsened by living with families that did not accept them and being away from friends and other important sources of support [19]. These stress factors have had an impact on the sexuality of LGBT people.

Due to social distancing measures, dating apps have become a key means of connection, especially for young MSM [20]. Despite COVID restrictions, there was an increase, or no change, in the use of dating or hook-up apps to meet or connect with other men. In addition, GBMSM reported no change or increase in the number of casual sexual partners. It is possible that men were only looking at the perceived lower likelihood of transmission through sex, underestimating the threat of being in close physical contact. In addition, the lack of effective vaccines and medical treatment and distressing news reports had made people feel more threatened by having sex with a COVID-19 partner than with one with HIV.

The negative impact of quarantine on mental health [21] appears to have been more pronounced in lesbian, gay, bisexual, and transgender (LGBT) people. Previous research has shown that LGBT people were more likely to suffer from psychiatric illnesses such as anxiety disorders and depression [22] than heterosexual people.

The study by Cochran et al. [22] found that women with a homosexual orientation reported consuming alcohol more frequently and in greater quantities than heterosexual women. Likewise, homosexual and bisexual men appeared to be at greater risk of suicide and depressive symptoms than heterosexual men.

MSM also seemed more likely to be single, leading to an increase in mental distress and perceived loneliness.

The pandemic then influenced not only the frequency of porn viewing, but also the emergence of a new type of porn: coronavirus-themed porn. It is possible that this new trend is an expression of the need for sexual novelty and the ability to fetishise practically everything. The increasing engagement with the use of pornography could be due to boredom [23]. It seems that, in addition to having a recreational function, watching pornographic material could represent a strategy to cope with negative emotions, stress, loneliness, depressive feelings, and fear of death [24].

In this regard, a recent study by Gillespie et al. [18], examining sexual thoughts and behaviours with themes of rape and violence, found that younger, male participants (who, among other things, did not comply with social distancing measures and lived alone) were more likely to have entertained thoughts related to rape/violence.

The consumption of pornography on the Internet has been found to be higher: studies in the literature show that 46–74% of men and 16–41% of women actively use pornographic material. These data are supported by one of the most popular pornographic websites, PornHub, which reported over 39 billion searches and 42 billion visits in 2019, suggesting 115 million visits and 18,073 terabytes of data transferred per day [25].

Another reason for this increased consumption of pornography could be related to the use of genital sexuality as a survival mechanism to cope with loneliness, depressive symptoms, and even fear of death [8]. In one study, Peter et al. [26] reported that people mostly used porn to cope with negative relationships and to manage mood and stress disorders.

Research among others has shown that to the extent that the COVID-19 pandemic makes mortality more salient, it would make sense for a person to experience an increase in lust [27] and the need for pornographic devices.

Estimates indicate that while 18 per cent of adolescents have been exposed to pornography with affective themes, 18% have been exposed to pornography with themes of dominance and 10% have been exposed to violent pornography, with exposure to more extreme genres increasing with age [28].

Approximately half of the men who have sex with men reported the perception that pornography had contributed to their involvement in "riskier" sexual behaviour, while over 90% fantasized about engaging in acts similar to those seen in pornography [28]. Young people reported perceptions that pornography had an impact on their sexual relationships, including affecting their libido: young women, for example, reported feeling pressured to engage in anal intercourse with their partners [29].

Conclusion

Mood, Sexuality, Eating Disorder

The public health emergency caused by the COVID-19 pandemic and the measures taken to reduce its spread have had a major impact on health, economies, and societies worldwide. Post-traumatic stress, anxiety, depression, sleep disturbances, rejection, fear, guilt, grief, loss, confusion, and anger were found to be the most common psychological responses to the pandemic [30].

All of these outcomes were generated by lasting isolation, fear of contagion, frustration, boredom, lack of information, financial loss, and stigma. In addition, the similarity of COVID-19 symptoms to those of other diseases, concern for children, fear of losing loved ones, and lack of support for vulnerable people are other threats to psychological well-being. The COVID-19 pandemic has also had a strong impact on the sexuality of individuals and couples [31].

The outbreak of the 2019 coronavirus pandemic (COVID-19) with the consequent adoption of social and physical distancing measures to contain virus transmission resulted in people being exposed to different types of stressors, such as social isolation, deterioration of family and/or individual economic status, disruption to routine activities and daily life, and fear of being infected [32, 33]. As a consequence of such a stressful situation, while some stress-related reactions, such as difficulty in concentrating, irritability, insomnia, and interpersonal conflicts, emerged as physiological responses to the pandemic [34–36], in the general population there was a markedly higher prevalence of pathological anxiety and depression. In line with this, people with a pre-existing psychiatric disorder showed a greater vulnerability in terms of physical and mental distress [37–40], while people with Eating Disorders showed greater food restriction, an increase in excessive exercise, and more frequent episodes of binge eating/laxative use, as well as a worsening of other Eating Disorder-specific and internalizing symptoms (i.e. anxiety, depression, and post-traumatic stress symptoms). These data are supported by the increase observed during the pandemic in the number of urgent and routine referrals of individuals with Eating Disorders [41] as well as the increase in hospital admissions, particularly of adolescents with eating disorders [42, 43].

The study by Vuillier et al. [41] collected qualitative and quantitative data from 207 (76 male) self-selected UK residents with self-reported eating disorders, who described and classified the impact of the pandemic on their symptoms. Regression analysis examined whether emotion regulation strategies were associated with self-reported symptom change, eating disorder symptomatology, and negative emotional states. The thematic analysis explored the causes of erectile dysfunction, coping strategies used, and experiences of psychological intervention. The majority of participants (83.1%) reported a worsening of Eating Disorder symptoms, although the factors influencing the change in symptoms differed among those most recognized by patients in earlier periods.

Qualitative findings indicated that difficult emotions (such as fear and uncertainty), changes in routine, and unhelpful social messages were triggers for restricting or indulging in food. While some participants described using positive coping strategies (such as limiting exposure to social media), others reported resorting to alcohol use and then experiencing erectile dysfunction, obsessive masturbation, feelings of anxiety and frustration.

Apropos of psychological therapies in times of pandemic, "e-therapy" (video call therapies) seems to have had positive results.

The 713 participants in the study by Linardon et al. [44] were optimistic about the wide-ranging benefits of e-therapy. Although three-quarters of participants expressed a preference for face-to-face therapy, a significant proportion of participants (~50%) reported an intention to use an e-therapy programme for current or future eating problems, with higher intention ratings (70%) among those with probable bulimia nervosa (BN). Variables associated with a preference for e-therapy were associated with those who had not undertaken pre-bulimia psychotherapy, whereas more positive attitudes towards e-therapy were associated with professional help sought by healthcare workers and those who had recently experienced pathological eating symptoms.

> If this was the experience of the "healthy" population, how did the pandemic impact on patients suffering from chronic diseases? What price did they pay in addition to their normal therapeutic, social, emotional, and sexual limitations? Here is a compendium.

Caregiver: The Other Face of Chronic Pathology

The psychophysical burden on caregivers of patients with chronic conditions is well documented throughout the scientific literature. It is not uncommon for them to be prone to depression, anxiety, sleep disorders, and post-traumatic stress disorder (PTDS) [45].

Individuals with PTDS are not necessarily victims of an event: witnessing, being involved in, or being informed about the progression of a family member's chronic condition can trigger a major psychophysical traumatic process [46].

A study by Saunders [47] investigated 50 caregivers and 41 patients with heart failure by examining the association between caregiver characteristics and caregiver environment on caregiver burden. Caregivers were interviewed face-to-face using a caregiver characteristic/demographic instrument designed for this study, the Centers for Epidemiological Studies Short Depression Scale, the Caregiver Response Assessment Questionnaire, and the New York Heart Association Functional Classification Guide to obtain the caregiver's perception of the severity of the patient's illness. Patient records were assessed following caregiver interviews for patient demographics, comorbidities, and ejection fraction percentages. Significantly higher levels of burden were found among Caucasian caregivers, those caring for relatives other than the patient, unemployed caregivers, and single-family caregivers compared to two-family caregivers. Fifty-one percent of the variance in caregiver burden was accounted for by the variables of older caregiver age, longer caregiver working hours, more caregiver physical health problems, higher levels of caregiver depressive symptoms, and more patient comorbidities.

Reine [48] starting from the negative consequences of psychiatric disorders on caregivers, assessed not only the inherent burden of the psychiatric patient's symptoms (schizophrenia), their behaviour and socio-demographic characteristics, but also investigated changes in the home routine, in family or social relationships, in work, leisure time, physical health, etc.

The subjective burden concerns mental health and subjective distress among family members.

Hence, research has evaluated psychometric scales to assess caregivers' emotional distress. Among the instruments validated for the research: the Perceived Family Burden Scale (PFBS), the Involvement Evaluation Questionnaire (IEQ), and the Experience of Caregiving Inventory (ECI). A good approach to this domain can be found in the PFBS. It comprises 24 items and the analysis of principal components produces two factors ("active" and "passive"), explaining 35% of the variance, with good consistency and acceptable test-retest reliability. The assessment is both objective (presence or absence) and subjective (induced stress). The Behaviour Disturbance Scale (BDS) can also be considered, although it is less validated.

Furthermore, the ECI containing 66 items consists of ten factors (eight "negative" and two "positive") with good internal consistency. The introduction of two positive factors (rewarding personal experiences, positive aspects of the relationship with the patient) could form the basis of a useful outcome measure for an intervention to promote caregiver well-being. No instrument is yet available to evaluate therapies from the caregiver's perspective.

Ciakowska et al. [49] evaluated and proposed for research (on caregiver stress) the Involvement Evaluation Questionnaire (IEQ). The IEQ is a 31-item questionnaire that is completed by the caregiver. It contains 27 items that can be divided into four subscales (domains): tension (nine items), worry (six items), supervision (six items), and stress (eight items). Two items are displayed in more than one domain. The items are rated on a 5-point Likert scale (never, sometimes, regularly, often, and always). The IEQ has proven to be a reliable instrument to measure consequences for caregivers in mental health care.

Beyond psychometric validations, Adelman et al. [50] sought to delineate the epidemiology of caregiver burden; to provide strategies to diagnose, assess, and intervene to support caregivers in clinical practice; and to evaluate evidence on interventions to avert or mitigate caregiver burden and related caregiver distress. Studies on the relationship between demographic and social risk factors and adverse outcomes of caregiver burden were reviewed. It was investigated through Ovid MEDLINE, AgeLine, and the Cochrane Library.

It was found that risk factors for caregiver burden include being female, low level of education, residence with the caregiver, more hours spent with the sick family member, depression, social isolation, financial stress, and lack of choice in being a caregiver.

A variety of psychosocial and pharmacological interventions have shown mild to modest effectiveness in mitigating caregiver burden and associated manifestations of caregiver distress in high-quality meta-analyses. Psychosocial interventions include support groups or psychoeducational interventions for caregivers of patients with dementia (effect size, 0.09–0.23). Pharmacological interventions include the use of anticholinergic or antipsychotic drugs for dementia or dementia-related behaviours in the recipient (effect size, 0.18–0.27).

Moreover, there are an estimated 5.2 million patients with Alzheimer's disease (AD) in the United States with most receiving care from family and friends (Alzheimer's Association, 2013). A large body of literature shows that the stress and burden of providing care for a loved one with dementia can have negative physical and mental health effects on family members, particularly spouses [51]. At the same time, there is a small body of research that emphasizes the positive aspects of caregiving that can be protective of caregivers' health, such as self-efficacy, quality of relationship, feelings of accomplishment, enriching events in daily life, and a sense of purpose or meaning [52].

Compassionate Love

From here the concept of "compassionate love" emerges as "an attitude towards the other(s), neighbour or stranger or all of humanity; containing feelings, cognitions and behaviours centred on caring, tenderness and orientation to support, help and understand the other(s), particularly when the other(s) is (are) perceived to be suffering or in need" [53]. Although this concept has been applied to a variety of social contexts [52], little is known about how compassionate love is related to the psychological health of informal caregivers. One exception is a qualitative study of end-of-life patients and their caregivers that highlighted the importance of compassionate love or "compassionate care" during the dying process.

Although existing research with young adults demonstrates that feeling compassionate love for others appears to have more benefits for oneself than receiving compassionate love from others [53], compassionate love from caregivers may also benefit the psychological health of caregivers. However, there are consequences. On the one hand, compassionate love may reduce the burden of caring for a loved one, while on the other it represents increased psychological closeness or empathy, which may make caregivers more vigilant about their partner's suffering and cause depression to persist [54]. The fact that compassionate love is not significantly associated with a reduction in depressive symptoms is also consistent with theory and research indicating that despair is a common reaction to imminent loss.

Then again, data from structured interviews of 142 caregivers (98 wives, 44 husbands) indicate that more depressed caregivers are more likely to treat their spouses in potentially harmful ways. However, consistent with hypotheses derived from community relations theory, when the pre-illness relationship between caregiver and care recipient was characterized by mutual responsiveness to each other's needs (i.e. was more communal), caregivers were less depressed and less likely to engage in potentially harmful behaviour. These effects were not attributable to demographic factors, amount of care provided, dementia status of the care recipient, or duration of the caregiving role [55].

Apps for Carers

Attempts have been made to support caregivers through modern technology, although not always with good results. Despite the potential, no intervention for non-professional caregivers delivered via a smartphone app has been shown to prevent depression in caregivers of surgical patients. The aim of the pilot study by Otero P et al. [56] was to evaluate the efficacy and feasibility of an indicated depression prevention intervention for lay caregivers delivered via an app with the addition of teleconferencing.

The intervention was administered to 31 caregivers (mean age = 54.0 years, 93.5% women). An independent evaluation determined the incidence of depression, depressive symptoms, risk of developing depression and variables in the theoretical model (positive environmental reinforcement, negative automatic thoughts) at pre-intervention and post-intervention as well as at 1 and 3 months follow-up. The incidence of depression at 3-month follow-up was 6.5%. There was a significant reduction in depressive symptoms ($p < 0.001$) and in the risk of developing depression ($p < 0.001$) at post-intervention and at one- and three-month follow-up. Model variables improved significantly after the intervention and were associated with post-intervention depressive symptoms. The intervention was more effective in caregivers who had a lower level of depressive symptoms at pre-intervention. Adherence and satisfaction with the intervention were higher.

The same basis for intervention, significant risk of emotional and physical exhaustion of caregivers, informs the study by Ferrè-Grau et al. [57]. The inference is that this situation can negatively affect both caregiver and care receiver.

Intervention programmes can help empower non-professional caregivers of people with chronic illnesses and develop solutions to reduce the physical and psychological consequences of caregiving. The aim of this study was to evaluate the effectiveness of an app-based intervention programme for smartphones to increase positive mental health for lay caregivers. The randomized trial lasted 3 months.

A total of 152 caregivers over 18 years of age with a minimum of 4 months experience as lay caregivers (relatives) were recruited from primary healthcare institutions. Non-professional caregivers were randomized into two groups. In the intervention group, each caregiver installed a smartphone app and used it for 28 days. This app offered them daily activities based on 10 recommendations to promote positive mental health. A change in positive mental health, measured using the Positive Mental Health Questionnaire (PMHQ), and caregiver burden, measured using the 7-item shortened version of the Zarit Caregiver Burden Interview (ZBI-7), were the primary outcomes. User satisfaction was also measured.

In all, 113 of the caregivers completed the study. After the first month of intervention, only one factor of the PMHQ, F1-Personal satisfaction, showed a significant difference between the groups, but was not clinically relevant (0.96; $P = 0.03$). However, the intervention group achieved a higher mean change for the overall PMHQ score (mean change between the groups: 1.40; $P = 0.24$). The results after the third month of intervention showed an increase in PMHQ scores. The mean change in PMHQ score showed a significant difference between the groups (11.43; $P < 0.001$; $d = 0.82$). Significant changes were reported in 5 of the 6 factors, namely F5-Problem solving and self-actualization (5.69; $P < 0.001$; $d = 0.71$), F2-Prosocial attitude (2.47; $P < 0.001$; $d = 1.18$), and F3-Self-control (0.76; $P = 0.03$; $d = 0.50$). The results of the ZBI-7 showed a decrease in caregiver burden in the intervention group, although the results were inconclusive. Approximately 93.9% (46/49) of the app users indicated that they would recommend the app to other caregivers and 56.3% (27/49) agreed that an extension of the programme duration would be beneficial.

In conclusion, an app-based intervention programme was effective in promoting positive mental health and reducing caregiver burden and achieved a wide range of user satisfaction. This study provides evidence that app-based intervention programmes for mobile phones can be useful tools to increase the well-being of lay caregivers.

New technologies notwithstanding, many carers reject the psychophysical support tools available to them. Previous research suggested that the refusal of support services may result from an insufficient adaptation of available services to the unmet needs of caregivers. The study by Zwingmann et al. [58] investigated the needs of 226 carers.

Some 505 needs were identified. While caregivers' refusal rates regarding recommendations concerning mental health (3.6%), physical health (2.5%), and social, legal and financial affairs (0%) were low, caregivers' refusal rates concerning social integration (in particular caregiver support groups) were high (71.7%). Therefore, refusals of family dementia caregivers were mainly related to delegation to caregiver support groups. Caregiver refusals were mainly related to personal caregiver factors ($n = 66$), service-related factors ($n = 6$), relational factors ($n = 1$), and other factors ($n = 17$). Furthermore, the number of caregivers' refusals was mainly associated with the refusal of caregiver support groups. Thus, caregivers visit support groups more often when the PwD shows poor skills in the activities of day to day life.

Using support groups for caregivers would mean admitting their own inadequacy, the emotional and caring failure of the family member most active in the care of the chronic patient. Affective emotionality would seem to prevail over an objective examination of reality where the human limits of chronic caregiving could also represent the references of the caregiver's mental and physical health.

Finally, an Austrian scale, the Carers' Needs Assessment for Dementia, is now available to measure carers' needs. The Italian version: CNA-D (iCNA-D) [59].

Milena Zucca et al. [59] evaluated a sample of 214 volunteer caregivers of dementia patients recruited from the Department of Neuroscience, University of Turin (Italy). All participants were administered the iCNA-D. The validity and reliability of the instrument were assessed using the Beck Depression Inventory (BDI), the Beck Anxiety Inventory (BAI), Symptom Checklist-90 (SCL-90), and the Italian version of Zarit Burden Interview (I-ZBI).

The most common unmet need reported for the iCNA-D was "counseling and emotional support" (31.5%). This item demonstrates adequate reliability with moderate internal consistency for all iCNA-D "summary scores" ($\alpha \geq 0.75$) and a middivision correlation greater than 0.80 for two of them. A better understanding of the needs of family carers could improve the planning of local services and reduce carers' perception of distress and burden. Just as multidisciplinary intervention that takes care of the family system and not only the chronic patient and the caregiver could become a therapeutic approach for caregivers and the family system.

Conclusion

From these observations, it is easy to see how caregivers' stress and concern about the consequences of COVID-19 infection has increased in times of pandemic. This is especially so given the perceived threat of contagion to the chronic patient and the discontinuity in medical care. About 90% of caregivers reported (in the study by Zucca et al. [60, 61]) at least one symptom of stress and almost 30% reported four or more symptoms. The most prevalent symptoms were worry about the consequences of COVID-19 on the patient's health (75%) and anxiety (46%). The main risk factors for stress were identified as an adversarial relationship with the patient and discontinuity of care, but the caregivers being female, of younger age, lower education, and living with the patient also had an impact. The availability of help from institutions or private individuals showed a protective effect against feelings of abandonment, but a negative effect on the patient's risk of contracting COVID-19. The only protective factor was the level of dementia being mild, which was associated with a lower risk of feeling isolated and abandoned.

Involvement Evaluation Questionnaire (IEQ)

https://novopsych.com.au/assessments/diagnosis/international-trauma-questionnaire-itq/

Burden Assessment Scale (BAS)

https://novopsych.com.au/assessments/diagnosis/international-trauma-questionnaire-itq/

Mental Health Inventory (MHI)

https://novopsych.com.au/assessments/diagnosis/international-trauma-questionnaire-itq/

Worrying Sub-Scale

https://novopsych.com.au/assessments/diagnosis/international-trauma-questionnaire-itq/

References

1. Eleuteri S, Alessi F, Petruccelli F, Saladino V. The global impact of the COVID-19 pandemic on the sexuality of individuals and couples. Front Psychol. 2022;12:798260. https://doi.org/10.3389/fpsyg.2021.798260.
2. Salari N, Hosseinian-Far A, Jalali R, Vaisi-Raygani AR, Rasoulpoor S, Mohammadi M, et al. Prevalence of stress, anxiety, depression among the general population during the COVID-19 pandemic: a systematic and meta review. Glob Health. 2020;16:1–11.
3. Cellini N, Canale N, Mioni G, Costa S. Changes in the rhythm of sleep, in the sense of time and in the use of digital media during the COVID-19 blockade in Italy. J Ris Sleep. 2020;29(4):e13074.
4. Pear A. Cognitive, behavioral and emotional disturbances in populations affected by the COVID-19 epidemic. Front Psych. 2020;11:2263.
5. Gawai JP, Singh S, Taksande VD, Sebastian T, Kasturkar P, Ankar RS. Revisione critica sull'impatto del COVID 19 e sulla salute mentale. J Evolut Med Ammaccatura Sci. 2020;9:2158–63.
6. Brooks SK, Webster RK, Smith LE, Woodland L, Wessely S, Greenberg N, et al. The psychological impact of quarantine and how to reduce it: rapid review of the evidence. Lancet. 2020;395(10227):912–20.

7. Neria Y, Sullivan GM. Understanding the mental health effects of indirect exposure to mass trauma through the media. JAMA. 2011;306(12):1374–5.

8. Bao Y, Sun Y, Meng S, Shi J, Lu L. 2019-nCoV epidemic: addressing mental health care to empower society. Lancet. 2020;395(10224):e37–e8.

9. Luo M, Guo L, Yu M, Jiang W, Wang H. The psychological and mental impact of coronavirus disease 2019 (COVID-19) on medical staff and general public - A systematic review and meta-analysis. Psychiatry Res. 2020;291:113190. https://doi.org/10.1016/j.psychres.2020.113190. Epub 2020 Jun 7. PMID: 32563745; PMCID: PMC7276119.

10. Giorgi G, Lecca LI, Alessio F, Finstad GL, Bondanini G, Lulli LG, Arcangeli G, Mucci N. COVID-19-related mental health effects in the workplace: a narrative review. Int J Environ Res Public Health. 2020;17(21):7857. https://doi.org/10.3390/ijerph17217857. PMID: 33120930; PMCID: PMC7663773.

11. Preti E, Di Mattei V, Perego G, Ferrari F, Mazzetti M, Taranto P, Di Pierro R, Madeddu F, Calati R. The psychological impact of epidemic and pandemic outbreaks on healthcare workers: rapid review of the evidence. Curr Psychiatry Rep. 2020;22(8):43. https://doi.org/10.1007/s11920-020-01166-z. PMID: 32651717; PMCID: PMC7350408.

12. Sharif S, Amin F, Hafiz M, Costa F, Dahlan RH, Vaishya S, Peev N, Benzel E, World Spinal Column Society Executive Board. A year of pandemic-comparison of depression among neurosurgeons after the advent of the COVID-19 vaccine. World Neurosurg. 2022;159:e466–78. https://doi.org/10.1016/j.wneu.2021.12.076. Epub ahead of print. PMID: 34973442; PMCID: PMC8756812.

13. Coombe J, Kong FY, Bittleston H, Williams H, Tomnay J, Vaisey A, et al. Love during the lockdown: the results of an online survey examining the impact of COVID-19 on the sexual health of people living in Australia. Sex Transm Infect. 2021;97:357–62. https://doi.org/10.1136/sextrans-2020-054688.

14. Shilo G, Mor Z. COVID-19 and changes in sexual behavior of men who have sex with men: results of an online survey. J Sex Med. 2020;17:1827–34. https://doi.org/10.1016/j.jsxm.2020.07.085.

15. Shilo G, Mor Z. Sexual practices and risk behaviors of Israeli adult heterosexual men. Treat AIDS. 2020;32:567–71. https://doi.org/10.1080/09540121.2019.1634786.

16. Stephenson R, Chavanduka TM, Rosso MT, Sullivan SP, Pitter RA, Hunter AS, et al. Sex in the days of COVID-19: results of an online survey of gays, bisexuals and other men who have sex with male experience of sex and HIV. Behav AIDS. 2020;25:40–8. https://doi.org/10.1007/s10461-020-03024-8.

17. Banerjee D, Rai M. Social isolation in COVID-19: the impact of loneliness. int. J Soc Psychiatry. 2020;66:525–7.

18. Gillespie SM, Jones A, Uzieblo K, Garofalo C, Robinson E. Addressing the use of sex during the 2019 coronavirus (COVID-19) outbreak in the UK. J Sex Med. 2021;18:50–62. https://doi.org/10.1016/j.jsxm.2020.11.002.

19. Barrientos J, Guzmán-González M, Urzúa A, Ulloa F. Psychosocial impact of the COVID-19 pandemic on LGBT people in Chile. Theol Sex. 2021;30:e35–41. https://doi.org/10.1016/j.sexol.2020.12.006.
20. Sanchez TH, Zlotorzynska M, Rai M, Baral SD. Characterize the impact of COVID-19 on men having sex with men in the United States in April 2020. Behavior AIDS. 2020;24:2024–32. https://doi.org/10.1007/s10461-020-02894-2.
21. Cao W, Fang Z, Hou G, Han MX, Dong J, Zheng J. The psychological impact of the COVID-19 outbreak on university students in China. Res Psychiatry. 2020;287:112934. https://doi.org/10.1016/j.psychres.2020.112934.
22. Cochran SD, Mays VM. Lifetime prevalence of suicide symptoms and affective disorders among men reporting same-sex sexual partners: NHANES III results. Am J Public Health. 2000;90:573. https://doi.org/10.2105/AJPH.90.4.573.
23. Zattoni F, Gül M, Soligo M, Morlacco A, Motterle G, Collavino J, et al. The impact of the COVID-19 pandemic on pornography habits: a global trend analysis from Google. Int J Impot Res. 2020;33:824–31. https://doi.org/10.1038/s41443-020-00380-w.
24. Velotti P, Rogier G, Beomonte Zobel S, Castellano R, Tambelli R. Loneliness, emotional dysregulation, and internalizing symptoms during covid-19: a structural equation modeling approach. Front Psych. 2020;11:1498. https://doi.org/10.3389/fpsyt.2020.581494.
25. Zhang Y, Ma ZF. Impact of the COVID-19 pandemic on mental health and quality of life among local residents in Liaison Province, China: a cross-sectional study. Int J Environ Res Public Health. 2020;17:2381.
26. Peter J, Valkenburg PM. The use of sexually explicit Internet material and its antecedents: a longitudinal comparison between adolescents and adults. Sex Behav Bow. 2011;40:1015–25.
27. Goldenberg JL, McCoy SK, Pyszczynski T, Greenberg J, Solomon S. The body as a source of self-esteem: the effect of mortality saliency on body identification, interest in sex, and appearance tracking. J Pers Soc Psychol. 2000;79:118–30.
28. Schrimshaw EW, Antebi-Gruszka N, Downing MJ. View internet-based sexually explicit media as a risk factor for condomless anal sex among men who have sex with men in four U.S. cities. PLoS One. 2016;11(4):65–77.
29. Marston C, Lewis R. Anal heterosexuality among young people and implications for health promotion: a qualitative study in the UK. BMJ Open. 2014;4(8):e004996. https://doi.org/10.1136/bmjopen-2014-004996.
30. Gawai JP, Singh S, Taksande VD, Sebastian T, Kasturkar P, Ankar RS. Critical review on the impact of COVID 19 and mental health. J Evolut Med Dent Sci. 2020;9:2158–63.
31. Eleuteri S, Terzitta G. Sexuality during the COVID-19 pandemic: the importance of the Internet. Theol Sex. 2021;30:e55–60. https://doi.org/10.1016/j.sexol.2020.12.008.

32. Adhanom-Ghebreyesus T. Addressing mental health needs: an integral part of the COVID-19 response. World Psychiatry. 2020;19:129–30.
33. Wasserman D, Iosue M, Wuestefeld A, Carli V. Adaptation of evidence-based suicide prevention strategies during and after the COVID-19 pandemic. World Psychiatry. 2020;19:294–306.
34. Galea S, Merchant RM, Lurie N. The mental health consequences of COVID-19 and physical distancing: the need for prevention and early intervention. JAMA Int Med. 2020;180:817–8. https://doi.org/10.1001/jamainternmed.2020.1562.
35. Rooksby M, Furuhashi T, McLeod HJ. Hikikomori: a hidden need for mental health following the COVID-19 pandemic. World Psychiatry. 2020;19:399–400. https://doi.org/10.1002/wps.20804.
36. Vinkers CH, van Amelsvoort T, Bisson JI, Branchi I, Cryan JF, Domschke K, Howes OD, Manchia M, Pinto L, de Quervain D, et al. Stress resilience during the coronavirus pandemic. Eur Neuropsychopharmacol. 2020;35:12–6.
37. Stewart DE. Appelbaum PS COVID-19 and the responsibility of psychiatrists: a WPA summary paper. World Psychiatry. 2020;19:406–7.
38. Unützer J, Kimmel RJ, Snowden M. Psychiatry in the age of COVID-19. World Psychiatry. 2020;19:130–1. https://doi.org/10.1002/wps.20766.
39. Wang Q, Xu R, Volkow ND. Increased risk of COVID-19 infection and mortality in people with mental disorders: analysis from electronic health records in the United States. World Psychiatry. 2021;20:124–30.
40. Marazziti D, Stahl SM. The relevance of the COVID-19 pandemic in psychiatry. World Psychiatry. 2020;19:261.
41. Vuillier L, May L, Greville-Harris M, Surman R, Moseley RL. The impact of the COVID-19 pandemic on individuals with eating disorders: the role of regulating emotions and exploring online treatment experiences. J Eat Disord. 2021;9:1–18.
42. Frayn M, Fojtu C, Juarascio A. COVID-19 and binge eating: patients' perceptions of eating disorder symptoms; teletherapy; and therapeutic implications. Corr Psychic. 2021;40:6249–58.
43. Shaw H, Robertson S, Ranceva N. What has been the impact of a global pandemic blockade (COVID-19) period on experiences within an eating disorder service? A service assessment of the views of patients, parents/carers, and staff. J Eat Disord. 2021;9:14.
44. Linardon J, Shatte A, Tepper H, Fuller-Tyszkiewicz M. A survey study of attitudes toward, and preferences for, e-therapy interventions for eating disorder psychopathology. Int J Eat Disord. 2020;53(6):907–16.
45. Carmassi C, et al. Risk and protective factors for PTSD in caregivers of adult patients with illness: a systematic review. Int J Environ Res Public Health. 2020;17:5888.
46. Johnson H, et al. The development and maintenance of post traumatic stress disorder (PTDS) in adults. Clin Psychol Rev. 2008;28:36–47.

47. Saunders MM. Factors associated with caregiver burden in heart failure family caregivers. West J Nurs Res. 2008;30(8):943–59.
48. Reine G, Lancon C, Simeoni MC, Duplan S, Auquier P. La charge des aidants naturels de patients schizophrènes: revue critique des instruments d'évaluation [Caregiver burden in relatives of persons with schizophrenia: an overview of measure instruments]. Encéphale. 2003;29(2):137–47.
49. Ciakowska M, Hadryś T, Kiejna A. Kwestionariusz Oceny Zaangazowania (Involvement Evaluation Questionnaire)--charakterystyka i zastosowanie [Involvement Evaluation Questionnaire--description and application]. Psychiatr Pol. 2009;43(4):435–44.
50. Adelman RD, Tmanova LL, Delgado D, Dion S, Lachs MS. Caregiver burden: a clinical review. JAMA. 2014;311(10):1052–60.
51. Pinquart M, Sörensen S. Associations of caregiving stressors and elevation with caregiver burden and depressive mood: a meta-analysis. J Gerontol Psychol Sci. 2003;58:112–26.
52. Roberts LJ, Wise M, DuBenske LL. Compassionate family care in the light and shadow of death. In: Fehr B, Sprecher S, Underwood LG, Fehr B, Sprecher S, Underwood LG, editors. The science of compassionate love: theory, research, and applications. Malden, MA: Wiley-Blackwell; 2009. p. 311–44.
53. Sprecher S, Fehr B, Zimmerman C. Expectation for mood improvement as a result of help: the effects of gender and compassionate love. Sex Roles. 2007;56:543–9.
54. Monin JK, Schulz R, Kershaw TS. Attachment orientations of caregiving spouses and physical and psychological health of people with Alzheimer's disease. Aging Ment Health. 2013;17:508–16.
55. Williamson GM, Shaffer DR. Relationship quality and potentially harmful behaviors by spousal caregivers: how we were then, how we are now. The Family Relationships in Late Life Project. Psychol Aging. 2001;16(2):217–26.
56. Otero P, Hita I, Torres ÁJ, Vázquez FL. Brief psychological intervention through mobile app and conference calls for the prevention of depression in non-professional caregivers: a pilot study. Int J Environ Res Public Health. 2020;17(12):4578.
57. Ferré-Grau C, Raigal-Aran L, Lorca-Cabrera J, Lluch-Canut T, Ferré-Bergadà M, Lleixá-Fortuño M, Puig-Llobet M, Miguel-Ruiz MD, Albacar-Riobóo N. A mobile app-based intervention program for nonprofessional caregivers to promote positive mental health: randomized controlled trial. JMIR Mhealth Uhealth. 2021;9(1):e21708.
58. Zwingmann I, Dreier-Wolfgramm A, Esser A, Wucherer D, Thyrian JR, Eichler T, Kaczynski A, Monsees J, Keller A, Hertel J, Kilimann I, Teipel S, Michalowsky B, Hoffmann W. Why do family dementia caregivers reject caregiver support services? Analyzing types of rejection and associated health-impairments in a

cluster-randomized controlled intervention trial. BMC Health Serv Res. 2020;20(1):121.
59. Zucca M, Rubino E, Vacca A, De Martino P, Caglio M, Marcinnó A, Bo M, Rainero I. The Carers' Needs Assessment for Dementia (CNA-D): a validation study in the Italian population. Neurol Sci. 2022;43(1):275–84.
60. Zucca M, Isella V, Lorenzo RD, Marra C, Cagnin A, Cupidi C, Bonanni L, Laganà V, Rubino E, Vanacore N, Agosta F, Caffarra P, Sambati R, Quaranta D, Guglielmi V, Appollonio IM, Logroscino G, Filippi M, Tedeschi G, Ferrarese C, Rainero I, Bruni AC, SINdem COVID-19 Study Group. Being the family caregiver of a patient with dementia during the coronavirus disease 2019 lockdown. Front Aging Neurosci. 2021;43(1):275–84.
61. Yoder VC, Virden TB, Amin K. Pornography and loneliness on the Internet: an association? Compuls Drug Addict. 2005;12:19–44.

Department of Sexual Medical Center   Elena Vittoria Longhi
San Raffaele Hospital
Milano, Italy

Contents

Part XI Inflammatory Bowel Diseases

Part XII Hypogonadism

Part XIII Neurology

Part XIV Odontoiatry

Part XV Ophthalmology

Part XVI Orthopaedics and Traumatology

Contributors

Marco Agrifoglio, MD, PhD Centro Cardiologico Monzino IRCCS, Milan, Italy

Department of Biomedical Surgical and Dental Sciences, University of Milan, Milan, Italy

Chiara Annunziata Pasqualina Anghelone Breast Surgeon, Breast Unit, ASST Ospedale Maggiore di Lodi, Lodi, Italy

Breast Surgeon, Breast Unit, SC Chirurgia Generale 3 -Senologia, Fondazione IRCCS Policlinico San Matteo, Pavia, Italy

Simone Antonini Endocrinology Unit, IRCCS Humanitas Research Hospital, Rozzano, Italy

Department of Biomedical Sciences, Humanitas University, Rozzano, Italy

Graziano Barera, MD Department of Pediatrics, IRCCS San Raffaele Scientific Institute, Milan, Italy

Elena Bartoloni Rheumatology Unit, Department of Medicine and Surgery, University of Perugia, Perugia, Italy

Matteo Bassetti, MD, PhD Clinica Malattie Infettive, Università degli Studi di Genova e IRCCS Policlinico San Martino, Genova, Italy

Alessandra Bassotti IRCCS Policlinico, Ehlers-Danlos Center, Milan, Italy

Mauro Belluz, MD IRCCS Gavazzeni, Milan, Italy

Maria Francesca Birtolo Endocrinology Unit, IRCCS Humanitas Research Hospital, Rozzano, Italy

Department of Biomedical Sciences, Humanitas University, Rozzano, Italy

Chiara Bosisio, MD Maternal and Pediatric Department USSD Centro PMA, ASST Papa Giovanni XXIII, Bergamo, Italy

Maria Chiara Buscarinu Department of Neuroscience, Mental Health and Sense Organs (NESMOS), Sapienza University of Rome, Rome, Italy

Stefano Buttò "Surveillance and Pathogenesis of HIV Variants and Associated Co-infections"-National Center for HIV/AIDS Research-Istituto Superiore di Sanità, Roma, Italy

Flavia Caretto CulturAutismo Onlus, Rome, Italy

Raffaella Chionna Gynecology and Obstetrics Unit, Menopause Center, IRCCS San Raffaele, Milan, Italy

Bruno Colombo, MD Neurological Department, Headache and Pain Unit, San Raffaele Hospital, Vita-Salute University, Milan, Italy

Marco Comoglio Medical Diabetes Association, AMD Comunicazione, Turin, Italy

Salvato Damiano Orthopedics and Traumatology Unit, IRCCS San Raffaele Hospital, Vita - Salute San Raffalele University, Milan, Italy

Letizia Maria Fatti Department of Medical Biotechnologies and Translational Medicine, University of Milan, Milan, Italy

Luigi Ferini-Strambi Department of Clinical Neurosciences, Vita-Salute San Raffaele University, Milan, Italy

Department of Clinical Neurosciences, Neurology-Sleep Disorder Center, IRCCS San Raffaele Scientific Institute, Milan, Italy

Maria Teresa Fierro Dermatology Clinic, University of Turin, Turin, Italy

Federica Fossataro Eye Clinic, Melegnano Hospital, Milan, Italy

Fondazione Retina 3000, Milan, Italy

Ciro Franzese Radiotherapy and Radiosurgery Department, Humanitas Clinical and Research Center—IRCCS, Milan, Italy

Department of Biomedical Sciences, Humanitas University, Milan, Italy

Francesco Maria Fusi, MD Maternal and Pediatric Department USSD Centro PMA, ASST Papa Giovanni XXIII, Bergamo, Italy

School of Obstetrics University of Milano Bicocca, Milan, Italy

Mariano Galdiero Department of Internal Medicine, Endocrinology and Andrology Section, A. Rizzoli Hospital, Ischia Island, Naples, Italy

Marco Gennari, MD Centro Cardiologico Monzino IRCCS, Milan, Italy

Roberto Gerli Rheumatology Unit, Department of Medicine and Surgery, University of Perugia, Perugia, Italy

Placella Giacomo Orthopedics and Traumatology Unit, IRCCS San Raffaele Hospital, Vita - Salute San Raffalele University, Milan, Italy

Marco Giandotti Urology and Oncology Unit, Pio XI Institute, Rome, Italy

Raffeale Giannattasio PPS San Gennaro, ASL Napoli 1 Centro, Naples, Italy

Carlo Hanau Association Cimadori for Italian Research on Down Syndrome, Autism and Brain Damage (A.P.R.I.), OdV, ETS, Bologna, Italy

Programming of Social and Health Services, The University of Modena and Reggio Emilia, Modena, Italy

Rodolfo Hurle Department of Urology, Humanitas Research Hospital IRCCS, Rozzano, MI, Italy

Pierandrea De Iaco Division of Oncologic Gynecology Unit, IRCCS—Azienda Ospedaliero-Universitaria di Bologna, University of Bologna, Bologna, Italy

Irene Pinucci Department of Human Neurosciences, SAPIENZA University of Rome, Rome, Italy

Zsolt Kopa Andrology Centre, Department of Urology, Semmelweis University, Budapest, Hungary

Andrea Lania Endocrinology Unit, IRCCS Humanitas Research Hospital, Rozzano, Italy

Department of Biomedical Sciences, Humanitas University, Rozzano, Italy

Antonio Lanzone Department of Woman, Child Health and Public Health, Fondazione Policlinico Universitario Agostino Gemelli IRCCS, Università Cattolica del Sacro Cuore, Rome, Italy

Gaetano Lombardi Endocrinology, Federico II University, Naples, Italy

Elena Vittoria Longhi, MPH Department of Sexual Medical Center, San Raffaele Hospital, Milano, Italy

Leonardo Lopiano, PhD, MD Department of Neuroscience, 'Rita Levi Montalcini'—University of Turin, Turin, Italy

Carmen Maccagnano, MD, FEBU Urotechnology Center, Scientific Institute "Istituto Auxologico Italiano", Milan, Italy

Laura Magnasco Clinica Malattie Infettive, Università degli Studi di Genova e IRCCS Policlinico San Martino, Genova, Italy

Nicoletta Marazzi Experimental Laboratory for Auxo-endocrinological Research, Milan, Italy

Ometti Marco Orthopedics and Traumatology Unit, IRCCS San Raffaele Hospital, Vita - Salute San Raffalele University, Milan, Italy

Emilia Marrazzo Breast Surgeon, Breast Unit, ASST Ospedale Maggiore di Lodi, Lodi, Italy

Massimo Pasquini Department of Human Neurosciences, SAPIENZA University of Rome, Rome, Italy

Giorgio Mastroiacovo, MD Centro Cardiologico Monzino IRCCS, Milan, Italy

Silvani Mauro Urologist and Oncosurgery, Biella, Italy

Anna Mazzucchi Department for Acquired Brain Injury Rehabilitation, Don Carlo Gnocchi Foundation, Milan, Italy

Santo Raffaele Mercuri, MD Unit of Dermatology and Cosmetology, Scientific Institute San Raffaele (IRCCS), Milan, Italy

Anna Mercuriali Department of Endocrinology Unit, Ospedale di Circolo e Fondazione Macchi, Varese, Italy

Luca Monge SCU Endocrinology, Diabetology and Metabolism, AOU City of Health and Science, Turin, Italy

Marcella Montini Humanitas Gavazzeni, Bergamo, Italy

Giorgio Del Noce Promea Institute, Turin, Italy

Alessandra Ana Maria Pagani ASST Papa Giovanni XXIII, Bergamo, Italy

Giovanni Paolino, MD Unit of Dermatology and Cosmetology, Scientific Institute San Raffaele (IRCCS), Milan, Italy

Alfredo Pece Eye Clinic, Melegnano Hospital, Milan, Italy

Fondazione Retina 3000, Milan, Italy

Giulia Pellicciari Department of Neuroscience, Mental Health and Sense Organs (NESMOS), Sapienza University of Rome, Rome, Italy

Anna Myriam Perrone Division of Oncologic Gynecology Unit, IRCCS—Azienda Ospedaliero-Universitaria di Bologna, University of Bologna, Bologna, Italy

Luca Persani Department of Endocrine and Metabolic Disorders, Istituto Auxologico Italiano, Milan, Italy

Department of Medical Biotechnologies and Translational Medicine, University of Milan, Milan, Italy

Lorenzo Pinessi Neurological Clinic and Specialization School in Neurology, University of Turin, Turin, Italy

Department of Neuroscience and Mental Health, Molinette-Città della Salute, Turin, Italy

Federica Portunato Clinica Malattie Infettive, Università degli Studi di Genova e IRCCS Policlinico San Martino, Genova, Italy

Caterina Premoli Department of Endocrine and Metabolic Disorders, Istituto Auxologico Italiano, Milan, Italy

Department of Medical Biotechnologies and Translational Medicine, University of Milan, Milan, Italy

Alice Ramondetta Dermatology Clinic, University of Turin, Turin, Italy

Furio Ravera The Unit for the Diagnosis and Treatment of Personality Disorders and Addictions, Private Clinic "Le Betulle" Appiano Gentile, Como, Italy

Vittoria Ravera Bibliography Research, The Bicocca University Milan, Milan, Italy

Alessandra Redolfi Spalenza Rehabilitation Centre, Don Carlo Gnocchi Foundation, Rovato, Italy

Simone Ribero Dermatology Clinic, University of Turin, Turin, Italy

Mario G. Rizzone, MD Department of Neuroscience, 'Rita Levi Montalcini'—University of Turin, Turin, Italy

Giulia Roda IBD Center, Humanitas Research Hospital, Milan, Italy

Silvia Romano Department of Neuroscience, Mental Health and Sense Organs (NESMOS), Sapienza University of Rome, Rome, Italy

Daniela Romualdi Department of Woman, Child Health and Public Health, Fondazione Policlinico Universitario Agostino Gemelli IRCCS, Università Cattolica del Sacro Cuore, Rome, Italy

Pia Fondazione di Culto e Religione, Azienda Ospedaliera Cardinale Panico, Tricase, Italy

Maria Salsone Institute of Molecular Bioimaging and Physiology, National Research Council, Milan, Italy

Stefano Salvatore Gynecology and Obstetrics Unit, Vita and Salute University, IRCCS San Raffaele, Milan, Italy

Marco Salvetti Department of Neuroscience, Mental Health and Sense Organs (NESMOS), Sapienza University of Rome, Rome, Italy

Alessandro Sartorio Division of Auxology and Metabolic Diseases, Istituto Auxologico Italiano, IRCCS, Verbania, Italy

Experimental Laboratory for Auxo-endocrinological Research, Milan, Italy

Marta Scorsetti Radiotherapy and Radiosurgery Department, Humanitas Clinical and Research Center—IRCCS, Milan, Italy

Department of Biomedical Sciences, Humanitas University, Milan, Italy

Fabrizio Ildefonso Scroppo Andrology Service, Department of Urology, Istituto Clinico Villa Aprica, Como, Italy

Omidreza Sedigh Reconstructive Urology and Andrology of Humanitas, Gradenigo, Turin, Italy

Paola Sgaramella, MD Department of Pediatrics, IRCCS San Raffaele Scientific Institute, Milan, Italy

Silvio Sporeni San Matteo Hospital, Pavia, Italy

Marina Di Stefano, MD Department of Pediatrics, IRCCS San Raffaele Scientific Institute, Milan, Italy

Elena Stroppiana Dermatology Clinic, University of Turin, Turin, Italy

Sofia Tamini Experimental Laboratory for Auxo-endocrinological Research, Milan, Italy

Valeria Versace Department of Woman, Child Health and Public Health, Fondazione Policlinico Universitario Agostino Gemelli IRCCS, Università Cattolica del Sacro Cuore, Rome, Italy

Salini Vincenzo Orthopedics and Traumatology Unit, IRCCS San Raffaele Hospital, Vita - Salute San Raffalele University, Milan, Italy

Part I
Autoimmune Disease

Coeliac Disease in Children and Young Adults

Marina Di Stefano, Paola Sgaramella, Graziano Barera, and Elena Vittoria Longhi

Introduction

Coeliac disease (CD) is an autoimmune disorder that occurs in genetically predisposed individuals who develop an immune reaction to gluten. The disease primarily affects the small intestine; however, the clinical manifestations are broad, with both intestinal and extra-intestinal symptoms [1]. CD provides a model of an immune-based disease with strong genetic and environmental risk factors. The key environmental factor responsible for the development of CD is gluten. Gluten is incompletely digested by gastric, pancreatic and brush border peptidases, leaving large peptides up to 33 amino acids long. These peptides enter the lamina propria where, in predisponed people, an adaptive immune reaction occurs, is dependent on deamidation of gliadin molecules by the enzyme tissue transglutaminase (TTG), the predominant autoantigen of CD [2]. Deamidation increases the immunogenicity of gliadin, facilitating binding to the HLA-DQ2 or HLA-DQ8 molecules on antigen presenting cells. Gliadin peptides are then presented to gliadin-reactive CD4+ cells. During this process, antibodies against TTG, gliadin and actin are made through unclear mechanism. Almost 100% of patients with CD possess specific variants of the HLA class II genes HLA-DQA1 and HLA-DQB1 encoding the alpha and beta chains making up the coeliac-associated heterodimer proteins DQ2 and DQ8 expressed on the surface of antigen presenting cells. These HLA genes and gluten ingestion are quite common in Caucasian people but CD occurs only in about 1% of the population, suggesting that other environmental factors besides gluten are probably important.

M. Di Stefano · P. Sgaramella · G. Barera (✉)
Department of Pediatrics, IRCCS San Raffaele Scientific Institute, Milan, Italy
e-mail: distefano.marina@hsr.it; sgaramella.paola@hsr.it; barera.graziano@hsr.it

E. V. Longhi
Department of Sexual Medical Center, San Raffaele Hospital, Milano, Italy

© Springer Nature Switzerland AG 2023
E. V. Longhi (ed.), *Managing Psychosexual Consequences in Chronic Diseases*,
https://doi.org/10.1007/978-3-031-31307-3_1

CD Main Medical Characteristics

The recognition of the broad clinical presentation of CD has evolved during the last decades. It has shifted from the historically classic symptoms of malabsorption in childhood to non-classic symptoms, which can be present in childhood or adulthood. Classical symptoms of malabsorption seem to be more specific and include failure to thrive, weight loss and chronic diarrhoea. The more common, non-classical symptoms include iron deficiency, bloating, constipation, chronic fatigue, headache and abdominal pain [1, 2] (Table 1).

Diagnosis

If CD is suspected, total serum IgA and IgA-antibodies against transglutaminase 2 (TGA-IgA) should be measured. Deamidated gliadin peptide antibodies (DGP-IgG/IgA) should not be used for initial testing. In patients with low or undetectable total IgA concentrations, an IgG-based test (DGP or TGA) should be performed as a second step [2]. Patients with positive results should be referred to a paediatric gastroenterologist. If TGA-IgA is ≥10 times the upper limit of normal (10 × ULN), the no-biopsy diagnosis may be applied, provided endomysial antibodies (EMA-IgA) will test positive in a second blood sample. In this case, HLA DQ2-/DQ8 determination and the presence of overt symptoms are not compelling criteria [2]. In children with positive TGA-IgA but with value below 10 × ULN, an upper endoscopy should be performed in order to collect at least four biopsies specimen from the distal duodenum and one from the bulb. Discordant results between TGA-IgA and histopathology may require endoscopic re-evaluation. Patients with no or mild histological changes (Marsh-Oberhuber classification 0/1) but confirmed autoimmunity (TGA-IgA or EMA-IgA positivity) should be re-evaluated closely during follow-up.

Table 1 Symptoms and signs suggesting CD

Gastrointestinal	Chronic or intermittent diarrhoea
	Chronic constipation[a]
	Chronic abdominal pain[a]
	Distended abdomen[a]
	Recurrent nausea and vomiting
Extra-intestinal symptoms	Weight loss, failure-to-thrive, stunted growth/ short stature
	Delayed puberty, amenorrhea
	Irritability, chronic fatigue[a]
	Chronic iron-deficiency anaemia[a]
	Recurrent aphthous stomatitis
	Dermatitis herpetiformis-type rash Dental enamel defects Abnormal liver biochemistry

[a]Common symptoms

Treatment and Follow-Up of CD

The mainstay of treatment of CD remains adherence to a gluten-free diet (GFD). Improvement and resolution of symptoms typically occurs within weeks and often precedes normalization of serological markers of duodenal villous atrophy [3]. Despite its effectiveness in achieving normalization of these parameters in most patients, the GFD encounters many difficulties. Gluten-free substitute foods are substantially more expensive than their gluten containing counterparts and therefore patients with low incomes might be at particularly high risk of non-adherence to the diet [4]. The quality of information regarding the gluten-free status of food ingredients is variable in online resources, which can lead to confusion among patients. Potential gluten exposure when travelling or eating in restaurants can be a hazard and a source of concern. Social pressures, particularly in adolescence, can also be an impediment to strict adherence [5]. Uncertainty regarding the presence of gluten in trace amounts in medications and supplements is another concern. Patients with newly diagnosed CD should be referred to an expert dietitian, because the GFD requires knowledge not only of hidden sources of gluten, but also of healthy gluten-free substitute grains that provide adequate fibre and nutrients. Upon diagnosis, patients should be tested for micronutrient deficiencies, including iron, folic acid and vitamin D. Beyond the initial diagnosis period, traditional medical follow-up for coeliac patients consists of regular physician visits to evaluate health, including weight and height measurements, dietary adherence and serology (which usually normalizes within 2 year of starting the diet). Vit D status should be monitored, and possibly the study of bone mineralization should be performed when indicated.

Transition from Childhood

The Child and Adolescent Health Measurement Initiative estimates that one million US children with special health needs make the transition to adult care every year [6]. CD is one of the most common chronic disorders in childhood and children with CD and constitutes an important part of transition healthcare in the Western world. The overall prevalence of CD varies from 0.71% in the USA [7] to as high as 2.9% in certain age groups in Sweden [8]. Generally, the transition from paediatric to adult care should be a collaborative process involving patients, their parents, the physician and the dietician.

Paediatric patients with CD are usually evaluated in specialized centres by teams including paediatric gastroenterologists, dieticians and psychologists. In children, the delivery of care is mainly family-centred, whereas in adulthood responsibility becomes autonomous and dependent upon the needs of individuals. The physical, mental, psychosocial and self-control development during transition from adolescence to adulthood is therefore pivotal. Children with a chronic disease may develop autonomy later than their peers [9]. Both the family and the adolescent patient should be at the centre of transition process, and the clinician's purpose is to balance parental authority and the adolescent's need for autonomy. To parents, this means stepping back and allowing their adolescent children to make independent decisions. The physician should start a discussion about transition when the adolescent is 12–13 years old, develop a transition plan when the child is 14–15, with the actual transfer taking place at 18 years of age [6].

Growth and Puberty

Growth impairment is a known consequence of untreated CD [10] though many children with short stature diagnosed with CD in childhood demonstrate good catch-up growth [11]. However, catch-up growth may occur more predictably for those with a delayed bone age at diagnosis and where growth velocity acceleration during the first year of treatment for CD is clear [12]. Untreated CD, or CD diagnosed after attainment of adult height, results in shorter adult height than healthy controls, particularly among men [13]. Some adolescents and young adults with CD will experience a delay in pubertal development and may continue to grow and sexually mature beyond the expected age of pubertal completion; the pathophysiology is currently poorly understood, but a hormone disregulation could be involved [14]. This may have implications for emotional maturity, sexual health and menstrual regularity. At the time when transition is planned, the paediatrician should provide data regarding the patient's history of physical development and should note to the gastroenterologist whether the patient has achieved his or her final adult height. It may be advisable to coordinate transition to an adult provider at the completion of puberty, particularly if paediatric gastroenterologist is still taking care of the patient in order to manage growth failure. A bone age X-ray may add information in cases of patient's pubertal delay, to inform growth expectations and timing of transition.

The Actual Transfer of Care

For adult gastroenterologists, CD is also often perceived as a less serious disease compared with GI cancer or IBD, and knowledge may be limited with respect to complications, diet, inheritance, extra-intestinal manifestations and how to monitor patients. The actual transfer can take many forms. In some settings, the paediatric and adult gastroenterologists see the patient at the same visit; in others, paediatric and adult gastroenterologists meet annually to discuss patients in transition. Hopefully, joint transition clinics with paediatric and adult service clinicians can be established for information delivery and generating trust in the new physician. Structured transitional models and targeted education are important and, in other chronic diseases, have been linked to improved care, better health outcome and improved health-related quality of life (QoL) [15]. One path to facilitate transition and transfer of care is to create a 'transition document', which would allow a smooth transfer of individual medical care data. This transition document should be created by the paediatrician prior to transfer, containing details and information during follow-up such as serology, anthropometric data, comorbidities and dietary compliance.

Several issue may be discussed during the transition period. Dietary adherence and consequences of non-adherence are key components for discussion in a transition setting. In Europe, adherence to a GFD by children and adolescent varies from 44% to 97% and accidental transgression are common [16]. Adolescence report lower adherence than younger children, particularly at social events. The risk of osteoporosis and adverse pregnancy outcome may be big issues in individuals with poor adherence [17]. The implementation of a systematic transition policy in CD has been limited by a lack of clinical guidelines based on outcome-related research and clear and consistent definitions. Models of transition will eventually need to be evaluated in randomized controlled trials with clear patient outcome measures. It is crucial to know to what extent a well-structured and planned transition will influence adherence to a GFD, which in CD is imperative for restoration of health and well-being.

Sexuality and QoL

Among the extra-digestive complications associated with CD, unexplained infertility has been reported since the 1970s. The prevalence of CD among women with unexplained infertility is 2.5–3.5%, higher, although not always significantly so, than in the control population. To date, it is widely accepted that untreated CD poses a risk of miscarriage, low-birth weight babies, and a short breastfeeding period. These characteristics can be remediated by a GFD. With regard to a potential pathogenic mechanism, because CD causes malabsorption of folic acid and other nutrients, this pathway has been proposed to explain unfavourable pregnancy outcomes [18, 19].

The psychological aspects of CD should not be underestimated. The feelings of deprivation and failure, alongside the burden of an unchanging lifelong diet, remain difficult components to accept. Also in social life.

In the time of Covid 19, the scientific literature has also investigated the perceived risk of celiac patients contracting the virus.

Jamie Zhen et al. [20] conducted a survey in ten countries between March and June 2020 and collected information on demographics, diet, COVID-19 testing and perceived risk of COVID-19 in patients with CD.

Participants were recruited through various coeliac associations and via clinical visits and social media. Perception of risk was assessed by asking people whether they believed that patients with CD had a higher risk of contracting COVID-19 than the general population. Perception of COVID-19 risk was measured according to age, gender, adherence to a GFD and comorbidities such as cardiac conditions, respiratory conditions and diabetes.

10,737 patients diagnosed with celiac disease completed the survey.

Specifically, 6019 (56.1%) patients perceived themselves to be at higher risk or were unsure as to whether or not they had a higher risk of contracting COVID-19 than the non-coeliac population.

A higher percentage of patients perceived an increased risk of contracting COVID-19 compared with infections in general due to their disease. As a result, 34.8% reported taking additional precautions against COVID-19.

Members of coeliac associations were less likely to perceive an increased risk of COVID-19 than non-members (49.5% vs 57.4%). Being older, male and strict adherence to a GFD were all associated with lower perceived COVID-19 risk.

The scientific literature has also investigated other correlations.

Giorgetti et al. [21] showed that CD was more common in subjects with insulin-dependent diabetes mellitus than in normal people. The study was conducted on a group of 93 diabetic children and adolescents who had undergone determination of antigliadin and anti-endomysium antibodies. In the study, the prevalence of CD exceeded the data reported in the literature. Hence, immunological screening for CD in paediatric T1DM patients is advocated.

A recent study conducted in the US population showed the following prevalence:

- 3–6% in individuals with Type 1 diabetes,
- up to 20% in first-degree relatives of coeliac patients,
- 10–15% among symptomatic cases of sideropenic anemia and
- 1–3% among those with osteoporosis. [22].

Given the prevalence of CD and the impact on patients' lives, extensive research has been conducted in several countries on the following aspects:

1. dietary compliance
2. health status including anthropometric data (primarily BMI)
3. daily habits
4. perception of QoL and of one's mental and physical health
5. any limitations in major social activities
6. ability to find gluten-free products
7. mode of supply
8. comorbidities, including psychiatric comorbidities such as anxiety disorder and depression
9. the relationship with health professionals and
10. the level of information provided by said professionals [23].

Most of the literature has identified the following [24]:

- SMOKING: present in both sexes in 24%; 4% are occasional smokers and 72% on average are non-smokers.
- WINE, BEER AND ALCOHOL: 24% of patients of both sexes habitually drink wine, 4% of males and 24% of females say they rarely drink it; 10% of males say they drink beer and alcoholic beverages, such as aperitifs vs 9% of females who say they drink beer (gluten free) and only 3% alcoholic beverages [25].

- MEDICATION: 25% males vs. 48% females take medication.
- Only females, 16%, report taking psychotropic drugs while 12% take drugs for osteoarticular disorders (osteoporosis, rheumatic disease), 8% use anti-allergic drugs, 4% take drugs for diseases of both the nervous system (Parkinson's disease) and the respiratory system (asthma) and 16% take contraceptives. Medications against gastrointestinal disorders (reflux and colon disease) are taken by 8% of both sexes.
- GFD: It is strictly observed in 90% of females vs. 79% of males. 10% of females do not follow the diet because they state that they are not able to "hold back" on social occasions vs. 21% of males who in part report not liking the taste of foods and find it difficult to buy them [26].
- LEISURE TIME: 71% of men and 58% of women pursue a hobby. 25% on average of both sexes answered that they do not pursue any hobby (in males 21% have no hobby and 4% did not answer). 41% of patients of both sexes had a pet in their care.

A study published by Digestive Diseases and Sciences, coordinated by Randi Wolf of Columbia University in New York, 2021, showed that CD had a major/moderate impact on their dating life.

With regard to sexuality however, many patients with CD report reduced sexual potency.

Problems related to infertility and oligospermia, on the other hand, are often solved with supplements and a GFD, even though the therapy lasts for several years [27].

In some patients, low-circulating levels of testosterone and 5-dihydrotestosterone were also detected, while the plasma level of luteinizing hormone often appeared elevated. These hormonal alterations may explain, in part, the delay in pubertal development and the appearance of secondary sexual characteristics observed in male patients not receiving any treatment.

CD has also been associated with spontaneous abortions and an increased incidence of intrauterine growth retardation.

Although the pathogenetic mechanism of celiac disease has not yet been clarified, a state of general malnutrition and the deficiency of specific factors such as iron, zinc and folic acid are to be considered as one of the causes that can lead to miscarriage. Moreover, pregnancy requires a calcium intake moderately higher than normal; consequently, bone remodelling becomes more important especially in women in whom the diagnosis of CD was made in adulthood, when occult malabsorption had already reduced the body's natural stores [28].

On the other hand, data from the National Social Life, Health, and Aging Project have shown that the psychological burden of chronic disease is associated with the sexual frequency and sexual dysfunction for men ($N = 893$) and women ($N = 641$). The results indicate that CD induces lubrication problems for women and orgasm problems for men. Especially among elderly patients. [23].

The GFD and consequent proper nutrition can help sexuality. Scientific literature reports that 18% report low interest in sex, compared with 13% in the GFD group and 11% in the "transitional" GFD group. Specifically, it is impossible to kiss someone wearing gluten-containing lipstick without getting risk of falling sick if you have celiac disease, and it is wise to ask a partner who eats gluten (or drinks beer), to brush his or her teeth before kissing. Women suffer from a wide range of reproductive disorders related to celiac disease, including an increased risk of infertility, miscarriage and other pregnancy problems. Although much less research has been done to document the reproductive health effects of celiac disease on men, the few studies available indicate that male infertility is higher among undiagnosed celiac men.

Conclusion

Every patient with CD must face a process of self-learning about his or her own life: not only from a nutritional point of view, but also in terms of intimacy, social relationships and in not being held back by the limitations of the disease. "Familiarizing oneself with CD appears to be a path of progressive growth, where every apparent difficulty (in diet, sexuality, health) can become a <difference> to be highlighted and given the proper attention so that the individual does not feel marginalized and in a state of constant underestimation of their psychophysical abilities". Consistency in diet as well as in self-care, hobbies, social relationships and interaction with peers can make the therapeutic discipline that CD imposes less painful. The communication between the specialists and the patient can contribute greatly to a more durable therapeutic contract and less risk of drop-off.

References

1. Lebwohl B, Sanders D, Green P. Coeliac disease. Lancet. 2018;391:70–81.
2. Dieterich W, Ehnis T, Bauer M, et al. Identification of tissue transglutaminase as the autoantigen of coeliac disease. Nat Med. 1997;3:797–801.
3. Husby S, Koletzko S, Korponay-Szabó I, Kurppa K, Mearin LM, Ribes-Koninck C, et al. European Society Paediatric Gastroenterology, Hepatology and Nutrition guidelines for diagnosing coeliac disease. J Pediatr Gastroenterol Nutr. 2020;70(1):141–56.
4. Murray J, Watson T, Clearman B, Mitros F. Effect of a gluten-free diet on gastrointestinal symptoms in celiac disease. Am J Clin Nutr. 2004;79:669–73.
5. Shah S, Akbari M, Kelly C, et al. Celiac disease has higher treatment burden than common medical conditions. Gastroenterology. 2012;142.
6. Ludvigsson J, Agreus L, Ciacci C, et al. Transition from childhood to adulthood in coeliac disease: the Prague consensus report. Gut. 2016;65:1242–51.
7. Child and adolescent health measurement initiative. National Survey of Children's Health; 2012.
8. Rubio-Tapia A, Ludvigsson J, Brantner T. The prevalence of celiac disease in the United States. Am J Gastroenterol. 2012;107:1538–44.
9. Myleus A, Ivarsson A, Webb C. Celiac disease revealed in 3% of Swedish 12-years-olds born during an epidemic. J Pediatr Gastroenterol Nutr. 2009;49:170–6.

10. Stam H, Hartman E, Deurloo J, et al. Young adult patients with a history of pediatric disease: impact on course of life and transition into adulthood. J Adolesc Health. 2006;39:4–13.
11. Meazza C, Pagani S, Laarej K, et al. Short stature in children with coeliac disease. Pediatr Endocrinol Rev. 2009;6:457–63.
12. Troncone R, Kosova R. Short stature and catch-up growth in celiac disease. J Pediatr Gastroenterol Nutr. 2010;51:S137–8.
13. Salardi S, Cacciari E, Volta U, et al. Growth and adult height in atypical coeliac patient, with or without growth hormone deficiency. J Pediatr Endocrinol Metab. 2005:769–75.
14. Weiss B, Skourikhin Y, Modan-Moses D, et al. Is adult height of patients with celiac disease influenced by delayed diagnosis? Am J Gastroenterol. 2008;103:1770–4.
15. Kumar PJ, Walter-Smith J, Milla P, et al. The teenage coeliac: follow-up study of 102 patients. Arch Dis Child. 1988;63:916–20.
16. Zeisler B, Hyams J. Transition of management in adolescents with IBD. Nat Rev Gastroenterol Hepatol. 2014;11:109–15.
17. Ludvigsson JF, Montgomery SM, Ekbom A. Celiac disease and risk of adverse fetal outcome: a population-based cohort study. Gastroenterology. 2005;129:454–63.
18. Pellicano R, et al. Women and celiac disease: association with unexplained infertility. Minerva Med. 2007;98(3):217–9.
19. Jackson JE, et al. Prevalence of celiac disease in a cohort of women with unexplained infertility. Fertil Steril. 2008;89(4):1002–4. https://doi.org/10.1016/j.fertnstert.2007.04.053.
20. Zhen J, et al. Perception of risk and knowledge of COVID-19 in patients with celiac disease. World J Gastroenterol. 2021;27(12):1213–25.
21. Giorgetti R, et al. Diabetes and celiac disease: a study linked to the association of the two pathologies. Minerva Pediatra. 1996;48(3):85–8.
22. World Health Organization. Define sexual health. Report of a technical consultation on sexual health. Ginevra: OMS; 2002.
23. Black JL, Orfila C. Impact of coeliac disease on dietary habits and quality of life. J Hum Nutr Diet. 2011;24:582–5.
24. Edwards JB, George LDA, Dennis MD, Franko DL, Blom-Hofman J, Kelly CP. Psychological correlates of gluten-free diet adherence in adults with celiac disease. J Clin Gastroenterol. 2009;4(43):301–6.
25. Hopman GD, Koopman HM, Wit JM, Mearin ML. Dietary compliance and health-related quality of life in patients with celiac disease. Eur J Gastroenterol Hepatol. 2009;21:1056–61.
26. Rashtak S, Murray JA. Celiac disease in the elderly. Gastroenterol Clin North Am. 2009;38(3):433–46. https://doi.org/10.1016/j.gtc.2009.06.005.
27. Lee AR, Ng DL, Diamond B, Ciaccio EJ, Green PHR. Living with celiac disease: survey result from the USA. J Hum Nutr Diet. 2012:233–8.
28. Rashtak S, Murray JA. Celiac disease in the elderly. Gastroenterol Clin N Am. 2009;38(3):433–46.

Part II
Cancer

Breast Cancer

Emilia Marrazzo, Chiara Annunziata Pasqualina Anghelone, and Elena Vittoria Longhi

Introduction to Chronic Disease

Breast cancer is currently the most diagnosed cancer in the female population, with a prevalence of 1 in 8 women.

Advances in knowledge of tumor biology such as the role of HER2, the estrogen-progestin receptors, the degree of differentiation, the proliferation index, the presence or absence of lymphovascular invasion have made it possible to reduce the prognostic value of the size of the tumor and the number lymph nodes involved which, while remaining important data, must be integrated with the biological parameters of the neoplasm itself within a multidisciplinary multi-specialist approach and in dedicated centers (BREAST UNIT).

The mammography screening programs implemented throughout the country have allowed an increase in early diagnoses in asymptomatic women, young and old, and therefore suitable treatments that are less and less demolishing, respecting the female anatomical functionality and oncological radicality.

Several factors come into play in the risk of getting breast cancer [1–6].

- Age: the risk increases with increasing age, probably this could be linked to the continuous and progressive endocrine proliferative stimulus that the mammary epithelium undergoes over the years combined with the progressive damage of

E. Marrazzo (✉)
Breast Surgeon, Breast Unit, ASST Ospedale Maggiore di Lodi, Lodi, Italy

C. A. P. Anghelone
Breast Surgeon, Breast Unit, ASST Ospedale Maggiore di Lodi, Lodi, Italy

Breast Surgeon, Breast Unit, SC Chirurgia Generale 3 -Senologia, Fondazione IRCCS Policlinico San Matteo, Pavia, Italy

E. V. Longhi
Department of Sexual Medical Center, San Raffaele Hospital, Milano, Italy

© Springer Nature Switzerland AG 2023
E. V. Longhi (ed.), *Managing Psychosexual Consequences in Chronic Diseases*,
https://doi.org/10.1007/978-3-031-31307-3_2

DNA and the accumulation of epigenetic alterations with alteration the balance of expression between oncogenes and suppressor genes.

- Reproductive factors: long duration of the fertile period, with an early menarche and a late menopause and therefore with a longer exposure of the glandular epithelium to the proliferative stimuli of the ovarian estrogens; nulliparity, a first term pregnancy after 30 years, failure to breastfeed.
- Hormonal factors: increased risk in women taking hormone replacement therapy during menopause, especially if based on synthetic estrogen-progestagen with androgenic activity and for a long time.
- Dietary and metabolic factors: high consumption of alcohol and animal fats and low consumption of vegetable fibers, obesity and metabolic syndrome.
- Previous radiotherapy (at the thoracic level and especially if before the age of 30) and previous dysplasias or breast neoplasms.
- -Familiarity and heredity: although most breast cancers are sporadic forms, 5% -7% are linked to hereditary factors, 1/4 of which are determined by the mutation of two genes: BRCA-1 and BRCA-2. In women with BRCA-1 mutations the risk of getting breast cancer is 65% and in women with BRCA-2 mutations 40%.

Main Tools for the Diagnosis of Breast Cancer

Women in the 40–50 s age group: X-ray mammography should be performed with an interval of 12–18 months integrated with bilateral breast ultrasound. The two exams are completed, reaching an accuracy index of about 98%.

The X-ray mammography used as a screening test has shown to reduce the relative risk of mortality from breast cancer in most of the randomized studies and is therefore still considered the most effective screening test. It is also useful in performing stereotaxic biopsy in selected cases.

Bilateral breast ultrasound alone is not considered a diagnostic screening method. Recommended in young women with prevalent glandular parenchyma, in women at high risk in association with other methods (breast MRI), as a mammography completion exam, as a guide for fine needle aspiration or needle agobiopsy.

Main Medical Characteristics of Breast Cancer

In relation to the histopathological characteristics we distinguish [7]:

- ductal carcinoma, in situ (DCIS), is a pre-invasive lesion that, in the absence of treatment, has the potential to evolve towards a form of invasive carcinoma
- invasive or infiltrating carcinoma (IDC) of the non-special histotype type (NST), commonly known as ductal carcinoma of the type not otherwise specified, represents the most frequent histotype among invasive breast carcinomas (70–80%)
- the infiltrating lobular carcinoma (ILC) more often multifocal or multicentric (5–15%)

- other less frequent types (tubular, cribriform, mucinous, etc.)

Breast cancer is a heterogeneous disease. In relation to the biological profile we distinguish [8]:

- Luminali A: positive hormonal receptors, negative HER2 and low proliferative activity (of which some special histotypes such as tubular carcinoma, classic lobular carcinoma frequently belong). Luminal A breast tumors are represented by tumors with positive estrogenic receptors, with positive progestogen receptors with a positivity value greater than 20%, with negative HER2 and low Ki67
- Luminali B/HER2 negative: hormonal receptors positive, HER2 negative and high proliferative activity (ki67 > 20%);
- Luminali B/HER2 positive: hormone receptors positive, HER2 overexpressed (score 3+ of immunohistochemical reactions) or amplified, any proliferative activity value;
- HER2 positive (not luminal): HER2 overexpressed (score 3+) or amplified (FISH or other methods) and both negative hormone receptors
- Triple-negative: absence of hormone receptor expression and negativity of HER2

Main Surgical Treatments

DCIS

In the ductal carcinoma in situ, as IDC, the choice of surgery is conditioned by the extent of the disease and the size of the breast. The procedure of choice, when possible, is the quadrantectomy followed by Radiotherapy [9].

Mastectomy (nipple sparing as first choice) remains indicated if the disease is too extensive to have negative margins, to be conservatively resected with a good aesthetic result, or in case of contraindications to radiotherapy. If blood nipple discharge occurs then it is recommended skin sparing mastectomy. Sentinel lymph node biopsy is only indicated after mastectomy.

Systemic adjuvant therapy is not recommended.

IDC/ILC

In patients with invasive carcinoma, where possible, conservative surgery [10] associated with whole breast irradiation or nipple sparing—skin sparing mastectomy—are the first choice treatment.

The type of surgery (radical vs conservative surgery) depends on the site and the tumor/breast size ratio, the mammographic characteristics, the patient's preference and the presence or absence of contraindications to radiotherapy. Where possible, conservative surgery is preferable, even through more extensive resections and reconstruction with oncoplastic techniques, if necessary, to ensure a good aesthetic result.

After mastectomy, however, plastic reconstruction in one or double time with expander or prosthesis is currently recommended, with satisfactory aesthetic results and less psychological impact on the patient.

The sentinel lymph node biopsy is considered the standard of treatment for patients with clinically negative lymph nodes or with negative needle biopsy.

Axillary dissection (AD) is indicated:

- with clinically pathological axillary lymph nodes, confirmed by pre-operative positive needle biopsy
- in the presence of a positive sentinel lymph node with macrometastasis on extemporaneous histological examination. In this case, the AD can be omitted if the patient is enrolled in specific clinical trials or in the presence of local or systemic contraindications or if she refuses axillary dissection [11–13]
- if the sentinel lymph node is not found
- in T4 tumors and inflammatory carcinoma

Main Non-Surgical Treatments

All the patients are discussed in a multidisciplinary meeting between breast surgeon, oncologist, radiotherapist, radiologist, pathologist and breast nurse.

Radiotherapy treatment is recommended after conservative surgery and in case of axillary metastatic nodes (more than four metastatic nodes) because it reduces the risk of local recurrence and mortality.

Medical therapy is chosen based on the biological characteristics of the carcinoma. It includes endocrine therapy and/or chemotherapy.

Hormone therapy [14] is indicated for all patients with hormone-responsive infiltrating tumors, meaning for them the presence of at least ER-positive ($\geq 1\%$) or PgR-positive ($\geq 1\%$), based on the patient's menopausal status; it is not indicated in tumors with negative hormonal receptors (ER and PgR negative: $<1\%$).

In premenopausal women: therapy with tamoxifen 20 mg/os/day for 5 years with or without ovarian suppression taking into account the risk of disease recovery of the individual patient, risk assessed in relation to patient characteristics (age) and tumor.

In postmenopausal women: hormone therapy with aromatase inhibitors for 5 years or tamoxifen for 2 years followed by x aromatase inhibitors 3 years.

Chemotherapy is used for both neoadjuvant and adjuvant treatment; the choice is always based on the size of the tumor, the presence or absence of pathological lymph nodes and the biological characteristics of the carcinoma, the patient's age and performance status.

In patients with operated breast cancer candidates for adjuvant or neoadjuvant chemotherapy treatment, polychemotherapy should be considered, as compared to monochemotherapy, it has an advantage in DFS and OS [15].

According to reports in the meta-analysis EBCTCG of 2012 (Early Breast Cancer Trialists' Collaborative Group) [16], it is possible to classify the polychemotherapy regimens available for breast cancer regimens in first, second and third generation.

First generation regimens: based on the combination of cyclophosphamide, methotrexate, fluorouracil (CMF) which, if administered × 6–12 cycles, reduce the risk of recurrence at 10 years by 30% and overall mortality by 16% if administered × 6–12 cycles. They are little used today.

Second generation regimes: these are regimens containing anthracyclines. These schemes are on average more effective than first generation schemes. There are several regimes:

- EC × 4 cycles, mostly used in patients at moderate risk of recovery. These regimens are substantially equivalent to CMF in terms of therapeutic efficacy but have a different toxicity profile, inducing less gonadal toxicity but greater alopecia and cardiotoxicity;
- FEC/CEF; FAC/CAF usually administered for 6 cycles.

These regimens are more effective than CMF, producing a further 11% reduction in risk of recurrence and 16% mortality.

Third generation regimens: include regimens containing anthracycline and taxanes administered sequentially (AC/EC/FEC × 3–4 cycles followed by taxane) or in combination (TAC/TEC). These regimens are on average higher than those of the second generation and produce a further reduction in the risk of recurrence by 16% and death by 14%.

In recent years, immunotherapy with monoclonal antibodies (e.g. Trastuzumab) has also been used in patients with Her2 overexpression. The duration of the adjuvant trastuzumab should be 1 year [17–20].

Sexuality and Quality of Life

There is no doubt that the impact of the diagnosis of breast cancer affects female body image, the relationship with the partner and changes in pleasure during intimacy. There is no doubt that the impact of the diagnosis of breast cancer conditions women's body image, the relationship with the partner and changes in pleasure during intimacy.

A study by Natalie Malone et al., using a sample of 153 women, investigated for the first time the emotional and intrapsychic feelings regarding the perception of sexuality after breast cancer: sadness, anhedonia, sexual pain (depending on age) and the state of the relationship with the partner.

The results indicated significant differences in the cognitive and emotional responses of younger, single women to sexual pain compared with older, coupled women. Qualitative responses revealed that women engage in several proactive coping strategies to mitigate their sexual pain, including non-penetrating activities, foreplay, arousal-enhancing tools and increased verbalization with their partner regarding spontaneous wants and desires. [21].

Yet within the clinical setting, most health professionals fail to address sexuality and feel more comfortable focusing on treatment outcomes, such as the management of treatment side effects [22]. Perhaps, this is due to the fact that many health professionals feel uncomfortable asking patients questions about sexuality (past and present) after cancer treatments and surgery, often citing lack of knowledge about the topic.

Here the sexologist often has carte blanche: it is a pity that the treatment process is not always shared between the sexologist, the oncologist and the surgeon right from the initial diagnosis. By contrast, a sexological anamnesis could anticipate problems of complementation or abandonment by the partner or family members in the post-surgical phase or during chemotherapy protocols.

This is especially true if the breast cancer diagnosis is a recurrence or follows the cancer treatment of another family member (parent, sister, brother).

There is no doubt, however, that physical changes for a woman are significant: foremost, the tightening of the labia, the exposure of the clitoris, altered sensitivity and involuntary contractions after orgasm. Vaginal tissue becomes thinner, drier and more fragile. In addition to a reduced amount of natural lubrication and a shortening of the length and width of the vagina, libido may decrease, often exacerbated by the pain related to a poorly lubricated vagina and a decrease in the intensity and speed of the sexual response [23].

This is a subjective situation which is very complex for any woman to comprehend, experience and accept. All the more so because the partners of patients are often unprepared. They avoid touching their partner, some of them as a precaution ('I don't want to accidentally hurt you") sleep in another room. They avoid watching their partner in the shower. Sexual initiative is mostly left to the woman and intimacy is often reduced to emotional acceptance and passion. The erotic aspect disappears and the female partner reports feeling <different>, less feminine and not at all seductive [24].

What of single women?

Seeking new relationships after a breast cancer diagnosis can be a stress factor for single women. Very little has been written about supporting single women, women separating from their partners after a cancer diagnosis and women entering new relationships after breast cancer management. Single women may fear that a potential partner will reject them, either because of the physical changes they have undergone following breast cancer treatment, or because of the fear of a recurrence. It is often difficult for single women to know when to disclose a prior breast cancer diagnosis or to share their fears or health concerns with a new partner [25].

And single women often change partners.

This is no less true of patients in same sex relationships. They often feel compelled to love in secret and are often forced to face their own fear of a relapse alone.

Either out of shame or modesty, fear of not being accepted or fear of criticism and judgment. They often then step back in their relationship with oncologists and surgeons, in order to assign to their families a greater authority in the management of primary care.

There is more [26].

Chemotherapy often causes stomatitis and intermittent vaginal irritation (during and for several weeks after treatment). Not to mention premature menopausal symptoms such as hot flushes, reduced libido, vaginal and vulvar dryness and atrophy.

Conclusion

These symptoms are reported by patients to be much more intense than those reported by naturally menopausal women. In induced menopause, the vaginal mucosa will remain thin and fragile and be easily irritated during and after sexual intercourse [27].

Furthermore, women over 35 are more likely to have a permanent menopause after chemotherapy (particularly alkylating agent therapy) than younger women who have a higher number of oocytes.

The diagnosis of breast cancer encompasses the clinical, care and enhancement process of the patient during and after surgery, chemotherapy and cosmetic surgery. The fear of recurrence is always present in the psyche of patient. Healthcare professionals can include family members and partners in the healing process. Care should be a joint process between the healthcare system, the rehabilitation system and the family systems of reference. In this respect, the sexologist can be a facilitator of the relationship between the systems, shaping an honest process between the parties.

References

1. Beral V, Million Women Study Collaborators, Bull D, et al. Ovarian cancer and hormone replacement therapy in the Million Women Study. Lancet. 2007;369:1703–10.
2. Rossouw JE, Anderson GL, Prentice RL, et al. Risks and benefits of estrogen plus progestin in healthy postmenopausal women: principal results from the Women's Health Initiative randomized controlled trial. JAMA. 2002;288:321–33.
3. Ravdin PM, Cronin KA, Howlader N, et al. The decrease in breast cancer incidence in 2003 in Unites States. N Engl J Med. 2007;356:1670–4.
4. Petracci E, Decarli A, Schairer C, et al. Risk factor modification and projections of absolute breast cancer risk. J Natl Cancer Inst. 2011;103:1037–48.
5. Chen S, Parmigiani G. Meta-analysis of BRCA1 and BRCA2 penetrance. J Clin Oncol. 2007;25:1329–33.
6. Melchor L, Benitez J. The complex genetic landscape of familial breast cancer. Hum Genet. 2013;132:845–63.
7. Lakhani S, Ellis IO, Schnitt SJ, et al., editors. WHO classification of tumour of the breast. 4th ed. Lyon: IARC; 2012.
8. Goldhirsch A, Winer EP, Coates AS, et al. Personalizing the treatment of women with early breast cancer: highlights of the St Gallen International Expert Consensus on the Primary Therapy of Early Breast Cancer 2013. Ann Oncol. 2013;24:2206–23.
9. Morrow M. De-escalating and escalating surgery in the management of early breast cancer. Breast. 2017;34(Suppl 1):S1–4. https://doi.org/10.1016/j.breast.2017.06.018.

10. Pilewskie M, Morrow M. Margins in breast cancer: how much is enough? Cancer. 2018;124(7):1335–41.
11. Giuliano AE, Hunt KK, Ballman KV, et al. Axillary dissection vs no axillary dissection in women with invasive breast cancer and sentinel node metastases: a randomized clinical trial. JAMA. 2011;305:569–75.
12. Giuliano AE, Ballman K, McCall L, et al. Locoregional recurrence after sentinel lymph node dissection with or without axillary dissection in patients with sentinel lymph node metastases: long-term follow-up from the American College of Surgeons Oncology Group (Alliance) ACOSOG Z0011 randomized trial. Ann Surg. 2016;264:413–20.
13. Tinterri C, Canavese G, Bruzzi P, et al. SINODAR ONE, an ongoing randomized clinical trial to assess the role of axillary surgery in breast cancer patients with one or two macrometastatic sentinel nodes. Breast. 2016; https://doi.org/10.1016/j.breast.2016.06.016.
14. Early Breast Cancer Trialists' Collaborative Group (EBCTCG). Aromatase inhibitors versus tamoxifen in early breast cancer: patient-level meta-analysis of the randomised trials. Lancet. 2015;386:1341–52.
15. Early Breast Cancer Trialist' Collaborative Group. Effects of chemotherapy and hormonal therapy for early breast cancer on recurrence and 15-year survival: an overview of the randomised trials. Lancet. 2005;365:1687–717.
16. Peto R, Davies C, Godwin J, et al. Comparisons between different polychemotherapy regimens for early breast cancer: meta-analyses of long-term outcome among 100,000 women in 123 randomised trials. Lancet. 2012;379:432–44.
17. Romond E, Perez EA, Bryant J, et al. Trastuzumab plus adjuvant chemotherapy for operable HER2-positive breast cancer. N Engl J Med. 2005;353:1673–84.
18. Perez EA, Romond EH, Suman VJ, et al. Four-year follow-up of trastuzumab plus adjuvant chemotherapy for operable human epidermal growth factor receptor 2-positive breast cancer: joint analysis of data from NCCTG N9831 and NSABP B-31. J Clin Oncol. 2011;29:3366–73.
19. Buzdar AU, Ibrahim NK, Francis D, et al. Significantly higher pathologic complete remission rate after neoadjuvant therapy with trastuzumab, paclitaxel, and epirubicin chemotherapy: results of a randomized trial in human epidermal growth factor receptor 2-positive operable breast cancer. J Clin Oncol. 2005;23:3676–85.
20. Buzdar AU, Valero V, Ibrahim NK, et al. Neoadjuvant therapy with paclitaxel followed by 5-fluorouracil, epirubicin, and cyclophosphamide chemotherapy and concurrent trastuzumab in human epidermal growth factor receptor 2-positive operable breast cancer: an update of the initial randomized study population and data of additional patients treated with the same regimen. Clin Cancer Res. 2007;13:228–33.
21. Malone N, Thorpe S, Jester JK, Dogan JN, Stevens-Watkins D, Hargons CN. Pursuing pleasure despite pain: a mixed-methods investigation of black women's responses to sexual pain and coping. J Sex Marital Ther. 2021;48(6):552–66. https://doi.org/10.1080/0092623X.2021.2012309.
22. Hordern A. Intimacy and sexuality for women with breast cancer. Cancer Nursing. 2000;23(3):230–6.
23. Uysal E. Top classic articles cited in breast cancer research. Eur J Breast Health. 2017;13(3):129.
24. Harbeck N, et al. Breast cancer. Nat Rev Dis Primer. 2019;5(1):66.
25. Jackisch C. Cancer Treat Rev. 2021;99:102229.
26. Al-Masri M, Aljalabneh B, Al-Najjar H, et al. Effetto del tempo alla chirurgia del cancro al seno dopo la chemioterapia neoadiuvante sugli esiti di sopravvivenza. Breast Cancer Res Treat. 2021;186:7–13. https://doi.org/10.1007/s10549-020-06090-7.
27. Marklund A. JAMA Oncol. 2021;7(1):86–91. https://doi.org/10.1001/jamaoncol.2020.5957.

Prostate Cancer and Radiotherapy

Marta Scorsetti, Ciro Franzese, and Elena Vittoria Longhi

Prostate cancer represents the most common malignancy in males [1, 2] and its incidence increased in the last decades due to the introduction of the prostate-specific antigen (PSA) as valuable test for early diagnosis and screening. The large majority of prostate cancer is diagnosed in patients with 65 years or more of age and is associated with risk factors like ethnicity and family history.

Prostate cancer is classified in risk classes according to National Comprehensive Cancer Network guidelines [3]. Very low risk includes stage T1c, Gleason score $\leq$ 6, PSA < 10 ng/mL, fewer than three prostate biopsy cores positive, $\leq$50% cancer in each core, and PSA density <0.15 ng/mL/g. Low-risk patients have T1–T2a disease, Gleason score $\leq$ 6, and PSA < 10 ng/mL. Intermediate risk is characterized by T2b–T2c or Gleason score 7 or PSA 10–20 ng/m. High-risk patients have diagnosis of T3a disease or Gleason score 8–10 or PSA > 20 ng/mL. Recently, the International Society of Urological Pathologists released new guidelines and a revised grading system, called the ISUP Grade Groups. The ISUP Grade group specifies five grades, from 1 through 5 and differentiate favorable (Gleason score 3 + 4) from unfavorable (Gleason score 4 + 3) intermediate risk prostate cancer.

M. Scorsetti (✉) · C. Franzese
Radiotherapy and Radiosurgery Department, Humanitas Clinical and Research Center—IRCCS, Milan, Italy

Department of Biomedical Sciences, Humanitas University, Milan, Italy
e-mail: marta.scorsetti@hunimed.eu; ciro.franzese@hunimed.eu

E. V. Longhi
Department of Sexual Medical Center, San Raffaele Hospital, Milano, Italy

© Springer Nature Switzerland AG 2023
E. V. Longhi (ed.), *Managing Psychosexual Consequences in Chronic Diseases*,
https://doi.org/10.1007/978-3-031-31307-3_3

Treatment Options

Treatment options for prostate cancer depend on the stage of disease. For localized prostate cancer, curative management includes nowadays both surgery and radiotherapy, in the form of external beam or brachytherapy, and in case of low-risk disease also actives surveillance. In a recently published randomized trial conducted by Hamdy et al. [4] including 1643 patients, after a median follow-up of 10 years, surgery and radiotherapy were associated with lower incidences of progression of disease compared to active monitoring. Moreover, no difference was observed in patients' survival between surgery (0.9 per 1000 person-years; 95% CI, 0.4 to 2.2) and radiotherapy (0.7 per 1000 person-years; 95% CI, 0.3 to 2.0) approaches.

External beam radiotherapy is considered an effective option for low- and intermediate-risk prostate cancer, but also in the setting of high-risk disease, alone or in combination with androgen deprivation therapy. Irradiation of prostate cancer includes the whole gland due to the risk of multifocal disease and also the seminal vesicles in the presence [5] of one or more risk factor (PSA > 10, Gleason $\geq$7, >T2a) or more than 15% of risk of infiltration according to Roach's formula [6] that is PSA + ([Gleason score − 6] × 10).

Lymph node irradiation in clinically node negative prostate cancer continues to be debated. To date, three randomized trials have been published comparing elective whole pelvic irradiation vs prostate only radiotherapy. The RTOG 77–06 trial [7] included 445 patients and didn't show any difference between the two treatment arms in terms of disease control and overall survival. The four arms RTOG 94-13 trial [8] showed no benefit from pelvic irradiation after a median follow-up of 6.6 years. Also the more recent GETUG trial [9] did not demonstrate difference between the two arms. However, all this studies were conducted with old radiotherapy technique and different treatment volumes compared to modern standards.

Radiotherapy provides lethal DNA double-strand breaks to the tumoral cells with a total dose of about 80 Gy delivered with daily fraction of 1.8–2.0 Gy, 5 days per week. Conventional fractionation has been widely used in the last decades, and at the beginning of the twenty-first century saw the implementation of intensity modulated radiation therapy (IMRT) as an highly conformal technique able to optimize the shape of the dose distribution reducing the dose to the healthy tissue. Kupelian et al. [10] demonstrated a benefit from the use of IMRT compared to 3D conformal radiotherapy (3DCRT), with a significant reduction of acute rectal toxicity ($p = 0.002$). Later in 2007 Vora et al. [11] increased the curative dose from 68.4 Gy of 3DCRT to 76.5 Gy of IMRT and observed an improvement in biochemical-recurrence-free survival at 5 years (74.1% vs. 60.4%, $p < 0.0001$) without any significant increase in toxicity rates.

This radiotherapy technical evolution paved the way for hypofractionation studies with the aim of delivering a higher biological equivalent dose (BED) in a shorter time along with a potential improvement in patients' outcome. The rationale at the bases of this hypothesis is related to the radiobiological aspects of prostate cancer. Considering that the sensitivity of tissues to a radiotherapy fractionation is expressed by the α/β ratio, the literature suggests that prostate cancer is characterized by a low α/β ratio, ranging from 1 to 2 Gy [12]. This information translates into a high sensitivity of prostate cancer to larger dose per fraction compared to other tumors. The recently published HYPRO [13] and PROFIT [14] trials compared moderate hypofractionation (daily dose of 3 and 3.4 Gy) with conventional fractionation and demonstrated good results in terms of disease control and mild pattern of toxicity. The randomized CHHiP trial confirmed with 5-year follow-up that hypofractionated radiotherapy with 60 Gy in 20 fractions is non-inferior to conventional 74 Gy in 37 fractions [15].

More recently, extreme hypofractionation (use of maximum 5 fractions) in the form of stereotactic body radiation therapy (SBRT) has been investigated in several phase I-II studies [16, 17] and demonstrated favorable results in terms of toxicity compared to conventional fractionation and moderate hypofractionation [18, 19]. SBRT is nowadays clinically adopted for the management of low- and intermediate-risk prostate cancer [20].

Radiotherapy for prostate cancer is commonly well tolerated, although some toxicity related to bladder and rectal alteration could appear in the acute setting. Most common acute symptoms are tenesmus, urinary urgency, nocturia, and dysuria. Less frequent are late side effects, with only 0 to a maximum of 10% of patients reporting moderate or severe gastrointestinal or genitourinary toxicity [21].

Compared to prostatectomy, radiotherapy seems to be less impacting on urinary continence and sexual dysfunction. Always according to the PROTECT trial [4], the percentage of men reporting firm erections were 17% in the prostatectomy group, 27% in the radiotherapy group, and 30% in the surveillance group, while the use of pads was 17% in the prostatectomy group, compared with 8% in the surveillance group and 4% in the radiotherapy group.

Moreover, incidence of toxicity from prostate radiotherapy has been improved by the adoption of Image guidance (Image guided radiation therapy or IGRT). With this use of advanced imaging, radiation oncologist can precisely see the position of the prostate just before the irradiation and during the dose delivery with systems of real-time tracking. This is important as the prostate can move or rotate by as much as centimeter, depending on how full bladder and rectum are, or from the passage of air in the bowel. Daily imaging ensures a safe dose delivery on the target with sparing of healthy structures and therefore reducing the side effects.

Radiotherapy can be a useful treatment also in the post-operative setting. Biochemical recurrence is a common event after prostatectomy in patients with risk factors such as infiltration of the prostate capsule or seminal vesicles, positive lymph nodes, or positive surgical margins [22–24]. Radiotherapy can be delivered just after surgery as an adjuvant treatment or as salvage radiotherapy in case of persisting or rising PSA values. In men with aggressive prostate cancer, the role of adjuvant versus early salvage radiotherapy was historically investigated in three randomized clinical trials [25–27]. All the studies demonstrated an improvement in progression-free survival with immediate radiotherapy over salvage treatment, but not on overall survival according to the meta-analysis conducted by Shaikh et al. [28]. However, in 2020, the prospectively planned systematic review and meta-analysis [29] including 2153 patients treated between 2007 and 2016 suggested that adjuvant radiotherapy does not improve event-free survival and early salvage treatment would seem the preferable treatment option.

Quality of Life and Sexuality

Prostate cancer treatments have different impacts on patient quality of life and function. The magnitude of difference between treatment-related adverse effects may be important to patients when choosing therapy.

The most extensive study on these issues is by Tsz Kin Lee [30]: the author proposed a systematic review of articles in English including the use of the Expanded Prostate Cancer Index Composite (EPIC), the questionnaire that measures the quality of life of patients with prostate cancer. The baseline data are: bowel, urinary, and sexual symptoms. It appears that post treatment, surgical patients had a better bowel quality of life as well as less urinary incontinence. Radiotherapy patients had more severe incontinence with anal irritation. Sexuality resumed earlier with surgical treatment than with radiotherapy.

The study by Zhou [31] investigated the association of overall and disease-specific survival with the five standard treatment modalities for prostate cancer (CaP): radical prostatectomy (RP), brachytherapy (BT), external beam radiation therapy (EBRT), androgen deprivation therapy (ADT), and no treatment (NT) within 6 months of CaP diagnosis. The study population included 10,179 men aged 65 years and over with an incidence of CaP diagnosed between 1999 and 2001. Using the linked Ohio Cancer Incidence Surveillance System Medicare, clinicians analyzed overall and disease-specific survival up to 2005 among the five clinically accepted therapies.

The disease-specific survival rates were 92.3% and 23.9% for patients with localized disease compared to those with distant disease at 7 years, respectively.

However, this is not all. A recent study by Guan Ting [32] investigated how disease uncertainty negatively affected patients' physical well-being ($P < 0.001$) and mental well-being ($P < 0.05$). Kurita and colleagues had already found, years earlier, that avoidant coping strategies fully explained the effects of disease uncertainty on non-somatic depressive symptoms and emotional well-being [33].

However, in Ting's study, men with prostate cancer report high levels of distress such as uncertainty, both at diagnosis and over time, regarding different treatment options, even though all treatments show substantial risk of physical disability.

This shows how the diagnosis and treatment of cancer is a stressful experience and uncertainty about the disease is itself a source of great stress. Added to this is the strain of adhering to protocols prior to radiotherapy such as the use of drugs to cleanse the bowels before each session, asthenia, and anal burning [34]. In many patients, the possibility of further "androgenic deprivation" after radiotherapy modifies, in no small way, the patients' virility, their motivation in life, their social role, the balance between partners, their relationships with their own bodies, and their relationship in general with the opposite sex.

Furthermore, Susan Bergius' study [35] observed patients with prostate cancer (PC) undergoing active surveillance ($n = 226$), radiotherapy ($n = 280$), surgery ($n = 299$), or hormone treatment ($n = 62$), who answered the 15-dimensional (15D) generic HRQoL questionnaire at the time of diagnosis, were followed up 3, 6, 12, and 24 months later.

Results: HRQoL was stable during the first 2 years after diagnosis in all treatment groups, except for patients treated with hormone therapy. Overall survival within 6.5 years of follow-up was 84.4%. The number of QALYs (Quality Adjusted Life Years) experienced during the 2-year follow-up was comparable in the active surveillance (1790), surgery (1784), and radiation groups (1767), but significantly lower in the hormone therapy group (1665).

The study by Groarke [36] also showed that the quality of life of prostate cancer patients is affected by stress and the constant threat to male identity (from cancer treatments).

A total of 204 men aged 44–88 years ($M = 65.24 \pm 7.51$) who had been diagnosed with localized prostate cancer within the previous 5 years were recruited. The measures used included the Perceived Stress Scale, the Cancer-Related Masculine Threat Scale, and the Conor-Davidson Resilience Scale. An online survey model was also utilized. The patients' perceived stress accounted for 26–44% of variance on quality of life and adjustment indices, with high stress associated with low mood and poor quality of life accompanied by asthenia, depression, insomnia, and hypoactive sexual desire.

Moreover, the study by Beckendorf [37], first in 1996 and later in 2020, assessed the sexual function before and after definitive irradiation for the treatment of prostate cancer in 67 patients (average age 68 years) treated in five radiotherapy departments and assessed with repeated questionnaires on their libido, arousal, frequency, and quality of intercourse and sexual satisfaction.

Interviews were conducted before radiotherapy and at the end of the first year after treatment. Sixty-three patients were married and 50 had a sexually active relationship. Forty-six patients presented with another medical condition or treatment that could induce sexual dysfunction. Before radiotherapy, 40 patients were sexually active, reporting good to acceptable relationships.

Between 10 and 24 months after the end of radiotherapy, no disease progression was observed and PSA levels remained elevated in only two patients. Sexual function was preserved in 67% of patients, although only 50% observed no change. The functional prognosis seemed to be related to the initial frequency and quality of intercourse; more than three times a month, the prognosis remained good, less than three times a month was considered inauspicious. The patient's age was a predictive factor for the frequency of intercourse.

Conclusions

Several causes of impaired sexual function may be associated and may change over the long term. Not without the anamnestic and sexual assessment of the partner, the conditioning of a partner who is younger than the patient, or a woman with a previous oncological diagnosis, or a partner who is menopausal, cardiopathic, diabetic, etc. will be different.

References

1. Soerjomataram I, Lortet-Tieulent J, Parkin DM, et al. Global burden of cancer in 2008: a systematic analysis of disability-adjusted life-years in 12 world regions. Lancet. 2012;380(9856):1840–50.
2. Miller KD, Siegel RL, Lin CC, et al. Cancer treatment and survivorship statistics, 2016. CA Cancer J Clin. 2016;66:271–89.
3. https://www.nccn.org/professionals/physician_gls/pdf/prostate.pdf
4. Hamdy FC, Donovan JL, Lane JA, et al. 10-year outcomes after monitoring, surgery, or radiotherapy for localized prostate cancer. N Engl J Med. 2016;375(15):1415–24. https://doi.org/10.1056/NEJMoa1606220. Epub 2016 Sep 14.
5. Bayman NA, Wylie JP. When should the seminal vesicles be included in the target volume in prostate radiotherapy? Clin Oncol (R Coll Radiol). 2007;19(5):302–7. Epub 2007 Apr 19.
6. Roach M 3rd. Re: the use of prostate specific antigen, clinical stage and Gleason score to predict pathological stage in men with localized prostate cancer. J Urol. 1993;150:1923–4.
7. Asbell SO, Martz KL, Shin KH, et al. Impact of surgical staging in evaluating the radiotherapeutic outcome in RTOP 77-06, a phase III study for T1bN0M0 (A2) and T2N0M0 (B) prostate carcinoma. Int J Radiat Oncol Biol Phys. 1998;40:769–82.
8. Roach M, DeSilvio M, Lawton C, et al. Phase III trial comparing whole-pelvic versus prostate-only radiotherapy and neo-adjuvant versus adjuvant combined androgen suppression: radiation therapy oncology group 9413. J Clin Oncol. 2003;21:1904–11.
9. Pommier P, Chabaud S, Lagrange JL, et al. Is there a role for pelvic irradiation in localized prostate adenocarcinoma? Preliminary results of GETUG-01. J Clin Oncol. 2007;25:5366–73.
10. Kupelian PA, Reddy CA, Carlson TP, et al. Preliminary observations on biochemical relapse-free survival rates after short-course intensity-modulated radiotherapy (70 Gy at 2.5 Gy/fraction) for localized prostate cancer. Int J Radiat Oncol Biol Phys. 2002;53(4):904–12.
11. Vora SA, Wong WW, Schild SE, et al. Analysis of biochemical control and prognostic factors in patients treated with either low-dose three-dimensional conformal radiation therapy or high-dose intensity- modulated radiotherapy for localized prostate cancer. Int J Radiat Oncol Biol Phys. 2007;68(4):1053–8.
12. Proust-Lima C, Taylor JMG, Sécher S, et al. Confirmation of a low α/βratio for prostate cancer treated by external beam radiation therapy alone using a post-treatment repeated-measures model for PSA dynamics. Int J Radiat Oncol Biol Phys. 2011;79(1):195–201.
13. Incrocci L, Wortel RC, Alemayehu WG, et al. Hypofractionated versus conventionally fractionated radiotherapy for patients with localised prostate cancer (HYPRO): final efficacy results from a randomised, multicentre, open- label, phase 3 trial. Lancet Oncol. 2016;17(8):1061–9.
14. Catton CN, Lukka H, Gu CS, et al. Randomized trial of a hypofractionated radiation regimen for the treatment of localized prostate cancer. J Clin Oncol. 2017;35(17):1884–90.
15. Dearnaley D, Syndikus I, Mossop H, et al. Conventional versus hypofractionated high-dose intensity-modulated radiotherapy for prostate cancer: 5-year outcomes of the randomised, non-inferiority, phase 3 CHHiP trial. Lancet Oncol. 2016;17(8):1047–60.
16. D'Agostino G, Franzese C, De Rose F, et al. High-quality linac-based stereotactic body radiation therapy with flattening filter free beams and volumetric modulated arc therapy for low-intermediate risk prostate cancer. a mono-institutional experience with 90 patients. Clin Oncol (R Coll Radiol). 2016;28(12):e173–8. https://doi.org/10.1016/j.clon.2016.06.013. Epub 2016 Jul 4.
17. Katz AJ, Santoro M, Diblasio F, et al. Stereotactic body radiotherapy for localized prostate cancer: disease control and quality of life at 6 years. Radiat Oncol. 2013;8(1):118.
18. Franzese C, D'agostino G, Di Brina L, et al. Linac-based stereotactic body radiation therapy vs moderate hypofractionated radiotherapy in prostate cancer: propensity-score based comparison of outcome and toxicity. Br J Radiol. 2019;92(1097):20190021. https://doi.org/10.1259/bjr.20190021.

19. Michalski JM, Winter K, Purdy JA, et al. Toxicity after three-dimensional radiotherapy for prostate cancer on RTOG 9406 dose level V. Int J Radiat Oncol Biol Phys. 2005;62:706–13.
20. Morgan SC, Hoffman K, Loblaw DA. Hypofractionated radiation therapy for localized prostate cancer: executive summary of an ASTRO, ASCO, and AUA evidence-based guideline. Pract Radiat Oncol. 2018;8(6):354–60.
21. Zelefsky MJ, Levin EJ, Hunt M, et al. Incidence of late rectal and urinary toxicities after three-dimensional conformal radiotherapy and intensity-modulated radiotherapy for localized prostate cancer. Int J Radiat Oncol Biol Phys. 2008;70:1124–9.
22. Chun FK, Graefen M, Zacharias M, et al. Anatomic radical retropubic prostatectomy-long-term recurrence-free survival rates for localized prostate cancer. World J Urol. 2006;24:273–80.
23. Swindle P, Eastham JA, Ohori M, et al. Do margins matter? The prognostic significance of positive surgical margins in radical prostatectomy specimens. J Urol. 2005;174:903–7.
24. Pinto F, Prayer-Galetti T, Gardiman M, et al. Clinical and pathological characteristics of patients presenting with biochemical progression after radical retropubic prostatectomy for pathologically organ-confined prostate cancer. Urol Int. 2006;76:202–8.
25. Thompson IM Jr, Tangen CM, Paradelo J, et al. Adjuvant radiotherapy for pathologically advanced prostate cancer: a randomized clinical trial. JAMA. 2006;296(19):2329–35.
26. Bolla M, van Poppel H, Tombal B, et al. European Organisation for Research and Treatment of Cancer, Radiation Oncology and Genito-Urinary Groups. Postoperative radiotherapy after radical prostatectomy for high-risk prostate cancer: long-term results of a randomised controlled trial (EORTC trial 22911). Lancet. 2012;380(9858):2018–27.
27. Thompson IM, Tangen CM, Paradelo J, et al. Adjuvant radiotherapy for pathological T3N0M0 prostate cancer significantly reduces risk of metastases and improves survival: long-term follow-up of a randomized clinical trial. J Urol. 2009;181(3):956–62.
28. Shaikh MP, Alite F, Wu M-J, Solanki AA, Harkenrider MM. Adjuvant radiotherapy versus wait-and-see strategy for pathologic T3 or margin-positive prostate cancer: a meta-analysis [published online February 20, 2017]. Am J Clin Oncol. 2017;41:730.
29. Vale CL, Fisher D, Kneebone A, et al. Adjuvant or early salvage radiotherapy for the treatment of localised and locally advanced prostate cancer: a prospectively planned systematic review and meta-analysis of aggregate data. Lancet. 2020;396(10260):1422–31.
30. Lee TK, et al. A systematic review of quality of life with prostate cancer index (EPIC) after surgery or radiation treatment. Can J. Urol. 2015;22(1):7599–606.
31. Zhou EH, et al. Radiation therapy and survival in prostate cancer patients: a population-based study. Int J Radiat Oncol Biol Phys. 2009;73(1):15–23.
32. Ting G. Uncertainty of disease, coping and quality of life among prostate cancer patients. Pshycooncology. 2020;29(6):1019–25.
33. Kurita K, Garon EB, Stanton AL, Meyerowitz BE. Uncertainty and psychological adjustment in patients with lung and prostate cancer. Pshycooncology. 2013;22(6):1396–401.
34. Canzone L, Northouse LL, Braun TM, et al. Assessing longitudinal quality of life in prostate cancer patients and their spouses: a multilevel modeling approach. Qual Life Ris. 2011;20(3):371–81.
35. Bergius S. Health-related quality of life and survival in prostate cancer patients in a real-world context. Urol Int. 2020;104(11–12):939–47.
36. Groarke AM. Quality of life and adaptation in men with prostate cancer: interaction of stress, threat, and resilience. PLoS One. 2020;15(9):e0239469.
37. Beckendorf V, et al. Prostate irradiation-induced sexual dysfunction: a review and multidisciplinary management guide in the age of radical radiation therapy (part II on urologic management). Rep Pract Oncol Radiother. 2020;25(4):619–24.

Cancers of the Female Genital Tract

Anna Myriam Perrone, Pierandrea De Iaco, and Elena Vittoria Longhi

Female genital cancers consist of neoplasms with different characteristics for age of incidence, frequency, symptoms, aggressiveness, and prognosis. Each neoplasm is characterized by a specific molecular pattern that makes it particularly sensitive to chemotherapy or radiation therapy, so the combination of various therapies (surgery, chemotherapy, hormone therapy, radiotherapy, and brachytherapy) is specific for every neoplasia (Fig. 1).

Gynecological cancers affect women of different ages. Cervical cancer (CC) may already be present in young women in their third decade of life, while ovarian or endometrial tumors occur, most frequently, in patients over 75 years of age. Clearly related issues, such as impairment of fertility, changes in hormone production, and sexual disorders, have different levels of impact in women at the extremes of age. The chronic tissue changes induced by therapies therefore cause variable deteriorations in the quality of life depending on the age and organ affected.

A. M. Perrone · P. De Iaco (✉)
Division of Oncologic Gynecology Unit, IRCCS—Azienda Ospedaliero-Universitaria di Bologna, University of Bologna, Bologna, Italy
e-mail: myriam.perrone@unibo.it; pierandrea.deiaco@unibo.it

E. V. Longhi
Department of Sexual Medical Center, San Raffaele Hospital, Milano, Italy

© Springer Nature Switzerland AG 2023
E. V. Longhi (ed.), *Managing Psychosexual Consequences in Chronic Diseases*,
https://doi.org/10.1007/978-3-031-31307-3_4

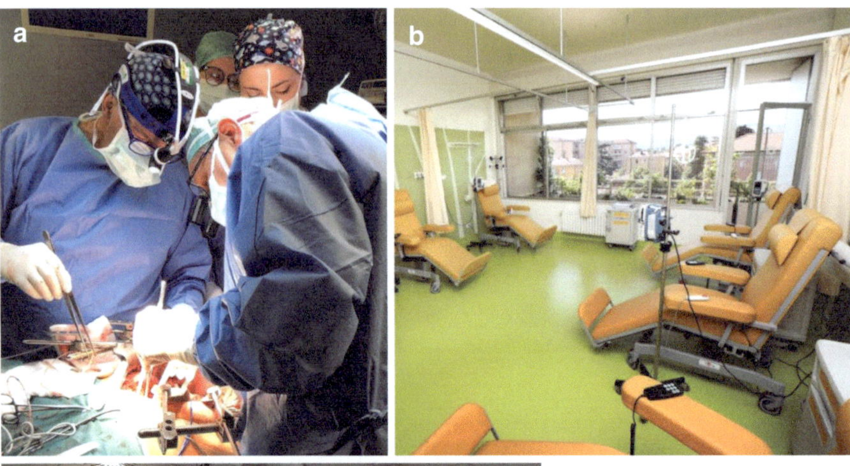

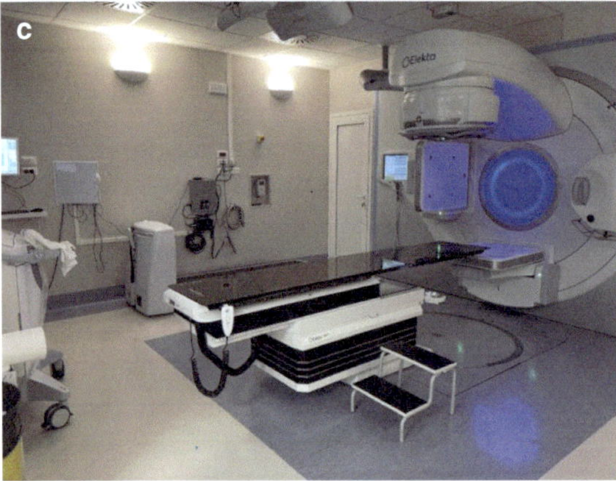

Fig. 1 The therapeutic options in gynecologic oncology. Surgery (**a**), Chemotherapy (**b**), Radiotherapy (**c**)

Endometrial Cancer

Endometrial cancer (EC), commonly referred to as uterine cancer, is the most common female genital cancer in the Western world and represents the fourth most frequent female cancer in women. The trend in the incidence of the disease was stable in the past but has increased since the 1980s. EC is generally present in postmenopausal women and has a peak incidence between 50 and 70 years of age. In 4% of cases, it occurs in women under the age of 40, who may not have completed their reproductive programs [1, 2].

EC has an important association with environmental risk factors: obesity, arterial hypertension, and fat-rich diet are responsible for increased estrogen production, which is the main cause of type I neoplasms. Type I neoplasms are hormone-dependent and account for 80–90% of cases; they are less aggressive, slower-growing, and better-prognosis cancers (5-year overall survival: 85%). Type II cancers are present in 10–20% of cases, are not linked to known risk factors, and do not present slow-developing pre-tumor forms (atypical hyperplasia). They have a higher frequency of advanced stages and a higher mortality (overall 5-year survival: 45–55%) [2]. A new classification has recently been introduced following the work of the Cancer Genome Atlas Research Network (TCGA) which identifies four risk classes (1. POLE ultramutated; 2. Hypermutated MSI; 3. Copy number low; 4. Copy number high) and will form the basis for selecting therapies in the coming years [3].

Hormone therapy is a risk factor for EC; treatment with estrogen without the addition of progestins to mitigate the symptoms of menopause leads to a twofold to tenfold increased risk [4]. Treatment with tamoxifen, a partial estrogen agonist also used as adjuvant therapy for breast cancer, causes an increased risk of EC. On the contrary, the use of estro-progestins for contraceptive purposes reduces the risk by 50% and the protective effect lasts for more than 20 years after the end of therapy. EC is associated with Lynch syndrome, which also involves an increased risk of cancer of the colon, breast, and ovaries [5].

No screening programs for the female population are available for this neoplasia. The symptoms that most frequently lead to diagnosis are the presence of atypical bleeding from the vagina, especially in menopausal women. The disease is rarely asymptomatic. The diagnosis of EC is obtained with transvaginal ultrasound, which evaluates endometrial thickness (suspected if >5 mm in post-menopause) and endometrial biopsy, usually performed during a diagnostic hysteroscopy [6].

The treatment of EC is generally surgical and consists of the removal of the uterus, ovaries, and regional lymph nodes. Recently, the sentinel lymph node technique has been proposed, which removes only the first draining lymph node; the technique is reliable and significantly reduces the morbidity caused by the removal of a large number of lymph nodes [7] (Fig. 2). Generally, surgery is performed with minimally invasive techniques (laparoscopy or robotics) resulting in improved aesthetic results and functional recovery. In rare cases, the use of laparotomy is still necessary, especially for patients who have undergone several abdominal procedures and in advanced stage disease. Adjuvant therapies (radiotherapy or chemotherapy) are established based on risk factors assessed after surgical pathological staging. Therefore, patients are divided into low, intermediate, and high risk of metastasis. In the case of lymph node metastases or particularly aggressive tumor histological types (serous histotype), patients receive platinum-based chemotherapy and external radiotherapy. In "fragile" women due to poor health conditions and/or advanced age, surgery is not performed, and external radiotherapy is offered with satisfactory results. Finally, in young women, with small tumors, with non-aggressive histological characteristics, a hormone-based therapy can be performed (often by means of intrauterine device with local progestins release) with the aim of preserving the uterus and allowing for a possible future pregnancy [8].

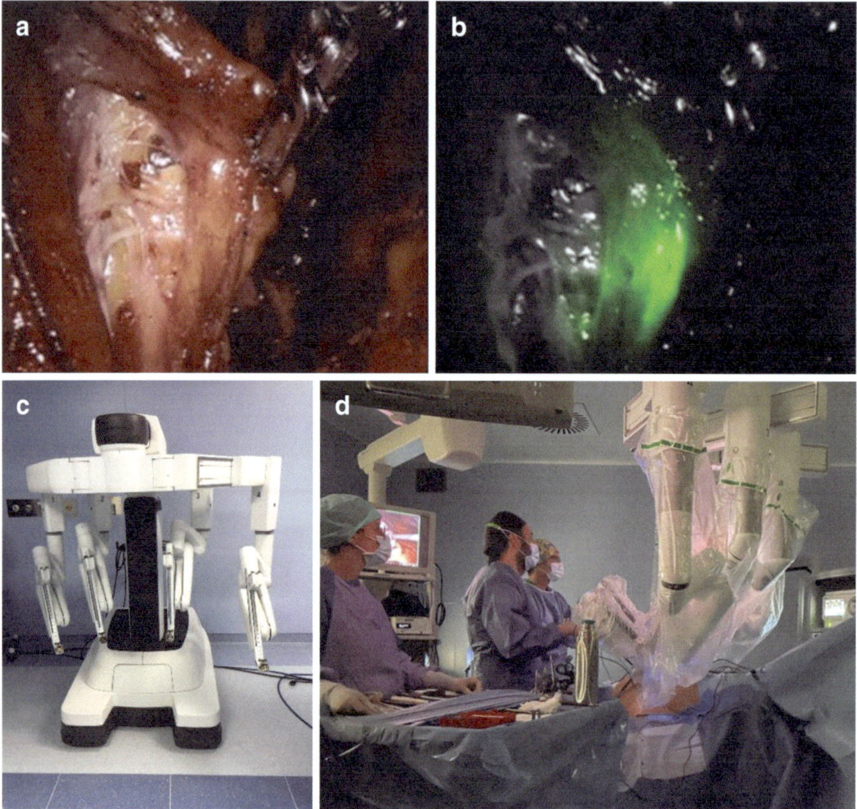

Fig. 2 The sentinel lymph node technique by robotic surgery. Sentinel pelvic lymph node observed by means of high resolution camera (**a**) and with indocyanine green fluorescence detection (**b**). The procedure is performed with the use of the Robotic Surgical System (da Vinci™ surgical system) (**c, d**)

Cervical Cancer

Cervical cancer (CC) is the second most common cancer among women in many developing countries. In Western countries, the frequency is very low due to screening programs (pap tests, HPV tests) that detect pre-tumoral forms. This cancer has a maximum incidence in women between 40 and 65 years, but it can also occur in young women (incidence of 4.5 per 100,000 women between 20 and 30 years). Risk factors are genital infections, early sexual activity, high number of partners, cigarette smoking, and low socio-economic status. Human papillomavirus infection (HPV) plays a crucial role in the development of cancer; virus DNA is present in cancer cells in 99.7% of cases. HPV infection is widespread in 80% of the population, but the virus is cleared by the immune system in 80% of cases within 1–2 years of first contact. The persistence of the virus and the presence of associated risk factors (other sexually transmitted infections, immunodepression, and use of estro-progestins) may induce the onset of CC [9].

Screening for CC is based on a cytological examination (pap smear test); the high reliability of the test, the low cost, and the high compliance by patients, makes it the ideal screening test to detect dysplasia and thus reduce the incidence of infiltrating tumors. The screening programs introduced since the 1960s in industrialized countries resulted in a 70% reduction in mortality (from 7.4 per 100,000 women to 2.4 per 100,000 women). Recently, in many countries the screening test has been replaced by an HPV test which, in combination with the pap test, presents higher sensitivity [10, 11].

CC is generally asymptomatic, especially in the early stages of disease; sometimes the only symptom is unexpected vaginal bleeding, often appearing after sexual intercourse. Only in case of advanced disease the patient complains of other symptoms, such as pelvic pain, or diffused lumbar and thigh pain. The diagnosis is obtained with a precise sequence of steps as the use of a pap smear test, colposcopy, and biopsy performed on the suspected area. In case of a doubtful early lesion, a large cervical biopsy (conization) is performed for diagnostic and sometimes therapeutic purposes [12].

The treatment of CC in the early stages is surgical: the removal of the uterus, cervix and paracervical tissue (parametrium) is warranted. This technique is called radical hysterectomy, which is modulated regarding the amount of parametrium removed based on pathologic risk factors (tumor size, neoplastic cells present in the lymphovascular spaces, type of invasion of the cervical stroma). The modulation of the surgical radicality frequently grants to preserve the nervous plexuses (parasympathetic and orthosympathetic). Such plexuses are near the uterine cervix and innervate the bladder, vagina, and rectum. Lesions of the peri-cervical nervous plexus can cause dysfunction in these areas. Surgery also consists of removing pelvic lymph nodes that receive lymph from the cervix (external, internal, and common iliac lymph nodes). Recently, the removal of the sentinel lymph node has been introduced, reducing post-operative complications [13].

After surgery, the presence of specific risk of recurrence requires postoperative external radiotherapy; it is generally administered in conjunction with a dose of chemotherapy for sensitizing purposes (concomitant chemo-radiotherapy). In the more advanced cases, the use of chemo-radiotherapy without surgery is required; the external radiotherapy is completed by brachytherapy, which consists an additional dose to the cervical and peri-cervical tissue [14, 15].

In rare cases of early stage cancer in young women who wish to become pregnant, the surgical removal of part of the cervix (conization or cervicectomy) and pelvic lymph nodes may be proposed. This allows the preservation of the uterus and the possibility of pregnancy at the end of the follow-up period [16].

Ovarian Cancer

Ovarian cancer (OC) represents a very complex entity because it collects numerous types of tumors (epithelial, germinal, and stromal) with different levels of incidence, aggressiveness, and prognosis. The most common cancer is malignant epithelial cancer, and it is the fourth leading cause of death from malignant neoplasm in women in industrialized countries. The incidence varies in different areas of the world, with the highest incidence in Europe (14 cases per 100,000 women) and minimal in Africa (4 per 100,000 women). The neoplasm is generally diagnosed at advanced stages, so overall 5-year survival is less than 50% [17].

OC is asymptomatic, especially at early stages of the disease. When the neoplasm has spread to the abdomen and to the peritoneum, intestinal loops, and omentum, the patient experiences vague abdominal pain, abdominal bloating, feeding difficulties, irregular bowel function, and asthenia. Unfortunately, these symptoms correspond to advanced stages of the disease with severe prognosis (5-year mortality over 70%) [18].

Multiparity, breastfeeding, and prolonged use of oral contraceptives reduce the risk of OC. Scientifically unproven risk factors include exposure to asbestos and talcum powder, alcohol abuse, and a high-fat diet. An increased incidence of endometrioid and clear cell tumors is reported in women with endometriosis after a long-term clinical history. Higher risk of OC was reported in cases of hormone therapy in menopause with the use of unopposed estrogen (without the addition of progestins). Family genetic factors are extremely important, as more than 10% of patients with OC have the genetic alteration of breast-ovarian cancer syndrome (BRCA type 1 and 2), and further patients are positive for other genetic factors (Lynch syndrome, Cowden syndrome, and Gorlin syndrome) [19].

Currently, no screening programs and adequate diagnostic procedures for malignant OC are available. An English randomized study (United Kingdom Collaborative Trial of Ovarian Cancer Screening—UKCTOCS) using the annual CA125 dosage and trans-vaginal ultrasound showed a reduction in mortality of 23% only after 14 years from the start of screening. However, a longer follow-up is currently considered necessary to define the effectiveness of this screening program [20].

The diagnosis of OC is based on pelvic ultrasound: the presence of an ovarian mass with specific ultrasound characteristics (presence of thick septa, vascularization, papillae, solid parts) is the first step in the diagnosis of the disease [21]. The tumor spread is then assessed with more complex imaging methods (computed tomography, magnetic resonance imaging, and positron emission tomography).

The OC is generally treated with the association of surgery and chemotherapy: surgery must be radical and must remove all the tumor nodules in the abdomen; therefore, multi-visceral interventions are often required. In addition to the removal of the genital organs (hysterectomy and bilateral salpingo-oophorectomy), it may be necessary to remove a tract of colon, ileum, an area of the diaphragm, or the spleen [22]. In less than 20% of cases, surgery requires only hysterectomy and salpingo-oophorectomy. In rare cases of young patients with early stage disease, a fertility-sparing surgery for a future pregnancy can be proposed (preservation of at least one ovary and the uterus) [23].

Usually, surgery is followed by systemic chemotherapy: carboplatin and paclitaxel are generally administered every 21 days for 6 cycles. Then a maintenance therapy is added with anti-angiogenetic drugs (bevacizumab) or PARP inhibitors (poly ADP ribose polymerase inhibitors) [24].

The quality of life can be severely altered in patients treated for gynecological neoplasms; surgery, radiation therapy, and chemotherapy, alone or in combination, can lead to short- and long-term damage. Demolitive surgery always involves a functional damage: hysterectomy is associated with the possible onset of pelvic pain from post-operative adhesions, changes in intestinal function in 30% of cases, dyspareunia from scarring reactions, and bladder dysfunction in 20% of cases. Oophorectomy may be associated with chronic pain ("phantom ovary") and/or adhesion pain. In the case of difficult removal of the ovary, "remnant ovary" syndrome may appear with persistence of pain associated with the function of an unknown ovarian residual. Bilateral salpingo-oophorectomy involves the complete disappearance of hormonal production that in women in pre-menopause causes the early onset of menopausal symptoms (hot-flushes, sleep disorders, mood changes, vaginal dryness, osteo-articular pain, osteoporosis, cognitive alterations) [25].

In case of radical hysterectomy due to CC, the lesion of the parasympathetic and orthosympathetic nervous plexuses can cause damage to urinary function (failure to empty the bladder until the need for self-catheterization), intestinal function (difficult evacuation, fecal incontinence, constipation, painful evacuation in 20–50% of cases), and sexual function (dyspareunia and alteration of sexual sensations, altered vaginal lubrication) [26].

Clearly, ultra-radical surgery, which is often performed in the case of advanced OC, entails a greater risk of complications and changes in quality of life. The following scenarios illustrate the most typical complications. The removal of large tracts of intestine (sigmoidectomy, hemi-colectomy, total colectomy) is associated with alterations of bowel function, intestinal pain, and changes in intestinal resorption, resulting in changes in nutrition and disvitaminosis; the image of the patient is severely altered in case of bowel stoma (ileostomy or colostomy) [27]. The removal of large tracts of peritoneum (peritonectomy) can cause chronic pain and intestinal function disorders from scar retractions. Omentectomy can cause in the immediate post-surgical period a temporary gastric paresis. Removal of the diaphragmatic peritoneum and of diaphragm may be associated with chronic abdominal and thoracic pain, while failure to regain function of part of the diaphragm may be associated with dyspnea [28].

Pelvic and peri-aortic lymphadenectomy is not complication-free: lymphatic collections (lymphocele) with compression pain and infections are common; in 10–20% of cases lymphedema appears in the lower limbs and common symptoms are: heaviness, altered movement, skin fragility and ulceration, erythema and pigmentation [29].

Modern radiotherapy has been developed to achieve the best oncological results by reducing complications to the surrounding organs. Currently, treatment planning uses radiological images and takes advantage of complex beam shaping. However, early and late reactions may develop and depend on dose, volume, type of fractionation, and technique. The skin may have inflammatory and fibrous reactions, especially at the vulva and groin. Acute gastrointestinal complications are common: diarrhea, rectal discomfort, abdominal cramps, and proctitis. Proctitis can cause alteration of bowel function and rectal bleeding; late reactions are frequently observed: small intestinal bacterial overgrowth, bile acid malabsorption, carbohydrate malabsorption, bowel strictures, pancreatic insufficiency, and changes in gastrointestinal transit. An uncommon chronic complication is fecal incontinence [30].

The urinary tract can also be affected by radiotherapy: acute cystitis, bladder bleeding; late complications are dysuria, nocturia, and frequency [31].

Lastly, we must remember the vaginal complications from radiotherapy, such as dryness, fibrosis, and stenosis that often hinder sexual intercourse and follow-up visits.

Chemotherapy presents various acute side effects (nausea, vomiting, asthenia, and alopecia) that are influenced by individual characteristics and type of drugs. Mucositis, esophagitis, and lower gastrointestinal tract infections with diarrhea, sometimes severe, are commonly seen. Some drugs, such as taxans, are neurotoxic and can cause major neurological deficits that are predominantly sensitive (especially to the hands and feet) and can last for years. Toxic effects on other organs (liver, heart, lung, and kidney) according to the type of drug are reported; in case of persistence of these long-lasting complications, a reduction in the quality of life is observed [32].

Finally, anti-neoplastic drugs can have a toxic effect on ovarian function and therefore lead to premature menopause and the appearance of sterility in young women [33].

The impact of gynecological cancer on women's lives is therefore extremely variable and multiform; besides the possibility of compromising various organs, the impact of therapies on the reproductive and sexual function cannot be neglected. Modification of the vagina after surgery or radiation therapy alters the ability for normal sexual intercourse. Removal of the ovaries or chemically induced toxicity causes severe estrogen-deprivation symptoms. Ultra-radical surgery with stoma placement alters the perception of body image and interpersonal relationships.

Sexuality and Quality of Life in Gynecological Cancer Patients

When we talk about sexuality and the quality of life of these patients, we must also include the sensitivity and reactions of the partner. Particularly as by "sexuality" we do not only mean coital intercourse but everything that intimacy includes: the relationship with one's own body, the confrontation with the disease, the sexual experience prior to the neoplastic diagnosis, the relationship with one's partner, sociability, and plans for the future. There has been no lack of specific studies in this area.

Casey M Hay [34] examined the needs of patients and caregivers. The survey explored doctor–patient interactions regarding sexuality across three domains (experiences, preferences, and barriers) and four stages of cancer care (diagnosis, treatment, completion of treatment, and follow-up). The mean age was 63 years. Most patients had been diagnosed with ovarian cancer (38%) or endometrial cancer (32%). 37% had received treatment in the last month, 55% were in a relationship, and 35%

were sexually active. 34% stated that sexuality was somewhat or very important, while 27% felt that it was somewhat or very important to discuss it. Importance of sexuality was associated with age, relationship status, and sexual activity, but not with cancer type. 57% reported that they had never discussed sexuality. The most common barrier to discussion was the patient's discomfort in talking about sexuality with doctors and nurses who were not interested or avoided questions on the topic. Follow-up was identified as the best time for discussion. But there is more.

Partner disorientation and a tendency to make intimacy a loving approach rather than an erotic one were evident in all interviewees.

But what tools do we have to assess post-diagnosis? Tim Luckett [35] identified one generic questionnaire (SF-36/SF-12), three specific ones (European Organization for the Research and Treatment of Cancer Quality of Life Questionnaire [EORTC QLQ] C30, Functional Assessment of Cancer Therapy-General [FACT-G], and Short Form Cancer Rehabilitation Assessment System [CARES-SF]), one disease-specific HRQoL questionnaire (QOL-Ovarian Cancer Patient Version), and five disease-specific (QLQ-OV28, FACT-O for ovarian, QLQ-CX24, FACT-Cx for cervical, and FACT-V for vulvar), one treatment-specific (FACT and Gynecologic Oncology Group-Ntx for neurotoxicity), and two symptom-specific (FACT-Anemia and Functional Assessment of Chronic Disease and Therapy [FACIT]-Fatigue) modules. Twenty-seven articles reported the results of 26 studies in which an MCID was identified [36]. Let us consider in detail.

Illness, Psyche, and Sexuality

Jona Ingibjorg Jonsdottir [37] studied women in ongoing cancer treatment and their partners. An experimental group of 30 couples was assigned to a nurse-managed intervention and a control group of 37 couples to a waiting list (delayed intervention) ($n = 27$ couples). Participants also had access to online evidence-based educational information. Data were collected before the intervention (T1, baseline), 1–2 weeks after the intervention (T2) and after a three-month follow-up session (T3). Data from 60 couples ($N = 120$) were analyzed.

What emerged? Positive communication, the perception of a good relationship, and the ability to redefine the meaning of sexual intimacy facilitated the sexual adaptation of each individual couple facing cancer [38]. Three different pathways of sexual adjustment could thus be identified: as a grieving process, as a cognitive restructuring process, and as a rehabilitation process. All three pathways appeared to be part of a rehabilitation process that doctors and nurses can positively connote a <new life project> for the individual and the couple. In another study, Abbott Anderson et al. identified the Illness Belief Model as a powerful tool for identifying and addressing constraining beliefs pertaining to the couple's sexual health, thus encouraging sexual adjustment [39].

Not surprisingly, partners of gynecological cancer patients reported that the onset of cancer negatively affected their sexual relationship, including cessation or decrease in frequency of sex and renegotiation of sexual and non-sexual intimacy. In addition, partners also linked sexual changes following cancer with stress, fatigue, revised priorities involving coping and survival, and their role of caregiver rather than that of lover.

A further difficulty for the partners seems to be how to awaken their interest in and desire for their partner as a 'woman' and not as a patient. It is no accident that some of them complained of erectile dysfunction, hypoactive desire, and premature ejaculation. And what of coitus? During the first penetrations, it seemed difficult for any couple to accept a new sexuality that included penetration. The one partner for fear of pain, pelvic burning, and poor lubrication, the other for fear of penetrating a physical space already damaged by surgery and consequently more conditioned by discomfort than by pleasure [40].

Sexuality and Follow-Up

The MD Anderson Symptom Inventory (MDASI) [41] captures the severity of common cancer symptoms of ovarian cancer from the patient's perspective.

The MDASI specifically assesses the severity of 13 common (core) cancer-related symptoms: pain, fatigue (tiredness), nausea, disturbed sleep, distress, shortness of breath, difficulty remembering, lack of appetite, feeling drowsy, dry mouth, feeling sad, vomiting, and numbness or tingling.

Mary H. Sailors [40] recruited 128 patients with invasive epithelial, peritoneal, or fallopian tube ovarian cancer treated at the MD Anderson Cancer Centre at the University of Texas. Patients completed the MDASI-OC, socio-demographic questionnaires, the Functional Assessment of Cancer Therapy-Ovary (FACT-O), and a global quality of life (QOL) item.

The sample was predominantly white (85.2%), with a mean age of 57.5 years (±12.7 years) and having previously been treated with chemotherapy (75.0%) and/ or surgery (93.8%). Approximately 30% of patients reported sleep disturbance, fatigue, or numbness/shaking of at least moderate severity ($\geq = 5$ on a scale of 0 to 10). Concerning ovarian cancer-specific symptoms, about 20% reported back pain, bloating, or constipation of moderate severity. Factor analysis revealed six underlying constructs (pain/sleep; cognitive; disease-related and numbness; treatment-related; affective; and gastrointestinal specific). The MDASI-OC symptom and interference had Cronbach α values of 0.90 and 0.89, respectively. MDASI-OC was sensitive to symptom severity based on performance status (p 0.009), QOL ($p = 0.002$), and FACT-O scores ($p < 0.001$) [42, 43].

Not only during the course of treatment, but also during follow-up. Laura Simonelli et al. [44] studied 260 patients with a previous diagnosis of gynecological cancer 2–10 years after the end of treatment and in follow-up. They investigated the gynecological symptoms reported by the patients, the essence of the new quality of life (in terms of harmony, motivation, planning, spirituality and, on the other hand, confusion and loss), and depressive symptoms. Several questionnaires were used to

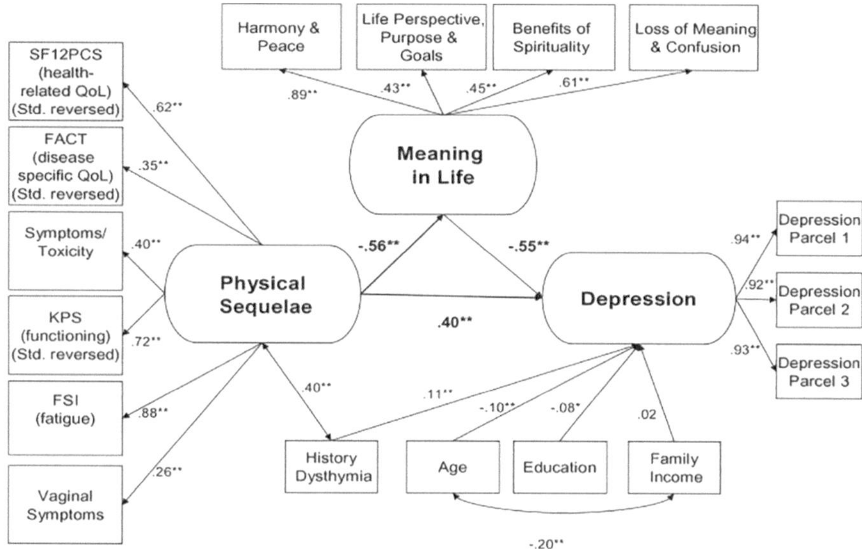

Fig. 3 The model of the hypothesized relationships tested by structural equation modelling (with permission from [44])

understand the complementarity of these elements: the Centre for Epidemiological Studies Depression Scale (CES-D), the SF-12 MCS (for mental health), the Short Profile of Mood States (POMS), and the Post-Traumatic Stress Disorder (PTSD) symptom checklist. The scheme in Fig. 3 shows the results of this study.

As can be seen, the physical consequences of the disease and depression were the major factors in loss of motivation. Individuals seeking meaning after cancer appeared discouraged as their physical symptoms worsened or persisted. Limitations to their ability to resume life as it had been (or as it had been anticipated to be) could lead to a lack of fulfilment, feelings of dissatisfaction with their current life, and disappointment when physical limitations or debilitation interfered with daily life. Patients diagnosed with gynecological cancer, in common with other cancer patients, also reported life-interrupting fatigue but their higher incidence of sexual difficulties distinguished their survival, vaginal changes, and decreased sexual function, and could adversely affect female self-perception and their role as a lover [45].

Conclusion

The persistence of symptoms in patients diagnosed with gynecological cancer affects their interest in life, their social life, and their plans for the future. The unpreparedness of the partner to take on the role of caregiver deadens the psycho-physical and sexual rehabilitation of the woman. This highlights how the psycho-sexological approach to the couple must begin alongside the surgeon–oncologist–gynecologist at the time of diagnosis. Showing the couple that the whole medical and nursing team is involved in positive and purposeful communication ensures that the couple do not find themselves alone, excluded from social life and deprived of all the pleasures of life [46].

References

1. Ferlay J, Colombet M, Soerjomataram I, Dyba T, Randi G, Bettio M, Gavin A, Visser O, Bray F. Cancer incidence and mortality patterns in Europe: estimates for 40 countries and 25 major cancers in 2018. Eur J Cancer. 2018;103:356–87. https://doi.org/10.1016/j.ejca.2018.07.005. Epub 2018 Aug 9. PMID: 30100160.
2. Setiawan VW, Yang HP, Pike MC, et al. Type I and II endometrial cancers: have they different risk factors? J Clin Oncol. 2013;31:2607–18. https://doi.org/10.1200/JCO.2012.48.2596.
3. Cancer Genome Atlas Research Network, Kandoth C, Schultz N, Cherniack AD, Akbani R, Liu Y, Shen H, Robertson AG, Pashtan I, Shen R, Benz CC, Yau C, Laird PW, Ding L, Zhang W, Mills GB, Kucherlapati R, Mardis ER, Levine DA. Integrated genomic characterization of endometrial carcinoma. Nature. 2013;497(7447):67–73. https://doi.org/10.1038/nature12113. Erratum in: Nature. 2013 Aug 8;500(7461):242. PMID: 23636398; PMCID: PMC3704730.
4. Crosbie EJ, Zwahlen M, Kitchener HC, Egger M, Renehan AG. Body mass index, hormone replacement therapy, and endometrial cancer risk: a meta-analysis. Cancer Epidemiol Biomark Prev. 2010;19(12):3119–30. https://doi.org/10.1158/1055-9965.EPI-10-0832. Epub 2010 Oct 28. PMID: 21030602.
5. Dondi G, Coluccelli S, De Leo A, et al. An analysis of clinical, surgical, pathological and molecular characteristics of endometrial cancer according to mismatch repair status. A multidisciplinary approach. Int J Mol Sci. 2020;21:1–17. https://doi.org/10.3390/ijms21197188.
6. Savelli L, Ceccarini M, Ludovisi M, Fruscella E, De Iaco PA, Salizzoni E, Mabrouk M, Manfredi R, Testa AC, Ferrandina G. Preoperative local staging of endometrial cancer: transvaginal sonography vs. magnetic resonance imaging. Ultrasound Obstet Gynecol. 2008;31(5):560–6. https://doi.org/10.1002/uog.5295. PMID: 18398926.
7. Bogani G, Papadia A, Buda A, et al. Sentinel node mapping vs. sentinel node mapping plus back-up lymphadenectomy in high-risk endometrial cancer patients: results from a multi-institutional study. Gynecol Oncol. 2021;161:122–9. https://doi.org/10.1016/j.ygyno.2021.01.008.
8. Concin N, Matias-Guiu X, Vergote I, et al. ESGO/ESTRO/ESP guidelines for the management of patients with endometrial carcinoma. Int J Gynecol Cancer. 2021;31:12–39. https://doi.org/10.1136/ijgc-2020-002230.
9. Bogani G, Sopracordevole F, Di Donato V, Ciavattini A, Ghelardi A, Lopez S, Simoncini T, Plotti F, Casarin J, Serati M, Pinelli C, Valenti G, Bergamini A, Gardella B, Dell'acqua A, Monti E, Vercellini P, Fischetti M, D'ippolito G, Aguzzoli L, Mandato VD, Carunchio P, Carlinfante G, Giannella L, Scaffa C, Falcone F, Borghi C, Ditto A, Malzoni M, Giannini A, Salerno MG, Liberale V, Contino B, Donfrancesco C, Desiato M, Perrone AM, Dondi G, De Iaco P, Chiappa V, Ferrero S, Sarpietro G, Matarazzo MG, Cianci A, Bosio S, Ruisi S, Guerrisi R, Brusadelli C, Mosca L, Lagana' AS, Tinelli R, Signorelli M, De Vincenzo R, Zannoni GF, Ferrandina G, Lovati S, Petrillo M, Dessole S, Carlea A, Zullo F, Angioli R, Greggi S, Spinillo A, Ghezzi F, Colacurci N, Muzii L, Benedetti Panici P, Scambia G, Raspagliesi F. High-risk HPV-positive and -negative high-grade cervical dysplasia: analysis of 5-year outcomes. Gynecol Oncol. 2021;161(1):173–8. https://doi.org/10.1016/j.ygyno.2021.01.020. Epub 2021 Jan 26. PMID: 33514481.
10. Koliopoulos G, Arbyn M, Martin-Hirsch P, Kyrgiou M, Prendiville W, Paraskevaidis E. Diagnostic accuracy of human papillomavirus testing in primary cervical screen-

ing: a systematic review and meta-analysis of non-randomized studies. Gynecol Oncol. 2007;104(1):232–46. https://doi.org/10.1016/j.ygyno.2006.08.053. Epub 2006 Nov 3. PMID: 17084886.

11. Paraskevaidis E, Arbyn M, Sotiriadis A, Diakomanolis E, Martin-Hirsch P, Koliopoulos G, Makrydimas G, Tofoski J, Roukos DH. The role of HPV DNA testing in the follow-up period after treatment for CIN: a systematic review of the literature. Cancer Treat Rev. 2004;30(2):205–11. https://doi.org/10.1016/j.ctrv.2003.07.008. PMID: 15023438.

12. Colombo N, Carinelli S, Colombo A, Marini C, Rollo D, Sessa C, ESMO Guidelines Working Group. Cervical cancer: ESMO Clinical Practice Guidelines for diagnosis, treatment and follow-up. Ann Oncol. 2012;23(Suppl 7):27–32. https://doi.org/10.1093/annonc/mds268. PMID: 22997451.

13. Olthof EP, van der Aa MA, Adam JA, Stalpers LJA, Wenzel HHB, van der Velden J, Mom CH. The role of lymph nodes in cervical cancer: incidence and identification of lymph node metastases-a literature review. Int J Clin Oncol. 2021;26:1600. https://doi.org/10.1007/s10147-021-01980-2.

14. Cima S, Perrone AM, Castellucci P, Macchia G, Buwenge M, Cammelli S, Cilla S, Ferioli M, Ferrandina G, Galuppi A, Salizzoni E, Rubino D, Fanti S, De Iaco P, Morganti AG. Prognostic impact of pretreatment fluorodeoxyglucose positron emission tomography/computed tomography SUVmax in patients with locally advanced cervical cancer. Int J Gynecol Cancer. 2018;28(3):575–80. https://doi.org/10.1097/IGC.0000000000001207. PMID: 29372911.

15. Perrone AM, Tesei M, Ferioli M, De Terlizzi F, Della Gatta AN, Boussedra S, Dondi G, Galuppi A, Morganti AG, De Iaco P. Results of a phase I-II study on laser therapy for vaginal side effects after radiotherapy for cancer of uterine cervix or endometrium. Cancers (Basel). 2020;12(6):1639. https://doi.org/10.3390/cancers12061639. PMID: 32575821; PMCID: PMC7352893.

16. Perrone AM, Bovicelli A, D'Andrilli G, Borghese G, Giordano A, De Iaco P. Cervical cancer in pregnancy: analysis of the literature and innovative approaches. J Cell Physiol. 2019;234(9):14975–90. https://doi.org/10.1002/jcp.28340. Epub 2019 Feb 20. PMID: 30790275.

17. Colombo N, Sessa C, Bois AD, Ledermann J, McCluggage WG, McNeish I, Morice P, Pignata S, Ray-Coquard I, Vergote I, Baert T, Belaroussi I, Dashora A, Olbrecht S, Planchamp F, Querleu D. ESMO–ESGO Ovarian Cancer Consensus Conference Working Group. ESMO-ESGO consensus conference recommendations on ovarian cancer: pathology and molecular biology, early and advanced stages, borderline tumours and recurrent disease. Int J Gynecol Cancer 2019:ijgc-2019-000308. https://doi.org/10.1136/ijgc-2019-000308. Epub ahead of print. PMID: 31048403.

18. Bankhead CR, Kehoe ST, Austoker J. Symptoms associated with diagnosis of ovarian cancer: a systematic review. BJOG. 2005;112(7):857–65. https://doi.org/10.1111/j.1471-0528.2005.00572.x. PMID: 15957984.

19. Sekine M, Nishino K, Enomoto T. *BRCA* genetic test and risk-reducing Salpingo-oophorectomy for hereditary breast and ovarian cancer: state-of-the-art. Cancers (Basel). 2021;13(11):2562. https://doi.org/10.3390/cancers13112562. PMID: 34071148; PMCID: PMC8197088.

20. Menon U, Gentry-Maharaj A, Burnell M, Singh N, Ryan A, Karpinskyj C, Carlino G, Taylor J, Massingham SK, Raikou M, Kalsi JK, Woolas R, Manchanda R, Arora R, Casey L, Dawnay A, Dobbs S, Leeson S, Mould T, Seif MW, Sharma A, Williamson K, Liu Y, Fallowfield L, McGuire AJ, Campbell S, Skates SJ, Jacobs IJ, Parmar M. Ovarian cancer population screening and mortality after long-term follow-up in the UK Collaborative Trial of Ovarian Cancer Screening (UKCTOCS): a randomised controlled trial. Lancet. 2021;397(10290):2182–93. https://doi.org/10.1016/S0140-6736(21)00731-5. Epub 2021 May 12. PMID: 33991479; PMCID: PMC8192829.

21. Timmerman D, Planchamp F, Bourne T, Landolfo C, du Bois A, Chiva L, Cibula D, Concin N, Fischerova D, Froyman W, Gallardo G, Lemley B, Loft A, Mereu L, Morice P, Querleu D, Testa C, Vergote I, Vandecaveye V, Scambia G, Fotopoulou C. ESGO/ISUOG/IOTA/ESGE consensus statement on preoperative diagnosis of ovarian tumours. Facts Views Vis Obgyn.

2021;13(2):107–30. https://doi.org/10.52054/FVVO.13.2.016. Epub 2021 Jun 10. PMID: 34107646.

22. Vergote I, Amant F, Kristensen G, Ehlen T, Reed NS, Casado A. Primary surgery or neoadjuvant chemotherapy followed by interval debulking surgery in advanced ovarian cancer. Eur J Cancer. 2011;47(Suppl 3):S88–92. https://doi.org/10.1016/S0959-8049(11)70152-6. PMID: 21944035.

23. Necula D, Istrate D, Mathis J. Fertility preservation in women with early ovarian cancer. Horm Mol Biol Clin Investig. 2020;43:163. https://doi.org/10.1515/hmbci-2020-0026. PMID: 34187159.

24. Wilson MK, Pujade-Lauraine E, Aoki D, Mirza MR, Lorusso D, Oza AM, du Bois A, Vergote I, Reuss A, Bacon M, Friedlander M, Gallardo-Rincon D, Joly F, Chang SJ, Ferrero AM, Edmondson RJ, Wimberger P, Maenpaa J, Gaffney D, Zang R, Okamoto A, Stuart G, Ochiai K. Participants of the fifth ovarian cancer consensus conference. Fifth ovarian cancer consensus conference of the gynecologic cancer InterGroup: recurrent disease. Ann Oncol. 2017;28(4):727–32. https://doi.org/10.1093/annonc/mdw663. PMID: 27993805; PMCID: PMC6246494.

25. Cianci S, Tarascio M, Rosati A, Caruso S, Uccella S, Cosentino F, Scaletta G, Gueli Alletti S, Scambia G. Sexual function and quality of life of patients affected by ovarian cancer. Minerva Med. 2019;110(4):320–9. https://doi.org/10.23736/S0026-4806.19.06080-4. Epub 2019 May 6. PMID: 31081305.

26. Kyo S, Kato T, Nakayama K. Current concepts and practical techniques of nerve-sparing laparoscopic radical hysterectomy. Eur J Obstet Gynecol Reprod Biol. 2016;207:80–8. https://doi.org/10.1016/j.ejogrb.2016.10.033. Epub 2016 Oct 28. PMID: 27825032.

27. Son JH, Chang SJ. Extrapelvic bowel resection and anastomosis in cytoreductive surgery for ovarian cancer. Gland Surg. 2021;10(3):1207–11. https://doi.org/10.21037/gs-2019-ursoc-01. PMID: 33842266; PMCID: PMC8033058.

28. Shin W, Mun J, Park SY, Lim MC. Narrative review of liver mobilization, diaphragm peritonectomy, full-thickness diaphragm resection, and reconstruction. Gland Surg. 2021;10(3):1212–7. https://doi.org/10.21037/gs-20-422. PMID: 33842267; PMCID: PMC8033081.

29. Bogani G, Borghi C, Ditto A, Signorelli M, Martinelli F, Chiappa V, Scaffa C, Perotto S, Leone Roberti Maggiore U, Montanelli L, Di Donato V, Infantino C, Lorusso D, Raspagliesi F. Impact of surgical route in influencing the risk of lymphatic complications after ovarian cancer staging. J Minim Invasive Gynecol. 2017;24(5):739–46. https://doi.org/10.1016/j.jmig.2017.03.014. Epub 2017 Mar 24. PMID: 28347880.

30. Huh JW, Tanksley J, Chino J, Willett CG, Dewhirst MW. Long-term consequences of pelvic irradiation: toxicities, challenges, and therapeutic opportunities with pharmacologic Mitigators. Clin Cancer Res. 2020;26(13):3079–90. https://doi.org/10.1158/1078-0432.CCR-19-2744. Epub 2020 Feb 25. PMID: 32098770.

31. Vilos GA, Reyes-MuÑoz E, Riemma G, Kahramanoglu I, Lin LT, Chiofalo B, Lordelo P, Della Corte L, Vitagliano A, Valenti G. Gynecological cancers and urinary dysfunction: a comparison between endometrial cancer and other gynecological malignancies. Minerva Med. 2021;112(1):96–110. https://doi.org/10.23736/S0026-4806.20.06770-1. Epub 2020 Jul 22. PMID: 32700863.

32. Woopen H, Richter R, Chekerov R, Siepmann T, Ismaeel F, Sehouli J. The influence of comorbidity and comedication on grade III/IV toxicity and prior discontinuation of chemotherapy in recurrent ovarian cancer patients: an individual participant data meta-analysis of the North-Eastern German Society of Gynecological Oncology (NOGGO). Gynecol Oncol. 2015;138(3):735–40. https://doi.org/10.1016/j.ygyno.2015.07.007. Epub 2015 Jul 13. PMID: 26185017.

33. Sun B, Yeh J. Onco-fertility and personalized testing for potential for loss of ovarian reserve in patients undergoing chemotherapy: proposed next steps for development of genetic testing to predict changes in ovarian reserve. Fertil Res Pract. 2021;7(1):13. https://doi.org/10.1186/s40738-021-00105-7. PMID: 34193292; PMCID: PMC8244159.

34. Hay CM, et al. Sexual health as part of gynecological cancer treatment: what do patients want? Int J. Gynecoll Cancer. 2018;28(9):1737–42.
35. Lukett T, et al. Health-related quality of life assessment in gynecological oncology: a systematic review of questionnaires and their ability to detect clinically important differences and changes. Int J. Gynecol Cancer. 2010;20(4):664–84.
36. White ID, Tennant A, Taylor C. Assessment of sexual morbidity in gynecological follow-up: development of sexual Well-being after cervical or endometrial cancer (SWELL-CE) patient-reported outcome measure. J Sex Med. 2020;17:2005–15.
37. Jonsdottir JI, et al. The efficacy of a couple intervention based on sexuality and intimacy among women in the treatment of active cancer: a quasi-experimental study. Eur J Oncol Nurs. 2021;52:101975.
38. Abbott-Anderson K, et al. Adjust to sex and intimacy: gynecological cancer survivors share their relationships with partners. Aging Women. 2020;32:329.
39. Abbott-Anderson K, et al. Sexual concerns of gynecological cancer survivors: development of the gynecological sexual concerns-cancer questionnaire. Master's thesis, 2020.
40. Albers LF, et al. Sexual health needs: how do breast cancer patients and their partners want information? J Marital Sex Ther. 2020;46:205.
41. Sailors MH, et al. Validation of the MD Anderson Symptom Inventory (MDASI) for use in ovarian cancer patients. Gynecol Oncol. 2013;130(2):323–8.
42. Fadol A, Mendoza T, Gning I, Kernicki J, Symes L, Cleeland CS, et al. MDASI-HF psychometric testing: a symptom assessment tool for patients with cancer and concomitant heart failure. J Card Fallire. 2008;14:497–507.
43. Wang XS, Cleeland CS, Mendoza TR, Yun YH, Wang Y, Okuyama T, et al. Impact of cultural and linguistic factors on the reporting of symptoms by cancer patients. J Natl Inst Canc. 2010;102:732–8.
44. Simonelli LE, et al. Article navigation physical consequences and depressive symptoms in gynecological cancer survivors: meaning of life as a mediator. Ann Behav Med. 2008;35(3):275–84.
45. Fisherman B, Graham K, Duffecy J. Chronic diseases, disabilities and sexuality. In: McAnulty R, Burnette M, editors. Sexual function and dysfunction. Westport, CT: Praeger; 2006. p. 233–60.
46. Longhi EV, et al. Psychosexual approach in andrological surgical. Springer; 2019.

Part III
Cardiology

Chronic Coronary Artery Disease

Marco Agrifoglio, Giorgio Mastroiacovo, Marco Gennari,
and Elena Vittoria Longhi

Abbreviations

BNP	Brain natriuretiuc peptide
CABG	Coronary artery bypass graft
CIHD	Chronic ischemic heart disease
CPK	Creatine phosphor kinase
CT	Computed tomography
Hs-TnI	High sensitive troponine I
PTCA	Percutaneous transluminal coronary angioplasty
TIA	Transient ischemic attack
WHO	World Health Organization

Introduction to Chronic Ischemic Heart Disease

Atherosclerosis is a chronic arterial disease and represents the first leading cause of vascular disease worldwide [1]. In addition, forecast estimated that by 2020 cardiovascular diseases, especially atherosclerosis, will become the most widespread

M. Agrifoglio (✉)
Centro Cardiologico Monzino IRCCS, Milan, Italy

Department of Biomedical Surgical and Dental Sciences, University of Milan, Milan, Italy
e-mail: marco.agrifoglio@unimi.it

G. Mastroiacovo · M. Gennari
Centro Cardiologico Monzino IRCCS, Milan, Italy
e-mail: giorgio.mastroiacovo@ccfm.it; marco.gennari@ccfm.it

E. V. Longhi
Department of Sexual Medical Center, San Raffaele Hospital, Milano, Italy

© Springer Nature Switzerland AG 2023
E. V. Longhi (ed.), *Managing Psychosexual Consequences in Chronic Diseases*,
https://doi.org/10.1007/978-3-031-31307-3_5

diseases in the world [2]. Atherosclerosis is at the basis of the most frequent cardiovascular disease: chronic ischemic heart disease (CIHD) [3]. In Europe (WHO data 2014), CIHD is responsible for almost half (46%) of all deaths (30% in individuals <65 years old and 37% in those <75 years old) [4]. Atherogenesis (i.e. the formation of atheromatic plaques) takes place at the endothelium level, involving arteries of the all human body and their growth lasts for decades [5]. After a silent and prolonged period, the atherosclerotic plaque tends to cause the obstruction to the passage of blood downstream the stenosis (a process called ischemia) either by a reduction in lumen vessel's size (chronic process) or by the rupture of the plaque itself with consequent embolization of atherogenic material (acute process) and subsequent acute ischemia, in most cases [6]. If different arteries of our body are affected, the signs and symptoms of atherosclerosis will depend on the affected sites; more frequently, atheromasic plaques are formed at the level of coronary arteries whose principal symptom is represented by chest pain ("angina"); if plaques involve carotid arteries the main manifestation will be a transient ischemic attack (TIA) or a cerebral stroke; finally if plaque forms at peripheral arteries' level, patients will experience pain during the march ("claudicatio intermittens") [6].

Although in developing countries CIHD is continuously increasing, its mortality and morbidity are dramatically decreasing over time since the middle of the twentieth century. For example, in the United Kingdom, the probability of death from vascular disease in middle-aged men (35–69 years) has decreased from 22% in 1950 to 6% in 2010 [7].

The total cost of CIHD in 2014 consisted of €81.1 billion in healthcare costs; by 2020 healthcare costs attributable to CIHD has expected to rise to €9 8.7 billion [8].

Main Clinical Features of CIHD

From a pathogenetic point of view, atherogenesis is the basis of CIHD.

The risk factors for this pathology are nowadays well established and identified, and are divided into two main categories: the modifiable and the unmodifiable [9]. The modifiable risk factors are represented by a series of pathologies or conditions on which it is possible to intervene pharmacologically or by changing patient's lifestyle to reduce them; the non-modifiable are instead intrinsic conditions that cannot be influenced by external actions.

The principals among the first category are: smoking, systemic arterial hypertension, high plasma cholesterol levels, obesity, and diabetes mellitus. The second category includes: male sex, age, and some genetic disorders [9].

CIHD is called the "silent killer," because it remains asymptomatic for decades without manifestation of itself, until the atherosclerotic plaque reaches the size which causes a significant obstruction of blood flow downstream the stenosis (this generally occurs when the plaque determines an obstruction of blood stream of more than 70% of its physiological flow) or, following an acute rupture, causes local thrombosis leading to partial or total occlusion of the affected artery [10]. The site, size, and velocity of vessel occlusion are intrinsic characteristics of atheromasic plaque on which the clinical consequences of ischemic heart disease depend [11]. As already mentioned, the most relevant clinical manifestation of ischemic heart disease is represented by acute myocardial infarction, which means irreversible death or necrosis of a portion of myocardial tissue. The main symptom is angina, which is defined as a retrosternal constricting or oppressive pain that can radiate to the jugular or right arm and less frequently to the upper left limb or retroscapolar level [6]. Another extremely frequent symptom is the difficulty in breathing or lack of air (dyspnoea) which can occur either under stress or at rest. Less frequent symptoms are paresthesias of the upper limbs, gastric burning or dyspepsia, and algid sweating. In some cases, acute myocardial infarction occurs directly with syncope, cardiac arrhythmias, and sudden cardiac death.

Main Tools for the Diagnosis

The diagnostic algorithm of CIHD is divided into first, second, and third level examinations. Laboratory tests such as hs-TnI, CPK, and BNP values are certainly useful even if they are not always illustrative [12].

Among the first level exams, the former to include is certainly the resting electrocardiogram which consists of a peripheral voltages recording that reflect cardiac electrical activity, permitting to understand if the patient is affected by myocardial ischemia, and suggesting about the coronary lesion's location responsible for the ischemia. Specific electrocardiographic changes such as ST segment upper or under elevation >1 mm in two or more contiguous leads the appearance of a new left bundle-branch block or a Q wave with a depth >1/3 of the subsequent QRS complex are highly indicative of myocardial infarction [13]. Unfortunately, the electrocardiogram does not have 100%; this means that it cannot identify all the subject suffering from CIHD.

Exercise electrocardiography consists of an electrocardiographic recording of a patient while he/she is making a physical effort (e.g. cycling or running) and simultaneously monitoring his/her blood pressure. This test has a sensitivity of 68% and a specificity of 77% [12].

The echocardiography represents another non-invasive first level exam, easy to perform, which enables doctors to directly visualize alterations in cardiac motion; however, it remains a qualitative more than quantitative exam in CIHD evaluation, highly operator dependent so that it does not give sufficient data to decide whether to treat a patient with CIHD or not.

In recent years, among the second level imaging techniques, cardiac CT-scan is gaining a growing consensus in the scientific community for its ability to determine the size reduction of coronary vessels [14]. CT-scan's main advantage is the non-invasiveness and the relatively low cost. The main limitation for CT-scan, to be assumed as gold standard technique to diagnose CIHD, is the unreliable results when it is applied on extremely calcified coronary arteries; since calcium deposits in the atheromasic plaque interfere with CT acquisition sequences.

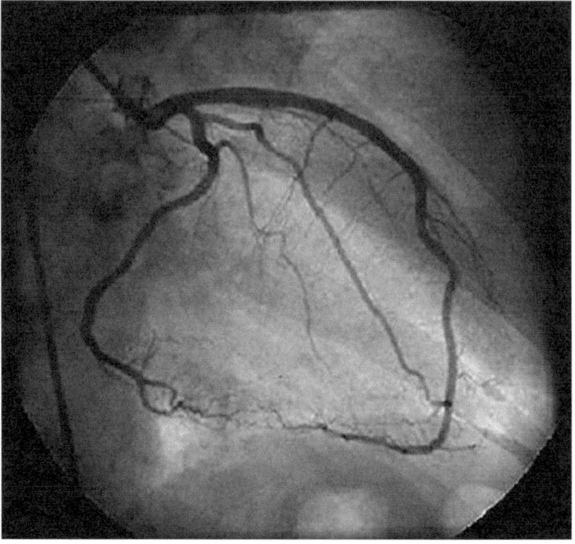

Fig. 1 Normal angiographic coronary aspect

Nowadays, the gold standard imaging technique for the diagnosis of CIHD is accounted by invasive coronary angiogram, which consists in imaging acquisition, under fluoroscopic vision, of the coronary artery tree after somministration of contrast medium enhancement via percutaneous catheter inserted in the radial or femoral artery (Fig. 1). The main disadvantage of this procedure is the inherent risk of coronary or aortic dissection, anaphylaxis to the contrast medium and, ultimately, death [15].

Main Non-invasive Treatments

Firstly, it is mandatory to intervene on the eliminable risk factors: quitting smoking, implementing a correct Mediterranean diet, weight loss, and physical activity. In some cases, it is required to combine these measures of modification in patient lifestyle with a pharmacological therapy [16]. The pharmacological armamentarium for the treatment of CIHD includes several drugs. The main medication is represented by the category of anti-platelets (the most widely used of which is Cardioaspirin) which, by inhibiting platelet aggregation, prevents, on the one hand, the increase in the size of the atheromasic plaque and, on the other hand, its rupture otherwise increasing the risk of bleeding [17].

Among these, those that have been identified as drugs capable of having a protective effect on the progression of ischemic damage, beta-blockers occupy certainly the first place. These medications act by reducing heart rate and blood pressure by blocking $\beta2$ receptors action. Ace inhibitors or sartans and aldosterone antagonists are commonly used in clinical practice because randomized controlled trials have shown that they increase survival in patients with CIHD [18]. In addition to these drugs, others are also commonly used to relieve the symptoms of CIHD itself. These include nitrates with the function of increasing venous return and vasodilating the coronary arteries and Ranolazine (a recently marketed drug).

Main Invasive Treatments

The invasive treatment of CIHD is divided into two main branches of action: (1) the percutaneous and (2) the surgical ones.

The percutaneous coronary approach consists in the release of a medicated or non-medicated stent which is inflated inside the coronary vessel at the level of the plaque. This procedure named percutaneous transluminal coronary angioplasty (PTCA) involves the delivery of the stent using catheters inserted by peripheral arteries (radial or femoral artery).

It is mostly used in single or multiple coronary artery lesions in non-diabetic patients. The main risk of coronary stents is their thrombosis and therefore the risk of intrastent restenosis [19]. In case of coronary lesions that cannot be treated by PTCA (for anatomical characteristics), in patients who have to undergo cardiac surgery for other reasons (e.g. for heart valve surgery) with associated coronary lesions or in diabetic patients with multiple coronary artery disease, coronary artery bypass graft (CABG) surgery is indicated [20]. CABG consists in bypassing the atherosclerotic plaque with arterial or venous ducts capable of conveying blood flow from the aorta directly beyond the coronary artery injury, through direct suturing of the duct with the coronary artery. The main advantage of CABG over PTCA is its longer duration (the patency of the anastomosis between the left internal thoracic artery and anterior interventricular artery has been demonstrated to be 90% at 20 years of age) (Fig. 2) [21].

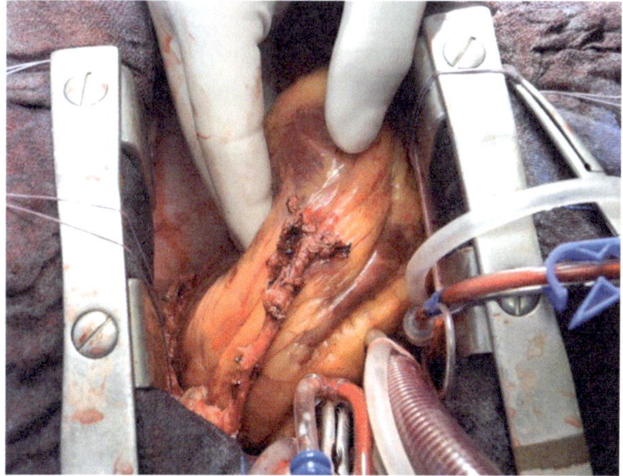

Fig. 2 An anastomosis between the left internal mammary artery and the interventricular artery

Among the major drawbacks of CABG, it has to be mentioned: the necessity for the patient to be subjected to a general anaesthesia and median sternotomy (i.e. the opening of the sternum to access the heart).

Psychological Point of View

CHID must be considered as a stressful psychological event for the patient's life [22].

First of all, it is necessary to take into consideration the aspect of the disease itself and the difficulty in taking into account the change of one's health status from "healthy" to "sick," from which comes the consideration of being fragile and approaching the normal activities of daily life with fear and apprehension. On the other hand, it is also needed to consider the change in lifestyle and quality of life that the diagnosis of ischemic heart disease entails [23]. First of all, it is required to start taking medication to reduce CIHD progression. On the other hand, angina limits a patient's daily life from sports activities (in the mildest cases) up to simpler everyday activities (such as walking or tying shoes) in the most serious instances.

In addition to these aspects, other factors related to drug therapy and its adverse effects must also be considered.

Sex life in coronary heart patients is severely limited for three main reasons [24, 25]:

1. Physical activity elicits chest pain that forces the patient to rest.
2. The drugs used in the treatment of CIHD such as nitrates contraindicate the use of other vasodilator drugs including Sildenafil, commonly used for erectile dysfunction.
3. Other drugs such as beta-blockers have an inherent risk (due to their mechanism of action) of depression and sexual impotence in men.

Last but certainly not least, it must be considered that many of these patients receive a diagnosis of ischemic heart disease in a "sudden" way for the appearance of symptoms even though the disease has been going on for years; many of them are forced to suddenly undergo a very heavy surgery such as CABG without having the time to realize and arriving psychologically unprepared at the time of surgery. In our clinical experience, this is extrinsic with phases of mood reduction in the first post-operative days up to cases of diagnosed depression. In our clinical practice, there have also been cases of patients who have put in place important removal mechanisms during the post-operative stay for which they were no longer able to remember the intervention or the acute episode that had led them to hospital admission.

In conclusion, for the above mentioned reasons, it is essential to provide a full psychological support within the health facilities of a psychologist consultant who can accompany patients both in the path of "realize" of their "sick" condition either in the difficult post-operative period following open heart surgery.

Sexuality and Quality of Life

Patients with ischemic heart disease (IHD) may report difficulties with sexual function and in marital relationships.

Shervin Assari et al. [26] conducted a study of 551 patients with IHD investigating both their sexual function and the quality of their marital relationship.

The questionnaires Relation and Sexuality Scale (RSS) and Revised Dyadic Adjustment Scale (RDAS) were used. The association between marital relationship quality and sexual function was assessed with respect to gender, educational level, and marital distress.

The majority of participants (72%) were men with a mean age of 57 ± 11 (range = 36–80) years. Total sexual function was significantly correlated with marital quality, marital accord, marital cohesion, relationship quality, and marital satisfaction.

The relationship of the couple, in patients with chronic diseases, seems to be very important given its influence on patients' quality of life, [27] adaptation to the disease, compliance, and long-term outcomes. The quality of patients' marital relationship also influences the quality of life and the psychological well-being of their children and spouses [28, 29].

At the Baqiyatallah Hospital in Tehran in 2006, a study of 630 men and 155 women with documented IHD was conducted.

The patients' relationships and sexuality since the onset of IHD were assessed using a version of the Relation and Sexuality Scale (RSS) questionnaire [30]. The RSS was developed for women but items in this questionnaire are not gender dependent and have been used previously to assess relationship and sexuality in both sexes [31].

All subjects were also asked to complete a version [32] of the Revised Dyadic Adjustment Scale (RDAS). The RDAS consists of 14 items that assess the couple's agreement on decisions, satisfaction, and marital complicity.

The results showed that male sexual dysfunction, in particular, is accompanied by anxiety and distress around intimacy, quarrels within the couple, misunderstanding, instability and lack of trust between partners. Hypoactive desire seems to be more frequent in the female population who report a lack of understanding by their partners towards female ischemic pathology [33, 34].

Delia Johnson et al. [35] studied the female ischemia syndrome (WISE) of menopausal hormone status to determine premenopausal, perimenopausal, and postmenopausal status using menstrual and reproductive history and reproductive hormone levels obtained in a single clinical visit.

The study population consisted of 515 women (329 clearly postmenopausal) enrolled in the WISE study: undergoing coronarography for suspected ischemia, they were compared with a subgroup of 186 women, not clearly postmenopausal.

Results showed that depressive symptoms and anxiety were more severe among the postmenopausal female subjects than among non-menopausal women. Panic attacks and mood disorders accompanied poor lubrication, arousal disorder, and anorgasmia in the postmenopausal sample. In contrast, a higher frequency of intercourse was present in the sample of non-menopausal women.

There is more. In women, processes of vascular endothelial dysfunction can lead to impaired genital blood flow that is essential for sexual arousal [36].

In a survey of 2763 postmenopausal women with coronary heart disease (CHD), 65% of the 39% of women who were sexually active complained of at least one sexual problem. Additionally, in patients with heart failure, 47% to 73% reported a marked loss of sexual interest and 48% to 76% reported a marked decrease in the frequency of sexual activity caused by their disease. [37].

Nor should it be underestimated that sexual problems experienced by patients with heart disease and their partners may also result from fear of a cardiovascular event or sudden death during sexual activity [38] and from loss of self-esteem, anxiety, and depression, commonly observed after cardiac events.

How Do Cardiologists Treat the Sexual Problems of Patients with Ischemia?

A national cross-sectional questionnaire of cardiologists was conducted in the Netherlands. The sample consisted of all active Dutch cardiologists and cardiology residents (1054) who were members of the Dutch Society of Cardiology in the fall of 2011.

A pilot study was conducted at the Department of Cardiology, Leiden University Medical Center; 40 anonymous pilot questionnaires were distributed, and 23 were completed and returned (response rate 57.5%).

The questionnaire included 31 questions focused on:

1. Level of knowledge and awareness of sexual problems in cardiac patients.
2. Current practice in addressing patients' sexual problems.
3. Assumed responsibility for sexual health care.
4. Perceived barriers (emotional, context, and character) to addressing sexual issues. Twenty barriers were listed and cardiologists were asked to rate their agreement with each barrier.

The mean age of respondents was 45.5 years and 75.8% were male. Of these respondents, 80.9% were cardiologists and 19.1% were residents. Female respondents were significantly younger than male respondents: mean age 42.31 years.

When asked, "How often do you discuss sexual health with your patients?" 2.9% of cardiologists responded "never," 29.6% said "rarely," 48.7% said "sometimes," 16.9% said "regularly," and 2.0% said "often."

Thus, it is estimated that approximately 2.2% (SD 4.2) were referred to another specialist (Sexologist, Endocrinologist, Andrologist, and Gynaecologist) for treatment of sexual problems.

Furthermore, 38.5% of respondents sustained that cardiologists have the responsibility to discuss sexual issues with their patients. In contrast, 41.5% claimed that caring for the quality of patients' sex lives is someone else's responsibility: nearly 70% (69.4%) of respondents answered that the primary care physician is responsible for this part of patient care, while 51.6% said that the patient should initiate a conversation about it. In addition, 16.9% indicated the psychologist/sexologist, 9.3% the rehabilitation physician, 8% the nurse practitioner, and 5.8% the social worker.

Twenty-eight percent of respondents said that lack of knowledge was a reason for not investigating sexual problems, and 35.2% said that lack of education was one reason they did not ask. Nearly 27% of respondents did not know if there was a specialist at their medical centre to whom they would refer patients with sexual dysfunction.

When asked, "Do you need training to increase your knowledge so you can discuss sexual issues with your patients?" 41.9% of respondents answered in the affirmative. Sixty-three percent indicated that it would be helpful to have a list of health care providers to whom they could refer patients with sexual issues.

More than two-thirds of respondents rarely (49.4%) or never (20.1%) advised patients when to resume sexual activity after myocardial infarction or heart failure. In patients aged 20 to 35 years and in patients older than 76 years, cardiologists asked about sexual function less often than in patients aged 36 to 75 years.

Why? One of the most recurring reasons for not discussing sexual function was, "I don't have a point of view or a reason to start talking about it," 45.9% agreed. A time constraint was mentioned by 42.9%. 35.2% agreed with "a lack of training to deal with sexual issues" and 33.8% agreed with "reasons related to language and ethnicity." The least agreed reasons were "embarrassment" (5.7%), "no connection to the patient" (6.2%), "age difference between me and the patient" (6.4%), and "fear of offending patients" (7.4%) especially if they were women.

The literature supports these data: in fact, more than 65% of hypertensive men with ED remain undiagnosed even though the majority report a desire for treatment. [39].

Conclusion

Over the past 30 years, recommendations and guidelines have emphasized the importance of assessing sexual function in patients with cardiovascular disease. Yet, it is still difficult to find the figure of a Sexologist in a Cardiac Surgery Department. The apparent lack of interest on the part of cardiologists should also be evaluated in relation to the absence of sufficiently confidential contexts in which to talk to patients about their sexuality. In addition, the time restriction of the visit often represents a limitation to extending the interview with the patient beyond discussion of physical symptoms and ongoing therapy.

In a progression of improvement, training that is not strictly clinical for cardiologists in sexuality and sexological counselling that accompanies the patient and partners through the first visit and follow-ups is desirable.

References

1. Herrington W, Lacey B, Sherliker P, Armitage J, Lewington S. Epidemiology of atherosclerosis and the potential to reduce the global burden of atherothrombotic disease. Circ Res. 2016;118(4):535–46.
2. Longo DL, Fauci AS, Kasper DL, Hauser SL, Jameson JL, Loscalzo J. Harrison, Internal medicine principles, vol. 2, part 10, chap. 243, 18th ed.
3. Moran AE. 1990-2010 global cardiovascular disease atlas. Glob Heart. 2014;9:3–16.
4. Nichols M. Cardiovascular disease in Europe 2014: epidemiological update. Eur Heart J. 2014;35:2950–9.
5. Bentzon JF, Otsuka F, Virmani R, Falk E. Mechanisms of plaque formation and rupture. Circ Res. 2014;114:1852–66. https://doi.org/10.1161/CIRCRESAHA.114.302721.
6. Braunwald E. Disease of the heart. 7th ed. Milan: Elsevier Masson; 2007.
7. Moran AE, Forouzanfar MH, Roth GA, Mensah GA, Ezzati M, Murray CJ, Naghavi M. Temporal trends in ischemic heart disease mortality in 21 world regions, 1980 to 2010: the Global Burden of Disease 2010 study. Circulation. 2014;129:1483–92. https://doi.org/10.1161/CIRCULATIONAHA.113.004042.
8. Centre for Economics and Business Research. The economic cost of cardiovascular disease from 2014–2020 in six European economies, August 2014.
9. Bennett DA, Krishnamurthi RV, Barker-Collo S, Forouzanfar MH, Naghavi M, Connor M, Lawes CM, Moran AE, Anderson LM, Roth GA, Mensah GA, Ezzati M, Murray CJ, Feigin VL, Global Burden of Diseases, Injuries, and Risk Factors. Study Stroke Expert Group. The global burden of ischemic stroke: findings of the GBD 2010 study. Glob Heart. 2010;2014(9):107–12.
10. Stern S, Tzivoni D. Early detection of silent ischemic heart disease by 24-hour electrocardiographic monitoring of active subjects. Br Heart J. 1974;35:481–6.
11. Moreno PR. Vulnerable plaque: definition, diagnosis, and treatment. Cardiol Clin. 2010;28:1.
12. Cassar A, Holmes DR Jr, Rihal CS, Gersh BJ. Chronic coronary artery disease: diagnosis and management. Mayo Clin Proc. 2009;84(12):1130–46.
13. Connolly DC, Elveback LR, Oxman HA. Coronary heart disease in residents of Rochester, Minnesota: IV, prognostic value of the resting electrocardiogram at the time of initial diagnosis of angina pectoris. Mayo Clin Proc. 1984;59(4):247–50.
14. Sun Z. Cardiac CT imaging in coronary artery disease: Current status and future directions. Quant Imaging Med Surg. 2012;2(2):98–105.
15. Čaluk J. Procedural techniques of coronary angiography. In: Kirac S, editor. Advances in the diagnosis of coronary atherosclerosis. InTech; 2011. ISBN: 978-953-307-286-9.
16. Burns P, Lima E, Bradbury AW. Second best medical therapy. Eur J Vas Endovasc Surg. 2002;24(5):400–4.
17. Santilli F, Davì G, et al. Thromboxane and prostacyclin biosynthesis in heart failure of ischemic origin: effects of disease severity and aspirin treatment. J Thromb Haemost. 2010;8(5):914–22.
18. McDonald K, Ledwidge M, Cahill J, et al. Elimination of early rehospitalization in a randomized, controlled trial of multidisciplinary care in a high-risk, elderly heart failure population: the potential contributions of specialist care, clinical swtability and optimal angiotensin-converting enzyme inhibitor dose at discharge. Eur J Heart Fail. 2001 Mar;3(2):209–15.
19. Smith Jr SC, Dove JT, Jacobs AK, Ward Kennedy J, Kereiakes D, Kern MJ, Kuntz RE, Popma JJ, Schaff HV, Williams DO, Gibbons RJ, Alpert JP, Eagle KA, Faxon DP, Fuster V, Gardner TJ, Gregoratos G, Russell RO, Smith SC. ACC/AHA guidelines for percutaneous

coronary intervention (revision of the 1993 PTCA guidelines)—executive summary A report of the American College of Cardiology/American Heart Association Task Force on practice guidelines (Committee to revise the 1993 guidelines for percutaneous transluminal coronary angioplasty) endorsed by the Society for Cardiac Angiography and Interventions. J Am Coll Cardiol. 2001;37(8):2215.

20. Neumann F-J, Sousa-Uva M, Ahlsson A, Alfonso F, Banning AP, Benedetto U, Byrne RA, Collet J-P, Falk V, Head SJ. 2018 ESC/EACTS Guidelines on myocardial revascularization. European Heart J. 2019;40(2):87–165.

21. Zamir AG, Pervaiz F, Iqbal M, et al. Outcome of long segmental reconstruction (LSR), of the left anterior descending artery (LAD) with the left internal mammary artery (LIMA), in patients undergoing coronary artery bypass graft (cabg) surgery for diffuse coronary artery disease (CAD). Pakistan Armed Forces Med J. 2019;69(Suppl-3):AFIC.

22. Majani AP, Giardini A, Callegari S, Opasich C, Cobelli F, Tavazzi L. Relationship between psychological profile and cardiological variables in chronic heart failure. The role of patient subjectivity G. Eur Heart J. 1999;20(21):1579–86.

23. Krantz DS, McCeney MK. Effects of psychological and social factors on organic disease: a critical assessment of research on coronary heart disease. Annu Rev Psychol. 2002;53:341–69.

24. Mandras SA, Uber PA, Mehra MR. Sexual activity and chronic heart failure. Mayo Clin Proc. 2007;82(10):1203–10.

25. Rieckmann N, Neumann K, Feger S. Health-related qualify of life, angina type and coronary artery disease in patients with stable chest pain. Health Qual Life Outcomes. 2020;18(1):140.

26. Assari S, et al. Association between sexual function and marital relationship in patients with ischemic heart disease. J Tehran Heart Cent. 2014;9(3):124–31.

27. Berman L, Berman J, Miles M, Pollets D, Powell JA. Genital self-image as a component of sexual health: relationship between genital self-image, female sexual function, and quality of life measures. J Marital Sex Ther. 2003;29:11–21.

28. Danoff A, Khan O, Wan DW, Hurst L, Cohen D, Tenner CT, Bini EJ. Sexual dysfunction is highly prevalent among men with chronic hepatitis C virus infection and negatively impacts health-related quality of life. Am J Gastroenterol. 2006;101:1235–43.

29. Hartman LM. Effects of sexual and marital therapy on sexual interaction and marital happiness. J Sex Marital Ther. 1983;9:137–51.

30. The ladder of relationship and sexuality. The medical algorithm project. Institute of Algorithmic Medicine; 2013. http://www.medal.org/visitor/www%5CActive%5Cch15%5Cch15.28%5Cch15.28.02.aspx.

31. Tavallaii SA, Fathi-Ashtiani A, Nasiri M, Assari S, Maleki P, Einollahi B. Correlation between sexual function and post-renal quality of life: does gender matter? J Sex Med. 2007;4:1610–8.

32. Crane KC, Middleton RA, Bean D. Determination of criteria scores for the Kansas marital satisfaction scale and the revised dyadic adjustment scale. Am J Fam Ther. 2000;28:53–60.

33. Brezsnyak M, Whisman MA. Sexual desire and relationship functioning: the effects of marital satisfaction and power. J Marital Sex Ther. 2004;30:199–217.

34. Shi H, Zhang FR, Zhu CX, Wang S, Li S, Chen SW. Incidence of changes and predictors for sexual function after coronary stenting. Andrology. 2007;39:16–21.

35. Johnson D, et al. Determining menopausal status in women: the NHLBI-sponsored Women's Ischemia Syndrome Assessment Study (WISE). Giornale di salute delle donnevol. 2004;13(8). doi:https://doi.org/10.1089/jwh.2004.13.872.

36. Miner M, Esposito K, Guay A, Montorsi P, Goldstein I. Cardiometabolic risk and female sexual health: the Princeton III summary. J Sex Med. 2012;9(3):641–51.

37. Taylor HA Jr. Sexual activity and the cardiovascular patient: guidelines. Am J Cardiol. 1999;84(5B):6N–10N.

38. Roose SP, Seidman SN. Sexual activity and heart risk: is depression a contributing factor? Am J Cardiol. 2000;86(2A):38F–40F.

39. Giuliano FA, Leriche A, Jaudinot EO, De Gendre AS. Prevalence of erectile dysfunction among 7689 patients with diabetes or hypertension, or both. Urology. 2004;64(6):1196–201.

Chronic Valvular Heart Disease

Marco Agrifoglio, Giorgio Mastroiacovo, Marco Gennari, and Elena Vittoria Longhi

Abbreviations

AVS   Aortic valve stenosis
COPD   Chronic obstructive pulmonary disease
MVI   Mitral valve insufficiency
MVP   Mitral valve plasty
TAVI   Transcatheter aortic valve implantation
VHD   Valvular heart disease

Introduction

Valvular heart disease (VHD) refers to a series of disorders that affect the heart valves by altering their correct functioning; they are divided into two main categories: stenosis (defined as a narrowing of the valve orifice) and insufficiency (which causes a lack of coaptation of the valvular leaflets leading to a retrograde blood regurgitation) [1]. VHD encompasses several common cardiovascular conditions that account for 10% to 20% of all cardiac surgical procedures in the United States.

M. Agrifoglio (✉)
Centro Cardiologico Monzino IRCCS, Milan, Italy

Department of Biomedical Surgical and Dental Sciences, University of Milan, Milan, Italy
e-mail: marco.agrifoglio@unimi.it

G. Mastroiacovo · M. Gennari
Centro Cardiologico Monzino IRCCS, Milan, Italy
e-mail: giorgio.mastroiacovo@ccfm.it; marco.gennari@ccfm.it

E. V. Longhi
Department of Sexual Medical Center, San Raffaele Hospital, Milano, Italy

© Springer Nature Switzerland AG 2023
E. V. Longhi (ed.), *Managing Psychosexual Consequences in Chronic Diseases*,
https://doi.org/10.1007/978-3-031-31307-3_6

The most frequent VHD occurs in the so-called left heart and therefore affects the aortic and mitral valves. With regard to the former, aortic valve stenosis (AVS) represents the most widespread valvulopathy in Western countries, mostly determined by the development of calcifications linked to ageing processes, reaching a prevalence of 3% in the population over 70 years of age [2]; the age of onset of severe AVS stenosis is 50 years for patients with bicuspid aortic valve and 30 years for patients with unicuspid aortic valve. In developing countries, rheumatic disease remains the leading cause of aortic valvulopathy [2].

Mitral valve insufficiency (MVI) is the second most frequent and prevalent valvulopathy in Western countries and is caused in most cases by primary or degenerative/organic abnormalities of the valvular tissue that is either too abundant or too scarce. In developing countries, on the other hand, MVI is the first valvulopathy in order of prevalence and is mainly caused by rheumatic pathology [3].

Main Medical Characteristic of VHD

The AVS causes an obstruction to the outflow of blood from the left ventricle, which in turn causes an increase in the thickness of the heart muscle at the expense of the ventricular chamber's volume, which tends to shrink (a process known as concentric ventricular hypertrophy). This leads to a decrease in the volume of blood delivered in the large arterial circulation at each systole [4].

The main symptoms of AVS are: angina pectoris (which is an infarct-like chest pain), syncope and dyspnea (defined as shortness of breath or "hunger for air") which generally occur when the aortic valvular area is reduced below 1 cm^2 (indexed for body surface area 0.65 cm^2/m^2); from the onset of these symptoms, the prognosis is 3 years for the first two and 2 years for dyspnea, respectively [4].

MVI causes a retrograde regurgitation of blood in the left atrium; this leads from one side to a continuous increase in blood volume in the left ventricle after each ventricular contraction (systole) which will lead to a stretching of the cardiac muscle fibers with a consequent increase in ventricular volume (eccentric hypertrophy) and on the other side to an atrial enlargement or stretching which over time may determine the onset of atrial fibrillation [5].

MVI is symptomatically manifested by dyspnea at first under stress and then also at rest, palpitations (secondary to arrhythmias that occur following atrial enlargement) that can also be confused with anxiety disorders, up to acute pulmonary edema [5].

Main Tools for the Diagnosis

It is mandatory to follow several steps for VHD diagnostics.

First, the physical examination of the patient is essential.

The auscultation of a patient with aortic valvular stenosis will present a systolic ejective murmur on aortic focus that will irradiate to the neck, while a patient with MVI will present a gentler systolic murmur at mitral level with irradiation to the left axilla [6].

The electrocardiogram allows, through the measurement of cardiac electrical voltages, to investigate the electrical activity of the heart; its specific alterations are indirect signs of ventricular hypertrophy.

Chest X-ray is routinely performed in patients with VHD to check if there are already signs of heart failure with lung congestion.

Certainly, however, neither the objective examination nor the electrocardiogram and the chest X-ray are diriment for the diagnosis of AVS or MVI.

The gold standard and essential instrumental examination for a correct and timely diagnosis is the Echocardiogram. This consists in the use of an external probe that by means of ultrasound allows the direct visualization of the heart through the rib cage and evaluates both the general cardiac contractility and heart valves in a qualitative and quantitative way. The Echocardiogram allows to extrinsic through mathematical calculations data on the basis of which VHD are classified into mild, moderate, or severe and is a fundamental and irreplaceable tool to place surgical indication at the right time.

Main Non-surgical Treatment

Medical treatment of VHD is purely symptomatic. This means that there are still no drugs on the market today that can reverse the pathological process underlying VHD; in this scenario, surgery is the only definitive and decisive treatment.

The pivotal drug in the treatment of MVI is the diuretic; its use is intended to prevent congestion of patient's pulmonary circulation and acute pulmonary edema.

Main Surgical Treatment

For years the surgical treatment of choice of VHD has been the removal of patient's native valve and its replacement with a prosthesis.

There are two main types of prosthesis on the market: the biological and the mechanical one.

The former is made by bovine or porcine pericardium treated with glutaraldehyde with the function of shielding antigenic residues from the response of the patient's immune system. The main advantage of bioprostheses is that they are not linked to an oral anticoagulation regimen, while their disadvantage is to be subjected to continuous and constant wear and tear over time until they degenerate and have to be surgically replaced by a new one [7].

Mechanical prostheses, on the other hand, do not tend to degenerate over time but, since they are made by non-biological material, they are linked to a life-long oral anticoagulant regime, which in turn is linked to an increased risk of thrombus-embolic and hemorrhagic bleeding over time [8].

Valve replacement surgery with prosthesis involves the use of the heart-lung machine to establish extracorporeal circulation, allowing the surgeon to work with a still, bloodless heart. The procedure is performed via a longitudinal median sternotomy. The major risks associated with this type of procedure are post-surgical bleeding, infections, prosthetic leakage, cerebrovascular events, malignant arrhythmias, coronary arteries injuries, and death [9].

Regarding specifically the treatment of AVS since 2001 are commercially available on market a series of bioprostheses with the possibility of being implanted directly into the native aortic valve by means of catheters that are inserted percutaneously from the femoral arteries; this type of procedure is named Transcatheter Aortic Valve Implantation (TAVI). This type of operation has the great advantages of avoiding the opening of patient's chest and the establishment of extracorporeal circulation, reducing the operating room time and working on a beating heart. It is now common clinical practice to subject elderly patients (age > 70 years) or patients with important comorbidities (e.g. neoplasms, COPD, particularly calcific aorta, etc.) to TAVI rather than traditional valve replacement surgery. The main disadvantage of TAVI is that a long time period follow-up on implanted valves is missing, so that the long-term bioprosthetic valve duration implanted via transcatheter approach is unknown [10].

Finally, for about 10 years now, Doctor Shigeyuki Ozaki from Japan has brought in aortic valve surgery field a great innovation for aortic valve treatment consisting in the reconstructing of a neo-aortic valve using the patient's autologous pericardium [11]. The huge advantage of Ozaki's technique is to create a neovalve with autologous tissue, which, for not being an "external" material does not eliciting an immune system response, considered the main actors of bioprosthesis's deterioration and failure in the long-term period; last but not least autologous tissue is more resistant to infection than other valves commercially available [11]. Figure 1 shows an aortic valve from the surgeon's point of view.

Considering specifically mitral valve therapy, the great innovation in the treatment of this pathology was the invention and systematization of surgical techniques by Alain Carpentier [12] in the 1980s, for repairing mitral valve defects responsible of its failure, preserving the valve without the necessity of replacing it with prostheses. Carpentier gave the name Mitral Valve Plasty (MVP) to his techniques. The enormous advantage of MVP is exactly the possibility of repairing the valve defect by preserving the native valve, which, in this way, represents a definitive procedure for the patient without the need either of a future intervention and of a life-long oral anticoagulants therapy.

With the development of new technologies, it is now possible to repair the mitral valve using a video thoracoscope inserted in the patient's chest through a 3-cm peri areolar incision, thus avoiding the traditional sternotomy (Fig. 2).

Fig. 1 Aortic valve

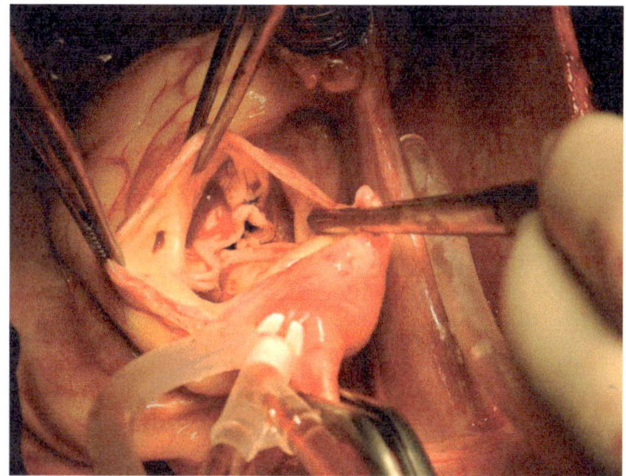

Fig. 2 Mitral valve
endoscopic view

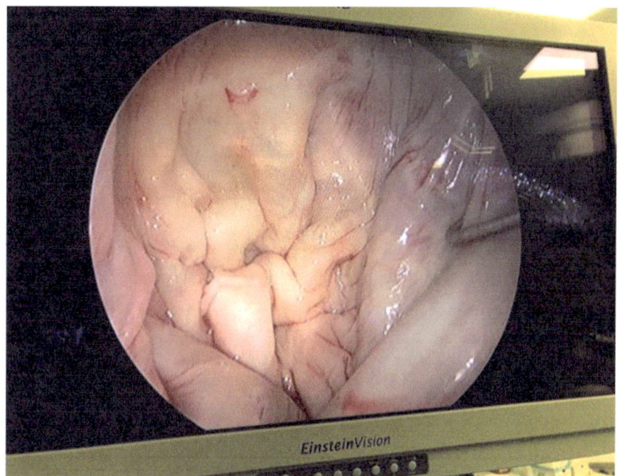

The surgical treatment of VHD remains a fascinating chapter in modern medicine; with scientific progress, new techniques and surgical instruments will certainly be available, allowing faster, more precise and less traumatic cardiac interventions.

Psychological Point of View

MVI is a pathology often associated with anxiety disorders [13]. Physiopathologically speaking, at the basis of this phenomenon there is an atrial stretching which determines the onset of supraventricular tachycardia (whose the most frequent are the supraventricular ectopic beats).

Often, therefore, the symptoms of onset in patients suffering from MVI are palpitations, panic attacks, and other similar anxious states. In some cases, patients suffering from mitral insufficiency first turn to psychiatric colleagues and are treated with anxiolytic drugs, delaying the true diagnosis.

It is also necessary to always keep in mind that patients who are diagnosed with severe VHD will necessarily have to undergo major surgery. Doctor's role is fundamental in clearly explaining to the patient the pathology he suffers from, the necessary treatment and what it consists of, having the arduous task of supporting him psychologically. Therefore, one of the most important danger for patients undergoing cardiac surgery is post-surgery depression: a formidable enemy because it prevents the patient from filling the post-operative period with the right forces, lengthening the hospitalization's time. We are convinced that giving the patient all the explanations and answers to his questions is a fundamental part of the medical work and improves the post-operative period; it is also important to prepare the patient to deal with any possible post-operative complications because knowing them helps to face them without fear.

Sexuality and Quality of Life

Patients with VHD often dread physical exertion for fear of triggering a flare-up of the disease, and as a result they often eliminate sexuality from being a factor in their quality of life. Doctors and nurses often show discomfort or embarrassment in providing useful guidance in this regard and patients, cowed by the pathology, do not have the courage to broach the subject [14].

Some patients claim to have tried to provoke erection through autoeroticism, but in the face of failure have abdicated the role of lover. ED therefore negatively affects the quality of life and well-being of patients and, the more severe and prolonged it is, the more it affects their self-esteem leading to depression, mood disorders, and insomnia. Right up to the point of ending relationships and cohabitation. [15].

Although guidance on limiting physical activity for patients with valvular disease is available, there are no studies that have specifically investigated the risk associated with sexual activity. However, it is possible to derive common sense indications from the existing evidence and clinical practice: patients with non-severe valvular disease can safely cope with non-intensive physical activity, and it is therefore reasonable to assume that they can undertake an active sexual life without concern.

In contrast, for patients with severe, symptomatic valvular disease, resumption of intimate relations should be postponed until after careful medical evaluation or surgical treatment.

In subjects in whom the severity and symptomaticity of the disease is doubtful, performing an inductive test allows assessment of hemodynamic response, symptoms, and the possible occurrence of arrhythmias.

There is no reason to preclude normal sexual activity for patients with normal functioning valve prostheses by at least 6 to 8 weeks after cardiac surgery. [16].

Conclusion

Certainly, the anxiety aspect modifies in no small way the male and female sexual response but there are no specific international studies on patients with valvulopathies that could offer us further data.

One tool, however, that might be useful in assessing psychogenic, character, or pathological levels of anxiety is State-Trait Anxiety Inventory for Adults-Self-Evaluation Questionnaire STAI Form Y-1 and Form Y-2.

References

1. Longo D, Fauci A, Kasper D, Hauser S, Jameson J, Loscalzo J. Harrison: principles of internal medicine, 18th ed., chap. 237.
2. Nkomo VT, Gardin JM, Skelton TN, Gottdiener JS, Scott CG, Enriquez-Sarano M. Burden of valvular heart diseases: a population-based study. Lancet. 2006;368(9540):1005–11.
3. World Health Organization. Rheumatic fever and rheumatic heart disease. World Health Organ Tech Rep Ser. 2004;923:1.
4. Rosenhek R, Baumgartner H. Aortic stenosis. In: Otto CM, Bonow RO, editors. Valvular heart disease. 4th ed. Philadelphia: Saunders/Elsevier; 2013. p. 139–62.
5. Virmani R, Atkinson JB, Forman MB. The pathology of mitral valve prolapse. Herz. 1988;13(4):215–26.
6. Mayo Clinic Proceedings. The Mayo Foundation for Medical Education and Research.
7. Mettler FA, Guiberteau MJ. Cardiovascular system mitral valve disorders essentials of nuclear medicine and molecular imaging, 7th ed. 2019.
8. Pibarot P, Dumesnil JG. Prosthetic heart valves: selection of the optimal prosthesis and long-term management. Circulation. 2009;119(7):1034–48.
9. Hote M. Cardiac surgery risk scoring systems: in quest for the best. Heart Asia. 2018;10(1):e011017.
10. Díez JG. Transcatheter aortic valve implantation (TAVI): the hype and the hope. Tex Heart Inst J. 2013;40(3):298–301.
11. Ozaki S, Kawase I, Yamashita H, Uchida S, Nozawa Y, Matsuyama T, et al. Aortic valve reconstruction using self-developed aortic valve plasty system in aortic valve disease. Interact Cardiovasc Thorac Surg. 2011;12(4):550–3.
12. Carpentier A. Carpentier's reconstructive valve surgery, 1st ed. 2010.
13. Dager SR, Saal AK, Comess KA, et al. Mitral valve prolapse and the anxiety disorders. Hosp Community Psychiatry. 1988;39(5):517–27.
14. Colombi I. Cardiovascular diseases: the issue of sexual counseling and the role of nursing in the management of problems related to the user's sexual health. Bachelor thesis, University of Applied Sciences and Arts of Southern Switzerland (SUPSI). 2019.
15. Taylor Nelson AGB Healthcare. Impotence association survey: 2000–2001.
16. Hermann C, Brand-Driehorst S, Buss U, Ruger U. Effect of anxiety and depression on five-years mortality in 5,057 patients referred for exercise testing. J Psychosom Res. 2000;48:455–62.

Part IV
Endocrinology

The Chronic Thyroid Diseases

Raffeale Giannattasio, Gaetano Lombardi, and Elena Vittoria Longhi

The classification of thyroid diseases (TD) has substantially remained the same in the last 30 years despite the fact that the molecular mechanisms of numerous conditions have been discovered and better characterized. Thyroid hormone dysfunctions can be linked to alterations of the target organs, at the receptor and post-receptor level. Some times during diseases evolution, a change in thyroid function is observed with the passage from hyperthyroidism to hypothyroidism and vice versa, while in other conditions it can be a remission after a quite long-term interval or not. Many TD are influenced by the iodine content of the diet which often affects its evolution.

Introduction

The structure of thyroid hormones is characterized by the presence of iodine (IO) and it is, therefore, evident that its deficiency increases the incidence of thyroid diseases (TD). In the early stages of the life, it causes a reduced physical and intellectual development; in adults entails many chronic TD, namely goiter (GO) and hypothyroidism (HY) [1]. Furthermore, in areas of GO endemia, the correction of the poor reduced in IO diet intake can lead to an increased frequency of hyperthyroidism (HP) only in Toxic Multinodular Goiter (MNG) but not in Graves' disease

R. Giannattasio
PPS San Gennaro, ASL Napoli 1 Centro, Naples, Italy
e-mail: raffegia2002@libero.it

G. Lombardi (✉)
Endocrinology, Federico II University, Naples, Italy
e-mail: gaelomba@unina.it

E. V. Longhi
Department of Sexual Medical Center, San Raffaele Hospital, Milano, Italy

© Springer Nature Switzerland AG 2023
E. V. Longhi (ed.), *Managing Psychosexual Consequences in Chronic Diseases*,
https://doi.org/10.1007/978-3-031-31307-3_7

(GD) [2]. In these areas, oral supplementation with IO compounds also induces a higher incidence of subclinical hypothyroidism and autoimmune TD.

The increase in the thyroid volume, called GO, certainly represents the most frequent thyroid pathology. The GO is so widely diffused in some populations that it can be defined as endemic; nevertheless, in most cases, the production of thyroid hormones is normal (euthyroidism).

The functional state of thyroid is identified by the clinical signs of HY and HP; in this way, it is possible to start the right therapy after the assay of the thyroid hormone serum levels. Currently, it is necessary to distinguish if the changes in the serum levels of thyroid hormones are linked to an alteration of their synthesis, or to the losses of the thyroid cells, iatrogenic causes or modification in target organs. The variations of the thyroid function are then categorized as transient, whose duration is up to a year, or chronic, when they persist throughout life. They are polar, when the clinical and functional characteristics change over time.

Goiter

GO is defined as an increase in the thyroid volume which maintains normal hormonal secretion; in the GO, the inflammatory, immune, and tumour processes are absent. GO is defined as endemic in geographic areas where in children between 6 and 12 years of age it has a frequency greater than 5%, sporadic when the incidence is less than 5% [3]. If the thyroid maintains its anatomical location in the neck it is indicated as cervical while it is defined as cervico-mediastinal when it extends to the anterior mediastinum. In some cases, the GO is transient (puberty, pregnancy, breastfeeding, etc.). The increase in the thyroid volume is generally secondary to a reduced IO intake in the diet. Additionally, it can arise from an increased intake of exogenous IO (amiodarone, iodine tincture, etc.) or from a diet rich in nutrients able to propitiate thyroid tumefaction. If GO is particularly voluminous, it causes compression phenomena on the adjacent structures: dislocation of the trachea and oesophagus and compression of the jugular veins which are sometimes responsible for choking and cough, as well as for dysphagia and headache, the latter related to venous stasis. The recurrent nerve compression can induce dysphonia and dyspnoea; similarly, compression of the phrenic nerve can elicit hiccups; however, in clinical practice such complications are rare. If pain occurs with a rapid increase in GO volume, the presence of intra-nodular haemorrhage should be considered. The main purpose of GO monitoring is the possible occurrence of thyroid carcinoma, since thyroid nodules are malignant tumours in 5% of cases [4]. Thyroid ultrasound examination represents the most useful tool to identify "suspect" nodules to be subjected to cytological examination (fine-needle aspiration cytology, FNAC). In GO with euthyroidism, the levels of TSH, FT3, and FT4 are normal; however, when the TSH still has values within the normal range but around 0.5 (TSH "blocked"), in the presence of tachycardia and other clinical signs, the presence of subclinical hyperthyroidism must be assessed. If TSH is located at the high limits of the norm (>3.0), the use of low doses of L-Thyroxine may reduce the TSH levels which can stimulate the proliferation of thyroid cells. When the GO is very voluminous which leads to an aesthetic damage or important compression phenomena to patient, total or subtotal thyroidectomy is required. In nodular GO, if the indication for thyroid-ectomy is caused by the presence of one or a few nodules, it is possible to use the alternative methods, as intranodular percutaneous injection of ethanol or ablation with laser hyperthermia.

But the most useful therapy of GO is to prevent its occurrence, that can be realized through the IO prophylaxis (i.e., iodized salt). Consequently, it is registered as a significant reduction of GO in some geographical areas [5].

Thyroiditis

The term "thyroiditis" encompasses a heterogeneous group of TD in which inflammatory phenomena can be minimal or very impressive. Their evolution is acute, subacute, or chronic, and is ruled by their aetiology since they identify numerous pathogenetic mechanisms: infectious, autoimmune, traumatic, radiation, drugs, and idiopathic factors.

Thyroid function may be normal but HY or HP occur more frequently with the possibility of varying from one condition to another. For a correct diagnosis, an accurate medical history is essential as well as the serum measurements not only of TSH, FT3, and FT4 but also of anti-thyroglobulin antibodies (ABHTG), anti-peroxidase (ABTPO), and anti-TSH receptor (ABTSHR). In some thyroiditis forms, inflammation parameters are altered and must be investigated. The most frequent forms are GD and Hashimoto's thyroiditis (HD). The first occurs with HP and is characterized by an increase in ABTSHR. Approximately about 15% of patients have relatives with the same disease while about 50% of their families have high levels of ABHTG and ABTPO [6]. The HD or chronic lymphocytic thyroiditis is the most frequent cause of HY in the Western countries [7]. Particular forms are: (1) De Quervain's subacute thyroiditis (or granulomatous), which is associated with fever, transient HP, high VES, and normal levels of ABHTG and ABTPO; (2) acute thyroiditis, of infectious aetiology (bacterial or viral) [8], which occurs with pain in the thyroid region, more frequently in the left lobe, and fever, and whose therapy includes the use of antibiotics; (3) silent thyroiditis whose origin is autoimmune and similar to the subacute form (which it differs from the previous one, because of the lack of pain) [9]; (4) chronic Riedel thyroiditis with positive ABHTG and ABTPO, HY in 30% of patients, in which the thyroid tissue is replaced by fibrosis with an increase in the compactness of the gland, dysphonia, and dysphagia [10]; (5) post-partum thyroiditis, similar to the silent form, which occurs within the 12 months following the delivery [11], with high antibodies and a typical three-phase trend characterized by an initial phase of HP, a longer period of HY and a return to euthyroidism.

Hypothyroidism

In the pediatric age, the HY determines a delay in psychic (cretinism) and growth development; in adults, there is a slow-down in metabolic processes and accumulation of glycosaminoglycans in the intercellular spaces especially at the level of the skin and skeletal muscle (myxoedema). The symptoms are: hair loss, constipation, reduction of cardiovascular, and pulmonary performances.

The presence of high TSH with normal (subclinical hypothyroidism) or low FT3 and FT4 values confirms the diagnosis [12]. The dosage of ABHTG and ABTPO and of the indicators of inflammation (VES, PCR, etc.) together with the thyroid ultrasound allows to identify the disease that causes HY. The therapy consists in the administration of L-thyroxine (T4) at adequate doses, able to normalize the serum levels of TSH, FT3, and FT4. When possible, a specific therapy for the condition that underlies the HY should be carried out. In about 20% of cases, even in the presence of normal or almost normal TSH, FT3, and FT4 values, it would be useful to associate to administration of T4 also T3 in order to determine the complete disappearance of the symptoms of HY. In fact, in some patients, there is a genetic deficit of the activity of desiodase 2; this enzyme transforms T4, a partially active hormone, into T3, with an activity approximately four times greater than T4 [13].

Hyperthyroidism

HP determines an increase in all metabolic activities with the appearance of tachycardia, nervousness, hyperkinesia, fatigue, insomnia, sweating, and intolerance to heat. Sometimes there are ocular manifestations defined with the term thyroid ophthalmopathy related both to ocular (conjunctiva, cornea, etc.) and extraocular (exophthalmos, retraction of the upper eyelid, etc.) alterations.

The finding of low TSH with high FT3 and FT4 or high limits of the standard (subclinical hyperthyroidism) allows us to diagnose HP. Additionally, the determination of ABHTG, ABTPO, ABTSR, and thyroid ultrasound allow us to identify the disease causing HP [14]. In some cases, it is necessary to carry out also the thyroid Scintigraphy (with I131, I123, or Tc99m) to specify if HP is causally related to MNG or toxic adenoma of the thyroid gland (Plummer's disease).

In HP therapy, anti-thyroid drugs are indicated [15]; (1) methimazole which blocks the iodization of thyroid hormones, peroxidase mediated; (2) propylthiouracil which has the same activity as methimazole but also blocks the conversion of T4 to T3, a more metabolically active hormone. If HP persists over time, total or partial thyroidectomy or therapy with I131 is indicated. The latter destroys hyperfunctioning thyroid nodules through the emission of β particles. More recently, the elimination of hyperfunctioning nodules has been carried out by percutaneous intranodular injection of ethanol or ablation with laser hyperthermia.

Thyroid Neoplasm

The most frequent thyroid neoplasms are: (1) papillary carcinoma (with its follicular variant); (2) follicular carcinoma (including Hörtle cell carcinoma; (3) anaplastic carcinoma; and (4) medullary carcinoma of the thyroid. The latter is due to the neoplastic transformation of the thyroid cells secreting calcitonin and is often genetically transmitted in association with tumours and/or hyperplasia of another endocrine gland, thereby configuring particular clinical pictures indicated as Multiple Endocrine Adenomatosis (MEN) [16]. Hence, in most cases, this cancer is diagnosed by calcitonin dosing, baseline or after stimulation, during screening programs.

Thyroid ultrasound plays a fundamental role in the diagnosis of some thyroid cancer forms by identifying the thyroid nodules and classifying them according to their characteristics as low-, intermediate-, and high-risk nodules [17]. The latter must be subjected to ultrasound-guided cytological examination (FNAC); in suspected cases, it is also possible to perform the genetic analysis of the collected material. The previous analysis allows us to identify the mutations that are more frequent or rare in papillary carcinoma [18].

In all thyroid neoplasms, the therapy of choice is total thyroidectomy with emptying, if necessary, of the laterocervical lymphonodes and the central compartment of the neck. After surgery, the neoplastic forms that maintain the ability to capture the IO are subjected (if necessary) to therapy with I 131 at high doses, which destroys the thyroid cells residual. Subsequent thyroid-suppressive therapy with high-dose thyroid hormones results in satisfactory recovery in 95% of patients. In the more aggressive forms, tyrosine kinase inhibitors are also available, with at least partially cytotoxic action on thyroid-derived cells [19].

Since papillary carcinoma of the thyroid gland is deemed to be poorly aggressive, it has recently been suggested to resort to active surveillance for some of these forms, i.e., surgery should be deserved only to the most severe forms [20]. Similarly, the lobectomy should be preferred rather than total thyroidectomy. The main issue is that in the case of lobectomy or partial thyroidectomy, it is not possible to carry out metabolic therapy with I131. Thus, the active surveillance could also be chosen to decide which type of surgery (total or partial) is to be recommended.

Sexuality and Quality of Life

The scientific literature in these years of SARS-CoV-2 has addressed the extent to which this pandemic could *induce, usually reversibly, thyroid dysfunction, including subclinical and atypical thyroiditis* [21]. Patients with baseline TD do not appear to be at increased risk of contracting or transmitting SARS-CoV-2, and baseline thyroid dysfunction does not promote worse progression of COVID-19. However, it is unclear whether low levels of free triiodothyronine, observed in critically ill patients with COVID-19, may worsen the clinical progression of the disease and, consequently, whether triiodothyronine supplementation could be a tool to reduce this burden. Glucocorticoids and heparin may affect thyroid hormone secretion and measurement, respectively, leading to a possible misdiagnosis of thyroid dysfunction in severe cases of COVID-19.

In a sample of *191 confirmed mild-to-moderate cases of COVID-19, thyroid dysfunction was observed in about 15%* [22]. Patients with subnormal TSH levels compared to those with normal TSH levels (0, 21 mUI/L versus 1.2 mUI/L) more frequently had fever (89 versus 59%, $p = 0.03$) and a lower SARS-Cov-2 polymerase chain reaction threshold (20.9 versus 26.3, p 0.01) suggestive of a higher viral load.

In another retrospective study of *50 patients confirmed with COVID-19, more than half (56%) had transiently subnormal* TSH levels and those with lower TSH values had a poor prognosis [23].

SARS-COV-2 aside, thyroid dysfunction and sexual dysfunction are both common conditions that have a major impact on quality of life (QoL).

Recent publications have documented an increase in the prevalence of sexual dysfunction in people with hypothyroidism and hyperthyroidism. To get a more complete picture of this issue, Gabrielson and colleagues performed a review of all studies conducted in this field between 1978 and 2018 [24].

The aspects analysed in the articles, which were collected through specific bibliographic research, were: frequency, symptoms, mechanisms of development, diagnosis, and therapy of the sexual dysfunctions identified in the evaluation of people with impaired thyroid function. The data collected indicated that sexual dysfunctions have an estimated frequency of between *59% and 63% and between 22% and 46%, respectively, in men and women with hypothyroidism. In subjects with hyperthyroidism, the percentages were 48–77% and 44–60%,* respectively, for males and females. Both hyperthyroidism and hypothyroidism are associated with erection and ejaculation problems. In particular, delayed ejaculation is common in hypothyroidism and premature ejaculation in hyperthyroidism. Libido alterations are reported for both thyroid dysfunctions. In women with hypothyroidism and hyperthyroidism, hypoactive desire disorder, vaginal dryness, arousal and orgasm disorder, and vaginismus are reported [24].

However, the QoL of patients diagnosed with thyroid carcinoma differs. In the study by Giusti et al. [25], it was found that those patients with malignant tumours suffer a very significant deterioration in their QoL. Since 2010, however, a new QoL inventory has been available: ThyPRO for benign thyroid disorders. From 2012 to 2016, this tool was used for an annual assessment of QoL on 123 adult patients with DTC. The ThyPRO questionnaire consists of 13 scales in which higher scores represent a greater impact on QoL in areas affected by TD. Disease-specific morbidity due to possibly inadequate treatment with L-T4 was assessed using the Billewicz scale (BS). The same tests were conducted in 192 control subjects who had undergone surgery for benign TD.

ALSO DTC and control subjects had similar scores on all but one scale; scores on the hyperthyroid symptom scale were significantly higher in DTC patients than in controls. Over the 5-year period, scores did not change significantly in the DTC group. Overall, QoL and BS scores showed a slight, but not significant, improvement during the study period in DTC patients. BMI had an impact on several ThyPRO scales.

The ThyPRO questionnaire also found that the perception of disease was similar after thyroidectomy for malignant and benign disease. Only a marginal improvement in QoL was noted in DTC subjects over the 5-year study period. In both groups, females showed a higher perception of the disease than males [26].

To date, most studies have found that patients with DTC generally suffer from impaired QoL [27] and that this is comparable to that of patients with tumours at other sites [28].

Using the results of the North American Thyroid Cancer Survivorship Study (NATCSS), a large-scale survival study, clinical research [28] compared the QOL of thyroid cancer survivors with the QOL of survivors of other cancers. The NATCSS assessed QOL in general and in four subcategories: physical, psychological, social, and spiritual well-being using the QOL-Cancer Survivor tool (QOL-CS). Studies that used the QOL-CS to assess survivors of other cancers were compared with the NATCSS results using two-tailed t-tests.

Comparing the results of the NATCSS and QOL studies on survival of colon cancer, glioma, breast cancer, and gynaecological cancer, the overall mean QOL in NATCSS was 5.56 (on a scale of 0 to 10, with 10 being the best). The overall QOL of patients with thyroid cancer was similar to that of patients with colon cancer (mean 5.20, $p = 0.13$), glioma (mean 5.96, $p = 0.23$), and gynaecological cancer (mean 5.59, $p = 0.43$). It was worse than for breast cancer patients (mean 6.51, $p < 0.01$).

The result is that the self-reported QOL of thyroid cancer survivors appears, overall, similar to or worse than that of survivors of other cancers examined with the same instrument. This should increase awareness of the significance of a thyroid cancer diagnosis and highlights the need for a multi-specialist approach to improved QOL.

Furthermore, after administering four validated questionnaires to 153 recovered DTC patients with a median duration of care of 6.3 years and to a large group of healthy controls matched for age, sex, and socioeconomic status, Hoftijzer et al. [27] documented impairment of QoL in the DTC group. Furthermore, after a literature search, Singer et al. [28] reported various features of QoL impairment in patients with DTC (*sudden bouts of fatigue, exhaustion, sleep quality, employment, social support, fear of cancer progression, fear of a second operation, swallowing difficulties and general feeling*). In the same period, a literature review [29], in which 16 articles concerning QoL in DTC patients were selected, revealed that several factors (surgery, radioiodine therapy, discontinuation of thyroid hormone instead of rhTSH administration, access to behavioural help, doctor-patient relationship) had a positive impact on patients, both physically and psychologically.

Recently, McIntyre et al. [30] collected data from a 5-dimensional EuroQoL questionnaire (EQ-5D) from 83 cancer patients attending the first UK thyroid cancer doctor–patient forum and found that mean QoL was lower in DTC patients than in breast, colorectal, or prostate cancer patients. A large group of these DTC patients suffered from *fatigue and depression*. These findings appear to partially confirm a 2016 report by Applewhite et al. [28], who observed that the self-reported QoL of thyroid cancer survivors was similar to or worse than that of the patients with different cancer diagnoses.

We can generally state that TD include several types: non-toxic goitre, hyperthyroidism, thyroid ophthalmopathy, and hypothyroidism. *Goitre may be associated with neck discomfort and cosmetic problems. The classic symptoms of hypothyroidism are non-specific but well described, with fatigue, slow cerebration, constipation, weight gain, and depression being the main features. Typical symptoms of hyperthyroidism are rapid heartbeat, tremor, weight loss, anxiety, and increased sweating.*

22–35%percent of goitre patients, 18–66% of hyperthyroid patients, 7–99% of TAO patients, and 16–51% of hypothyroid patients experienced limitations in normal activities. Persistent impairment of HRQL was very frequent in patients with hyper- and hypothyroidism. Approximately half of the patients presented with reduced general health and QoL, limitations in normal activities, and social and emotional problems. *Two thirds were tired. Anxiety, cognitive, and sexual problems were present in about one-third of the patients* [31].

Meanwhile, scientific research has developed two new condition-specific questionnaires for use in hypothyroidism: the Thyroid Dependent Quality of Life Questionnaire (ThyDQoL) and the Thyroid Treatment Satisfaction Questionnaire (ThyTSQ).

Conclusion

The ThyPRO consists of 85 items: the scales cover physical and mental symptoms, well-being and function, as well as social and daily functions and aesthetic concerns. Responses ($N = 1810$) to the ThyPRO were collected from seven countries: the United Kingdom ($n = 166$), the Netherlands ($n = 147$), Serbia ($n = 150$), Italy ($n = 110$), India ($n = 148$), Denmark ($n = 902$), and Sweden ($n = 187$). The translated versions were compared in pairs with the English version by examining the uniform and non-uniform DIF, i.e., whether patients from different countries responded differently to a particular item [32, 33].

Although there is no shortage of tools for validating the QOL of patients diagnosed with thyroid pathology or thyroid carcinoma, there remains much to be done to increase multidisciplinary teams that take charge not only of the pathology but also of the whole individual/patient and family contexts of reference. The psycho-sexologist could be a facilitating figure in a therapeutic pathway where clinicians themselves complain of not having the tools to approach the psyche, sexuality, mood disorders, anhedonia, and patients' decline in therapeutic motivation.

References

1. Andersson M, Karumbunathan V, Zimmermann MB. Global iodine status in 2011 and trends over the past decade. J Nutr. 2012;142(4):744–50.
2. Laurberg P, Pedersen KM, Vestergaard H, Sigurdsson G. High incidence of multinodular toxic goitre in the elderly population in a low iodine intake area vs high incidence of Graves' disease in the young in a high iodine intake area: comparative surveys of thyrotoxicosis epidemiology in East – Jutland Denmark and Iceland. J Intern Med. 1991;229(5):415–20.
3. Hegedüs L, Bonnema SJ, Bennedbaek FN. Management of simple nodular goiter: current status and future perspectives. Endocr Rev. 2003;24(1):102–32.
4. Gharib H, Papini E, Valcavi R, Baskin HJ, Crescenzi A, Dottorini ME, Duick DS, Guglielmi R, Hamilton CR Jr, Zeiger MA, Zini M. AACE/AME Task Force on Thyroid Nodules. American Association of Clinical Endocrinologist and Associazione Medici Endocrinologi Medical guidelines for clinical practice for the diagnosis and management of thyroid nodules. Endocr Pract. 2006;12(1):63–102.
5. Zimmermann MB, Boelaert K. Iodine deficiency and thyroid disorders. Lancet Diabetes Endocrinol. 2015;3(4):286–95.
6. Gough SC. The genetics of Graves' disease. Endocrinol Metab Clin N Am. 2000;29(2):255–66.
7. Davies TF. Ord –Hashimoto's disease: renaming a common disorder – again. Thyroid. 2003;13(4):317.
8. Berger SA, Zonszein J, Villamena P, Mittman N. Infectious diseases of the thyroid gland. Rev Infect Dis. 1983;5(1):108–22.
9. Lazarus JH. Sporadic and postpartum thyroiditis. In: Braverman LE, Utiger RE, editors. Werner and Ingbar's the thyroid: a fundamental and clinical text. 9th ed. Lippincott; 2005. p. 536.
10. Guimares VC. Subacute and Riedel's thyroiditis. In: De Groot LJ, Jameson JL, editors. Endocrinology. 5th ed. Saunders; 2006. p. 2069.
11. Azizi F. The occurrence of permanent thyroid failure in patients with subclinical postpartum thyroiditis. Eur J Endocrinol. 2005;153(3):367–71.
12. Wiersinga WM. Hypothyroidism and myxedema coma. In: De Groot L, Jameson JL, editors. Endocrinology. 5th ed. Elsevier Saunders; 2006. p. 2081.
13. Guglielmi R, Frasoldati A, Zini M, Grimaldi F, Gharib H, Garber JR, Papini E. Italian Association of Clinical Endocrinologists statement – replacement therapy for primary hypothyroidism: a brief guide for clinical practice. Endocr Pract. 2016;22(11):1319–26.
14. Wallaschofski H, Orda C, Georgi P, Miehle K, Paschke R. Distinction between autoimmune and non-autoimmune thyrotoxicosis by determination of TSH–receptor antibodies in patients with the initial diagnosis of toxic multinodular goiter. Horm Metab Res. 2001;33(8):504–7.
15. Cooper DS. Antithyroid drugs. N Engl J Med. 2005;352(9):905–17.

16. Nix PA, Nicolaides A, Coatesworth AP. Thyroid cancer review 3: management of medullary and undifferentiated thyroid cancer. Int J Clin Pract. 2006;60(1):80–4.
17. Gharib H, Papini E, Garber JR, Duick DS, Harrel RM, Hegedös L, Paschke R, Valcavi R, Vitti P, AACE/ACE/AME Task Force on Thyroid Nodules. American Association of Clinical Endocrinologists, American College of Endocrinology, and Associazione Medici Endocrinologi medical guidelines for clinical practice for the diagnosis and management of thyroid nodules – 2016 update. Endocr Pract. 2016;22(5):622–39.
18. Bellevicine C, Sgariglia R, Migliaccio I, Vigliar E, D'Anna M, Nacchio MA, Serra N, Malapelle U, Bongiovanni M, Troncone G. Different qualifiers of AUS/FLUS thyroid FNA have distinct BRAF, RAS, RET/PTC, and PAX8/PPARg alterations. Cancer Cytopathol. 2018;126(5):317–25.
19. Jayarangaiah A, Sidhu G, Brown J, Barret-Campbell O, Bahtiyar G, Youssef I, Arora S, Skwiersky S, McFarlane SI. Therapeutic options for advanced thyroid cancer. Int J Clin Endocrinol Metab. 2019;5(1):2–34.
20. Ito Y, Miyauchi A, Oda H. Low – risk papillary microcarcinoma of the thyroid: a review of active surveillance trials. Eur J Surg Oncol. 2018;44(3):307–15.
21. Lisco G, De Tullio A, Jirillo E, Giagulli VA, De Pergola G, Guastamacchia E, Triggiani V. Thyroid and COVID-19: a review on pathophysiological, clinical and organizational aspects. J Endocrinol Investig. 2021;44(9):1801–14. https://doi.org/10.1007/s40618-021-01554-z. Epub 2021 Mar 25. PMID: 33765288; PMCID: PMC7992516.
22. Lui DTW, Lee CH, Chow WS, Lee ACH, Tam AR, Fong CHY, Law CY, Leung EKH, To KKW, Tan KCB, Woo YC, Lam CW, Hung IFN, Lam KSL. Thyroid dysfunction related to immune profile, disease status and outcome in 191 patients with COVID-19. J Clin Metab Endocrinol. 2021;106(2):e926–35. https://doi.org/10.1210/clinem/dgaa813.
23. Chen M, Zhou W, Xu W. Thyroid function analysis in 50 COVID-19 patients: a retrospective study. Thyroid. 2021;31(1):8–11. https://doi.org/10.1089/thy.2020.0363.
24. Gabrielson G, et al. The impact of thyroid disease on sexual dysfunction in men and women. Sex Med Rev. 2019;7(1):57–70.
25. Giusti M, Gay S, Conte L, et al. Assessment of quality of life in patients with differentiated thyroid cancer using the patient-reported thyroid-specific outcome questionnaire: a 5-year longitudinal study. Eur Thyroid J. 2020;9(5):247–55. https://doi.org/10.1159/000501201.
26. Gamper EM, Wintner LM, Rodrigues M, Buxbaum S, Nilica B, Singer S, et al. Persistent quality of life disturbances in patients with differentiated thyroid cancer: results of a monitoring program. Eur J Nucl Med Mol Imaging. 2015;42(8):1179–88.
27. Singer S, Lincke T, Gamper E, Bhaskaran K, Schreiber S, Hinz A, et al. Quality of life in patients with thyroid cancer compared to the general population. Thyroid. 2012;22(2):117–24.
28. Applewhite MK, James BC, Kaplan SP, Angelos P, Kaplan EL, Grogan RH, et al. The quality of life in thyroid cancer is similar to that of other cancers with worse survival. World J Surg. 2016;40(3):551–61.
29. Bărbuș E, Peștean C, Larg MI, Piciu D. Quality of life in patients with thyroid cancer: a review of the literature. Clujul Med. 2017;90(2):147–53.
30. Watt T, Bjorner JB, Groenvold M, et al. Establish construct validity for patient-reported outcome measurement specific to thyroid (ThyPRO): an initial exam. Qual Life Res. 2009;18:483–96.
31. McMillan CV, Bradley C, Woodcock A, Razvi S, Weaver JU. Design of new questionnaires to measure quality of life and treatment satisfaction in hypothyroidism. Thyroid. 2004;14(11):916–25.
32. Watt T, Barbesino G, Bjorner JB, et al. Cross-cultural validity of the patient-reported outcome measure on thyroid-specific quality of life, ThyPRO. Qual Life Res. 2015;24:769–80.
33. Hoftijzer HC, Heemstra KA, Corssmit EP, van der Klaauw AA, Romijn JA, Smit JW. Quality of life in cured patients with differentiated thyroid cancer. J Clin Metab Endocrinol. 2008;93(1):200–3.

Down Syndrome

Caterina Premoli, Letizia Maria Fatti, Luca Persani, and Elena Vittoria Longhi

Introduction

Down syndrome (DS) is the most commonly identified genetic form of mental retardation and the leading cause of specific birth defects and medical conditions (Table 1).

Live birth prevalence is influenced by changes in prenatal screening technologies and policies. In the United States, DS birth prevalence is estimated at 12.6 per 10,000 with around 5300 births annually [1]. According to EUROCAT registries, the prevalence of DS in Europe per 10,000 live births for the years 2010–2014 is 22.09 [2].

C. Premoli · L. Persani
Department of Endocrine and Metabolic Disorders, Istituto Auxologico Italiano, Milan, Italy

Department of Medical Biotechnologies and Translational Medicine, University of Milan, Milan, Italy
e-mail: persani@auxologico.it

L. M. Fatti (✉)
Department of Medical Biotechnologies and Translational Medicine, University of Milan, Milan, Italy
e-mail: l.fatti@auxologico.it

E. V. Longhi
Department of Sexual Medical Center, San Raffaele Hospital, Milano, Italy

© Springer Nature Switzerland AG 2023
E. V. Longhi (ed.), *Managing Psychosexual Consequences in Chronic Diseases*,
https://doi.org/10.1007/978-3-031-31307-3_8

Table 1 Incidence of comorbidity in DS

Congenital heart disease (including simple anatomic features)	up to 50%
Pulmonary hypertension	1.2–5.2%
OSA	57–73%
Hearing deficits	84%
Neutrophilia, thrombocytopenia, and polycythemia at birth	Respectively 80%, 66%, and 33%
Transient myeloproliferative disease	3–10%
Acute myeloid leukemia	20–30% (among patients with transient myeloproliferative disease)
Iron deficiency	45–66%
Thyroid abnormalities	50%
Obesity	23–70%
Neurodevelopmental disorders	18–38%
Epilepsy	8%
Autism spectrum disorders	7–16%

Table 2 Risk of DS in relation to maternal age

Maternal age	Risk of DS
20	1/1527
25	1/1352
28	1/1113
30	1/895
32	1/659
34	1/446
35	1/356
36	1/280
37	1/218
38	1/167
39	1/128
40	1/97
44	1/30

Geleherter TD et al, Principles of Medical Genetics, Elsevier, 1999

Genetic Features

The cause of DS has been recognized in the presence of a third copy of chromosome 21 which occurs sporadically in 90–95% of patients due to a meiotic nondisjunction. In approximately 2–4% of persons with DS phenotype, the trisomy occurs by unbalanced de novo or familial translocation between chromosome 21 and another acrocentric chromosome (usually cr. 14, 21 or 22). The remaining 2–4% of people with DS had a mosaicism, a condition characterized by both trisomic and euploid cell lines, usually associated with fewer clinical features of DS [3] The only known risk factor for DS is advanced maternal age [4] (Table 2).

Table 3 DS clinical features at birth

Clinical features	Presentation at birth (%)
Flat face	90
Absence of Moro reflex	85
General hypotonia	80
Ligament laxity	80
Abundant neck skin	80
Epicanthic eye-fold	80
Pelvic dysplasia	70
Dysplastic ear	60
Fifth finger clinodactyly	60

Hall B. Mongolism in newborn infants. An examination of the criteria for recognition and some speculations on the pathogenic activity of the chromosomal abnormality. Clin Pediatr (Phila). 1966 Jan;5(1):4–12.

Prenatal and Postnatal Diagnosis

The development of non-invasive prenatal screening (NIPS) using cell-free DNA has reduced the use of invasive testing showing a specificity of 99.7% in the prenatal detection of DS [5]. Nevertheless, genetic analysis of karyotype by amniocentesis and chorionic villus sampling is still required for a definitive prenatal diagnosis of DS. At delivery, physical examination is the most sensitive initial diagnostic assessment for DS. When DS is suspected post-natally (Table 3), karyotype is mandatory in order to confirm the diagnosis and to determine whether the cause is a non-disjunction or a translocation [6].

As life expectancy for individuals with DS has significantly improved, with a median age of 30 in 1973 to 60 as of 2020, the medical community is challenged with continuing to optimize medical treatments in order to reduce morbidity and maximize social function [7].

Cardiovascular Issues

Up to 50% of patients with DS are diagnosed with congenital heart diseases (CHD), with a prevalence of simple anatomic patterns showing no impact on morbidity and mortality. In the last years, genetics studies are trying to explain the high prevalence and the pathogenesis of CHD in DS. It is possible that the overexpression of genes mapping on chromosome 21 (i.e. COL6A1 and COL6A2) could be related to cardiac malformations [9].

The most frequent CHD diagnosed in DS is the atrioventricular septal defect (AVSD) representing the 30–50%. Other DS-associated CHD are atrial septal defects (ASD), ventricular septal defects (VSD), and tetralogy of Fallot [8]. Even in the absence of structural heart disease, neonates with DS are at risk of developing persistent pulmonary hypertension with a higher incidence (1.2–5.2%) compared with non-DS. This is due to other medical conditions that frequently affected DS people such as obstructive sleep apnea and obesity [10].

For these reasons, the American Academy of Pediatrics (AAP) guidelines recommend all neonates with DS to be screened for CHD with physical examination, ECG, chest radiography and echocardiography. DS people should be on cardiac surveillance through childhood and adulthood [6, 11].

Early surgical repair of CHD is the best strategy to prevent pulmonary hypertension and contribute to the increasing survival and to the better quality of life.

Despite premature aging and a tendency toward obesity, DS patients appear protected from atherosclerosis, arterial hypertension, and coronary artery disease [12].

Airways, Pulmonary, and Hearing Issues

Respiratory disorders are common causes of illness and death in DS children and adults. DS people are known to be affected by small airways for patient's age, micrognathia, relative macroglossia, tracheal stenosis due to complete tracheal rings, hypotonia, obstructive airway disease (OSA), increased risk of respiratory tract infection and serous otitis media and hearing impairment [13].

The prevalence of OSA in DS people has been underestimated frequently underrecognized. In recent reports, the prevalence ranges from 57% to 73% [14]. According to the AAP guidelines, polysomnography (PSG) has to be performed on all DS patients under 4 years of age [6]. The first line treatment is surgical and consists in adenotonsillectomy although it is not as effective in DS children as it is in non-affected children [15]. Continuous positive airway pressure (CPAP) is the mainstay of non- surgical treatment.

Adults with DS can have frequent ear wax impactions that may impair hearing, therefore ear examinations should be performed routinely.

The AAP recommends audiologic evaluation every 6 months for the first 5 years of life in patients with DS to evaluate for hearing loss [6]. Otolaryngologic and audiologic interventions are important to optimized speech and communication in order to achieve social integration and intellectual abilities.

Hematological Issues

DS is associated with a broad spectrum of hematological findings occurring at different ages. After birth, the altered hematopoiesis leads to peripheral blood abnormalities such as neutrophilia (in 80% of DS neonates), thrombocytopenia (in 66% of DS neonates), and polycythemia (in 33% of DS neonates) [16].

Within 1–2 months of life, 3–10% of DS infants develop transient myeloproliferative disease. Despite a spontaneous regression in most of the cases, TMD can be fatal or lead to the subsequent development of acute myeloid leukemia (AML) in 20% of DS children with a high sensitivity to chemotherapy and a favorable outcome. Children with DS also have an a 10–20-fold increased risk of developing acute lymphoblastic leukemia (ALL) compared to non-DS children associated to a higher rate of treatment-related toxicities [17].

To promptly recognize hematological disorders, various authors propose to perform a blood smear either in any DS child presenting with symptoms of TMD or leukemia or in every DS infant at approximately 2 months of life. In the absence of biological abnormalities, a blood smear should be performed yearly [16, 17]. In contrast, the risk of developing solid tumor except retinoblastoma and germ-cell tumors is lower in children and adults with DS [18].

Iron deficiency and vitamin B12 and folate deficiencies are frequent in DS persons as in general population. To this extent, current health supervision guidelines for children with DS recommend obtaining a complete blood count (CBC) in the newborn period and annually between ages of 13 and 21 years. Sufficient iron stores and adequate vitamin B12 and folate levels are of great importance to maximize learning and psychomotor development, particularly in children with baseline cognitive delay [19].

Endocrine Disorders

Endocrine disorders such as thyroid dysfunction, low bone mass, short stature, diabetes, and obesity are much more common in DS people rather than in general population.

Thyroid abnormalities include congenital hypothyroidism, acquired subclinical hypothyroidism, acquired overt hypothyroidism and hyperthyroidism, and thyroid autoimmunity [20]. The AAP guidelines recommend screening for thyroid dysfunction at birth, 6 months, 12 months, and annually thereafter [6]. Unlike the general population, there is no female predominance for any type of thyroid disorder. When looking at all types of thyroid disease, up to 50% of patients with DS are expected to have a diagnosis of thyroid disease by adulthood [21].

The incidence of congenital hypothyroidism is estimated between 1:113 and 1:141 DS live births being 14–21 fold more common among DS patients compared to the general population, as a likely consequence of the extra chromosome 21 and possibly to overexpression of the DYRK1A gene [22]. Most cases are associated with thyroid hypoplasia, whereas thyroid agenesis, ectopy, or goiter are infrequent. Subclinical hypothyroidism (SH) is the most frequent thyroid abnormality, with a prevalence ranging between 7% and 40%. SH before the age of 5 years may be a transient and self-limiting condition in >70% of DS cases. It has been postulated that mild TSH elevation in DS may be an inherent defect of the syndrome reflecting a resetting of the HPT axis. For these reasons, it has been suggested that SH may be over-diagnosed in DS patients, leading to unnecessary life-long treatment. Autoimmune hypothyroidism is the most frequent autoimmune disorder in DS. Anti-thyroid antibodies are found in 13–46% of patients showing no gender predilection, but with an increased prevalence of SH at presentation [23].

Skeletal maturation and bone-mass accrual in DS patients are impaired by hypogonadism, low vitamin D, low calcium intake, obesity, low physical activity, decreased muscle mass, decreased sun exposure, and anti-epileptic medication use [24]. Adults with DS have a high prevalence of osteoporosis [25] and present with lower bone mineral density (BMD) compared with persons with other intellectual disabilities but BMD can be underestimated due to short stature, and it has been suggested that volumetric BMD (vBMD). However, so far, data on fractures incidence are lacking in this population [26].

Adolescents with Down syndrome do not differ substantially from others in the age of onset of puberty, however DS male are sometimes affected by hypergonadotropic hypogonadism with evidence the Sertoli and Leydig cell dysfunction. The sperm count is abnormally low in men with DS; the resulting azoospermia or oligospermia may be associated with damaged spermatogenesis.

Women with DS are fertile, since many cases of maternity have been reported [27]. However, data in literature highlighted early menopause in women with DS (relative to a healthy population) and a marked decrease in levels of anti-Müllerian hormone. This premature ovarian failure might be associated with a reduced ovarian reserve due to oogenesis failure and/or lower levels of primordial cell maturation [28].

To this extent, infertility should not be assumed. It should be mandatory to discuss about sexuality and parenthood with DS patients and their families [20].

The combined prevalence of overweight and obesity varies between studies from 23% to 70%. Etiology of obesity is multifactorial including increased leptin, decreased resting energy expenditure, comorbidities, unfavorable diet, and low physical activity levels [29]. Obesity contributes to both reduced quality of life and to worse medical conditions such as OSA, cardiopulmonary disease, metabolic abnormalities, and mood disorders. To this extent, DS patients with BMI >30 has to be referred to a multicomponent behavioral intervention [30].

DS subjects are characterized by an acceleration of the ageing process leading to progeroid aspects and many age-associated diseases with an early onset including epidermal thickening, visual and hearing impairment, cognitive impairment, overweight, osteoporosis, early menopause, and diastolic dysfunction. The only exception is the incidence of solid cancer that in DS adult is lower with respect to age-matched controls. The main molecular mechanisms involved in the aging process are markedly altered in DS. These mechanisms include metabolism, stem cells and regeneration, macromolecular damage, inflammation, adaptation to stress, proteostasis, and epigenetics. So far, different biomarkers of age, such as telomere shortening, have been studied in DS in order to predict age-related functional decline and lifespan better than chronological age [31].

Autoimmune Disorders

Autoimmune diseases have a higher incidence and prevalence among individuals with DS than in people without this chromosomopathy. In particular, children with DS are at an increased risk for thyroid, gut, islet autoimmunity and alopecia, vitiligo, and juvenile idiopathic arthritis [32].

The immunological bases of relationships between DS and autoimmunity should be searched into thymic atrophy and diminished expansion of T and B lymphocytes, altered thymic expression of the autoimmune regulator (AIRE) gene located on chromosome 21q22.3, the genetic contribution of class II MHC genes, altered activity of enzymes that modulate inflammatory and immune processes and hyper-responsiveness to interferon [20, 23].

Neurodevelopment Disorders

Current prevalence estimates of neurobehavioral and psychiatric co-morbidity in children with DS range from 18% to 38% [33]. Decreased motor coordination, increased incidence of autism spectrum disorder (ASD), psychiatric problems, and, later in life, dementia are conditions that are frequently recognized in DS people [34]. The estimated prevalence of ASD among DS people ranges from 7% to 16% according to various studies [35]. The diagnosis of these problems is often delayed due to the overlap of DS-specific behaviors and autism. Epilepsy is seen in 8% of children with DS, with 40% occurring in infancy and often presenting as infantile spasms. Dementia that resembles Alzheimer's disease is common in adults with Down's syndrome [36]. Behavioral management is a challenge for families and caregivers of DS patient. Both pharmacological, counseling, and behavioral support have shown to have positive impact on quality of life.

In Conclusion

DS condition is complex and associated not only with health problems but also to psychological and social issues. Nowadays, people with DS have a better life expectancy; therefore, clinical research and development of evidence-based care guidelines for adults are needed with focus on probable changes in long-term DS morbidity. Involvement in community life has become increasingly important as persons with DS survive longer and achieve greater degrees of independence. An emphasis on transitions such as employment, source of health care, community involvement, as well as on legal issues and financial support, has been found to be essential for the long-term well-being of persons with DS and their families [33]. To this extent, in 2016, the Italian Parliament has promulgated the law no.112/2016 with the aim of promoting independence and providing support in daily life to people with disability that lose parental assistance.

Sexuality and Quality of Life

Individuals with DS and other mental disabilities who engage in sexual behaviors may encounter social prejudice and significant parental anxiety [37].

The emergence of sexual behaviors in the individual with DS alarms some parents and guardians who fear that the child may be particularly vulnerable to experiences such as unwanted pregnancies, sexual exploitation and abuse, and sexually transmitted diseases.

The incidence of masturbation in individuals with DS has been reported to be 40% in males and 52% in females [38]. Masturbation rates are not significantly higher in individuals with DS than in the general population [39]; reports show that incidence in the general population is 100% in males and 25% in females at age 15 years [40].

Certainly, the possibility of sexual abuse is not uncommon in these patients.

In a 1987 study by Elvik et al., following pelvic examination, 37% of women with mental disabilities showed signs that were thought to be consistent with previous vaginal penetration [41].

Schor's review of 87 non-institutionalized mentally disabled individuals indicated that 50% of mildly disabled individuals had engaged in sexual intercourse [42]. Rape or incest had occurred in 33% of mildly disabled and 25% of moderately disabled individuals. The mentally disabled individual is vulnerable to sexual maltreatment for several reasons: isolation; communication deficits; small peer group; and limited mutual support services. Loneliness and frustration may drive an individual to accept any form of individual attention whether negative or positive. Other contributing factors include multiple life situations and transient caregivers, some of whom may be pedophiles.

Sex education in these patients should begin in early childhood [43]. Young children and those individuals with DS who have severe cognitive or language impairment may learn best from a good/bad touch model: "Just say no to advances or unwanted touches" [44, 45]. Older children and individuals with mild language and cognitive impairment may be able to learn a physical and emotional distance paradigm [46] in which individuals learn appropriate behaviors for each circle of intimacy (space and physical distance) and are warned that "sometimes a friend may want to be closer to you than you want." You need to tell your friend to "STOP".

As adolescents with DS they require early sex education accompanied by open discussion. However, because of the significant variations within this population in cognitive levels, learning styles, living arrangements, and health problems, they require an individualized approach to sex education [37].

What About Contraception?

In general, adults with DS underutilize the healthcare system [47]. Women with DS demonstrate significantly lower utilization of gynecological and reproductive services than do women in the general population and while it is recommended that all women with DS have a baseline pelvic exam and pap test between the ages of 17 and 20, this recommendation is rarely followed [48].

Men with DS should learn testicular self-examination if their cognitive level permits; likewise, women should learn breast self-examination and undergo regular gynecological care [49, 50].

As in the general population, the only non-surgical contraceptive method available to males is the condom. There are, however, numerous methods available to women including condoms, spermicidal foams and gels, diaphragms, sponges, cervical caps, IUDs, oral contraceptives, Norplant, and Depo-Provera. No form of contraception is totally contraindicated for individuals with DS [45].

Oral contraceptives are frequently used by women with DS, and contraindications are similar to those reported by the rest of the female population.

The real difficulty detected by the scientific literature is: how to talk about sexuality to Down's syndrome patients in childhood and adolescence? Are caregivers—especially mothers—open in this sense?

> My husband still accepts our son as a child. When our son wishes to engage in masturbation, my husband is upset. Since our son cannot marry according to my husband's way of thinking, he chooses not to see my son's sexual needs or wants them to be unfulfilled. [51]

Mothers often report that they avoid talking about sexuality with their children because they do not feel comfortable with the topic. They blamed a lack of knowledge and of being conditioned by their cultural and religious approach to sexuality. In fact, some also reported that the traditional rules that defined sexuality as shame discouraged them from getting help to understand their children's sexual needs and they could not pass on their experiences to their child.

> My son doesn't know what fluid comes after masturbation, but he does wonder. I don't know how I can explain it to him because I can't talk openly about sexuality to anyone. I told him "You were urinating". [51]

Manor-Binyamini [52] study explored communication difficulties, for example, in a group of mothers in Turkey.

The mothers stated that they try to maintain control over their children's sexual behaviors, because they felt responsible for maintaining cultural and social values and expressed fear and anxiety related to public displays of sexual behavior, such as masturbation. However, labelling people with DS as eternal children [53] causes family members to act in a more controlling and traditionalist manner toward sexual needs and to focus only on caring responsibilities [54].

Parental pressure and control over children's sexuality can limit social interactions and reinforce social isolation [55].

Therefore, social, educational, and psychological support programs regarding their children's developmental characteristics could help mothers feel more competent and comfortable [56].

Teachers, among others, play an important role in children's sexual development, but they have limited knowledge and varying perspectives on communicating sexuality.

A study by LJ Scholes [57] researched teachers' knowledge and beliefs related to sex education. This research used a quantitative and qualitative (mixed method) approach. A total of 40 pre-school teachers were asked to complete a questionnaire describing teachers' knowledge and demographics, as well as a scale of beliefs about what teachers felt about teaching sex education.

Quantitative results showed that teachers had limited knowledge (M = 8.75, SD = 2.56) and low conviction (M = 2.75, SD = 0.28) as to the teaching of sexuality education to children. According to qualitative data, learning resources with regard to teaching sexuality were very limited.

There is more.

Individuals with DS also have an increased likelihood of a number of medical complications including those of the thyroid gland and the gastrointestinal, upper respiratory, audiological, haematological, and neurological systems [58].

Studies report that obesity is more prevalent in individuals with DS than in individuals with other types of intellectual disability (ID). However, no studies using a matched comparison group methodology were conducted, and results from previous studies are contradictory.

A detailed method was used to identify all adults with ID in Leicestershire. Individuals were invited to participate in a medical examination which included measurement of their height and weight, from which their body mass index (BMI) was calculated. For each person with DS, an individual matched for gender, age, and housing type was identified from the Leicestershire ID database.

Results

Women with DS had lower mean height and weight but higher mean BMI than paired pairs. Men with DS had lower mean height and weight, but there was no statistical difference in BMI compared with matched pairs. Using World Health Organization BMI categories, women with DS were more likely to be overweight or obese than their matched pairs (odds ratio = 2.17). Men with DS were more likely to be in the overweight category than their matched pairs but were less likely to be obese (odds ratio = 0.85).

It can be inferred that there is a higher prevalence of obesity among women with DS but not among men. As the impact on the health of people with DS of being overweight or obese is uncertain, this is an area that requires further study [59].

Conclusion

It is not easy for caregivers to approach the sexuality of their down's adolescent son/ daughter, especially for mothers. While fathers tend to deny the patient's sexual development and fear abuse or pregnancy, mothers often report the fear that their down's child could become a rapist. In no other pathology has the sexologist been able to accompany physicians, patients, and family members on various self-cultivating journeys into intimacy. The parent, gaining awareness in educating the patient with clear and neutral information, the patients, children, and adolescents, learning to experience the body and its urges as a normal process of growth. Adult patients experience intimacy as one of many acquired skills. The desire for a family and child in these patients should be welcomed and planned in stages according to the individual's mental and cognitive abilities. Physicians can incentivize patients and caregivers to experience the sexologist as an accomplice and positive specialist in the patient's quality of life.

Most parents noticed signs of physical sexual development. More than 60% of adolescents reacted to these changes by showing interest. About 70% of the girls had menarche. 91% of parents observed changes in behavior: mood instability, revolt, and shame. 37% of parents talked with their child about sexual topics, most of them responding to the child's interest. 47% of youth, particularly boys, showed interest in the opposite sex. Half of the youth planned to have a family; however, most parents did not approve of their children starting a family. When asked about means of contraception, parents preferred contraceptive pills and sterilization. 34% of parents would panic at the news of their children's pregnancy. 23% would not accept marriage between adults with DS, 66% were against having children by them.

The psychosexual development of people with DS is characterized by problems similar to those of puberty in healthy adolescents. The essential issue is the need for sex education and support for young people with DS, which will make it possible to avoid sexual abuse and asexual treatment of adolescents.

References

1. De Graaf G, Buckley F, Skotko BG. Estimates of the live births, natural losses, and elective terminations with down syndrome in the United States. Am J Med Genet Part A. 2015;167A:756–67.
2. Surveillance of congenital anomalies in Europe: epidemiology of Down syndrome. EUROCAT 1990–2014.
3. Papavassiliou P, Charalsawadi C, Rafferty K, Jackson-Cook C. Mosaicism for trisomy 21: a review. Am J Med Genet Part A. 2015;167A:26–39.
4. Hecht CA, Hook EB. Rates of Down syndrome at livebirth by one-year maternal age intervals in studies with apparent close to complete ascertainment in populations of European origin: a proposed revised rate schedule for use in genetic and prenatal screening. Am J Med Genet. 1996;62:376–85.
5. Gil MM, Quezada MS, Revello R, Akolekar R, Nicolaides KH. Analysis of cell-free DNA in maternal blood in screening for fetal aneuploidies: updated meta-analysis. Ultrasound Obstet Gynecol. 2015;45:249–66.
6. Bull MJ. Committee on genetics, Health supervision for children with Down syndrome. Pediatrics. 2011;128(2):393–406.
7. Tsou AY, Bulova P, Capone G, Chicoine B, Gelaro B, Harville TO, Martin BA, McGuire DE, McKelvey KD, Peterson M, Tyler C, Wells M, Whitten MS. Global Down syndrome foundation medical care guidelines for adults with Down syndrome workgroup. Medical care of adults with Down syndrome: a clinical guideline. JAMA. 2020;324(15):1543–56.
8. De Graaf G, Buckley F, Skokto B. Estimation of the number of people with Down syndrome in the United States. Genet Med. 2017;19(4):439–47.

9. Gittenberger-de Groot AC, Bartram U, Oosthoek PW, et al. Collagen type VI expression during cardiac development and in human fetuses with trisomy 21. Anat Rec A Discov Mol Cell Evol Biol. 2003;275:1109–16.

10. Weijerman ME, van Furth AM, van der Mooren MD, van Weissenbruch MM, Rammeloo L, Broers CJ, Gemke RJ. Prevalence of congenital heart defects and persistent pulmonary hypertension of the neonate with Down syndrome. Eur J Pediatr. 2010;169(10):1195–9.

11. Versacci P, Di Carlo D, Digilio MC, Marino B. Cardiovascular disease in Down syndrome. Curr Opin Pediatr. 2018;30(5):616–22.

12. Draheim CC, Geijer JR, Dengel DR. Comparison of intima–media thickness of the carotid artery and cardiovascular disease risk factors in adults with versus without the Down syndrome. Am J Cardiol. 2010;106:1512–6.

13. Bassett EC, Musso MF. Otolaryngologic management of Down syndrome patients: what is new? Curr Opin Otolaryngol Head Neck Surg. 2017;25(6):493–7.

14. Hill CM, Evans HJ, Elphick H, et al. Prevalence and predictors of obstructive sleep apnoea in young children with Down syndrome. Sleep Med. 2016;28:99–106.

15. Nation J, Brigger M. The efficacy of adenotonsillectomy for obstructive sleep apnea in children with Down syndrome: a systematic review. Otolaryngol Head Neck Surg. 2017;157:1–8.

16. Henry E, Walker D, Wiedmeier SE, Christensen RD. Hematological abnormalities during the first week of life among neonates with Down syndrome: data from a multihospital healthcare system. Am J Med Genet A. 2007;143:42–50.

17. Bruwier A, Chantrain CF. Hematological disorders and leukemia in children with Down syndrome. Eur J Pediatr. 2012;171(9):1301–7.

18. Hasle H. Pattern of malignant disorders in individuals with Down's syndrome. Lancet Oncol. 2001;2:429–36.

19. Dixon NE, Crissman BG, Smith PB, Zimmerman SA, Worley G, Kishnani PS. Prevalence of iron deficiency in children with Down syndrome. J Pediatr. 2010;157(6):967–71.

20. Whooten R, Schmitt J, Schwartz A. Endocrine manifestations of Down syndrome. Curr Opin Endocrinol Diabetes Obes. 2018;25(1):61–6.

21. Pierce MJ, LaFranchi SH, Pinter JD. Characterization of thyroid abnormalities in a large cohort of children with Down syndrome. Horm Res Paediatr. 2017;87(3):170–8.

22. van Trotsenburg P, Stoupa A, Léger J, Rohrer T, Peters C, Fugazzola L, Cassio A, Heinrichs C, Beauloye V, Pohlenz J, Rodien P, Coutant R, Szinnai G, Murray P, Bartés B, Luton D, Salerno M, de Sanctis L, Vigone M, Krude H, Persani L, Polak M. Congenital hypothyroidism: a 2020-2021 consensus guidelines update-an ENDO- European Reference Network initiative endorsed by the European Society for Pediatric Endocrinology and the European Society for Endocrinology. Thyroid. 2021;31(3):387–419.

23. Kyritsi EM, Kanaka-Gantenbein C. Autoimmune thyroid disease in specific genetic syndromes in childhood and adolescence. Front Endocrinol. 2020;11:543.

24. Hawli Y, Nasrallah M, El-Hajj Fuleihan G. Endocrine and musculoskeletal abnormalities in patients with Down syndrome. Nat Rev Endocrinol. 2009;5(6):327 34.

25. Baptista F, Varela A, Sardinha LB. Bone mineral mass in males and females with and without Down syndrome. Osteoporos Int. 2005;16:380–8.

26. Carfì A, Liperoti R, Fusco D, Giovannini S, Brandi V, Vetrano DL, Meloni E, Mascia D, Villani ER, Manes Gravina E, Bernabei R, Onder G. Bone mineral density in adults with Down syndrome. Osteoporos Int. 2017;28(10):2929–34.

27. Bovicelli L, Orsini LF, Rizzo N, Montacuti V, Bacchetta M. Reproduction in Down syndrome. Obstet Gynecol. 1982;59(6 Suppl):13S–7S.

28. Parizot E, Dard R, Janel N, Vialard F. Down syndrome and infertility: what support should we provide? J Assist Reprod Genet. 2019;36(6):1063–7.

29. Bertapelli F, Pitetti K, Agiovlasitis S, Guerra-Junior G. Overweight and obesity in children and adolescents with Down syndrome-prevalence, determinants, consequences, and interventions: a literature review. Res Dev Disabil. 2016;57:181–92.

30. Capone GT, Chicoine B, Bulova P, Stephens M, Hart S, Crissman B, Videlefsky A, Myers K, Roizen N, Esbensen A, Peterson M, Santoro S, Woodward J, Martin B, Smith D. Down

Syndrome Medical Interest Group DSMIG-USA Adult Health Care Workgroup. Co-occurring medical conditions in adults with Down syndrome: a systematic review toward the development of health care guidelines. Am J Med Genet A. 2018;176(1):116–33.
31. Franceschi C, Garagnani P, Gensous N, Bacalini MG, Conte M, Salvioli S. Accelerated biocognitive aging in Down syndrome: state of the art and possible deceleration strategies. Aging Cell. 2019;18(3):e12903.
32. Aversa T, Valenzise M, Corrias A, Salerno M, Iughetti L, Tessaris D, Capalbo D, Predieri B, De Luca F, Wasniewska M. In children with autoimmune thyroid diseases the association with Down syndrome can modify the clustering of extra-thyroidal autoimmune disorders. J Pediatr Endocrinol Metab. 2016;29(9):1041–6.
33. Weijerman ME, de Winter JP. Clinical practice: the care of children with Down syndrome. Eur J Pediatr. 2010;169:1445–52.
34. Capone G, Goyal P, Ares W, Lannigan E. Neurobehavioral disorders in children, adolescents, and young adults with Down syndrome. Am J Med Genet C Semin Med Genet. 2006;142C(3):158–72.
35. Di Guiseppi C, Hepburn S, Davis JM, Fidler DJ, Hartway S, Lee NR, Miller L, Ruttenber M, Robinson C. Screening for autism spectrum disorders in children with Down syndrome: population prevalence and screening test characteristics. J Dev Behav Pediatr. 2010;31(3):181–91.
36. Lott IT, Dierssen M. Cognitive deficits and associated neurological complications in individuals with Down's syndrome. Lancet Neurol. 2010;9(6):623–33.
37. Van Dyke DC, McBrien DM, Mattheis, PJ. Psychosexual behavior, sexuality and management problems in individuals with Down syndrome. Presentation, European Symposium on Down Syndrome. Majorca, Spain, 1995.
38. Pueschel SM. Masturbation in adolescence: Down syndrome. Paper and abstract for professionals, 9, 1. 1986.
39. Myers BA, Pueschel SM. Psychiatric disorders in a Down syndrome population. J Nerv Ment Dis. 1991;179:609–13.
40. Van Dyke D, McBrien D, Sherbondy A. Sexuality problems in Down syndrome. Down Syndr Res Pract. 1995;3(2):65–9. https://doi.org/10.3104/reviews.53.
41. Schwab US. Sexuality and community life. In: Down syndrome: advances in medical care. New York: Wiley-Liss; 1992. p. 157–66.
42. Elvik SL, Berkowitz CD, Nicholas E, Lipman JL, Inkelis SH. Sexual abuse in the developmentally disabled: diagnosis dilemmas. Child Abuse Negl. 1990;14:497–502.
43. Schor DP. Sex and sexual abuse in adolescents with developmental disabilities. Semin Adolesc Med. 1987;3(1):1–7.
44. Haka-Ikse K, Mian M. Sexuality in children. Pediatr Rev. 1993;14(10):401–7.
45. Heaton CJ. Providing reproductive health services to people with Down syndrome and other mental retardation. In: Redfern DE, editor. Caring for individuals with Down syndrome and their families, report of the third ross round table on cultural issues in family medicine. 1995.
46. Walker-Hirsch L, Champagne MP. Circles III: safer ways. In: Crocker AC, Cohen HJ, Kastner TA, editors. HIV infection and developmental disabilities. Baltimore: Paul H. Brookes Co.; 1992. p. 147–58.
47. Elkins TE, Spinnado J, Muram D. Sexuality and family interaction in Down syndrome: parental relationship. J Psychosom Obstet Gynecol. 1987;6:81–5.
48. Elkins TE. Gynecological care. In: Pueschel SM, Pueschel JK, editors. Biomedical problems in people with Down syndrome. Baltimore: Paul H. Brooks Co.; 1990. p. 131–46.
49. Doty S. Healthcare in adult life and aging. In: Redfern DE, editor. Caring for individuals with down syndrome and their families, report of the third ross round table on critical issues in family medicine, in print. 1995.
50. Edgerton RB. The report on contraception. Some socio-cultural research considerations. In: de la Cruz FF, Laveck GD, editors. Human sexuality and the mentally retarded. New York: Brunner/Mazel; 1993. p. 240–63.
51. Gokgoz C, Demirci AD, Kabukcuoglu K. Sexual behaviours and education in adolescents and young adults with Down syndrome: a grounded theory study of experiences and opin-

ions of their mothers in Turkey. Res Dev Disabil. 2021;112:103907. https://doi.org/10.1016/j.ridd.2021.103907.

52. Manor-Binyamini I, Schreiber-Divon M. Parental perceptions of the sexuality of adolescents with intellectual disabilities. Sex Disabil. 2019;37:599–612.

53. Pueschel SM, Scola PS. Parental perception of social and sexual functions in adolescents with Down syndrome. J Intellect Disabil Res. 1988;32(3):215–20.

54. Barg E, Bury M, Marczyk T, Pałac K, Wirth M. Psychosexual problem in young people with Down syndrome in parental opinion - personal experience. Pediatr Endocrinol Diabetes Metab. 2008;14(4):225–30.

55. Malovic A, Murphy G, Coulton S. Finding the right assessment measures for young people with intellectual disabilities who exhibit harmful sexual behavior. J Appl Res Intellect Disabil. 2020;33(1):101–10. https://doi.org/10.1111/jar.12299.

56. Michielsen K, Brockschmidt L. Barriers to sex education for children and young people with disabilities in the WHO European region: a scope review. Sex Educ. 2021;21(6):1–19. https://doi.org/10.1080/14681811.2020.185118.

57. Scholes LJ, Jones C, Stieler-Hunt C, Rolfe B, Pozzebon K. The role of teachers in child sexual abuse prevention programs: implications for teacher training Australian. J Teach Educ. 2012;37(11):104–31. https://doi.org/10.14221/ajte.2012v37n11.5.

58. Melville CA, Cooper S-A, McGrother CW, Thorp CF, Collacott R. Obesity in adults with Down syndrome: a case-control study. Res J Intellect Disabil. 2020. https://doi.org/10.1002/9781119432692.ch24

59. Song BRP, Manfredi P, de Souza IF. Nutritional status of children and adolescents with Down syndrome: a supplementary review. Revista Científica Multidisciplinar Núcleo do Conhecimento. 2020;19:55–70. ISSN: 2448-0959, Access link: https://www.nucleodoconhecimento.com.br/nutrition/stato-nutrizioni.

Hashimoto Thyroiditis

Simone Antonini, Maria Francesca Birtolo, Andrea Lania, and Elena Vittoria Longhi

Introduction

Hashimoto Thyroiditis is a chronic autoimmune disease clinically characterized by gradual thyroid failure due to the presence of specific antibodies directed to thyroid antigens. Haraku Hashimoto, a Japanese physician, first described in 1912 this condition, naming as *"struma lymphomatosa"* and referring to patients with goiter and intense lymphocytic infiltration of the thyroid gland [1]. Several studies have then stated that lymphocytic infiltration was the result of an immunological reaction to thyroid antigens and thyroid autoantibodies were identified [2]. Since then, Hashimoto thyroiditis has been considered an autoimmune disease characterized by the detection of serum thyroid autoantibodies, regardless of the presence of goiter.

Pathogenesis

Thyroid autoantibodies are detected in about 11% of the general population and in iodine sufficient areas, Hashimoto thyroiditis is considered the most common cause of hypothyroidism [3]. Hashimoto thyroiditis is more frequent in advanced age, in women, in iodine sufficient populations and in people moving from iodine sufficient to deficient areas. Its prevalence differs among races and geographical areas being more frequent in white race rather than black one and rare in Pacific Islanders.

S. Antonini · M. F. Birtolo · A. Lania (✉)
Endocrinology Unit, IRCCS Humanitas Research Hospital, Rozzano, Italy

Department of Biomedical Sciences, Humanitas University, Rozzano, Italy
e-mail: simone.antonini@humanitas.it; mariafrancesca.birtolo@humanitas.it;
andrea.lania@hunimed.eu

E. V. Longhi
Department of Sexual Medical Center, San Raffaele Hospital, Milano, Italy

© Springer Nature Switzerland AG 2023
E. V. Longhi (ed.), *Managing Psychosexual Consequences in Chronic Diseases*,
https://doi.org/10.1007/978-3-031-31307-3_9

Nevertheless, an increased incidence over time has been reported, particularly in the last three decades [4].

The pathogenic mechanisms underlying Hashimoto thyroiditis are still largely unknown, but it seems to be the result of a combination of genetic influences, environmental triggers, and epigenetic factors.

Genetic susceptibility has firstly been proven analyzing the impact of familial predisposition on the development of the disease and it has been demonstrated a concordance rate of more than 50% in monozygotic twins [5]. Several genes have been identified, particularly those involved in the immune response regulation, such as those coded in the Human Leukocyte Antigen complex (HLA). These genes could alternatively play a role of susceptibility or resistance in the development of the disease. HLA-A*02:07, HLA-DRB4, and HLA-B* 46:01 fall in the first group [6].

The main determinant in the rising incidence of autoimmune diseases, including Hashimoto Thyroiditis, appears to be a more hygienic environment with few microbial agents. Diet has also a central role: excess of iodine may cause the onset of the thyroiditis in predisposal individuals, while insufficient selenium and vitamin D deficiency may result in a worsening of the disease. In this context, the role of smoking and alcohol is still controversial of smoking and alcohol, but some studies report a moderate consumption of alcohol as a protective factor as well as lower peroxidase antibody levels in smokers rather than nonsmokers [3]. Eventually, viral infections could represent a risk factor in predisposed subjects, probably based on molecular mimicry mechanism between viral and self-antigens, but further studies are needed to clearly demonstrate a significant association.

Environment and genetic factors are mutually dependent, and the first ones can influence genes expression inducing epigenetic modifications, such as methylation and histone modifications.

Hashimoto thyroiditis is characterized by specific histopathology modifications, such as lymphocytic infiltration, lymphatic follicular formation, and replacement of glandular tissue in a fibrotic one, in a large spectrum of phenotypes including both goiter and gland atrophy. In pathogenesis, both humoral and cellular immunity play a role. The first event is a dysfunction of B cells with overproduction of thyroid autoantibodies. Nevertheless, hypothyroidism is due to the destruction of thyroid tissue which is realized by cellular immunity through cytotoxic and apoptotic mechanisms. Recent studies pointed out other factors involved in the pathogenesis such as alteration in the function of T cell suppressors [7].

Clinical Presentation and Diagnosis

Hashimoto thyroiditis has been associated with local and systemic symptoms (Table 1), even if more frequently is clinically silent leading to a condition named subclinical hypothyroidism.

Table 1 Clinical presentation and implications of hypothyroidism

Apparatus	Clinical evidence
Cardiovascular	Pericardial effusion, hyperhomocysteinemia, ECG changes, diastolic dysfunction, arterial hypertension, increased ITM
Metabolic	Increased BMI, high triglycerides, high cholesterol levels, low metabolic expenditure, fatigue
Neurological and psychological	Reduced or impaired cognitive functions (mostly memory), neuropathy, dementia, ataxia. In extremely severe cases myxedematous coma, depression
Endocrine	Sexual dysfunction and reduced fertility, increased prolactin, multinodular goiter
Dermatological	Dry skin, alopecia areata, macroglossia, Hertoghe sign, hair loss
Others	Cold intolerance, constipation, peripheral myxedema, macrocytic anemia, arthralgia, muscle weakness, muscle cramps

The local symptoms, occurring in case of goiter, are due to compression and include dyspnea, dysphagia, and dysphonia involving respectively trachea, esophagus, and recurrent laryngeal nerve. Systemic symptoms are due to primary hypothyroidism and may involve nearly all major organs, including a wide variety of symptoms from few and not severe to myxedematous coma. The latter is the result of severe and longstanding untreated hypothyroidism which leads to altered mental status, bradycardia, hypothermia, and progressive multiple organ dysfunction. Nowadays myxedema coma is a rare condition, while the most common systemic symptoms are weight gain, constipation, lethargy, fatigue, hair loss, and infertility in case of severe hypothyroidism [3]. Systemic symptoms are nonspecific, especially in elderly patients, and up to 15% of patients with autoimmune hypothyroidism are asymptomatic [8].

The diagnosis of chronic autoimmune thyroiditis is based on the presence of antithyroid autoantibodies and peculiar ultrasonography characteristics of the thyroid gland.

The antibodies routinely used in clinical practice are antithyroglobulin (AbTg) and antithyroid peroxidase (AbTPO) [9]. The former is a fundamental protein in the formation of thyroid hormones, acting as a scaffold for the incorporation of iodine, and the latter is the enzyme that fixes iodine in the Tg during the T4 synthesis [10, 11]. These antibodies show little, if any, functional activity but act as an important marker of the thyroiditic process that occurs in Hashimoto's disease. More than 90% of the patients have AbTg and/or AbTPO positivity, usually with AbTPO having a better sensibility than the AbTg.

Thyroid ultrasound can be useful in the differential diagnosis of Hashimoto's thyroiditis: the signature characteristics tend to be a diffusely enlarged gland with low echogenicity, a dishomogeneous structure, with low blood flow at the Color Doppler imaging (Fig. 1). Often these patients also show a multinodular goiter in the gland. Usually both the ultrasonographic characteristics and the AbTPO/AbTg positivity are present at the time of diagnosis.

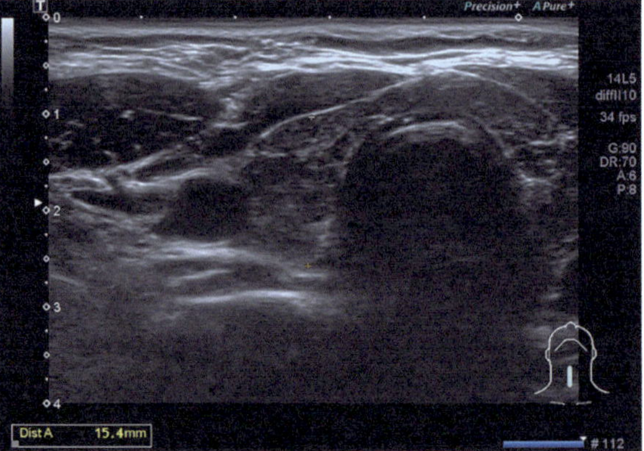

Fig. 1 Ultrasonography that shows the typical pattern of a Hashimoto thyroiditis, with hypoechoic and dishomogeneous ecostructure and the discrete presence of fibrous areas. No solid nodules were detected in this US [personal series]

There is no evidence that suggests the utility of repeating the antithyroid autoantibodies in the disease's follow-up, while the TSH levels must be periodically monitored every 9 to 12 months.

Treatment and Follow-Up

Hashimoto's disease needs no specific treatment in itself until a subclinical or overt hypothyroidism is developed by the patient. The follow-up process, once the diagnosis has been made, is based on an annual serum TSH evaluation, because approximately 5 percent per year evolve to overt hypothyroidism [12]. Thyroid ultrasonography must be repeated annually only when solid nodules are present. If TSH is less than 7 mUI/L, there is no need for specific therapy with levothyroxine. When TSH levels are between 7 and 10 mUI/L and/or hypothyroidism symptoms are developed, Hashimoto's thyroiditis can start to be treated with levothyroxine. If TSH is more than 10 mUI/l or the hypothyroidism is overt (fT4 lower than the LLR), treatment is recommended. Goals of the therapy are amelioration of symptoms and normalization of serum TSH.

The standard treatment for primary hypothyroidism is 1.2–1.6 mcg/kg/day of levothyroxine, administrated orally in a single dose in the morning, in a fasting state, at least 20 minutes before having breakfast. In patients with atherosclerotic coronary heart disease or older age (age over 60 years), the drug should be started gradually, receiving in the first weeks of treatment an increasing fraction of the full-dose therapy. Patients must be informed to avoid soy containing products and papaya during breakfast and avoid protonic pump inhibitors and mineral iron in the hours following levothyroxine to allow a better absorption of the drug. The half-life of T4 is 7 days, allowing different posology over a week to reach more accurate titration of the drug. Levothyroxine preparations can be tablets, liquid oral suspensions or gel capsules. Liquid and gel capsules formulation allow a shorter time between the administration and breakfast. Revaluation after starting levothyroxine therapy should be performed after 6 to 8 weeks with serum TSH levels that should be between 0.5 mUI/l and the URL, usually between 4 and 5 mUI/l.

If the serum TSH is too high, levothyroxine dose must be increased by 6 to 25 mcg/day, based on the serum TSH levels, and rechecked after 6–8 weeks; the patient should also be reminded the correct way to assume the drug to allow an ideal absorption. Keep gradual dose titration until TSH is normal.

If serum TSH is too low, levothyroxine dose must be reduced by 12 to 25 mcg/day, and rechecked at 6–8 weeks, then keep gradual dose titration until TSH is normal.

When serum TSH is normal, keep an annual serum TSH check. A closer follow-up must be performed if: the patients develop symptoms of hypothyroidism or hyperthyroidism, pregnancy, initiation or discontinuation of estrogen replacement therapy, and gain or loss of more than 10% of body weight.

Recent studies have analyzed long-term consequences of hypothyroidism in terms of quality of life and association with all-causes mortality, particularly in the subclinical setting to identify conditions worthy of treatment despite the presence of symptoms.

Great attention has been given to the implications of hypothyroidism on cardio-vascular system and several studies have confirmed a major risk of myocardial injuries and pericardial effusions in patients with hypothyroidism than in matched euthyroid controls. Also, subclinical hypothyroidism with TSH concentrations above 10 mUI/L has been associated with an increased risk of heart failure [13]. This is based on the evidence that low levels of thyroid hormones lead to increased vascular resistance, decreased cardiac output, and changes in markers of cardiovascular contractility.

Lastly, several studies have proposed a relationship between Hashimoto's thyroiditis and a possible malignant transformation, but this correlation is still debated and need to be further analyzed with prospective studies [14].

Sexuality and Quality of Life

Sexual dysfunction (SD), in both men and women, is a highly prevalent problem with multiple underlying etiologies. From a male perspective, SD can be classified into the categories of erectile dysfunction, ejaculation disorders (premature ejaculation (EP) and delayed ejaculation (ED)) and decreased libido.

PE is the most common male sexual disorder, occurring in 20–30% of men during their lifetime [15]. ED is a male sexual dysfunction that is highly age-dependent: it is 18% for the 50–59 age group, increasing to 37% for the 70–75 age group [16]. It is estimated that 5–15% of men suffer from decreased libido, many of whom have reported concomitant impairment in other domains of sexual functioning.

From a female perspective, SD is addressed from the domains of sexual desire, arousal/lubrication, orgasm, satisfaction, and pain with sexual activity. According to an international survey of women aged 40–80 years, 39% of women reported dysfunction in at least one of these areas [17]. There is also an element of age-dependent change in FSD, as genitourinary syndrome of menopause is said to cause discomfort, lack of lubrication, or pain in 40% of postmenopausal women [18].

According to the study Prevalence of Female Sexual Problems Associated with Distress and Determinants of Treatment Seeking, which surveyed 30,000 women in the United States, 43% of women experienced difficulties with these sexual problems. The most common symptom reported by women in the United States, at 39%, was reduced desire. Decreased arousal was reported by 26% of women and 21% had difficulty with orgasm [19].

In addition, alterations in the hypothalamic-pituitary-gonadal axis in thyroid disorders can affect fertility and stimulate recurrent pregnancy terminations.

Bear in mind that this pathology can be associated with symptoms of fatigue, weight gain, and a depressed mood, all of which contribute to reducing interest in sexual activity in both men and women.

This condition can have several major repercussions on the body and mind. Hyperthyroidism, the excessive production of thyroid hormones, often causes anxiety and irritability, tremors and weakness, sensitivity to heat, and problems gaining or maintaining one's weight. Hashimoto's syndrome can cause depression and mental confusion, soreness and inflammation, sensitivity to cold and weight changes. Severe hypothyroidism from Hashimoto thyroiditis can lead to fatigue, desensitization to the preliminaries of sexual intercourse, distraction, disturbance of arousal, inhibition of desire.

To make matters worse, the researchers admit that they did not particularly prioritize concerns regarding patients' sexual life and well-being. Recent studies suggest that, on average, at least 40 percent of people with the condition have experienced sexual consequences, whether caused directly by the change in hormone balance or as a secondary result of treatment (low-pain threshold, fatigue). Male patients report erectile dysfunction at a higher than average rate, premature ejaculation, and delayed ejaculation. People with vaginas report that they often have difficulty with lubrication and reaching orgasm.

To get pregnant, the thyroid hormones L-thyroxine (fT4 or T4) and triiodothyronine (fT3 or T3) must be in the normal range. These hormones affect, among other things, the cycle and ovulation, corpus luteum function, embryo implantation, and placental function.

Is the Desire for a Child Possible?

With Hashimoto's, these hormones get out of control. Hashimoto's disease is an autoimmune disease that attacks the body's defenses, particularly thyroid tissue, leading to chronic inflammation of the thyroid gland. In the short-term, there is the possibility of an overactive thyroid, that is, the gland secretes more hormones than usual. In general, overactive thyroid is not as bad as underactive thyroid, but it can lead to complications during pregnancy.

Infertility is not definitive. But during conception, it is important to monitor Hashimoto's disease to avoid consequences for the child. Physical or brain growth may be affected, and eventually, these changes or atrophy may affect the child's intelligence.

In these cases, the gynecologist and endocrinologist must work as a team, and the consultation of a neonatologist is not excluded.

Especially since cases of miscarriage during pregnancy are not uncommon.

Partners often suffer from the patient's fragility and show anxious-depressive symptoms, with alterations in aggression, impatience, anger.

Conclusion

Hashimoto's syndrome poses many risks to the health and quality of life of adult and adolescent patients.

The following factors are associated with an increased risk of Hashimoto's disease:

- **Sex:** Women are much more likely to get Hashimoto's disease.
- **Age:** Hashimoto's disease can occur at any age but most commonly occurs during middle age.
- **Other autoimmune diseases:** Having another autoimmune disease, such as rheumatoid arthritis, type 1 diabetes or lupus, increases the risk of developing Hashimoto's disease.
- **Genetics and family history:** You are at increased risk of getting Hashimoto's disease if other members of your family have thyroid disorders or other autoimmune diseases.
- **Pregnancy:** Typical changes in immune function during pregnancy may be a factor in Hashimoto's disease starting after pregnancy.
- **Excessive iodine intake:** Too much iodine in the diet can act as a trigger among people already at risk for Hashimoto's disease.
- **Radiation exposure:** People exposed to excessive levels of environmental radiation are more prone to Hashimoto's disease.

Moreover, although clinical research has found more adaptive therapies, *the emotional investment of the patient and caregiver is often underestimated.* From sexuality to mood disorders, from apathy to thermogenesis difficulties, every life experience seems to these patients to be an excessive burden and not always assessable in advance. The scientific diligence of clinicians often does not seem sufficient for the individual diagnosed with Hashimoto's and their partner. Often, the difficulties are emotional, from putting up with a partner's caresses, to inability to distinguish a caress from a passionate touch. *The psychosexologist can help these patients to construct a personalized approach that is not governed by the limitations of the pathology, but by alternative solutions, so that they need not give up on their life plans.*

References

1. Hashimoto H. Zur Kenntniss der lymphomatösen Veränderung der Schilddrüse (Struma lymphomatosa). Arch Klin Chir. 1912;97:219–48.
2. Roitt IM, Doniach D, Campbell PN, Hudson RV. Auto-antibodies in Hashimoto's disease (lymphadenoid goitre). Lancet. 1956;271(6947):820–1.
3. Chaker L, Bianco AC, Jonklaas J, Peeters RP. Hypothyroidism. Lancet. 2017;390(10101):1550–62.
4. McLeod DS, Caturegli P, Cooper DS, Matos PG, Hutfless S. Variation in rates of autoimmune thyroid disease by race/ethnicity in US military personnel. JAMA. 2014;311:1563–5.
5. Kust D, Matesa N. The impact of familial predisposition on the development of Hashimoto's thyroiditis. Acta Clin Belg. 2018;75(2):104–8.
6. Ueda S, Oryoji D, Yamamoto K, Noh JY, Okamura K, Noda M, Kashiwase K, Kosuga Y, Sekiya K, Inoue K, Yamada H, Oyamada A, Nishimura Y, Yoshikai Y, Ito K, Sasazuki T. Identification of independent susceptible and protective HLA alleles in Japanese autoimmune thyroid disease and their epistasis. J Clin Endocrinol Metab. 2014;99:E379–83.
7. Ralli M, Angeletti D, Fiore M, D'Aguanno V, Lambiase A, Artico M, de Vincentiis M, Greco A. Hashimoto's thyroiditis: an update on pathogenic mechanisms, diagnostic protocols, therapeutic strategies, and potential malignant transformation. Autoimmun Rev. 2020;19(10):102649.
8. Carlé A, Pedersen IB, Knudsen N, Perrild H, Ovesen L, Laurberg P. Hypothyroid symptoms and the likelihood of overt thyroid failure: a population-based case control study. Eur J Endocrinol. 2014;171:593–602.
9. Weetman AP, McGregor AM. Autoimmune thyroid disease: further developments in our understanding. Endocr Rev. 1994;15(6):788–830.
10. Mariotti S, Caturegli P, Piccolo P, Barbesino G, Pinchera A. Antithyroid peroxidase autoantibodies in thyroid diseases. J Clin Endocrinol Metab. 1990;71(3):661–9.
11. Nordyke RA, Gilbert FI Jr, Miyamoto LA, Fleury KA. The superiority of antimicrosomal over antithyroglobulin antibodies for detecting Hashimoto's thyroiditis. Arch Intern Med. 1993;153(7):862–5.
12. Huber G, Staub JJ, Meier C, Mitrache C, Guglielmetti M, Huber P, Braverman LE. Prospective study of the spontaneous course of subclinical hypothyroidism: prognostic value of thyrotropin, thyroid reserve, and thyroid antibodies. J Clin Endocrinol Metab. 2002 Jul;87(7):3221–6.
13. Rodondi N, den Elzen WPJ, Bauer DC, et al. for the Thyroid Studies Collaboration Study Group. Subclinical hypothyroidism and the risk of coronary heart disease and mortality. JAMA. 2010;304:1365–74.
14. Jankovic B, Le KT, Hershman JM. Clinical review: Hashimoto's thyroiditis and papillary thyroid carcinoma: is there a correlation? J Clin Endocrinol Metab. 2013;98:474–82.
15. Carson C, Gunn K. Premature ejaculation: definition and prevalence. Int J Impot Res. 2006;18(Suppl):S5–13.
16. Feldman HA, Goldstein I, Hatzichristou DG, et al. Impotence and its medical and psychosocial correlates: results from the Massachusetts Male Aging Study. J Urol. 1994;151:54–61.
17. Laumann EO, Nicolosi A, Glasser DB, et al. Sexual problems between women and men aged 40 to 80: prevalence and correlates identified in the Global Study of Sexual Attitudes and Behaviors. Int J Impot Res. 2005;17:39–57.
18. Santoro N, Komi J. Prevalence and impact of vaginal symptoms in postmenopausal women. J Sex Med. 2009;6:2133–42.
19. Shifren JL, Monz BU, Russo PA, et al. Sexual problems and discomfort in US women: prevalence and related. Obstet Gynecol. 2008;112:970–8.

Part V
Dermatology

Psoriasis in Adolescents and Adults

Santo Raffaele Mercuri, Giovanni Paolino, and Elena Vittoria Longhi

Introduction

Psoriasis is a common chronic immune-mediated inflammatory skin disorder, affecting the skin, nails, and joints in both children and adults. Depending on the studied population, psoriasis is estimated to affect 2.0–8.5% of the population [1]. The main causes of psoriasis remain unknown, although a complex of interactions between genetic, biochemical, and immunological abnormalities have been involved [1]. Regarding the genetic aspects, PSORS1 (at chromosome 6p21) is the major susceptibility locus for psoriasis [1–3]. Many HLA markers have been associated with psoriasis, but HLA-Cw6 is the highest relative risk for psoriasis in Caucasian population. However, as reported above, the onset of a psoriatic lesion is a complex and multicellular process that involves keratinocytes, T cells (above all CD4+ T cells in the upper dermis and CD8+ T cells in the epidermis), dendritic cells, macrophages, mast cells, endothelial cells, and neutrophils. While, at the same time, cytokines (e.g., TNF-alpha, IL-17, IL-23, etc.) and growth factor initiate and sustain inflammation in this process [1]. The cutaneous microbiota of patients with psoriasis is different to those without psoriasis, although the significance of this is unclear [4]. Indeed a wide range of microorganisms have been associated with psoriasis; however, the microorganism that is most associated with the onset of psoriasis is *Streptococcus*. Indeed, in some cases, psoriatic patients show a higher incidence of Beta-hemolytic streptococci of Lancefield groups A, C, and G, exacerbating the cutaneous symptomatology [5]. In this regard, Th1 cells recognize bacteria of the class of A streptococci and a HLA variation shows a specific effect on the immune

S. R. Mercuri · G. Paolino (✉)
Unit of Dermatology and Cosmetology, Scientific Institute San Raffaele (IRCCS), Milan, Italy
e-mail: mercuri.santoraffaele@hsr.it; paolino.giovanni@hsr.it

E. V. Longhi
Department of Sexual Medical Center, San Raffaele Hospital, Milano, Italy

© Springer Nature Switzerland AG 2023
E. V. Longhi (ed.), *Managing Psychosexual Consequences in Chronic Diseases*,
https://doi.org/10.1007/978-3-031-31307-3_10

response to group A streptococci [5]. Finally, also some drugs can induce the onset of psoriasis in some predisposed subjects, such as beta-blockers, lithium, antimalarials, terbinafine, calcium channel blockers, captopril, glyburide, granulocyte colony-stimulating factor, interleukins and interferons [5]. Finally, various studies highlighted a correlation between stress and severity of psoriasis, where stress seems to play a pivotal role for the onset and/or exacerbation of psoriasis [5].

Psoriasis causes a significant impairment in quality of life and the incidence of psoriasis is equal in women and men. The majority of patients (about 2/3 of affected patients) have a mild disease, while about 1/3 of patients show a more severe involvement. Although, psoriasis may appear at any age, usually arises between the ages of 15 and 30 [1]. The association with particular HLA I antigens (most notably HLA-Cw6) is particularly associated with an earlier age of onset of the disease [1]. In this regard and according to Henseler and Cristhophers, there are two main type of psoriasis: type I with an onset before 40 and type II with age of onset after the age 40 [1].

Visiting a patient with psoriasis is always necessary to have all the necessary information about the age of onset of the disease and whether psoriasis is present in family members. The presence or absence of joint symptoms should be recorded, as well as other comorbidities (smoking status, high blood pressure, hypercholesterolemia, hypertriglyceridemia, diabetes, obesity) as psoriasis is an independent risk factor above all for cardiovascular disorders. Finally, treatment history should be also recorded in order to identify patient's candidate for biologic treatments and/or for alternative treatments.

Main Medical Characteristics of Psoriasis

Psoriasis shows a very wide range of clinical manifestation and sometimes can be a diagnostic challenge for the clinician. There are different types of psoriasis that can show different clinical manifestations and that we report below.

Plaque psoriasis/Psoriasis vulgaris (PV) affects about 90% of psoriatic patients and it is the most common type of psoriasis. PV is characterized by demarcated erythematous plaques with whitish scales. After removing a scale, a small dripping of point blood is observed (Auspitz sign). Psoriatic lesions can arise after local trauma and this is known as "Koebner response" and typically appears after 7–14 days after the trauma (e.g., after a tattoo or trauma) [1].

Guttate psoriasis (GP) is a psoriasis characterized by multiple small psoriatic plaques in the trunk and limbs and typically arises in children, adolescents, and young adults (Fig. 1). It is often proceeded by a Streptococcal infection or by other infections [1, 5]. Usually, after an appropriate treatment of the of the eventual underlying infection, there is an improvement of the cutaneous symptoms, although up to date there is limited evidence that antimicrobial therapy is of direct benefit in preventing flares of psoriasis [1, 4]. Unfortunately, one-third of patients with GT develop a chronic plaque psoriasis [1].

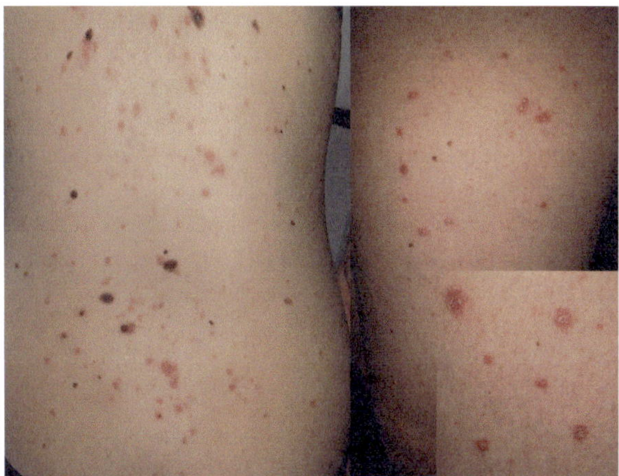

Fig. 1 Typical clinical aspects of a guttate psoriasis in an 18-year-old female patient. In the insert lower right, note the typical small, annular, erythematous, and scale papules. The patient had a concomitant dental infection. After the appropriate dental therapy, the cutaneous lesions disappeared

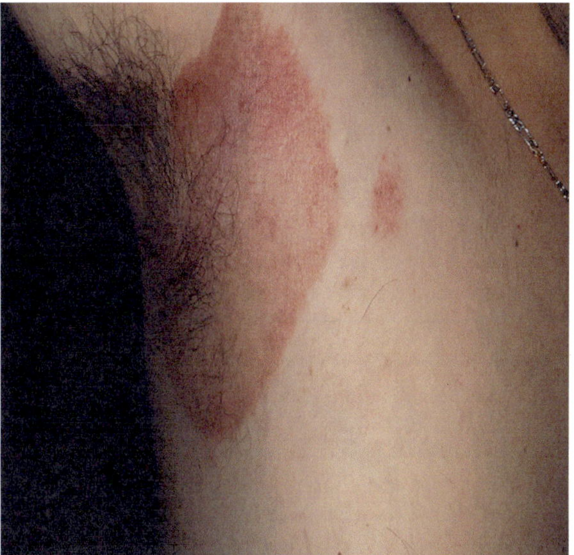

Fig. 2 A 16-year-old boy with an inverse psoriasis characterized by the presence of typical smooth and shiny bilateral axillary lesions

Inverse psoriasis (IP) arises in the major skin folds, as in axillae, inguinal creases, intergluteal clefts, umbilicus, and inframammary folds. Lesions are typically erythematous (bright appearance) and sharply demarcated, without the presence of any scale. Sweating is decreased in affected areas and localized fungal or bacterial infections may arise [1] (Fig. 2).

Erythrodermic psoriasis (EP) is the generalized form of psoriasis and may involve face, trunk, extremities, hands, and feet. EP is an inflammatory skin disease with redness and scaling that affects nearly the entire cutaneous surface. This term applies when 90% or more of the skin is affected. Patients lose their autonomic control of body temperature and may present systemic symptoms. Besides, the generalized vasodilatation puts patients at risk for high-output cardiac failure, impaired hepatic and renal function, and lower extremities edema [1].

Pustular psoriasis (PP) is characterized by the appearance of 2 to 3 mm sterile pustules that show subcorneal neutrophils on histopathology. There are four main clinical categories of PP: *generalized pustular psoriasis von Zumbusch* (involves the trunk and limbs and possible triggering factors include infections, irritating topical treatments, and withdrawal of systemic corticosteroids) that may have life-threatening complications including hypocalcemia, acute respiratory distress syndrome, bacterial superinfection, sepsis, and dehydration; *annular PP and impetigo herpetiformis (IH)* that are similar to gyrate erythemas and typically arise during pregnancy; *localized PP* that is characterized by two variants: *palmoplantar PP (PPP)* that involves palmoplantar regions and is characterized by sterile pustules with yellow-brown macules; and *acrodermatitis continua of Hallopeau* that is a rare eruption of sterile pustules on the fingers or toes that slowly extend proximally and may be associated to atrophy of digit and destruction of nail matrix [1].

Napkin psoriasis (NP) is a type of psoriasis that typically appears in the diaper (napkin) areas between the ages of 3 months and 6 months. Linear psoriasis (LP) is a rare form that typically presents as a linear plaque on an extremity or dermatome of the trunk [1].

Nail involvement is common in psoriasis and is present in about 40% of psoriatic patients and the involvement of the nails increase with age, extent of the disease, duration of the disease, and eventual presence of psoriatic arthritis. Psoriatic arthritis (PA) occurs in 5% to 30% of patients with cutaneous psoriasis. Cutaneous disease usually arises 10–12 years before the involvement of the joints. However, 10–15% of PA patients present also without any cutaneous involvement [1]. The diagnosis of PA is pretty difficult, since there are no serological markers and the radiographic alterations, erosive changes may occur years after the initial inflammation. The classic aspects of PA are characterized by both the involvement of the distal (DIP) and proximal (PIP) interphalangeal joints, in about 40% of patients [1]. Prolonged disease in the PIP and DIP of a single digit can lead to swelling (dactylitis) and the appearance of a "sausage" digit. Enthesitis (inflammation of the tendons into the bones) is also commonly present in PA and is seen in approximately 20% of patients with PA. Finally, arthritis mutilans is the most severe form of PA, characterized by severe joint damage and is seen in 5% of PA patients [1].

Psoriatic patients show an increased risk of several diseases and complication. According to a study, younger patients, such as 30-year-old psoriatic patients with a severe form of psoriasis have a relative risk of myocardial infarction, compared to healthy controls. As well as psoriatic patients have an increased risk to develop metabolic syndrome (obesity, hypertriglyceridemia, low high-density lipoprotein, hypertension, and diabetes), since they have in increased risk to develop each of the diseases included in metabolic syndrome [1]. In addition, there is an increased prevalence to develop rheumatoid arthritis, Chron disease, ulcerative colitis, Hodgkin lymphoma, and cutaneous T-cell lymphoma. Psoriasis shows also an important psychological impact. Indeed, cutaneous lesions lead to concerns about appearance, lowered self-esteem, guilt, social rejection. All these factors increase the risk to develop anxiety, depression, and suicidal ideations. Besides, pruritus and pain exacerbate all these psychological stressors [1].

Main Tools for the Diagnosis of Psoriasis

The vast majority of patients with psoriasis can be diagnosed according to the clinical features and based on their clinical history. However, a cutaneous biopsy with a relative histopathological evaluation is necessary to exclude other cutaneous differential diagnosis. The histology, in case of psoriasis, shows: acanthosis, thinning of the epidermis over elongated dermal papillae, increased mitosis of keratinocytes, parakeratosis, hyperkeratosis, inflammatory cells in the dermis (lymphocytes and monocytes) and in the epidermis (lymphocytes and polymorphonuclear cells) where they form Munroe microabscess [1–3].

The current gold standard for assessment of extensive psoriasis and relative severity is the Psoriasis Area and Severity Index (PASI). As PASI increases, the severity of the disease increases [2].

Currently, there are no serum markers specific for psoriasis. It is important to check laboratory investigations in patients with severe disease to assess for systemic complications [1]. Some patients may have a decrease of serum albumin or elevated uric acid, increasing the risk of developing gouty arthritis. Many psoriatic patients also manifest altered lipid profiles with an increase of high-density lipoproteins and elevated apolipoprotein A1 concentrations. These alterations of lipids contribute to increased cardiovascular risk. Finally, markers of systemic inflammation, such as C-reactive protein and erythrocyte sedimentation rate are elevated in a little percentage of psoriatic patients, suggesting an eventual underlying PA [1].

Treatments

The high percentage of therapeutic agents used for psoriasis are immunomodulatory medications. There is no definitive cure for psoriasis and the treatments can be long and frustrating. However, with the new era of biologic therapies with their relative increased treatment responses, patient's expectations increased in the last years. The dermatologist should always evaluate each patient and prescribe the most effective treatment for the target patient and in case of disease progression individualize the alternative treatment to achieve long-term control. The actual treatments for psoriasis can be divided in four main classes: topical treatments, phototherapy, systemic, and biologic therapies.

The vast majority of psoriatic patients are initially treated with only topical therapies. However, about 40% of patients report to be noncompliant with their topical treatments because they feel these treatments time-consuming and cosmetically unacceptable. The main local therapies include corticosteroids, vitamin D analogs, tazarotene, salicylic acid, and calcineurin inhibitors (such as tacrolimus and pimecrolimus) [1].

In 1970, photochemotherapy with psoralen and UVA light (named PUVA) was developed, but now is not so much used given increased risk to develop skin cancers.

Subsequently, in 1980, narrow band UVB (311–313 nm) was developed, showing efficacy [1]. Excimer laser is a high-intensity ultraviolet B (UVB) light, that emits dose of a very specific wavelength (308 nm) directly at the psoriasis plaques, resulting as a safe and effective alternative treatment for localized psoriasis [1].

In case of extended psoriasis, not responding to local treatments or where local treatments (due to the extension of the disease) cannot be prescribed, systemic therapy is needed. Systemic steroids, cyclosporine, acitretin, and methotrexate are classified as conventional systemic treatments and remain effective and inexpensive [1]. Recently, a novel oral phosphodiesterase 4 (PDE4) inhibitor (apremilast) has shown good responses in cutaneous psoriasis and PA. Subsequently, in case of nonresponse to these treatments, an alternative with biological therapy is being considered [1]. Indeed since 1998, there has been an explosion in the development of new biologic agents. These molecules are targeted and potent, with also an excellent safety profile. Multiple classes of biologics are available: TNF-alpha inhibitors, anti-p40 (IL-12/IL-23 antagonists), IL-17 inhibitors as well as the new anti-p-19 inhibitors (selective for IL-23). All these treatments are changing the treatment of patients with psoriasis, improving also clinical outcomes and quality of life of the patients [1].

Sexuality and Quality of Life

Notwithstanding the many therapies available to combat this condition, the resulting sexual discomfort and quality of life of patients appear to be significantly impaired. A recent study by Mohammed Mohammed Salem Selim et al. [6] evaluated female sexual dysfunction and the correlation with psoriasis severity.

The study involved two groups; 30 female patients with psoriasis, ranging in age from 20 to 60 years, and the control group comprising 20 age-matched healthy women. Disease severity was classified according to the Psoriasis Area and Severity Index (PASI) score. Female sexual function was assessed by the Female Sexual Function Index (FSFI).

It was found that the mean of all six FSFI domains was lower in the psoriatic group than in the control group, except that pain was increased although with no statistically significant difference between the two groups. It was found that orgasm appeared significantly reduced in female patients with psoriasis compared with the control group. There was a significant negative correlation between female sexual function index (FSFI) and psoriasis severity (PASI). In contrast to the psoriasis group, there was no correlation between FSFI and age or disease duration in the control.

Maunder and Hunter [7], researchers at the University of Toronto and Mount Sinai Hospital in Toronto (part of the Integrated Medicine Project) conducted a program of research on the aspects of psychiatric health and pathology that lie at the interface between psychology, psychiatry, and biomedicine. Specifically, they examined the well-known hypothesis that adverse events occurring during childhood influence health in adulthood and facilitate the processes of adult disease onset and chronicization. The relationship is not absolute (not all individuals who experienced childhood adverse events become ill with certain diseases as adults, and vice versa), but affective (e.g., depression) and neurobiological (e.g., hypothalamic dysfunction) predispositions and/or association with contextual factors (e.g., poor health care and inadequate nutrition) are often associated with the chronic disease process.

They surmised that attachment style may be associated with biological indicators of disease in diabetes and ulcerative colitis. In fact, in diabetic patients, distancing attachment (avoidant parent-child relationship) is associated with glycosylated hemoglobin levels while in patients with ulcerative colitis, anxious attachment mediates the association between depression and active disease status.

Ultimately, the authors identified mechanisms through which attachment can affect health status:

1. Alteration of stress physiology
2. Assumption of certain illness behaviors
3. Interaction between disease indices and attachment behavior
4. Alteration of affective behavior

Robert G. Maunder and Jonathan J. Hunter [8] (University of Toronto and Mount Sinai Hospital, Toronto, Canada) also support the hypothesis that chronic disease, particularly psoriasis, may appear as a consequence of factors related to low socio-economic status and suboptimal health care, nutrition, and education. Adverse events in childhood may consist, for example, of parental substance abuse. If a child grows up with an adult who abuses alcohol, tobacco, or other drugs, the risk increases as a result of the genetic or experiential influence that parents pass on. A third pathway in the link between adversity in childhood and illness in the adult relates to the effects of adversity such as a propensity for depression, poor self-care caused by a sense of powerlessness, or dysregulation of affect and pituitary function in the hypothalamus. These traumas are severe and persistent.

Metaphorically speaking, psoriasis could be a system of defense and control of the individual in order to oppose a reality that is perceived to be too heavy and disturbing. A <shell> in which to hide impotence, inadequacy, depression, and mood and eating disorders.

In addition to psychological aspects, scientific studies also reveal psychiatric factors [9].

Psychosocial factors are important in the onset and/or exacerbation of psoriasis in 40–80% of cases. A subset of psoriatic patients appears to be "stress reactors" and these patients may have a better long-term prognosis. Identifying such patients early in treatment and incorporating specific psychosocial interventions into their overall treatment regimen may improve the course of the disease. Psoriasis has also been associated with suicide and a higher prevalence of alcoholism. Disturbances in body image perception and the effect of psoriasis on interpersonal, social, and occupational functioning may further contribute to overall morbidity, especially if psoriasis first occurs during a critical developmental period such as adolescence.

Multiple comorbidities such as diabetes mellitus, atherosclerotic disease, metabolic syndrome, and symptoms such as anxiety as well as smoking are often associated with psoriasis [10]. Feelings of embarrassment and low self-esteem are common in patients with psoriasis and contribute to their avoiding starting a family or having children because of the possibility of passing on the disease [11]. In addition, numerous studies suggest that depression plays a significant role in increasing morbidity among patients [12]. What's more, the physical, social, and psychological impact of psoriasis may contribute to sexual dysfunction. Indeed, many women report some degree of difficulty in their sex lives, which ultimately results in intense personal distress and decreased quality of life [13].

Of the 102 British women with psoriasis evaluated using the Female Sexual Function Index (FSFI), sexual dysfunction was found in 48.7% [14]. All domains of the FSFI, with the exception of lubrication and pain, appear to be significantly affected in patients with psoriasis [15]; however, of all domains, sexual desire may be the most affected [16]. Which part of the body affected by psoriasis may play an important role in the development of sexual dysfunction: skin lesions in the genital areas, thighs, abdomen, and back are significantly associated with sexual dysfunction [17]. The prevalence of genital lesions at any time during the course of psoriasis, noted by physicians during examination or reported by patients ranged from 33% to 63%. Baseline data from two randomized controlled trials showed a prevalence of psoriatic lesions in the genital area of 35% and 42% [18].

Genital Psoriasis 35–42%

In male patients with psoriasis, approximately 60% report erectile dysfunction (using the International Index of Erectile Dysfunction questionnaire) [19]. Risk factors for erectile dysfunction tend to be confused with other conditions observed in psoriasis patients such as dyslipidemia, hypertension, diabetes, obesity, metabolic syndrome, and depression, as well as with the effects of a very sedentary lifestyle [20].

Finally, there is a bidirectional relationship between psoriasis and periodontitis, in which systemic inflammation produced by psoriasis can increase the severity of periodontitis, and this outbreak of infection serves as a trigger for psoriasis [21]. Furthermore, periodontal disease causes infection of the vascular endothelium, a local increase in white blood cells, tissue growth factors, and endotoxins, promoting atherosclerosis and erectile dysfunction [20].

Conclusion

Psoriasis appears to be a stigmatizing disease that impairs quality of life and damages self-esteem through its effects on social relationships and self-esteem, negatively impacting physical, mental, and sexual health. Patients with psoriasis, both male and female, are known to be at increased risk for impaired sexual function.

The form of male psoriasis that most commonly affects the genital area is psoriasis inverse. However, even in other cases, genital lesions should be treated promptly, even when they initially appear in a very mild form. Generally, the appearance first occurs at the level of the inguinal folds and then spreads to the genitals in the form of reddish patches that tend to be more prominent after sexual intercourse.

In males, these lesions can affect the glans and the balanopreputial groove, which is the area between the glans and the shaft normally covered by the foreskin of uncircumcised males. Here, small, reddened, sometimes shiny patches may occur, causing severe itching: this prompts affected individuals to scratch, with the risk of small cuts forming.

Many people, even in good faith, may initially fear that the lesions are related to sexually transmitted infections. In the course of a stable relationship, it is also important to make it clear that the condition itself does not interfere with sexual life: this is the only way to regain confidence in oneself and one's partner, overcoming inhibitions that, if not addressed immediately, could undermine the couple's serenity.

Psychosexual counseling, coupled with the dermatologist's diagnostic and therapeutic process, could become an element in the greater understanding of the sexual response mechanisms of both the patient and the partner, tracing psychological and relational components of the individual and the couple that may negatively affect the therapeutic success or improve compliance.Conflict of InterestsNone to declare.

References

1. Kelly-Sell M, Gudjonsson JE. Overview of psoriasis. In: Wu JJ, Feldman SR, Lebwohl MG, editors. Therapy for severe psoriasis. Philadelphia: Elsevier; 2017.
2. Feldman SR, Krueger GG. Psoriasis assessment tools in clinical trials. Ann Rheum Dis. 2005;64(Suppl 2):ii65–73.
3. Kutzner H, Hantschke M, WHC B, Kempf W. Dermatopathology. Dresden: Steinkopff Darmstadt; 2008.
4. Rademaker M, Agnew K, Anagnostou N, Andrews M, Armour K, Baker C, Foley P, Gebauer K, Gupta M, Marshman G, Rubel D, Sullivan J, Wong LC. Psoriasis and infection. A clinical practice narrative. Australas J Dermatol. 2019;60:91–8.
5. James W, Berger T, Elston D. Andrews' diseases of the skin. 11th ed. Amsterdam: Elsevier; 2011.
6. Salem MM, Nassar AA, Ibrahim AM. The effect of psoriasis on female sexual function. Egypt J Hosp Med. 2021;84:1686–9.
7. Maunder R, Hunter J. Attachment relationships as determinants of physical health. J Am Acad Psychoanal Dyn Psychiatry. 2008;36(1):11–32.
8. Maunder RG, Hunter J. An integrated approach to the formulation and psychotherapy of medically unexplained symptoms: meaning- and attachment-based intervention. Am J Psychother. 2004;58:17–33.
9. Gupta MA, Gupta AK, Haberman HF. Psoriasis and psychiatry: an update. Gen Hosp Psychiatry. 1987;9(3):157–66.
10. Lowes MA, Bowcock AM, Krueger JG. Pathogenesis and therapy of psoriasis. Nature. 2007;445(7130):866–73.
11. Kdes S, Eatda S. Psoríase and its relação with psychological aspects, stress and life events. Psychol Stud. 2007;24(2):257–66.

12. Mesquita PMA. Psoríase: physiopathology and Therapêutica [dissertação]. Porto: Universidade Fernando Pessoa; 2013. p. 31.
13. Kurizky PS, Mota LM. Sexual dysfunction in patients with psoriasis and psoriatic arthritis: a systematic review. Rev Bras Rheumatol. 2012;52(6):943–8.
14. Meeuwis KA, de Hullu JA, van de Nieuwenhof HP, et al. Qualità della vita e salute sessuale nei pazienti con psoriasi genitale. Br J Dermatol. 2011;164.
15. Türel Ermertcan A, Temeltaş G, Deveci A, Dinç G, Güler HB, Oztürk-can S. Sexual dysfunction in patients with psoriasis. J Dermatol. 2006;33(11):772.
16. Kurizky PS. Warning for sexual disorders in patients with psoriasis and psoriatic arthritis: in this case, control of 150 mulheres brasileiras. Tese (mestrado em Ciências Médicas) - Faculdade de Medicine, Universidade de Brasília; Brasilia; 2013.
17. Meeuwis KAP, Potts Bleakman A, van de Kerkhof PCM, et al. Prevalence of genital psoriasis in patients with psoriasis. Dermatolog Treat J. 2018;29:1–7.
18. Sarbu MI, Tampa M, Sarbu AE, Georgescu SR. Sexual dysfunction in psoriatic patients. J Mind Med Sci. 2014;1:1.
19. Goulding JM, Price CL, Defty CL, Hulangamuwa CS, Bader E, Ahmed I. Erectile dysfunction in patients with psoriasis: higher prevalence, unmet need and the possibility of intervention. Br J Dermatol. 2011;164(1):103–9.
20. Mehta NN, Azfar RS, Shin DB, et al. Patients with severe psoriasis are at increased risk of cardiovascular mortality: cohort study using the general practice research database. Eur Heart J. 2010;31(8):1000–6.
21. Gelfand JM, Neimann AL, Shin DB, et al. Risk of myocardial infarction in patients with psoriasis. JAMA. 2006;296(14):1735–41.

Part VI
Diabetology

Type 1 and Type 2 Diabetes Mellitus

Marco Comoglio, Luca Monge, and Elena Vittoria Longhi

Epidemiology of Diabetes

Diabetes is now a rapidly growing global health problem. The number of people with diabetes has risen from 180 million in 1980 to 422 million in 2014. The global prevalence of diabetes among the adult population over 18 has increased from 4.7% in 1980 to 8.5% in 2014 [1, 2].

The International Diabetes Federation (IDF) in the ninth edition of the Diabetes Atlas of 2019, a publication that occurs every 2 years, estimated that in 2019 in the world 463 million people between the ages of 20 and 79 would be affected by diabetes, equal to 9.3% of the population in this age range, and this number should reach 578 million in 2030 and 700 million in 2045, and one million and one hundred thousand children under 20 will be affected by diabetes. Data are updated every 2 years (Fig. 1). Two-thirds of people with diabetes live in urban areas, and three of four are of working age. Global annual spending on diabetes treatment is $ 760 billion and will reach $ 845 billion by 2045. In 2019, four million people aged 20 to 79 years died from diabetes-related causes and the number of children and adolescents with diabetes is increasing every year. It is estimated that 136 million people over the age of 65 have diabetes and the prevalence in this age group varies widely in different regions of the world.

Gestational diabetes mellitus (GDM) is diagnosed in one of six pregnancies.

M. Comoglio (⊠)
Medical Diabetes Association, AMD Comunicazione, Turin, Italy

L. Monge
SCU Endocrinology, Diabetology and Metabolism, AOU City of Health and Science,
Turin, Italy
e-mail: amd-to.monge@alma.it

E. V. Longhi
Department of Sexual Medical Center, San Raffaele Hospital, Milano, Italy

© Springer Nature Switzerland AG 2023

117

E. V. Longhi (ed.), *Managing Psychosexual Consequences in Chronic Diseases*,
https://doi.org/10.1007/978-3-031-31307-3_11

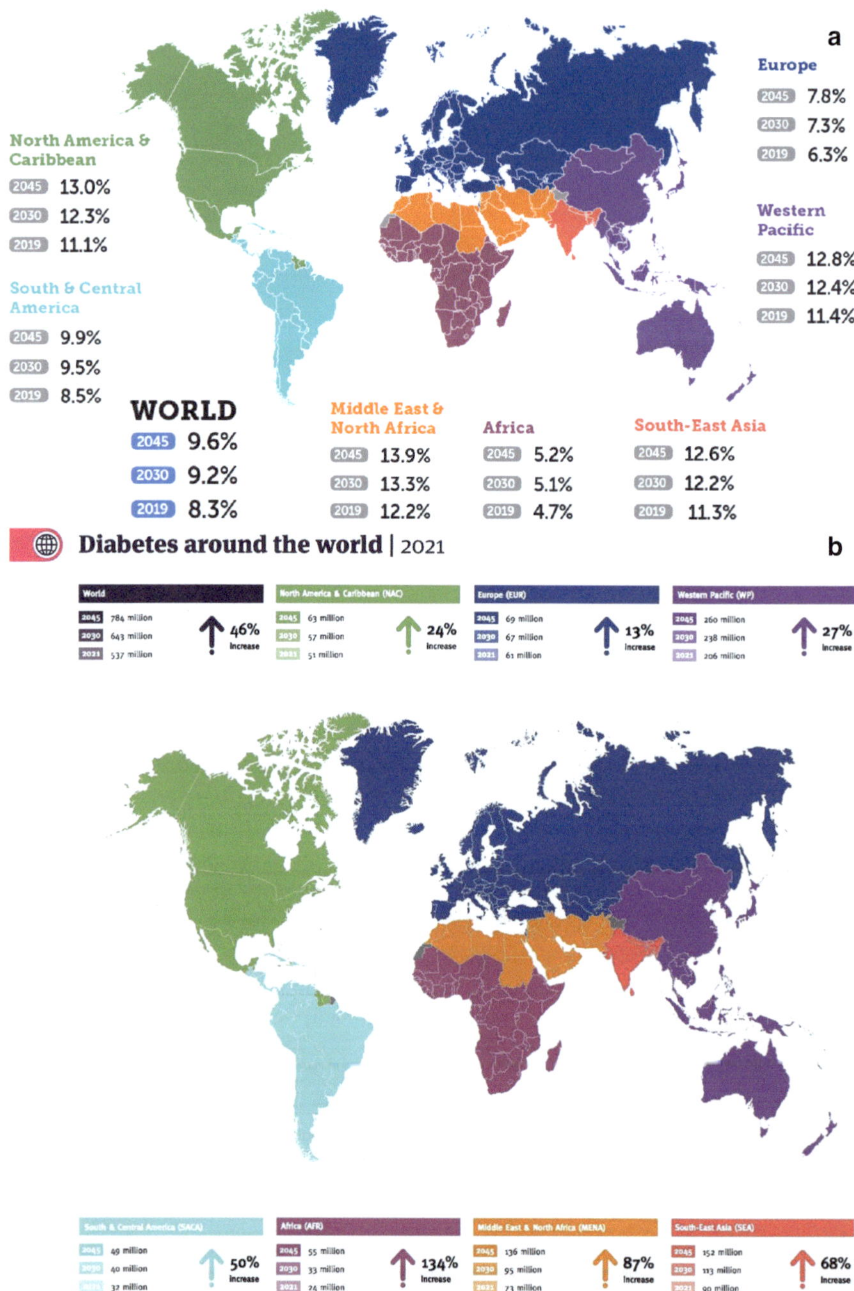

Fig. 1 Prevalence of diabetes in adults (20–79 years) in IDF regions, by age-adjusted comparative diabetes prevalence. (**a**) 2019. (Modified from International Diabetes Federation. *Diabetes Atlas.* ninth Edition 2019. https://www.diabetesatlas.org/en/.) (**b**) *2021, 966 billion* dollars in health expenditure—a 316% increase over the last 15 years. (Modified from International Diabetes Federation *Diabetes Atlas.* tenth Edition 2021. https://www.diabetesatlas.org/en/)

Another problem identified by the IDF Atlas is the high number of people with undiagnosed diabetes, mainly type 2 diabetes (T2D), with the consequent need to diagnose people with the disease as quickly as possible in order to start treatment as soon as possible.

The IDF still defines the diabetes situation in the seven different regions of the world: Africa, Europe; Middle East and North Africa; North America and Caribbean; South and Central America; South-East Asia; and Western Pacific (Fig. 1). Diabetes in the African region is expected to increase by 48% by 2030 and by 143% by 2045, the highest increase expected among all IDF regions. The European region has the largest number of children and adolescents (0–19 years) with type 1 diabetes (T1D)—296,500 in total. The Middle East and the North African region have the highest age-adjusted diabetes prevalence of all IDF regions—nearly 12%. Forty-three percent of global diabetes-related spending occurs in North America and the Caribbean region. In the Central and South American region, 44% of diabetes-related deaths occur in people under the age of 60. In the Southeast Asian region, 57% of adults aged 20 to 79 with diabetes are undiagnosed. The largest number of diabetes-related deaths in 2019 occurred in the Western Pacific region—well over one million [3].

Finally, as regards Italy, the Istituto Nazionale di Statistica website reports that in 2016 there were over three million 200 thousand people in Italy who declared to be affected by diabetes, 5.3% of the entire population (16.5% among people aged 65 and over) [4].

A healthy diet, regular physical activity, maintaining a correct body weight, and quitting smoking can prevent or delay the onset of diabetes. Diabetes can be treated, and its consequences are avoided or delayed with diet, physical activity, therapy, and regular screening and treatment for complications.

Classification of Diabetes

Diabetes mellitus is actually classified into the following general categories:

1. T1D: It is due to autoimmune β-cell destruction, usually leading to absolute insulin deficiency. It can develop at any age, but usually occurs in children and adolescents. The subtype latent autoimmune diabetes in adults (LADA) evolves slowly and manifests itself in the adult.
2. T2D: It is due to a progressive loss of adequate β-cell insulin secretion, which typically progresses over time but never leads to absolute insulin deficiency, frequently on the background of insulin resistance on a multifactorial basis. It is often presents a reduced incretin effect. It is more common in adults and accounts for about 90% of all diabetes cases.
3. GDM: It is diagnosed in the second or third trimester of pregnancy that is not clearly overt diabetes prior to gestation. It is caused by defects similar to those of T2D; is associated with complications to both mother and child; and usually regresses after childbirth but increases the risk of T2D later in life.

4. Specific types of diabetes occur due to other causes, e.g., monogenic diabetes syndromes (such as neonatal diabetes and maturity-onset diabetes of the young, MODY), diseases of the exocrine pancreas (such as cystic fibrosis and pancreatitis), endocrinopathies (such as Cushing's disease and acromegaly), and drug- or chemical-induced diabetes (such as with glucocorticoid use, in the treatment of HIV/AIDS, or after organ transplantation) [5–7].

Criteria Defining Diabetes

- Fasting[1] plasma glucose (FPG) $\geq$126 mg/dL ($\geq$7 mmol/L).
- *or*
- 2-h plasma glucose (PG) $\geq$200 mg/dL (11.1 mmol/L) during 75-g oral glucose tolerance test.[2]
- *or*
- HbA_{1C}[3] $\geq$6.5% (48 mmol/mol).
- *or*
- In a patient with classical symptoms of hyperglycemia or hyperglycemic crisis, a random PG >200 mg/dL (11.1 mmol/L).

In the absence of unequivocal hyperglycemia, diagnosis requires two abnormal test results (PG and HbA_{1C}) from the same sample or in two separate test samples [7].

Dysglycemic State

Dysglycemia—or intermediate hyperglycemia [6] or prediabetes [7]—is the term used for individuals whose PG levels do not meet the criteria for diabetes but are too high to be considered normal. Dysglycemia should not be viewed as a clinical entity in its own right but rather as an increased risk for diabetes and cardiovascular (CV) disease. Dysglycemia is often associated with overweight/obesity, atherogenic dyslipidemia, and hypertension [6, 7].

---

[1] Fasting for at least 8 h.

[2] Glucose load of 75 g glucose.

[3] Glycated hemoglobin.

Table 1 Clinical differential characteristics between T1D and T2D

	T1D	T2D
Population prevalence[a]	About 0.3%	About 5%
Symptomatology	Usually present, often impressive, and abrupt onset	Often moderate or absent
Propensity to ketosis	Present	Absent
Weight	Generally normal	Generally overweight
Age at onset	Most commonly <30 years	Most commonly >40 years
Appearance of chronic complications	Not earlier than a few years after diagnosis	Often present at diagnosis
Circulating insulin	Reduced or absent	Normal or increased
Autoimmunity	Positive	Negative
Therapy	Insulin often at onset, diet, SGLT2 inhibitors	Diet, physical activity, oral hypoglycemic agents, GLP-1 receptor agonists, insulin

T1D type 1 diabetes, *T2D* type 2 diabetes
Modified from Associazione Medici Diabeteologi, Società Italiana di Diabetologia. *Standard italiani per la cura del diabete mellito 2019*. http://aemmedi.it/wp-content/uploads/2009/06/AMD-Standard-unico1.pdf
[a]In Italy

Criteria Defining Dysglycemia

- Impaired Fasting Glucose (IFG): FPG 100 mg/dL (5.6 mmol/L) to 125 mg/dL (6.9 mmol/L).

- *or*
- Impaired Glucose Tolerance (IGT): 2-h PG during 75-g OGTT 140 mg/dL (7.8 mmol/L) to 199 mg/dL.
- *or*
- HbA_{1C} 5.7–6.4% (39–47 mmol/mol) [7].

In Table 1, we present the main clinical differential characteristics between the two main forms of diabetes mellitus: T1D and T2D [5].

Acute Complications

Hyperglycemic Complications

- **Diabetic Ketoacidosis (DKA):** It occurs with high blood glucose levels with an accumulation of ketone bodies in the blood, sometimes at onset in T1D if not recognized, and can also occur, with some drugs, in T2D and other forms of diabetes. It can be life-threatening if not treated properly according to coded fluid, electrolyte, and insulin protocols [8]. With adequate therapy, the results are

generally satisfactory. There is also recent evidence that DKA can cause adverse neurocognitive outcomes in the medium term [8, 9].
- **Hyperosmolar Hyperglycemic State (HHS):** It is a metabolic complication of diabetes mellitus characterized by severe hyperglycemia, extreme dehydration, high plasmatic osmolarity without significant ketoacidosis, and often altered consciousness. It most frequently occurs in T2D.

Hypoglycemia

It is common in T1D and also in T2D when using insulin or sulfonylureas. It is divided into mild when the intake of fast-acting carbohydrates such as sugary drink, glucose tablets, or sweets is sufficient to resolve it and severe when the person with diabetes needs external assistance. Prompt treatment with glucagon or dextrose is required intravenously, and if not treated properly, it can quickly lead to convulsions, coma, and death. It occurs due to an imbalance between hypoglycemic drugs, food intake, and exercise [10]. Severe hypoglycemia is a common but life-threatening complication associated in T2D with increased CV disease [11] and in older T1D with poorer cognition [12].

Complications of Pregnancy

Women with any type of diabetes during pregnancy have a risk of complications if they do not monitor and manage their blood glucose levels carefully. To prevent possible fetal organ damage, women with T1D or T2D should reach glucose levels close to normal before conception. All women with T1D, T2D, or GDM during pregnancy should try to achieve optimal glucose levels all the time to minimize complications. High blood sugar during pregnancy can cause the fetus to gain weight due to hyperinsulinemia induced by maternal hyperglycemia. This can lead to problems in childbirth, trauma to the baby and the mother, and may cause significant hypoglycemia to the baby after birth. Babies who are exposed for a long time to high blood glucose levels in the womb are at increased risk of developing diabetes in the future [13].

Chronic Complications

Diabetes can lead to serious complications with damage to the heart, blood vessels, eyes, kidneys, nerves, and teeth. We can divide the complications into micro- and macrovascular, the former induced by hyperglycemia, which causes damage to the small vessels, and the latter linked to atherosclerotic damage to the large vessels. In DT2, they are sometimes already present at onset due to the long asymptomatic period of the disease already present.

Cardiovascular Disease

Atherosclerotic cardiovascular disease (ASCVD), defined as coronary artery disease (CHD), cerebrovascular disease, or peripheral arterial disease presumed to be of atherosclerotic origin, is the leading cause of morbidity and mortality for individuals with diabetes and translates into an estimated $ 37.3 billion in annual expenditure related to the CV system associated with diabetes [14]. Common conditions that coexist with T2D (e.g., hypertension and dyslipidemia) are clear risk factors for ASCVD, and diabetes itself confers independent risk. Numerous studies have shown the effectiveness of controlling individual CV risk factors in preventing or slowing ASCVD in people with diabetes. Furthermore, great benefits are achieved when multiple CV risk factors are addressed simultaneously. In the current paradigm of aggressive risk factor modification in patients with diabetes, there is evidence that measures of 10-year CHD risk among adults with diabetes have improved significantly over the past decade [15] and that mortality decreased [16, 17]. Heart failure (HF) is another major cause of CV disease morbidity and mortality. Recent studies found that hospitalization rates for incident HF (adjusted for age and sex) were twice higher in patients with diabetes than in those without [18, 19]. People with diabetes may have HF with preserved ejection fraction or with reduced ejection fraction (HFrEF). Hypertension is often a precursor to HF of both types, and ASCVD can coexist with both types [20], while a previous myocardial infarction is often a major factor in HFrEF.

Kidney Disease (Diabetic Nephropathy)

It occurs in 20–40% of patients with diabetes. Microalbuminuria is considered the earliest stage of diabetic nephropathy in T1D and a marker for the development of nephropathy in T2D. The increased urinary albumin excretion, already in the high-normal range, is also a risk marker of CV disease in diabetes and in the general population [21]. Patients with impaired urinary albumin excretion who progress to macroalbuminuria ($\geq$300 mg/24 h) have a high probability of developing end-stage chronic renal failure over the years [22, 23]. However, several therapeutic interventions have been shown to be effective in reducing the risk and slowing the progression of kidney disease.

Eye Disease (Diabetic Retinopathy)

It is the most important ocular complication of diabetes and is the main cause of legal blindness among people of working age in industrialized countries. Symptoms related to it often appear late, when the lesions are already advanced, and this often limits the effectiveness of the treatment. Diabetic retinopathy (RD) progresses from microvascular lesions (microaneurysms) to forms of neovascular proliferation and macular edema (most important cause of blindness) induced by retinal ischemia. Today, the prevalence of RD is clearly decreasing thanks to improved glycemic control and closer eye monitoring of patients and the new techniques of diagnosis and therapy (optical coherence tomography, fundus camera, and new laser).

Nerve Disease (Diabetic Polyneuropathy)

Is a heterogeneous disease with different clinical forms. Diabetic polyneuropathy (DPN) has recently been redefined as a length-dependent symmetric motor-sensory polyneuropathy in patients with diabetes, attributable to metabolic and microvascular alterations resulting from exposure to chronic hyperglycemia and to cofactors CV risk. DPN is a common complication with a prevalence of 50% in adult diabetics with a range of disease of 10–20 years [24]. Among the areas most affected are the lower limbs, especially the feet. Damage to the nerves in these areas is called peripheral neuropathy and can lead to pain, tingling, and loss of sensation. Loss of sensation is especially important because it can allow injuries to go unnoticed, leading to serious infections and possible amputations. Another aspect of DNP is erectile dysfunction (ED). Diabetes is one of the organic conditions most involved in the pathogenesis of ED. The prevalence of ED in the diabetic population varies from 35 to 90% and is closely linked to the duration of the disease and the presence of micro- and macrovascular complications. Furthermore, ED in the diabetic population appears on average earlier than in the nondiabetic population (10–15 years earlier) and is associated with a reduced quality of life and the presence of depressive symptoms. ED has a predictive value for CV event equal to or greater than other traditional risk factors such as family history of ischemic heart disease, cigarette smoking, or dyslipidemia.

Diabetic Foot

It is defined as infection, wound, or destruction of tissue of the foot associated with neurological abnormalities and/or various degrees of peripheral artery disease in the lower limb. Loss of sensation due to neuropathy is especially important because it can allow injuries to go unnoticed. Diabetic foot is a major public health issue, which may lead to leg amputation, thus resulting in severe disability, reduced quality of life, and high health costs. People with diabetes carry a risk of amputation that can be 25 times greater than that of people without diabetes [3]; however, with careful management by a multidisciplinary foot care team, a large percentage of diabetes-related amputations can be prevented [25].

Oral Complications

People with diabetes have an increased risk of inflammation of the gums (periodontitis) if their blood sugar is not properly managed. Periodontitis is a leading cause of tooth loss and is associated with an increased risk of CV disease. Regular oral checkups should be established to ensure early diagnosis, particularly among people with previously undiagnosed diabetes and prompt management of any oral complications in people with diabetes.

Therapy

T1D, Insulin Therapy

Because the hallmark of T1D is absence or near-absence of β-cell function, in these patients insulin treatment is essential. In addition to hyperglycemia, insulinopenia can contribute to other metabolic disturbances like hypertriglyceridemia and ketoacidosis and tissue catabolism that can be life-threatening. In the past three decades, evidence has accumulated supporting more intensive insulin replacement, using multiple daily insulin injections or continuous subcutaneous insulin infusion (CSII) through a pump, as providing the best combination of effectiveness and safety for people with T1D. The Diabetes Control and Complications Trial demonstrated that intensive therapy reduced HbA_{1C} and was associated with improved long-term outcomes [26–28].

Over the last 25 years, rapid-acting and long-acting insulin analogs have been developed that have distinct pharmacokinetics compared with recombinant human insulins: Basal insulin analogs have a longer duration of action with flat, constant plasma concentrations, and activity profiles. In people with T1D, treatment with analog insulins is associated with reduced hypoglycemia and weight gain and lower HbA_{1C}. More recently, two new injectable insulin formulations with enhanced rapid action profiles have been introduced: faster-acting insulin aspart and insulin lispro-aabc may reduce prandial excursions. In addition, new longer-acting basal analogs (U-300 glargine and degludec) may confer a lower hypoglycemia risk compared with glargine U-100 [29, 30]. Despite the advantages of insulin analogs in patients with T1D, for some patients the burden of treatment required for their use is very heavy. There are multiple approaches to insulin treatment, and the central precept in the management of T1D is that some form of insulin is given in a planned regimen tailored to the individual patient to keep them safe and out of diabetic ketoacidosis and to avoid significant hypoglycemia, with every effort made to reach the patient's glycemic targets.

T2D Therapy

T2D therapy, unlike what is written for T1D, which has insulin as its only therapy, has been enriched in recent years by a large number of new drugs belonging to different classes that affect the various etiopathogenetic moments of T2D.

Secretagogues

Sulfonylureas and glinides

Insulin Sensitizers

Metformin; thiazolidinediones

Agents on the Incretin Axis.

Dipeptidyl peptidase-4 (DDP-4) inhibitors; glucagon-like peptide-1 receptor agonists (GLP-1 RAs)

Agents on the Renal Reabsorption of Glucose

Sodium-glucose cotransporter-2 (SGLT-2) inhibitors

Agents on the Intestinal Absorption of Glucose

Acarbose

Insulins

The guidelines of all scientific societies recommend a personalized patient-centered approach to choose the most appropriate pharmacological treatment aimed at obtaining the best possible glycemic control taking into account possible side effects and the patient's overall clinical picture.

It will be necessary to consider the presence of important comorbidities such as ASCVD and high-risk indicators of ASCVD, HF and chronic kidney disease (CKD), risk of hypoglycemia, effects on body weight, side effects, cost, and patient preferences.

Not least are lifestyle changes that help improve glycemic control and quality of life.

Initial Therapy

Metformin should be started at the time of T2D diagnosis unless there are contraindications; for many patients, this will be monotherapy in combination with lifestyle modifications. Metformin is effective and safe, is inexpensive, and is available in an immediate-release form or in an extended release form. As a first-line therapy, it has beneficial effects on HbA_{1C}, weight, and CV mortality [31]. The main side effects of metformin are gastrointestinal intolerance due to bloating, abdominal discomfort, and diarrhea; these can be mitigated by gradual dose titration. The drug is eliminated by renal filtration, and very high circulating levels (e.g., following overdose or acute renal failure) have been associated with lactic acidosis. Metformin can be used safely in patients with reduced glomerular filtration rate (eGFR); the U.S. Food and Drug Administration has confirmed its safety at appropriate doses up to an eGFR $\geq$30 mL/min/1.73m^2 [32]. In patients with contraindications or intolerance to metformin, initial therapy should be based on the patient's characteristics; a drug of another class must be considered.

Combination Therapy

Because T2D is a progressive disease in many patients, maintenance of glycemic goals with monotherapy is often only possible for a few years, after which combination therapy is required. Current recommendations advise us to gradually add medications to metformin to maintain HbA_{1C} at target. However, there are data to support initial combination therapy for faster achievement of glycemic goals [33, 34]. There are data to suggest that more intensive early treatment has some benefits and should be considered through shared decision-making with patients, as appropriate. The choice of drug added to metformin is based on the patient's clinical characteristics and their preferences. If the HbA_{1C} goal is not achieved after approximately 3 months, metformin can be combined with any of the possible treatment options available: SGLT-2 inhibitors, GLP-1 RAs, DPP-4 inhibitors, thiazolidinediones, sulfonylureas, or basal insulins; the choice of the agent to add is based on the specific effects of the drug and the patient's factors (Table 2). For patients with established ASCVD or high-risk indicators of ASCVD, HF, or CKD, an SGLT-2 inhibitor and/or GLP-1 RA that has demonstrated benefit on the CV system is recommended, independent of HbA_{1C} [35]. For patients without ASCVD, drug choice is based on efficacy, prevention of side effects (particularly hypoglycemia and weight gain), cost, and patient preference [36]. Similar considerations apply in patients who require a third agent to achieve glycemic goals.

Finally, the addition of basal insulin in addition to oral therapy is an established and effective approach for many patients. Insulin has the advantage of being effective where other agents are not and should be considered as part of any combination regimen when hyperglycemia is severe, especially if symptoms of hyperglycemia (i.e., polyuria or polydipsia) and/or catabolic features (weight loss, hypertriglyceridemia, and ketosis) are present.

Table 2 Drug-specific and patient factors to consider when selecting antihyperglycemic treatment in adults with T2D

	Efficacy	Hypoglycemia	Weight change	CV effects		Cost	Oral/SQ	Renal effects		Additional consideration
				ASCVD	HF			Progression of DKD	Dosing/use considerations[a]	
Metformin	High	No	Neutral (potential for modest loss)	Potential benefit	Neutral	Low	Oral	Neutral	• Contraindicates with eGFR <30 mL/min/1.73 m^2	• Gastrointestinal side effects common (diarrhea, nausea) • Potential for B12 deficiency
SGLT-2i	Intermediate	No	Loss	Benefit: Empagliflozin[b] Canagliflozin[b]	Benefit: Empagliflozin[b] Canagliflozin Dapagliflozin[c]	High	Oral	Benefit: Canagliflozin[d] Empagliflozin Dapagliflozin	• Renal dose adjustment required (canagliflozin, dapagliflozin Empagliflozin, ertugliflozin)	• Should be discontinued before any scheduled surgery to avoid potential risk for DKA • DKA risk (all agents, rare in T2D) • Risk for bone fractures (canagliflozin) • Genitourinary infections • Risk of volume depletion, hypotension • LDL cholesterol • Risk of Fournier's gangrene

| GLP-1 RAs | High | No | Loss | Benefit: dulaglutide[b] liraglutide[b] Semaglutide (SQ)[b] Neutral: Exenatide once weekly lixisenatide | Neutral | High | SQ; oral (semaglutide) | Benefit on renal end points in CVOTs, driven by albuminuria outcomes: Liraglutide, semaglutide, dulaglutide | • Exenatide, lixisenatide: Avoid for eGFR <30 mL/min/1.73 m^2 • No dose adjustment for dulaglutide, liraglutide, semaglutide • Caution when initiating or increasing dose due to potential risk of nausea, vomiting, diarrhea, or dehydration. Monitor renal function in patients reporting severe adverse gastrointestinal reactions when initiating or increasing dose of therapy | • *FDA black box*: Risk of thyroid C-cell tumors in rodents; human relevance not determined (*liraglutide, dulaglutide, exenatide extended release, semaglutide*) • Gastrointestinal side effects common (nausea, vomiting, diarrhea) • Injection site reactions • Pancreatitis has been reported in clinical trials but causality has not been established. Discontinue if pancreatitis is suspected |

(continued)

Table 2 (continued)

	Efficacy	Hypoglycemia	Weight change	CV effects		Cost	Oral/SQ	Renal effects		Additional consideration
				ASCVD	HF			Progression of DKD	Dosing/use considerations[a]	
DPP-4i	Intermediate	No	Neutral	Neutral	Potential risk: Saxagliptin	High	Oral	Neutral	• Renal dose adjustment required (sitagliptin, saxagliptin, alogliptin); can be used in renal impairment • No dose adjustment required for linagliptin	• Pancreatitis has been reported in clinical trials but causality has not been established. Discontinue if pancreatitis is suspected • Joint pain
Thiazolidinediones	High	No	Gain	Potential benefit: Pioglitazone	Increased risk	High	Oral	Neutral	• No dose adjustment required • Generally, not recommended in renal impairment due to potential for fluid retention	• *FDA black box*: Congestive heart failure (*pioglitazone, rosiglitazone*) • Fluid retention (edema, heart failure) • Benefit in NASH • Risk of bone fracture • Bladder cancer (pioglitazone) • 〈 LDL cholesterol (rosiglitazone)

Sulfonylureas (second generation)		High	Yes	Gain	Neutral	Neutral	Low	Oral	Neutral	• Glyburide: Generally, not recommended in chronic kidney disease • Glipizide and glimepiride: Initiate conservatively to avoid hypoglycemia	• *FDA special warning* on increased risk of cardiovascular mortality based on studies of an older sulfonylurea (tolbutamide)
Insulin	Human	High	Yes	Gain	Neutral	Neutral	Low (SQ)	SQ; inhaled	Neutral	• Lower insulin doses required with a decrease in eGFR; titrate per clinical response	• Injection site reactions • Higher risk of hypoglycemia with human insulin (NPH or premixed formulations) vs analogs
	Analogs						High	SQ			

ASCVD atherosclerotic cardiovascular disease, *CV* cardiovascular, *CVOT* cardiovascular outcomes trial, *DPP-4i* dipeptidyl peptidase-4 inhibitors, *DKA* diabetic ketoacidosis, *DKD* diabetic kidney disease, *eGFR* estimated glomerular filtration rate, *GI* gastrointestinal, *GLP-1 RAs* glucagon-like peptide 1 receptor agonists, *HF* heart failure, *NASH* nonalcoholic steatohepatitis, *SGLT2i* sodium–glucose cotransporter 2 inhibitors, *SQ* subcutaneous, *T2D* type 2 diabetes

Modified from American Diabetes Association. *Standard of medical care in diabetes* 2021. https://care.diabetesjournals.org/content/44/Supplement_1

[a]For agent-specific dosing recommendations, please refer to the manufacturers' prescribing information

[b]FDA-approved for cardiovascular disease benefit

[c]FDA-approved for heart failure indication

[d]FDA-approved for chronic kidney disease indication

Diabetes Technology

It is the term used to describe the hardware, devices, and software that people with diabetes use to manage their conditions, from lifestyle to blood glucose levels. Historically, diabetes technology has been divided into two main categories: insulin delivery devices (syringe, pen, or pump) and blood glucose monitoring as assessed by the meter or continuous glucose monitoring. More recently, diabetes technology has expanded to include hybrid devices that monitor glucose and deliver insulin, some automatically. Major clinical trials in insulin-treated patients have included self-monitoring of blood glucose (SMBG) as part of multifactorial interventions to demonstrate the benefit of intensive glycemic control on diabetes complications [37]. SMBG is therefore an integral component of effective therapy for patients taking insulin. In recent years, flash monitoring and continuous glucose monitoring (CGM) has emerged as a method for assessing glucose levels [38]. Glucose monitoring allows patients to assess their individual response to therapy and assess whether glycemic goals are safely achieved. Integrating the findings into diabetes management can be a useful tool to guide medical nutrition therapy and physical activity, prevent hypoglycemia, or adjust medications (particularly mealtime insulin doses). The patient's specific needs and objectives should guide the use of the SMBG or CGM.

Sexuality and Quality of Life

Sexual lifestyles, encompassing sexual activity, problems, satisfaction, and relationship formation and maintenance, are strongly influenced by physical health. Data on the sexual lifestyles of adolescents and young adults with type 1 diabetes mellitus (DM1) are limited. Fear of hypoglycemic episodes during intercourse and intimacy problems may have a conditioning impact on people living with T1DM.

A study by Pinhas-Hamiel et al. [39] assessed the sexual lifestyles of individuals with T1DM.

Fifty-three patients with T1DM were recruited, 27 (51%) males, with mean age ± SD 27.9 ± 8.3 years completed the Hypoglycemia Fear Survey II and Sex Practices and Concerns questionnaire.

Results Thirty-seven patients (70%) reported never or almost never having diabetes-related concerns about their sexual lifestyle. None experienced severe hypoglycemia during intercourse, but 21 (40%) reported occasional mild hypoglycemic events. More than two-thirds took no measures to prevent hypoglycemia before intercourse (decreasing insulin dose, snacking, and measuring blood glucose levels). Fear of hypoglycemia during sex was reported by 18 (35%); those who reported greater fear experienced mild hypoglycemic events during sex (61.1% vs 26.5%, $P = 0.01$), were single (94.4% vs 64.7%, $P = 0.02$), and had higher scores on the subscale.

Thus, we could say that among young people with T1DM, most do not have diabetes-related concerns about sex, and most do not take specific measures before or after sex. One-third, however, fear hypoglycemia during sex, mostly singles, and those who have suffered from hypoglycemia in the past. Caregivers should be aware of and address these concerns.

Comparing the literature, the study by Gjerløw and Bjørgaas et al. [40] investigated specific fears related to hypoglycemia in adults with type 1 diabetes and which aspects of fear of hypoglycemia may differ between the sexes.

Six hundred and thirty-six patients with type 1 diabetes, aged 18 to 75 years, and who had attended the outpatient clinic at St. Olavs Hospital, Trondheim, Norway, were recruited. Fears related to hypoglycemia were assessed using the Hypoglycemia Fear Survey II Worry (HFS-II-Worry) subscale. The response rate was 70% ($N = 445$, 216 women and 229 men). The mean HFS-II-Worry score was higher in women than in men (2.46 [SD = 0.80] vs. 2.22 [SD = 0.74], respectively; $p < 0.001$). Women scored higher than men in all items on the HFS-II-Worry, and women's mean scores were statistically significantly higher in 5 of 18 items after adjusting for multiple comparisons. The largest gender differences in mean scores occurred in the items "low blood sugar interfering with important things," "becoming upset and difficult," "difficulty thinking clearly," and "feeling lightheaded or dizzy." In both women and men, the highest mean scores appeared in the worry items "becoming hypoglycemic during sleep." From this, feelings of low self-esteem, inadequacy, and fear of "not controlling" changes in the condition also emerged.

What influence can caregivers have on patients with type 1 diabetes? [41] The study by Haugstvedt et al. did in fact address parents' fear of hypoglycemia, as this can influence treatment management and blood glucose regulation in children. The availability of appropriate instruments to assess parents' fear of hypoglycemia is thus critical. The psychometric properties of the Hypoglycemia Fear Survey-Parent Version (HFS-P) were evaluated.

176 parents representing 102 children with type 1 diabetes (6–15 years) were recruited. Questionnaire results showed that subscales matched moderately to weakly with symptoms of emotional distress, from the Hopkins Symptom Checklist—25 items. Mothers showed higher scores than fathers on both HFS-P subscales. This confirms that the caregivers most at risk are mothers whose caregiving responsibility for children can turn into a form of underlying distress and fear of the unexpected episode of hypoglycemia.

In contrast, the survey [42] by Abitbol et al. investigated associated anxiety among parents of children with T1D within the Canadian Diabetes Association and identified factors associated with increased FOH. Two hundred and sixty-four parents of juveniles (2 to 18 years of age; mean ± standard deviation, 12.4 ± 3.5 years) with T1D were recruited and completed a survey that included demographic and disease-specific questions, the Spielberger State-Trait Anxiety Inventory, and the Fear of Hypoglycemia Survey-Parent Version (HFS-P).

Results: Of the 264 participants, 207 completed the full HFS-P, with a mean score of 67 ± 19 (range, 31 to 119). The most frequent concerns related to the child's hypoglycemia while alone or asleep. Higher HFS-P scores were also associated with more frequent and severe hypoglycemic episodes, higher state-trait anxiety scores, use of a continuous glycemic monitor, and more frequent blood glucose checks. Higher HFS-P scores were also associated with worse parental sleep quality and less parental involvement in treatment plans, which shows that as much as mothers are the most anxious caregivers, fathers associate night-time sleep with uncertainty and an inadequate monitoring role.

How do juveniles experience the pathological and family situation? The clinical investigation [43] by Shapira et al. assessed this in depth. A total of 601 juveniles with type 1 diabetes were recruited and followed up with a proxy report from parents.

Juveniles with type 1 diabetes, aged 5 to 18 years, and their parents completed the PedsQL 4.0 Generic Core Scales self-report and parent-proxy report, respectively. Indeed, health-related quality of life appears to be preserved in juveniles with type 1 diabetes unless they face multiple comorbidities as reported by youth and their parents. The findings highlight the importance of tracking the presence of multiple comorbid conditions, possibly revising problem and medication lists in the medical record, as well as screening and addressing mental health conditions in routine diabetes care.

Is there a difference in quality of life between patients diagnosed with type 1 and type 2 diabetes? [44].

Yi-Frazier et al. investigated potential differences between self-reported and parent-proxy reports of Pediatric Quality of Life Inventory (PedsQL) scores of juveniles with type 1 (T1D) or type 2 (T2D) diabetes and assessed associations between discrepancies, PedsQL scores, and glycemic control (HbA1c).

Juveniles and parents in the SEARCH for Diabetes in Youth Study (T1D: ages 5–18, $n = 3402$; T2D: ages 8–18, $n = 353$) completed the PedsQL Generic and Diabetes modules and juveniles provided a blood sample to assess HbA1c. Discrepancies (juvenile minus parent PedsQL assessments) were calculated and examined according to age and type of diabetes, and associations with youth PedsQL and HbA1c scores were assessed.

It emerged that there were differences between juvenile and parent-proxy reports of generic and PedsQL in both T1D and T2D (all p values <0.01). Higher (more favorable) ratings were reported by juveniles with the exception of those aged 5–7 years, where parent scores appeared higher. When parent-proxy scores were higher, discrepancies were highest when the child reported low PedsQL scores. Higher HbA1c was associated with greater discrepancies (higher juvenile scores) for adolescents with T1D.

It follows that discrepant PedsQL ratings suggest that parents may often underestimate the HRQOL of juveniles except in younger children. While examination of both reports is optimal, that of the juvenile should be prioritized, particularly for young children with T1D and adolescents with T1D or T2D.

Schreiner-Engel et al. [45] assessed the sexual dysfunction of patients with type 2 diabetes. Although diabetes is associated with a high prevalence of erectile insufficiency in men, she wanted to investigate patients' sexual functioning and marital satisfaction.

To examine this possibility, 35 married type 1 diabetic women were recruited and compared with 42 healthy married controls and 23 type 2 diabetic women and 23 other controls. Assessments were made on all aspects of sexual response, activity, dysfunction, and satisfaction; cognitive and psychological dimensions of sexuality; and marital adjustment.

Results indicated that diabetes type is highly associated with sexual responsiveness and marital satisfaction. Type I diabetes was found to have little or no effect on women, *whereas type II diabetes had a pervasively negative impact on sexual desire, orgasmic capacity, lubrication, sexual satisfaction, sexual activity, and the relationship with the sexual partner.*

However, for comparison, the study by Esposito et al. [46] investigated the prevalence and correlations of female sexual function in a sample of 595 women with type 2 diabetes Their age was 57.9 ± 6.9 (mean and sd), duration of diabetes was 5.2 ± 1.5 years, and mean hemoglobin A1c (HbA1c) level was $8.3 \pm 1.3\%$. Female sexual dysfunction (FSD) was assessed using the Female Sexual Function Index instrument with a cutoff score of 23. The overall prevalence of FSD among diabetic women was 53.4% and was significantly higher in postmenopausal women (63.9%), compared with those in the postmenopausal control group (41.0%, $P < 0.001$). There was no association between HbA1c, duration of diabetes, hypertension, or cigarette smoking status and FSD; in contrast, age, metabolic syndrome, and atherogenic dyslipidemia were significantly associated with FSD. Both depression and marital status were independent predictors of FSD, whereas physical activity was protective.

Furthermore, it seems that in type 1 diabetes sexual dysfunction is related more directly to psychological factors, [47] an interpretation recently confirmed by the results of a large prospective study of 625 women with type 1 diabetes (Epidemiology of Diabetes Interventions and Complications study), in which depression was found to be the main predictor of sexual dysfunction [48]. The majority of diabetic patients had an HbA1c level above 7% and by recent guidelines would be considered out of good glycemic control. The prevalence of obesity (BMI > 30), metabolic syndrome, hypertension, and atherogenic dyslipidemia was 29.4, 70.0, 53.9, and 19.7%, respectively [49].

In the largest study published to date, Abu Ali et al. [50] evaluated 613 diabetic and 524 nondiabetic women in Jordan and found a prevalence of FSD of 59.6% in diabetic women aged 50 years or older compared with 45.6% found in nondiabetic women of the same age ($P < 0.05$). Interestingly, the prevalence of FSD in the diabetic sample aged <50 years was approximately 41%; the mean FSFI score was 20.8. FSFI scores reported in other studies were 29.3 (72 women), [51] 20.5 (51 women), [52] 23.6 (23 women) [53], and 16.2 (58 women) [54].

Although both sexes share a similar risk of cardiovascular and neurological complications of diabetes, which presumably may result from similar pathogenetic mechanisms, the pattern of diabetes-specific effects may differ in men and women. Erectile dysfunction in diabetic men is associated with glycemic control and other classic cardiovascular and neuropathic complications of diabetes [47]; in addition, the prevalence of other cardiovascular risk factors (obesity, hypertension, and dyslipidemia) is high, especially in type 2 diabetes. Moreover, ED is an independent risk factor for new-onset cardiovascular disease and a powerful predictor of the development of major cardiovascular events in diabetic patients with known coronary artery disease [55].

On the other hand, FSD in women with type 1 diabetes appears to be the most unrelated to cardiovascular risk factors: Neuropathy [56], vascular damage [57], and psychological disorders [58] have been implicated in the pathogenesis of decreased libido, low excitability, reduced vaginal lubrication, orgasmic dysfunction, and dyspareunia among diabetic women.

Lastly, studies suggest that diabetes is a state of imbalance in sex hormone levels; in the context of type 1 or type 2 diabetes, however, there appears to be no difference in the incidence and/or rate of progression of kidney disease between men and women [59]. Much research reports that being male is still a risk factor for the development of kidney disease in diabetes [60] and that being female appears to accelerate disease progression [61]. This observation, together with the fact that diabetic kidney complications rarely develop before puberty, implies that sex hormones contribute to the evolution of the pathophysiology of diabetic kidney disease.

Conclusion

Delving into the impact of type 1 and type 2 diabetic disease on patients (children, adolescents, and adults) and caregivers involves a complex system of clinical, psychological, relational, and sexual assessments. If parental anxiety can affect a child's quality of life, sexual dysfunction in the adult diabetic patient compromises his or her lifestyle and body pattern. Metaphorically, therefore, "being obese" can become for the patient an unconscious defense against an uncomfortable reality filled with therapies, food deprivation, inadequacy in relationships, and sexual frustration.

Unfortunately, even now few diabetologists integrate the clinical history of diabetes 1 and 2 with the evaluation of these factors. The psychosexologist is often the easiest to turn to and frequently at the request of the patient. A team approach, even in the definition and respect of individual skills, would not only offer patients and caregivers an integrated approach, but would increase the value of therapy, lowering the levels of anxiety, depression, impotence, inadequacy, and social isolation. (The Impact of Externally Worn Diabetes Technology on Sexual Behavior and Activity, Body Image, and Anxiety in Type 1 Diabetes https://www.ncbi.nlm.nih.gov/pmc/articles/PMC7196867/ 2- Sexual activity in diabetic patients treated by continuous subcutaneous insulin infusion therapy https://pubmed.ncbi.nlm.nih.gov/20303814/ 3- You, me, and diabetes: Intimacy and technology among adults with T1D and their Partners https://pubmed.ncbi.nlm.nih.gov/33591783/ 4- Sleep and diabetes-specific psycho-behavioral outcomes of a new automated insulin delivery system in young children with type 1 diabetes and their parents https://pubmed.ncbi.nlm.nih.gov/33289242/)

References

1. World Health Organization. https://www.who.int/news-room/fact-sheets/detail/diabetes. Accessed 15 Mar 2021.
2. Emerging Risk Factors Collaboration, Sarwar N, Gao P, Seshasai SR, Gobin R, Kaptoge S, et al. Diabetes mellitus, fasting blood glucose concentration, and risk of vascular disease: a collaborative meta-analysis of 102 prospective studies. Lancet. 2010;375(9733):2215–22.
3. International Diabetes Federation. Diabetes atlas, 9th ed. 2019. https://www.diabetesatlas.org/en/. Accessed 15 Mar 2021.
4. Istituto Nazionale di Statistica. https://www.istat.it/it/archivio/202600. Accessed 15 Mar 2021.
5. Associazione Medici Diabetologi, Società Italiana di Diabetologia. Standard italiani per la cura del diabete mellito. 2019. http://aemmedi.it/wp-content/uploads/2009/06/AMD-Standard-unico1.pdf. Accessed 15 Mar 2021.
6. World Health Organization, International Diabetes Federation. Definition and diagnosis of diabetes mellitus and intermediate hyperglycaemia. 2006. https://www.who.int/publications/i/item/definition-and-diagnosis-of-diabetes-mellitus-and-intermediatehyperglycaemia. Accessed 11 Jun 2023.
7. American Diabetes Association. 2. Classification and diagnosis of diabetes: Standards of Medical Care in Diabetes-2021. Diabetes Care. 2021;44(Suppl 1):S15–33.
8. Wolfsdorf JI, Glaser N, Agus M, Fritsch M, Hanas R, Rewers A, Sperling MA, Codner E. ISPAD Clinical Practice Consensus Guidelines 2018: diabetic ketoacidosis and the hyperglycemic hyperosmolar state. Pediatr Diabetes. 2018 Oct;19(Suppl 27):155–77.
9. Cameron FJ, Scratch SE, Nadebaum C, Northam EA, Koves I, Jennings J, Finney K, Neil JJ, Wellard RM, Mackay M, Inder TE, DKA Brain Injury Study Group. Neurological consequences of diabetic ketoacidosis at initial presentation of type 1 diabetes in a prospective cohort study of children. Diabetes Care. 2014;37(6):1554–62.
10. Abraham MB, Jones TW, Naranjo D, Karges B, Oduwole A, Tauschmann M, Maahs DM. ISPAD Clinical Practice Consensus Guidelines 2018: assessment and management of hypoglycemia in children and adolescents with diabetes. Pediatr Diabetes. 2018;19(Suppl 27):178–92.
11. Duckworth W, Abraira C, Moritz T, Reda D, Emanuele N, Reaven PD, Zieve FJ, Marks J, Davis SN, Hayward R, Warren SR, Goldman S, McCarren M, Vitek ME, Henderson WG, Huang GD, Investigators VADT. Glucose control and vascular complications in veterans with type 2 diabetes. N Engl J Med. 2009;360(2):129–39.
12. Lacy ME, Gilsanz P, Eng C, Beeri MS, Karter AJ, Whitmer RA. Severe hypoglycemia and cognitive function in older adults with type 1 diabetes: the Study of Longevity in Diabetes (SOLID). Diabetes Care. 2020;43(3):541–8.
13. Wicklow BA, Sellers EAC, Sharma AK, Kroeker K, Nickel NC, Philips-Beck W, Shen GX. Association of gestational diabetes and type 2 diabetes exposure in utero with the development of type 2 diabetes in first nations and non-first nations offspring. JAMA Pediatr. 2018;172(8):724–31.
14. American Diabetes Association. Economic costs of diabetes in the U.S. in 2017. Diabetes Care. 2018;41:917–28.
15. Ali MK, Bullard KM, Saaddine JB, Cowie CC, Imperatore G, Gregg EW. Achievement of goals in U.S. diabetes care, 1999-2010. N Engl J Med. 2013;368:1613–24.
16. Buse JB, Ginsberg HN, Bakris GL, Clark NG, Costa F, Eckel R, Fonseca V, Gerstein HC, Grundy S, Nesto RW, Pignone MP, Plutzky J, Porte D, Redberg R, Stitzel KF, Stone NJ, American Heart Association, American Diabetes Association. Primary prevention of cardiovascular diseases in people with diabetes mellitus: a scientific statement from the American Heart Association and the American Diabetes Association. Diabetes Care. 2007;30(1):162–72.
17. Gaede P, Lund-Andersen H, Parving H-H, Pedersen O. Effect of a multifactorial intervention on mortality in type 2 diabetes. N Engl J Med. 2008;358:580–91.

18. Cavender MA, Steg PG, Smith SC Jr, Eagle K, Ohman EM, Goto S, Kuder J, Im K, Wilson PW, Bhatt DL, Registry REACH, Investigators. Impact of diabetes mellitus on hospitalization for heart failure, cardiovascular events, and death: outcomes at 4 years from the Reduction of Atherothrombosis for Continued Health (REACH) Registry. Circulation. 2015;132(10):923–31.
19. McAllister DA, Read SH, Kerssens J, Livingstone S, McGurnaghan S, Jhund P, Petrie J, Sattar N, Fischbacher C, Kristensen SL, McMurray J, Colhoun HM, Wild SH. Incidence of hospitalization for heart failure and case-fatality among 3.25 million people with and without diabetes mellitus. Circulation. 2018;138(24):2774–86.
20. Lam CSP, Voors AA, de Boer RA, Solomon SD, van Veldhuisen DJ. Heart failure with preserved ejection fraction: from mechanisms to therapies. Eur Heart J. 2018;39:2780–92.
21. Klausen K, Borch-Johnsen K, Feldt-Rasmussen B, Jensen G, Clausen P, Scharling H, Appleyard M, Jensen JS. Very low levels of microalbuminuria are associated with increased risk of coronary heart disease and death independently of renal function, hypertension, and diabetes. Circulation. 2004;110(1):32–5.
22. Gall MA, Hougaard P, Borch-Johnsen K, Parving HH. Risk factors for development of incipient and overt diabetic nephropathy in patients with non-insulin dependent diabetes mellitus: prospective, observational study. BMJ. 1997;314(7083):783–8.
23. Ninomiya T, Perkovic V, de Galan BE, Zoungas S, Pillai A, Jardine M, Patel A, Cass A, Neal B, Poulter N, Mogensen CE, Cooper M, Marre M, Williams B, Hamet P, Mancia G, Woodward M, Macmahon S, Chalmers J, ADVANCE Collaborative Group. Albuminuria and kidney function independently predict cardiovascular and renal outcomes in diabetes. J Am Soc Nephrol. 2009 Aug;20(8):1813–21.
24. Tesfaye S, Boulton AJ, Dyck PJ, Freeman R, Horowitz M, Kempler P, Lauria G, Malik RA, Spallone V, Vinik A, Bernardi L, Valensi P, Toronto Diabetic Neuropathy Expert Group. Diabetic neuropathies: update on definitions, diagnostic criteria, estimation of severity, and treatments. Diabetes Care. 2010;33(10):2285–93.
25. International Working Group on the Diabetic Foot. Guidelines on the prevention and management of diabetic foot disease. 2019. Practical Guidelines. https://iwgdfguidelines.org/practical-guidelines/. Accessed 17 Apr 2021.
26. Cleary PA, Orchard TJ, Genuth S, Wong ND, Detrano R, Backlund JY, Zinman B, Jacobson A, Sun W, Lachin JM, Nathan DM, DCCT/EDIC Research Group. The effect of intensive glycemic treatment on coronary artery calcification in type 1 diabetic participants of the Diabetes Control and Complications Trial/Epidemiology of Diabetes Interventions and Complications (DCCT/EDIC) Study. Diabetes. 2006;55(12):3556–65.
27. Nathan DM, Cleary PA, Backlund JY, Genuth SM, Lachin JM, Orchard TJ, Raskin P, Zinman B, Diabetes Control and Complications Trial/Epidemiology of Diabetes Interventions and Complications (DCCT/EDIC) Study Research Group. Intensive diabetes treatment and cardiovascular disease in patients with type 1 diabetes. N Engl J Med. 2005;353(25):2643–53.
28. Diabetes Control and Complications Trial (DCCT)/Epidemiology of Diabetes Interventions and Complications (EDIC) Study Research Group. Mortality in type 1 diabetes in the DCCT/EDIC versus the general population. Diabetes Care. 2016;39(8):1378–83.
29. Lane W, Bailey TS, Gerety G, Gumprecht J, Philis-Tsimikas A, Hansen CT, Nielsen TSS, Warren M, Group Information; SWITCH 1. Effect of insulin degludec vs insulin glargine u100 on hypoglycemia in patients with type 1 diabetes: the SWITCH 1 randomized clinical trial. JAMA. 2017;318(1):33–44.
30. Home PD, Bergenstal RM, Bolli GB, Ziemen M, Rojeski M, Espinasse M, Riddle MC. New insulin glargine 300 units/mL versus glargine 100 units/mL in people with type 1 diabetes: a randomized, phase 3a, open-label clinical trial (EDITION 4). Diabetes Care. 2015;38(12):2217–25.
31. Maruthur NM, Tseng E, Hutfless S, Wilson LM, Suarez-Cuervo C, Berger Z, Chu Y, Iyoha E, Segal JB, Bolen S. Diabetes medications as monotherapy or metformin-based combina-

tion therapy for type 2 diabetes: a systematic review and meta-analysis. Ann Intern Med. 2016;164(11):740–51.

32. U.S. Food and Drug Administration. FDA Drug Safety Communication: FDA revises warnings regarding use of the diabetes medicine metformin in certain patients with reduced kidney function. Available from https://www.fda.gov/drugs/drug-safety-and-availability/fda-drug-safety-communication-fda-revises-warnings-regarding-use-diabetes-medicine-metformin-certain. Accessed 6 Mar 2020.

33. Abdul-Ghani MA, Puckett C, Triplitt C, Maggs D, Adams J, Cersosimo E, DeFronzo RA. Initial combination therapy with metformin, pioglitazone and exenatide is more effective than sequential add-on therapy in subjects with new-onset diabetes. Results from the Efficacy and Durability of Initial Combination Therapy for Type 2 Diabetes (EDICT): a randomized trial. Diabetes Obes Metab. 2015;17(3):268–75.

34. Phung OJ, Sobieraj DM, Engel SS, Rajpathak SN. Early combination therapy for the treatment of type 2 diabetes mellitus: systematic review and meta-analysis. Diabetes Obes Metab. 2014;16(5):410–7.

35. Palmer SC, Tendal B, Mustafa RA, Vandvik PO, Li S, Hao Q, Tunnicliffe D, Ruospo M, Natale P, Saglimbene V, Nicolucci A, Johnson DW, Tonelli M, Rossi MC, Badve SV, Cho Y, Nadeau-Fredette AC, Burke M, Faruque LI, Lloyd A, Ahmad N, Liu Y, Tiv S, Millard T, Gagliardi L, Kolanu N, Barmanray RD, McMorrow R, Raygoza Cortez AK, White H, Chen X, Zhou X, Liu J, Rodríguez AF, González-Colmenero AD, Wang Y, Li L, Sutanto S, Solis RC, Díaz González-Colmenero F, Rodriguez-Gutierrez R, Walsh M, Guyatt G, Strippoli GFM. Sodium-glucose cotransporter protein-2 (SGLT-2) inhibitors and glucagon-like peptide-1 (GLP-1) receptor agonists for type 2 diabetes: systematic review and network meta-analysis of randomised controlled trials. BMJ. 2021;372:m4573.

36. Vijan S, Sussman JB, Yudkin JS, Hayward RA. Effect of patients' risks and preferences on health gains with plasma glucose level lowering in type 2 diabetes mellitus. JAMA Intern Med. 2014;174(8):1227–34.

37. Diabetes Control and Complications Trial Research Group, Nathan DM, Genuth S, Lachin J, Cleary P, Crofford O, Davis M, Rand L, Siebert C. The effect of intensive treatment of diabetes on the development and progression of long-term complications in insulin-dependent diabetes mellitus. N Engl J Med. 1993;329(14):977–86.

38. Battelino T, Danne T, Bergenstal RM, Amiel SA, Beck R, Biester T, Bosi E, Buckingham BA, Cefalu WT, Close KL, Cobelli C, Dassau E, DeVries JH, Donaghue KC, Dovc K, Doyle FJ 3rd, Garg S, Grunberger G, Heller S, Heinemann L, Hirsch IB, Hovorka R, Jia W, Kordonouri O, Kovatchev B, Kowalski A, Laffel L, Levine B, Mayorov A, Mathieu C, Murphy HR, Nimri R, Nørgaard K, Parkin CG, Renard E, Rodbard D, Saboo B, Schatz D, Stoner K, Urakami T, Weinzimer SA, Phillip M. Clinical targets for continuous glucose monitoring data interpretation: recommendations from the International Consensus on Time in Range. Diabetes Care. 2019;42(8):1593–603.

39. Pinhas-Hamiel O, Tisch E, Levek N, Ben-David RF, Graf-Bar-El C, Yaron M, Boyko V, Lerner-Geva L. Sexual lifestyle among young adults with type 1 diabetes. Diabetes Metab Res Rev. 2017;33(2). https://doi.org/10.1002/dmrr.2837. Epub 2016 Aug 16. PMID: 27385271.

40. Gjerløw E, Bjørgaas MR, Nielsen EW, Olsen SE, Asvold BO. Fear of hypoglycemia in women and men with type 1 diabetes. Nurs Res. 2014;63(2):143–9. https://doi.org/10.1097/NNR.0000000000000020. PMID: 24589650.

41. Haugstvedt A, Wentzel-Larsen T, Aarflot M, Rokne B, Graue M. Assessing fear of hypoglycemia in a population-based study among parents of children with type 1 diabetes - psychometric properties of the hypoglycemia fear survey - parent version. BMC Endocr Disord. 2015;19(15):2. https://doi.org/10.1186/1472-6823-15-2. PMID: 25599725; PMCID: PMC4324848.

42. Abitbol L, Palmert MR. When low blood sugars cause high anxiety: fear of hypoglycemia among parents of youth with type 1 diabetes mellitus. Can J Diabetes. 2021;45(5):403–410.e2. https://doi.org/10.1016/j.jcjd.2020.08.098. Epub 2020 Aug 20. PMID: 33046404.

43. Shapira A, Harrington KR, Goethals ER, Volkening LK, Laffel LM. Health-related quality of life in youth with type 1 diabetes: associations with multiple comorbidities and mental health conditions. Diabet Med. 2021;38(10):e14617. https://doi.org/10.1111/dme.14617. Epub 2021 Jun 19. PMID: 34060668; PMCID: PMC8429188.

44. Yi-Frazier JP, Hilliard ME, Fino NF, Naughton MJ, Liese AD, Hockett CW, Hood KK, Pihoker C, Seid M, Lang W, Lawrence JM. Whose quality of life is it anyway? Discrepancies between youth and parent health-related quality of life ratings in type 1 and type 2 diabetes. Qual Life Res. 2016;25(5):1113–21. https://doi.org/10.1007/s11136-015-1158-5. Epub 2015 Oct 14. PMID: 26466834; PMCID: PMC4936832.

45. Schreiner-Engel P, Vietorisz D, Smith H. The differential impact of diabetes type on female sexuality. J Psychosom Res. 1987;31(1):23–33.

46. Esposito K, Maiorino M, Bellastella G, et al. Determinanti della disfunzione sessuale femminile nel diabete di tipo 2. Int J Impot Res. 2010;22:179–84.

47. Hisasue S, Kumamoto Y, Sato Y, Masumori N, Horita H, Kato R, et al. Prevalence of symptoms of female sexual dysfunction and its relationship to quality of life: a Japanese female cohort study. Urology. 2005;65:143–8.

48. Esposito K, Giugliano D. Obesity, metabolic syndrome and sexual dysfunction. Int J Impot Res. 2005;17:391–8.

49. Nathan DM, Buse JB, Davidson MB, Ferrannini E, Holman RR, Sherman R, et al. Medical management of hyperglycemia in type 2 diabetes: a consensus algorithm for initiation and adjustment of therapy: a consensus statement from the American Diabetes Association and the European Association for the Study of diabetes. Diabetes Care. 2009;32(1):193–203.

50. Abu Ali RM, Al Hajeri RM, Khader YS, Shegem NS, Ajlouni KM. Sexual dysfunction in Jordanian diabetic women. Diabetes Care. 2008;31:1580–1.

51. Salman F, Dincag N, Kadioglu A, et al. Sexual dysfunction in type II diabetic women: a comparative study. J Marital Sex Ther. 2002;28(Suppl 1):55–62.

52. Olarinoye J, Olarinoye A. Determinants of sexual function among women with type 2 diabetes in a Nigerian population. J Sex Med. 2008;5:878–86.

53. Letme SS, Tachavi SM. Assessment of sexual function in women with type 2 diabetes mellitus. Diabetes Vasc Dis Res. 2009;6:38–9.

54. Ogbera AO, Chinenye S, Akinlade A, Eregie A, Awobusuyi J. Frequency and correlates of sexual dysfunction in women with diabetes mellitus. J Sex Med. 2009;6:3401–6.

55. Gazzaruso C, Solerte SB, Pujia A, Coppola A, Vezzoli M, Salvucci F, et al. La disfunzione erettile come predittore di eventi cardiovascolari e morte nei pazienti diabetici con malattia coronarica asintomatica accertata angiograficamente: un potenziale ruolo protettivo per statine e inibitori della 5-fosfodiesterasi. J Am Coll Cardiol. 2008;51:2040–4.

56. Erol B, Tefekli A, Sanli O, Ziylan O, Armagan A, Kendirci M, et al. Is sexual dysfunction related to deterioration of the somatic sensory system in diabetic women? Int J Impot Res. 2003;15:198–202.

57. Enzlin P, Rosen R, Wiegel M, Brown J, Wessells H, Gatcomb P, et al. Sexual dysfunction in women with type 1 diabetes. Long-term results from the DCCT / EDIC study cohort. Diabetes Care. 2009;32:780–5.

58. Erol B, Tefekli A, Ozbey I, Salman F, Dincag N, Kadioglu A, et al. Sexual dysfunction in type II diabetic women: a comparative study. J Marital Sex Ther. 2002;28(Suppl 1):55–62.

59. Monti MC, Lonsdale JT, Montomoli C, Montross R, Schlag E, Greenberg DA. Familial risk factors for microvascular complications and male-female differential risk in a large cohort of American families with type 1 diabetes. J Clin Metab Endocrinol. 2007;92:4650–5.

60. Sibley SD, Thomas W, de Boer I, Brunzell JD, Steffes MW. Gender and high albumin excretion in the Diabetes Control and Complications Trial/Epidemiology of Diabetes Interventions and Complications (DCCT/EDIC) cohort: role of central obesity. Am J Kidney Dis. 2006;47:223–32.

61. Laron-Kenet T, Shamis I, Weitzman S, Rosen S, Laron ZV. Mortality of patients with childhood onset (0–17 years) Type I diabetes in Israel: a population-based study. Diabetologia. 2001;44(Suppl 3):B81–6.

Part VII
Eating Disorders

Eating Disorders

Furio Ravera, Vittoria Ravera, and Elena Vittoria Longhi

Introduction

Nowadays, eating disorders plague both the feminine and masculine population, and they show new and different peculiarities compared to the past patterns. Especially concerning males, this phenomenon occurs to a lesser extent, even if it is increasing considerably.

As a matter of fact, eating disorders evolved together with young culture, in which young patients are dipped.

The renunciation/rejection of food has been replaced mainly by bulimic behaviours, which are complemented by compensatory behaviours, such as self-induced vomit, which represents the first solution for hunger grief and does not represent anymore a way to expiate and deny personal needs.

The needs for purity, which are searched through the rejection of food, has become need for purity and emptying, so it is necessary to separate the relationship with food into two phases: in the first phase, the patient is completely overwhelmed by the desire of being filled, of devouring, of destroying and of succumbing to a need; the second phase occurs at the edge of the first one, when the need has reached its peak, and the necessity of devouring, of swallowing and of self-filling up to the limit is temporarily quieted. At this moment, a feeling of disgust and heaviness is manifested, which can occur at the same time because of a leaf of lettuce or a whole biscuits' box, which can both be scarfed in a trance state.

F. Ravera (✉)
The Unit for the Diagnosis and Treatment of Personality Disorders and Addictions, Private Clinic "Le Betulle" Appiano Gentile, Como, Italy

V. Ravera
Bibliography Research, The Bicocca University Milan, Milan, Italy

E. V. Longhi
Department of Sexual Medical Center, San Raffaele Hospital, Milano, Italy

Whatever it may be, gastric contents are intolerable; the disgust is associated with a feeling of fear and danger, similar to the feeling experimented on by someone who has drunk poison. That is, when the solution arrives, the self-induced vomit that the more time passes the more it becomes easier to produce; sometimes, the whole thing is accompanied by drinking water, in order to execute a sort of gastric lavage. This kind of loop can be episodic and sporadic, but in severe cases it can happen several times during the day until the patient lies completely exhausted and aching because of the repetition of the binge eating/vomit loop.

The Internal Medicine consequences related to these behavioural patterns can be really severe and they include electrolytes' alteration, especially a loss of potassium that causes huge impairments to the electrogenesis of the wave of cardiac contraction. It causes damage to the plasma proteins as well: damaged plasma proteins can produce pericardial effusion, anaemia and oedemas. The combined action of hormonal alterations and malnutrition, which are reported by amenorrhoea in the first place, underlies the deficiencies of ossification processes that cause osteoporosis because of the lack of osteocytes, which cannot be easily reverted. This phenomenon is associated with angular stomatitis, glossitis, hypertrichosis and loss and thinning of hair. I am insisting on amenorrhoea because it is the main marker for the organic suffering, the signals of which are gathered by hypothalamus, which influences the hypophysial activity. Hypercholesterolaemia is common as well, and it is caused by lipometabolism's disorder; salivary amylasaemia can also occur, which is caused by salivary glands' hyperactivity triggered by the vomit. In particular, the increase in salivary amylase differentiated from pancreatic amylase is a revealing signal of self-induced vomit. It is possible to observe asthenia, cephalea, muscular and bones' pain, torpor and difficulty in focusing.

Eating Disorder Diagnosis

It is required to make a reflection on the diagnosis. The well-known DSM-V offers the possibility to classify eating disorders in order to configure a successful therapy, but the disorder is so intricate that it is necessary to develop a "therapeutically spendable" diagnosis, which can provide information to the patient about beliefs and meanings related to the body and to the object food and about their role in the attachment system. In my opinion, eating disorders are linked to a combination of very specific and personal perception and beliefs on the body, attachment's patterns, attributions of meaning and beliefs on food. Beliefs, meanings and representations underlie the distortion of eating habits.

It is necessary to develop an accurate diagnosis about these three factors: food, body, attachment pattern and the related attributions of meaning and beliefs. In this way, it is possible to draw a detailed map of their features.

Food's first prerogative should be to be nourishing, digestible, assimilable, not toxic and, last but not least, enjoyable. Its pleasantness helps to select it as preferable in a perspective of choice. For thousands of years, human beings have searched for food as just food, no one used to think about the amount of calories, carbs and proteins and having a vegetarian diet or not. No one used to worry about if food was healthy or not, and food should only feed. It was essential for life.

Even today should be like that, but things have imperceptibly but inexorably changed. Culturally, together with medical development and greater availability of food in the most evolved areas of the planet, we passed from the pursuit of food's availability to the pursuit of the quality of food, which inevitably caused a classification of food and its features. We started to be suspicious about food, in part also because of medical restrictions for some diseases like diabetes, hypercholesterolaemia and celiac condition: "will it be healthy?" "Maybe is this too much?" "Does it contain too many calories or too many carbs?" until we built a society based on choosing and rationing food according to a possible danger. From essential nourishment for life, food became something to discuss and be aware of. An entity that is able to produce effects modifies its representation, pulling on itself new attributions of meaning. Trivially, if you eat too much, you are not just someone who has a large availability of food, which can be considered opulent, instead you are someone who does not respect himself, someone who does not take care about his physical conditions, someone without temper, which is not able to control his impulses, slave of his own needs and someone that is needy. This is a list of meanings.

At this point, it is possible to consider that an eating disorder develops from the moment in which food keeps a distance from its original function and meaning to assume another one, the one the patient specifically adopts. Likewise, we can consider that an eating disorder rises when the feeding act breaks with its biological meaning to embrace a new one. Exploring this kind of patient, it is really important to avoid preconceived notions, because each patient can attribute a different and personal meaning to the food and to the nourishing, even if it is possible to observe a recurrent pattern. Some patients, through an accurate selection of food, implement a sort of ritual selection of what they can accept to "get into" themselves. About that, we must remember a crucial aspect of food: it is something we put inside ourselves, and at the same time, something we cannot live without. We depend on it.

At this point, we can make another consideration. If we consider these two aspects of food, what do we need to improve the diagnosis? We need to know how the person feels putting something inside himself and likewise how he accepts the dependence condition. We must examine accurately the relationship with parents to get an answer, in particular the one with the mother, which, we must remember, represents the origin of offspring's life: the mother has a body that is physiologically organized to nourish, she has mammaries full of milk and in the majority of cases she is the person who takes care about her children's nutrition. The concept of the mother is strongly associated with nourishment and to dependence on what concerns humankind.

In this perspective, we can easily understand that food can quickly become an object that allows a ritualization of fear of putting something maternal inside ourselves, which can provoke unwanted consequences; equally, it is possible to ritualize a rejection or an ambivalence towards the dependence. The verification of these elements establishes a base from which we can organize the investigation about beliefs generated by these two possibilities of ritualization. The diagnosis on the attachment's pattern that reveals an insecure or chaotic attachment lets us understand easily how it can be hard for a young girl to accept the dependence on a parent that she does not trust but whom she needs.

Different patterns of binge eating followed by self-induced vomit are related to an insecure attachment, and binge eating represents accurately the abandonment of a voracious need to be filled and to fill a void (of reassuring and supportive parental introjection). When the stomach is stuffed, the fear rises up, and it is described as a real terror for what can happen because of what has been introduced inside the body, which shows vomiting as a good solution, as a liberating act, as an action that achieves the illusion of "delete what we have done" and "restore everything as it was before". This rewind effect associated with the purification effect is so important that it makes the vomit the fundamental centre of an eating disorder. We binge eat to vomit instead of we vomit because we binge ate.

In these cases, the theme of purification and the theme of getting back to the time before something happened for the patient result prevailing.

This particular shade of the binge eating/vomit circle is often related to cases that show sexual violence traumas during the anamnesis. Frequently, patients avoid the narration about sexual abuses they suffered, because they feel guilty for what they went through. It is a defence mechanism that is built on the illusory idea of having had a control on the abuse, which could make this fact more bearable instead of considering themselves powerless victims. If we look into vomit as a way to cancel what has been done or what happened, it suggests to gently insist on the research of traumas; it is necessary to create conditions of confidence and acceptance in order to reveal crucial details.

Until now, we did not talk about thinness, not because it is not important but because I think that the approach we have followed makes us understand that the exasperated pursuit of thinness should be explored and detected in terms of beliefs and functions.

We often talk about the alteration of body image, but this is just a definition that requires a specific diagnosis, which should involve purposes and functions related to thinness.

Superficially and originally, the aesthetic factor is on the line, but particularly in the most severe cases it fades away. There is something else that patients see in thinness. A patient used to talk about herself like a target of a shooting gallery. If you are tiny, it is harder to hit you.

Another patient used to talk about thinness in terms of military fortifications. I feel myself sharp and hard because there is nothing smooth in my body. In this way, I feel safer.

A male patient used to reject food and to reassure himself through his extreme thinness. In this way, I feel weak and I am sure I do not have the energy to assault my father.

Another patient used to reject food for this reason. I cannot tell the difference between food and sexual pleasure, and I am ashamed for that, and I cannot stand it.

This is a short list of beliefs that is not exhaustive. The therapist must not apply to the patient his beliefs' knowledge mechanically: the therapist must know that there are beliefs that support some behaviours and he/she must discover their features.

On that note, I am going to say a few words about the different kinds of intervention.

Intervention

It is necessary to distinguish between the medical actions adopted to make the patient safe and the strategies and the therapeutic specialized methods.

The nutritionist doctor has to make the patient safe, and he/she has to remember that he/she is working with a patient for whom the nourishing represents a source of intense fear. So, wisely, he has to negotiate on the diet, and the normalization of the most alarming parameters has to be put as the primary goal (electrolytes, anaemia, serum protein, the elimination of the eventual pericardial effusion and the restoration of the normal cardiac rhythm). Menstruations get normal in a longer time compared to the achievement of a satisfying BMI.[1]

Residential therapies offer the advantage of separating the patient from the familiar dynamics and the setting has to give facilitations for the achievement of appropriate eating habits: not accessible food, food served on a tray depending on the diet, a common dining room, an accurate assistance from the educators during the meals, the bathroom can be used only before the meal or at least 2 h after the meal and remaining in a living room in which the educators assist the patients using techniques of emotional control for the after meal.

A mindfulness' session can be useful in order to prepare the patient for the meal. The most useful therapeutic methods are as follows:

- DBT: dialectical and behavioural therapy enables problem-solving techniques, through proper teaching modules related to consciousness and the control of emotions. It also enables the development of better relational resources. It provides an examination of the sheet of impulsive behaviours' dynamics and the possibility of examining contingencies, of achieving a higher mastery together with a sort of alphabetization for observing and describing the inner world in the interest of the therapy and self-control.
- EMDR (eye movement desensitization and reprocessing): this technique is extremely efficient in the desensitization of traumatic experiences that are present with a significant frequency in the story of eating disorders.

---

[1] BMI, body mass index, is calculated by this formula: kg/height squared in meters. Below 18.5 is an underweight condition, between 18.5 and 24.9 is the range of normality and over 30 begins obesity.

- Mindfulness: it is a meditation practice developed by Jon Kabat-Zinn, who is the founder of the Stress Reduction Clinic and of the Center for Mindfulness in Medicine at the University of Massachusetts Medical School. This technique enables the patients to achieve a higher consciousness about their emotions and about their body signals that are at the base of the emotions, contributing to better self-comprehension and to a control of their feelings.

Psychotherapy initially has an explorative function, and it has to use the complementarity of other techniques. We can say that the ability to engage in an efficient psychotherapy for this kind of patient is a moving target that includes the growth of the capability of benefit from a technique, which at the start represents support and over time it reaches an expressive level that allows the patient to work on the integration of partial transferal segments.

Pharmacological therapy has the only purpose of adjusting depressive conditions, fluctuation of the emotional mood, anxiety disorders and panic attacks, dissociative crisis or psychotic traits.

We should not use just one strategy to handle these disorders, and it is necessary an eclectic strategy that combines the aforementioned methods.

Sexuality and Quality of Life

Pinheiro et al. [1] conducted a study on physical intimacy, libido, sexual anxiety, partner status and sexual relationships in 242 women with eating disorders, as part of the International Price Foundation Genetic Studies.

Results: 55.3% were sexually active and 52.7% had a partner, while 66.9% reported decreased sexual desire and 59.2% increased sexual anxiety. Patients diagnosed with restrictive anorexia nervosa and purging had a higher prevalence of libido loss than women with bulimia nervosa and an eating disorder not otherwise specified (75%, 74.6%, 39% and 45.4%, respectively). Sexual absence was associated with lower lifetime body mass index (BMI) and earlier age of onset; loss of libido with lower lifetime BMI, greater interoceptive awareness and trait anxiety; and sexual anxiety with lower lifetime BMI, greater avoidance of harm and inefficacy. Sexual dysfunction in eating disorders was greater than in the normative sample.

We must consider that eating disorders constitute a wide range of individual behaviours in dealing with food. In addition to bulimia and anorexia nervosa, we include eating compulsivity and obsessive–compulsive disorder that immediately leads us to the connection between eating disorders and personality traits [2].

According to a review of the literature, obsessive–compulsive personality disorder is the most common axis II disorder in individuals with eating disorders with restrictive eating behaviour, whereas borderline personality disorder is the most common axis II disorder in those with impulsive eating pathology. Because personality disorders evolutionarily precede eating disorders and personality disorder characteristics often mirror the style of eating pathology (e.g. highly controlled personality styles and highly controlled eating patterns; and impulsive personality styles and impulsive eating pathology), it is reasonable to assume that personality disorders influence subsequent eating pathology. Thus, it is likely that personality disorders function, to some extent, as risk factors for the development of specific types of eating disorders.

The Diagnostic and Statistical Manual of Mental Disorders (DSM-V) tells us that criteria 1 eating disorders belong on axis I. Axis I disorders represent the major psychiatric disorders and include major depression, panic disorder, bipolar disorder and schizophrenia. (Unlike axis I disorders, axis II disorders represent both personality and developmental disorders.)

Studies by Sansone et al. [3] showed that the most common personality disorder found is obsessive–compulsive personality disorder. Among the study samples reviewed, this disorder was present in approximately 22% of individuals. These patients regularly engage in food restriction behaviours and misuse of laxatives, diuretics or enemas. The perfectionist trait of these patients (higher female than male frequency of this disorder) is manifested in the tendency to set rigid life standards (maximum performance in study or work, maximum sports performance, etc.) and very high life goals. Because of its self-defeating nature in individuals with eating disorders, perfectionism is described in this context by some authors as "maladaptive perfectionism" [4, 5].

In disorders in which the individual regularly engages in binge eating, self-induced vomiting and/or abuse of laxatives, diuretics or enemas (axis II disorder) is linked with borderline personality disorder, with a prevalence rate of approximately 25%. The presence of impulsive eating disorder behaviours such as binge eating and purging shows a clear association with impulsive personality disorder, with clear up-and-down mood disorders.

Like obsessive–compulsive personality disorder, borderline personality disorder also tends to have a genetically influenced temperamental basis. In a recent study by Distel and colleagues, [6] genetic factors accounted for 42% of the variance in this disorder. However, in addition to genetic influences, borderline personality disorder has strong associations with childhood histories of repeated abuse and maltreatment (e.g. sexual, physical and emotional abuse) [7]. In an exemplary study, Zanarini and colleagues [8] found, in a large sample of patients with borderline personality disorder, that over 90% reported both childhood abuse and neglect.

It is often assumed that preoccupation (excessive and constant thoughts) with shape/weight and food/eating is prominent in individuals with eating disorders. Lydecker et al. [9] evaluated 1363 individuals for a web-based survey (with measures of eating disorder psychopathology and depression), comparing preoccupation among individuals with prominent features of bulimia nervosa (BN; $n = 144$), uncontrolled eating disorder (BED; $n = 576$), anorexia nervosa (AN; $n = 48$) and higher body weight (body mass index [BMI] ≥ 25) without eating disorder features (higher weight [HW]; $n = 595$).

The preoccupation with shape/weight and preoccupation with food/eating showed a stepwise pattern of statistically significant differences: AN and BN had greater preoccupation than BED, which was greater than HW. Within the BN, BED and AN study groups, the magnitudes of correlation of shape/weight and preoccupation with food/eating with eating disorder psychopathology and depression did not differ significantly. Within the HW group, the preoccupation with shape/weight was significantly more strongly correlated than the preoccupation with food/eating with overestimation, body dissatisfaction and depression.

The sexual sphere is particularly important when attempting to elucidate the unique characteristics of eating disorders in males [10]. The clinical picture of anorexia nervosa and bulimia nervosa appears to differ for men and women in this area, with more men with eating disorders exhibiting gender dysphoria and/or a homosexual orientation than female counterparts.

There is a typical overrepresentation of homosexual males in eating disorder clinical samples.

The study by Hospers et al. [11] investigated the role of gender orientation, peer pressure, self-esteem and body dissatisfaction in relation to eating disorder symptoms among a sample of homosexual men and a sample of heterosexual men.

The results show that body dissatisfaction, and not self-esteem, was the dominant predictor of eating disorder symptoms. For both heterosexual and homosexual men, a higher level of body dissatisfaction was related to a higher body mass index (BMI), greater competition with peers and lower masculinity scores. Furthermore, an interaction between sexual orientation and peer rivalry was found: the relationship between peer pressure and body dissatisfaction was substantially more pronounced among homosexual men.

Finally, the results show the central role of body dissatisfaction in the relationship between homosexuality and eating disorder symptoms, as well as the contribution of peer rivalry.

With regard to the lack of self-esteem and expectations in love and sexual relationships with partners, female patients with eating disorders have given rise to various scientific investigations [12].

The study by Maria Raciti et al. [13] evaluated a sample of 232 women (82% white non-Hispanic, 12% white Hispanic, 4% black, 2% oriental and others): the patients reported that the eating disorder was related to possessiveness towards the partner and fear of sudden abandonment (by the partner) due to low self-esteem.

Within the range of eating disorders, late-onset types of anorexia nervosa have been identified. While most cases of anorexia nervosa begin in adolescence, a considerable number can develop the condition at any advanced age [14]. The term late anorexia nervosa is reintroduced to describe women who develop anorexia nervosa at or after their marriage.

The study by Peter Dally [14] (Department of Psychological Medicine, Westminster Hospital, London) investigated 50 patients and their partners. The patients were divided into four groups: those who developed late-onset anorexia:

1. During the engagement period
2. After marriage and before pregnancy

3. After childbirth
4. During or after menopause

In the first three groups, late-onset anorexia developed as a maladaptive solution to a growing marital crisis. Many of the husbands were immature men who readily accepted a sick-dependent wife. The women in group 4 differed in several respects and their weight loss eventually came to express a desire to die, to separate from everything and everyone through depression, mood swings and anhedonia.

Furthermore, a recent study by Perko et al. [15] investigated the intimacy of sexual minorities on the assumption that they are at greater risk of developing eating disorder (ED) psychopathology.

Despite the importance of understanding the symptoms of ED in sexual minority men, most measures of ED have been developed and validated in heterosexuals, young adults and white men. The psychometric properties of ED measures in different populations remain largely unknown. The aim of Perko's study was to verify the following:

1. Whether the eight-factor structure of the Eating Disorder Symptom Inventory (EPSI) is replicated in sexual minority men.
2. Average group-level differences between gay and bisexual men on the eight EPSI scales.

International participants (=722 sexual minority men from 20 countries) were recruited via the smartphone application Grindr. Group differences in eating pathology between homosexual and bisexual men were tested using independent-samples t-tests.

Results: Homosexual and bisexual men differed only on the EPSI Binge Eating Scale. The results of this investigation suggest that the EPSI may be a useful tool for understanding eating pathology in this population. The use of psychometrically valid assessment tools for sexual minority men is a key element of treatment planning and clinical decision-making.

Conclusions

Food and sex depend on the five senses and presuppose, for healthy balance, distribution by quality, quantity and distribution.

Excessive or insufficient caloric intake can affect the body's activity, consuming muscle tissue, including heart tissue. Complementary complications include endocrine disruption, osteoporosis, insulin resistance and gastric problems including gastroparesis, constipation or pancreatitis. The altered biochemical processes and psychological changes must therefore be addressed in a single programme where food is not the priority and the solution to the problem, but is approached in conjunction with the individual's inadequacy, fear of relationships, body dysmorphism and often the individual's excessive perfectionism.

References

1. Pinheiro AP, et al. Sexual function in women with eating disorder. Int J Eat Disord. 2010;43:123–9.
2. Sansone RA, et al. Personality disorders as risk factors for eating disorders. Nutr Clin Pract. 2010;25:116. https://doi.org/10.1177/0884533609357563.
3. Sansone RA, Levitt JL, Sansone LA. The prevalence of personality disorders in individuals with eating disorders. In: Sansone RA, Levitt JL, editors. Personality disorders and eating disorders: exploring the frontier. New York: Routledge; 2006. p. 23–39.
4. Halmi KA, Tozzi F, Thornton LM, et al. The relationship between perfectionism, obsessive-compulsive personality disorder, and obsessive-compulsive disorder in individuals with eating disorders. Int J Eat Disord. 2005;38:371–4.
5. Soenens B, Nevelsteen W, Vandereycken W. The significance of perfectionism in eating disorders: a comparative study. Tijdschr Psychiatr. 2007;49:709–18.
6. Distel MA, Trull TJ, Derom CA, et al. The inheritance of borderline personality disorder characteristics is similar in three countries. Psychol Med. 2008;38:1219–29.
7. Sansone RA, Sansone LA. Borderline personality disorder: the enigma. Prim Care Represent. 2000;6:219–26.
8. Zanarini MC, Williams AA, Lewis RE, et al. Report pathological childhood experiences associated with the development of borderline personality disorder. Am J Psychiatry. 1997;154:1101–6.
9. Lydecker JA, et al. Concern for bulimia nervosa, binge eating disorder, anorexia nervosa and higher weight. J Eat Disord. 2021;55:76. https://doi.org/10.1002/eat.23630.
10. Herzog DB, Bradbum IS, Newman K. Males with eating disorders. 2014. taylorfrancis.com.
11. Hospers HJ, Jansen A. Why homosexuality is a risk factor for eating disorders in males. J Soc Clin Psychol. 2006;24:1188. https://doi.org/10.1521/jscp.2005.24.8.1188.
12. Wiederman MW, Hurst SR. Physical attraction, body image, and sexual self-pattern of women. Women's Psychol Quart. 1997;21(4):567–80.
13. Raciti M, Hendrick SS. Relations between eating disorder characteristics and amorous and sexual attitudes. Sex Roles. 1992;27:553–64.
14. Dally P. Anorexia tardive—late onset marital anorexia nervosa. J Psychosom Res. 1984;28(5):423–8.
15. Perko VL, Forbush KT, Christensen KA, Richson BN, Chapa DAN, Bohrer BK, Griffiths S. Validation of the factor structure of the Eating Pathology Symptoms Inventory in an international sample of sexual minority men. Eat Behav. 2021;42:101511.

Part VIII
Obesity

Obesity

**Alessandro Sartorio, Sofia Tamini, Nicoletta Marazzi,
and Elena Vittoria Longhi**

The global epidemic of obesity is widespread in almost all countries in the world, and further development is expected in the future [1]. Despite the fact that a genetic predisposition to obesity is unquestionably involved, various environmental factors are also implied [2], such as excess portion size, dietary macronutrient composition, and sedentary lifestyle in the setting of modern-day habits.

For the definition of obesity body mass index (BMI) is classically used, however, this simple index is actually an imperfect measure of excessive or abnormal body fat accumulation [3]. As reported in Table 1, waist circumference has been suggested as a more precise predictor of comorbidities, because it allows to identify different degrees of health risk.

A. Sartorio (✉) · S. Tamini · N. Marazzi
Istituto Auxologico Italiano, IRCCS, Experimental Laboratory for Auxo-endocrinological Research, Milan and Verbania, Italy
e-mail: sartorio@auxologico.it; n.marazzi@auxologico.it

E. V. Longhi
Department of Sexual Medical Center, San Raffaele Hospital, Milano, Italy

© Springer Nature Switzerland AG 2023

E. V. Longhi (ed.), *Managing Psychosexual Consequences in Chronic Diseases*,
https://doi.org/10.1007/978-3-031-31307-3_13

Table 1 Classification of overweight and obesity by BMI and waist circumference

	BMI			Waist	
				Waist circumference and comorbidity risk	
Classification	BMI (kg/m²)	Comorbidity risk		Men ≤102 cm Women ≤88 cm	Men >102 cm Women >88 cm
Underweight	<18.5	Low (with other problems)			
Normal weight	18.5–24.9	Average			
Overweight	25–29.9	Increased		Increased	High
Obese class 1	30–34.9	Moderate		High	Very high
Obese class 2	35–39.9	Severe		Very high	Very high
Obese class 3	≥40	Very severe		Extremely high	Extremely high

Main Medical Characteristics

Obesity is a risk factor for a number of chronic diseases, most notably type 2 diabetes (T2DM), cardiovascular diseases (CVD), and certain types of cancer [4, 5]. Taken all together, obesity-related comorbidities incur significant healthcare costs, which represent approximately 2.4% of the whole healthcare expenditure.

The neologism "diabesity" has been created to define the overlap between T2DM and obesity [6]. The risk of T2DM rises by 100% with a BMI between 27 and 29 kg/m² and by about 300% for BMI >29 kg/m² [7, 8]. Since the long-term complications of T2DM include CVD, stroke, peripheral vascular diseases, retinopathy, nephropathy, and neuropathy, prevention or at least control of T2DM is reported to reduce the obesity-related complications and hold down the direct healthcare costs.

Obesity is frequently associated with metabolic syndrome (i.e., the combination of at least three of the following features: central obesity, high serum triglyceride levels, low serum high-density lipoprotein, cholesterol levels, hypertension, and elevated fasting blood glucose levels), and this concomitant condition also determines an increased CVD risk.

Subjects with severe obesity frequently suffer from obesity hypoventilation syndrome, with its prevalence being 10–20% in obese patients with associated obstructive sleep apnea and almost 50% in hospitalized patients with a BMI greater than 50 kg/m².

BMI shows a strong, independent, and positive correlation with asthma, not only because of the impact of adipose tissue on the chest wall, which causes restrictive lung disease, but also because of the chronic inflammatory state of obesity.

Insulin resistance related to obesity represents the major causative factor of non-alcoholic fatty liver disease (NAFLD), resulting in progressive fibrosis (38%) and hepatocellular carcinoma (4–10%) as the years go on.

The frequent occurrence of subfertility in obese subjects has been attributed to androgen excess, insulin resistance, and hyper-insulinism [9]. Obesity is associated with an increased peripheral aromatization of androgens to estrogens and with reduced hepatic synthesis of sex hormone-binding globulin, causing an increase in free estradiol and testosterone, which leads to abnormal folliculogenesis and follicular atresia.

In the last 20 years, obesity has been reported to be a relevant risk factor for the development of different types of cancer (mammary, renal, esophageal, gastrointestinal, reproductive, etc.) [5].

Considering the prevalence of obesity worldwide, it is not surprising that obesity now competes with smoking tobacco as the leading preventable risk factor for cancer, being responsible for approximately 14% and 20% of all cancer-related deaths in male and female subjects, respectively [10].

Significant clinical symptoms of depression, poor self-esteem, and body image distortions occur in around 25–30% of obese subjects, who, moreover, feel and are frequently socially isolated and discriminated. In addition to these psychological problems, the severely obese subjects show marked impairment in their daily living activities (such as walking, climbing stairs, and bathing) and decreased postural control and stability, all these limitations causing marked distress and disability.

The main economic repercussions of obesity are low productivity, unemployment, and direct healthcare costs [11]. The latter refer to money spent on hospitalization, medical consultations in outpatient clinics, and the consumption of medications in order to treat health problems related to obesity, and the former are indirect costs related to loss of productivity or to the economy outside of the health sector.

The association between BMI and mortality substantially varies between populations and causes of death and can change over time.

The study of Flegal et al. [12] reported that grade 2 obesity and grade 3 obesity were both related to significantly higher all-cause mortality, while grade 1 was not associated with higher mortality, thus indicating that the excess mortality in obesity is predominantly due to the elevated mortality at higher BMI levels. In another study [13], over a BMI of 25 each 5 kg/m^2 increment was associated with significantly increased all-cause mortality (40% higher vascular, 120% higher diabetes, 80% higher kidney, and 10% higher neoplastic mortality).

Retrospectively applying the Edmonton obesity staging system (EOSS) [14] to the National Health and Nutrition Examination Survey (NHANES) data, patients in stages 2–4 of EOSS have increased all-cause mortality compared to stage 0 or 1. These authors concluded that the severity of the medical complication(s) exerted a more negative effect on survival than BMI itself [15] (Table 2).

Table 2 Edmonton obesity staging system

Stage	Obesity-related risk factors	Physical symptoms, psychopathology, functional limitations, and impairment of well-being
0	None (normal blood pressure, serum lipids, fasting glucose, etc.)	None
1	Subclinical (borderline hypertension, impaired fasting glucose, elevated liver enzymes, etc.)	Mild
2	Established (hypertension, type 2 diabetes mellitus, sleep apnea, osteoarthritis, reflux disease, polycystic ovary syndrome, anxiety disorder, etc.)	Moderate
3	Established end-organ damage (myocardial infarction, heart failure, diabetic complications, incapacitating osteoarthritis, etc.)	Significant
4	Severe disabilities (potentially end-stage disabilities, etc.)	Severe

Main Treatments

A comprehensive or multicomponent lifestyle intervention (i.e., lifestyle or behavioral training, dietary change with energy intake reduction, and physical activity increase) is the starting point for obesity management [16].

A schematic guide to selecting treatment for obesity, based on BMI categories and comorbidities, is reported in Table 3.

Despite the great number of weight loss diets available (all based on the reduction in the total energy intake), few of them have been actually studied in a systematic way.

The most popular dietary programs include low calorie (i.e., a deficit of 500 calories per day), very low calorie (i.e., a total daily calorie intake of less than or equal to 800 kcal/day), high protein, and low carbohydrate and low fat.

Adherence is difficult for most of the participants on any diet. Despite weight loss in individuals who were able to adhere to the diet, no single diet actually results in a satisfactory long-term adherence rate.

Interestingly, diet adherence is the most important predictor of weight loss and reduction in cardiovascular risk factors than the specific diet. Potentially, improvements in dietary adherence may be carried out by offering the patients a variety of dietary options and matching their preference, lifestyle, and cardiovascular profile to optimize weight loss and thus health benefits [17].

Increased physical activity is a basic element of the comprehensive lifestyle intervention for obesity management. Although some reports indicate that exercise alone can determine a 2–3% BMI reduction [18], a more effective (and long-term persistent) weight loss is reported to occur when exercise is associated with dietary changes.

Table 3 A guide to selecting treatment

	BMI category				
Treatment	25–26.9 kg/m²	27–29.9 kg/m²	30–34 kg/m²	35–39.9 kg/m²	≥ 40 kg/m²
Diet, exercise and behavior therapy	With comorbidities	With comorbidities	+	+	+
Pharmacotherapy		With comorbidities	+	+	+
Surgery			With comorbidities		

Adapted from the National Institutes of Health and North American Association for the Study of Obesity.

A starting program of 30–45 min of moderate exercise (i.e., brisk walking) at least 3 days per week is recommended, and this amount of physical exercise allows us to expend approximately 150 kcal/day (i.e., 500 to 1000 calories per week). However, some obese patients may need a loss of 2000 calories or more per week to ensure weight loss maintenance.

Behavioral strategies are designed to change patients' dietary and exercise habits. These strategies include eating habits and physical activity self-monitoring, stress management of situations that lead to overeating, avoiding situations that lead to incidental eating, cognitive restructuring to correct unrealistic goals and misconceptions about weight loss and body image, social support from family and friends, and relapse prevention after episodes of overeating or weight gain. Regular behavioral therapy and regular contact with treatment providers are crucial to achieve and maintain long-term weight loss.

As far as anti-obesity drug therapy is concerned [19, 20], a wide variety of weight loss agents have been tested and proposed for the use in the last decades. Currently, the major FDA-approved anti-obesity agents are as follows: phentermine, orlistat, phentermine/topiramate-extended release (ER), naltrexone-sustained release (SR)/bupropion SR, liraglutide, and semaglutide [20]. Although most of these drugs are reported to determine a significant weight loss in clinical trials, individual variations in response rates are frequently observed.

Drug therapy is indicated for those individuals who cannot achieve weight loss despite an adequate attempt at lifestyle modification. Pharmacotherapy should only be prescribed in association with changes in lifestyle and not as monotherapy for obesity.

Suitable candidates for pharmacological treatment may be those individuals with a BMI of 30 kg/m² or more without concomitant comorbidities and those with a BMI of 27.0 kg/m² to 29.9 kg/m² suffering from two of the following conditions (hypertension, dyslipidemia, coronary artery disease, T2DM, or sleep apnea).

Considering obesity as a chronic disease, pharmacologic treatment should be in the long term, as for the current management of T2DM. In this respect, multicenter trials are mandatory to evaluate the efficacy and safety of current and future medications on a long-term basis.

The weight loss effects obtained with endoscopically placed balloons appear to be transient and inconsistent [21]. This procedure consists of inserting a soft, saline-filled balloon intra-gastrically, able to induce satiety and restriction. Placement can be complicated by nausea, vomiting, abdominal pain, gastric erosions, ulcers, balloon deflation, and balloon migration, resulting in bowel obstruction.

Usually, balloons need to be removed and replaced every 3–6 months to prevent complications; if they are placed for longer periods, appropriate monitoring with imaging is required.

Patients with severe obesity may undergo weight loss surgeries (i.e., restrictive, malabsorptive, or combination procedures). Recent joint guidelines advise that the surgical approach should be reserved for patients with BMI over 40 kg/m^2 regardless of comorbidities, for patients with BMI of 35–40 kg/m^2 in the presence of a severe obesity-related comorbidity, and for patients with BMI 30–35 kg/m^2 in the presence of a severe obesity-related comorbidity, such as diabetes [22].

The rapid, marked, and long-lasting weight loss obtained with the surgical approach, associated with an acceptable safety profile [19, 23], is able to reduce effectively the multiple obesity-associated comorbidities [24], such as diabetes, CVD, stroke, heart failure, malignancy, and OSA [25, 26].

Sexuality and Quality of Life

Many studies have investigated the characteristics of male and female sexual dysfunction in patients diagnosed with obesity.

In particular, Kaneshiro et al. [27] investigated the possible connection between body mass and sexual behavior, investigating sexual orientation, age at first intercourse, experience of sexual intercourse with a male partner, number of partners, and frequency of intercourse.

The 2002 National Survey of Family Growth, a nationally representative, cross-sectional database in which women between the ages of 15 and 44 were interviewed and asked, among other things, whether they had ever been pregnant, was used.

Sexual behavior was compared between body mass index groups: normal (less than 25 m/kg), overweight (25–30 m/kg), and obese (greater than 30 m/kg), using self-reported height and weight. Results showed that body mass index was not significantly associated with sexual orientation, age at first intercourse, frequency of heterosexual intercourse, and number of lifetime or current male partners. Overweight and obese women were more likely to have never engaged in sexual intercourse with a partner, and their sexual behavior differed little between women with different body mass indexes.

However, a more recent study by Carretero Gómez et al. [28] reiterated the importance of the holistic approach in the diagnosis and treatment of obesity. Between September 2019 and January 2020, an online survey was distributed to members of the Spanish Society of Internal Medicine.

A total of 599 responses were obtained. The mean age of the respondents was 44.4 ± 11 years, and 52.1% were women. Approximately 91.8% of internists assessed their patients to exclude obesity-associated comorbidities, mainly type 2 diabetes mellitus (96.2%), cardiovascular disease (88.9%), and obesity-associated hypoventilation syndrome (73%). Approximately 79.9% gave indications for life-style changes. About 64.1% and 74.9% of the respondents were familiar with the indications for medication and bariatric surgery, respectively. About 93.8% and 83% of the respondents considered obesity and excess weight to be a chronic disease and 88.7% considered it to be a disease of specific interest to internists, who should take an active and leading role in its treatment (85.3%).

Changing one's body mass is not only a question of diagnosis and treatment: How do patients experience the change in image, quality of life, and sexual habits? Especially after surgical treatment?

Kinzl et al. [29] conducted a study to determine what consequences surgery for morbid obesity has on sexual attitudes and relationships in obese female patients.

To this end, semi-structured interviews concerning socio-demographic data, sexuality, and relationships were conducted with 82 patients before surgery and 1 year after surgery.

It would appear that physical appearance played the main role in the decision to undergo weight reduction surgery in only 17% of the patients in the study. After surgery, half of the patients were satisfied with their appearance 1 year after surgery, and the remaining 50% of patients expressed disappointment and inadequacy.

Before surgery, 44% of patients reported that their sexuality with their partner was satisfactory and the frequency of sexual intercourse was regular. After surgery, 63% of patients reported enjoying sex more, compared to 12% of patients who enjoyed sex less than before surgery. After surgery, 20% of patients reported that the partnership had changed positively and 10% negatively.

This shows the complexity of the psychological and relational aspects of obesity: lack of self-esteem, unsatisfactory relationships, or collective stigmatization of obese individuals. Uncontrolled eating, often found in patients with morbid obesity, seemed to be less conditioned by the extent of sexual problems, but more a result of psychosocial or psychological problems. While in every patient the desire and body ideal were for a slim individual well accepted by all, becoming obese showed the unpreparedness to face, through a desirable body, the judgment, the external criticism, the anxiety of not being accepted, and the frustration of competing with a world that demands a high performance in every sphere of life: profession, affections, social relations, and sexuality.

Sexual dysfunction does certainly appear to be related to obesity, but clinicians and patients rarely talk about it, neglecting an aspect suffered by the individual and the partner [30]. In particular, the scientific literature has investigated male sexual dysfunction related to sexuality, but there seems to be little research between the female sexual function index (FSFI) and body weight.

In particular, the following have been investigated: persistent or recurrent sexual interest/desire disorders, subjective and genital arousal disorders, orgasm disorders, and pain and difficulty with attempted or incomplete intercourse [31, 32].

The FSFI, which is a 19-item validated self-assessment tool, well described by Rosen et al. is the most widely used [33].

It is unclear whether obese women have sexual dysfunction more often than non-obese women. Data from clinical trials suggest an ambiguous association between obesity and sexual satisfaction in young women [34].

Veronelli et al. [35] reported that obese women had a lower FSFI questionnaire score than healthy women and a higher FSFI score was associated with healthier anthropometric and metabolic status. Furthermore, the FSFI global score was negatively correlated with known risk factors for cardiovascular disease, such as blood pressure, HbA1c, low-density lipoprotein cholesterol, and TSH, while it was positively correlated with high-density lipoprotein cholesterol [36].

Obesity researchers have a growing interest in measuring the impact of weight and weight reduction on quality of life. The Impact of Weight on Quality of Life (IWQOL) questionnaire was the first self-assessment tool specifically developed to assess the effect of obesity on quality of life. Although the IWQOL has demonstrated excellent psychometric properties, its length (74 items) makes it somewhat cumbersome as an outcome metric in clinical research. This report describes the development of a 31-item version of the IWQOL (IWQOL-Lite).

IWQOL-Lite consists of five scales:

1. Physical function (11 items)
2. Self-esteem (7 items)
3. Sexual life (4 items)
4. Public distress (5 items)
5. Work (4 items)

The correlation between the new 31-item instrument (IWQOL-Lite) and the longer 74-item instrument (IWQOL) was 0.97.

In this regard, the study by Fontaine et al. [37] examined for comparison the health-related quality of life (HRQL) as measured by the Medical Outcomes Study Short Form-36 Health Survey (SF-36) and the clinical characteristics of 312 consecutive individuals seeking outpatient care for obesity. SF-36 scores were adjusted for socio-demographic factors and various comorbidities, including depression, to better estimate the effect of obesity on HRQL. The health-related quality of life of obese patients was then compared with that of the general population and with a sample of patients with other chronic medical conditions.

Compared to general population norms, participants who had an average body mass index (BMI) of 38.1 reported significantly lower scores (i.e., more impairment) on all eight domains of quality of life, particularly physical pain and vitality. People with morbid obesity (mean BMI, 48.7) reported significantly worse physical, social, and role functioning, worse perceived general health, and more physical pain than people with mild obesity (mean BMI, 29.2) or moderately to severely obese (mean BMI, 34.5). The obese also reported significantly greater disability due to body pain than patients with other chronic medical conditions.

Conclusion

The epidemic of obesity has underlined the extent of the risks associated with this disease. A thorough medical assessment is required to identify patients who are obese or at risk for obesity or obesity-related complications.

The medical evaluation should entail a complete history (eating patterns, behavioral patterns, physical activity, weight history, attempts at weight loss, and obesity-related risk factors and complications) and a careful physical examination, as well as appropriate laboratory and diagnostic testing [38].

Selecting the appropriate obesity therapy can be guided by BMI and obesity-related complications [39].

The available therapeutic armamentarium ranges from non-pharmacological therapy, such as cognitive and behavioral treatment, physical activity, and diets, up to pharmacotherapy and to endoscopic/surgical procedures.

Since obesity is a multifactorial disease, combination treatment may be necessary to target more than one pathogenetic factor, as it occurs in T2DM and NAFLD management, both diseases being closely associated with obesity.

The multifactorial pathogenesis of obesity must render its management more personalized on an individual basis in the future, in order to be more effective in the long term.

Epidemiological studies suggest that modifiable health behaviors, including physical activity and slimness, are associated with a reduced risk of erectile dysfunction (ED) among men. Obesity, however, may be a risk factor for sexual dysfunction in both sexes; the high prevalence of ED in patients with cardiovascular risk factors suggests that abnormalities in the vasodilator system of penile arteries play an important role in the pathophysiology of ED. It has been shown that one third of obese men with erectile dysfunction can resume sexual activity 2 years after adopting healthy behaviors, mainly regular exercise and weight reduction.

Certainly, the multidisciplinary clinical approach, including the sexologist, would allow the patient's adherence to the therapeutic plan to be scanned according to their psychic state and their relationship with the outside world. Proposing only goals of weight loss and increased psycho-sexual performance could produce in the patient unbearable anxiety for goals that are too demanding. An individualized progression of the various therapies (nutritional, cardiological, physical, etc.) would make it possible to respect the patient's psychic downtime, feelings of tiredness, and discouragement. Introducing these aspects into a personalized plan would also allow the patient to accept these moments of fatigue and to live them as "normal" in any process of change in progress.

References

1. NCD Risk Factor Collaboration. Trends in adult body-mass index in 200 countries from 1975 to 2014: a pooled analysis of 1698 population-based measurement studies with 19.2 million participants. Lancet. 2016;387(10026):1377–96.

2. Young LR, et al. The contribution of expanding portion sizes to the US obesity epidemic. Am J Public Health. 2002;92(2):246–9.
3. Pischon T. Use of obesity biomarkers in cardiovascular epidemiology. Dis Markers. 2009;26(5–6):247–63.
4. Haslam DW, et al. Obesity. Lancet. 2005;366(9492):1197–209.
5. Nimptsch K, et al. Body fatness, related biomarkers and cancer risk: an epidemiological perspective. Horm Mol Biol Clin Investig. 2015;22(2):39–51.
6. Dixon JB. Obesity and diabetes: the impact of bariatric surgery on type-2 diabetes. World J Surg. 2009;33(10):2014–21.
7. Meisinger C, et al. Body fat distribution and risk of type 2 diabetes in the general population: are there differences between men and women? The MONICA/KORA Augsburg cohort study. Am J Clin Nutr. 2006;84(3):483–9.
8. Hartemink N, et al. Combining risk estimates from observational studies with different exposure cutpoints: a meta-analysis on body mass index and diabetes type 2. Am J Epidemiol. 2006;163(11):1042–52.
9. Pasquali R, et al. Obesity and infertility. Curr Opin Endocrinol Diabetes Obes. 2007;14(6): 482–7.
10. Quail DF. The obese adipose tissue microenvironment in cancer development and progression. Nat Rev Endocrinol. 2019;15(3):139–54.
11. Lehnert T, et al. Economic costs of overweight and obesity. Best Pract Res Clin Endocrinol Metab. 2013;27(2):105–15.
12. Flegal KM, et al. Association of all- cause mortality with overweight and obesity using standard body mass index categories: a systematic review and meta-analysis. JAMA. 2013;309(1):71–82.
13. Nimptsch K, et al. Diagnosis of obesity and use of obesity biomarkers in science and clinical medicine. Metabolism. 2019;92:61–70.
14. Kushner RF. Clinical assessment and management of adult obesity. Circulation. 2012;126(24):2870–7.
15. Kuk JL, et al. Edmonton obesity staging system: association with weight history and mortality risk. Appl Physiol Nutr Metab. 2011;36(4):570–6.
16. Sweeting AN. Approaches to obesity management. Intern Med J. 2017;47(7):734–9.
17. Gibson AA. Strategies to improve adherence to dietary weight loss interventions in research and real-world settings. Behav Sci. 2017;7(3):44.
18. Garrow JS, et al. Meta-analysis: effect of exercise, with or without dieting, on the body composition of overweight subjects. Eur J Clin Nutr. 1995;49(1):1–10.
19. Pilitsi E, et al. Pharmacotherapy of obesity: available medications and drugs under investigation. Metabolism. 2019;92:170–92.
20. Muller TD, et al. Anti-obesity drug discovery: advances and challenges. Nat Rev Drug Discov. 2021;21:1–23. https://doi.org/10.1038/s41573-021-00337-8. PMID: 34815532.
21. Mathus-Vliegen EM, et al. Intragastric balloon for treatment resistant obesity: safety, tolerance, and efficacy of 1-year balloon treatment followed by a 1-year balloon-free follow-up Gastrointest Endosc. 2005;61(1):19–27.
22. Mechanick JI, et al. Clinical practice guidelines for the perioperative nutritional, metabolic, and nonsurgical support of the bariatric surgery patient-2013 update: cosponsored by American Association of Clinical Endocrinologists, the Obesity Society, and American Society for Metabolic & Bariatric Surgery. Obesity. 2013;21(suppl 1):S1–27.
23. Courcoulas AP, et al. Seven-year weight trajectories and health outcomes in the longitudinal assessment of bariatric surgery (LABS) study. JAMA Surg. 2018;153(5):427–34.
24. Sjöström L, et al. Association of bariatric surgery with long-term remission of type 2 diabetes and with microvascular and macrovascular complications. JAMA. 2014;311(22):2297–304.
25. Sjöström L, et al. Effects of bariatric surgery on cancer incidence in obese patients in Sweden (Swedish Obese Subjects Study): a prospective, controlled intervention trial. Lancet Oncol. 2009;10(7):653–62.

26. Sjöström L, et al. Bariatric surgery and long-term cardiovascular events. JAMA. 2012;307(1):56–65.
27. Kaneshiro B, Jensen JT, Carlson NE, Harvey SM, Nichols MD, Edelman AB. Body mass index and sexual behavior. Obstet Gynecol. 2008;112(3):586–92. https://doi.org/10.1097/AOG.0b013e31818425ec.
28. Carretero Gómez J, Ena J, Arévalo Lorido JC, Seguí Ripoll JM, Carrasco-Sánchez FJ, Gómez-Huelgas R, Pérez Soto MI, Delgado Lista J, Pérez Martínez P. Obesity is a chronic disease. Positioning statement of the Diabetes, Obesity and Nutrition Workgroup of the Spanish Society of Internal Medicine (SEMI) for an approach centred on individuals with obesity. Revista Clínica Española (English Edition). 2021;221(9):509–16.
29. Kinzl JF, Trefalt E, Fiala M, et al. Sexual association, sexuality and sexual disorders in morbidly obese women: consequences of weight loss after gastric banding. Obes Surg. 2001;11:455–8.
30. Larsen SH, Wagner G, Heitmann BL. Sexual function and obesity. Int J Obes (London). 2007;31:1189–98.
31. Corona G, Jannini EA, Maggi M. Inventories for male and female sexual dysfunctions. Int J Impot Res. 2006;18:236–50.
32. World Health Organization. Obesity: preventing and managing the global epidemic. Report of a WHO consultation on obesity. Geneva: WHO; 1997.
33. Lue T, Bassoon R, Rosen R, Giuliano F, Khoury S, Montorsi F. Sexual medicine. Sexual dysfunction in men and women. 2nd International Consultation on Sexual Dysfunction. Health Publication: Paris; 2004.
34. Borges R, Temido P, Sousa L, Azinhais P, Conceição P, Pereira B, et al. Metabolic syndrome (dys) sexual function. J Sex Med. 2009;6:2958–75.
35. Rosen R, Brown C, Heiman J, Leiblum S, Meston C, Shabsign R, et al. The Female Sexual Function Index (FSFI): a multidimensional self-assessment tool for assessing female sexual function. J Sex Marit Ther. 2000;26:191–208.
36. Veronelli A, Mauri C, Zecchini B, Peca MG, Turri O, Valitutti MT, et al. Sexual dysfunction is common in premenopausal women with diabetes, obesity and hypothyroidism and correlates with markers of increased cardiovascular risk. A preliminary report. J Sex Med. 2009;6:1561–8.
37. Fontaine KR, Cheskin LJ, Barofsky I. Health-related quality of life in obese persons seeking treatment. J Fam Pract. 1996;43(3):265–70. PMID: 8797754.
38. Samaha FF, et al. A low-carbohydrate as compared with a low-fat diet in severe obesity. New Engl J Med. 2003;348(21):2074–81.
39. Serdula MK, et al. Prevalence of attempting weight loss and strategies for controlling weight. JAMA. 1999;282(14):1353–8.
40. Padwal RS, et al. Using the Edmonton obesity staging system to predict mortality in a population-representative cohort of people with overweight and obesity. CMAJ. 2011;183(14):E1059–66.
41. Esposito K, Giugliano D. Obesity, metabolic syndrome and sexual dysfunction. Int J Impot Res. 2005;17:391–8.

Part IX
Gynaecology

Premature Ovarian Failure

Raffaella Chionna, Stefano Salvatore, and Elena Vittoria Longhi

Natural menopause occurs at a median age of 51.4 years [1], and it is due to complete, or near-complete, ovarian follicular depletion, resulting in sex steroid deficiency and high follicle-stimulating hormone (FSH).

Primary hypogonadism is defined as an ovarian failure in the presence of high serum FSH concentration in women under the age of 40 years [1].

Premature ovarian failure is nowadays referred to as primary ovarian insufficiency (POI).

POI is characterized by infertility due to the loss of oocytes and deficiency of ovarian estrogen. POI affects 1% of women before age 40 and 0.1% before age 30. Diminished ovarian reserve is not a synonym for POI. Five to 10% of patients with POI can conceive and have regular pregnancies even several years after the diagnosis was performed [2].

Etiopathogenesis

There are multiple potential etiologies for POI. Some of them do not imply follicle depletion, some accelerate follicle depletion, and some are due to decreased steroid production. The cause of POI remains unknown in approximately 75% of cases.

R. Chionna (✉)
Gynecology and Obstetrics Unit, Menopause Center, IRCCS San Raffaele, Milan, Italy
e-mail: chionna.raffaella@hsr.it

S. Salvatore
Gynecology and Obstetrics Unit, Vita and Salute University, IRCCS San Raffaele, Milan, Italy
e-mail: salvatore.stefano@hsr.it

E. V. Longhi
Department of Sexual Medical Center, San Raffaele Hospital, Milano, Italy

© Springer Nature Switzerland AG 2023
E. V. Longhi (ed.), *Managing Psychosexual Consequences in Chronic Diseases*,
https://doi.org/10.1007/978-3-031-31307-3_14

Primary Hypogonadism without Follicle Depletion These disorders result in decreased estradiol and the absence of normal FSH-negative feedback. The main mechanisms of these types of primary hypogonadism without follicle depletion are the following:

- Endogenous activation of the gonadotropin receptor
- Steroidogenic enzyme defects that prevent estrogen production

FSH Receptor Mutation A mutation in the gene coding for the FSH receptor results in the production of receptors that bind FSH poorly. This does not stimulate the aromatization of the precursor to estradiol causing estrogen deficiency. LH receptor gene mutation has been reported too.

Genetic Disorders that Accelerate the Rate of Follicle Depletion

- *Turner's Syndrome:* Due to the lack of a second X chromosome (45X0), Tuner's syndrome is the most common cause of POI, occurring in up to 1 of 2500 live births. The ovaries in Turner's syndrome have no follicles or few atretic follicles, and this phenotype presents absent pubertal development, multiple morphologic defects, and primary amenorrhea. However, the dysfunctions and defects are variable, and most of these women have primary amenorrhea, although some of them develop normally and have secondary amenorrhea. Few have no morphologic defects [3, 4].
- *Other X Chromosome Deletion/Translocation.* X chromosome inversion, duplication, deletion, and balanced X chromosome to autosome translocations are the most frequent causes of POI.

Small deletions and breakpoints in translocated X chromosomes (like from Xq13 to Xq26) that are involved in ovarian function can cause POI [5].

- *Fragile X Syndrome*: Approximately 6% of cases of POI are associated with premutation in the FMR1 gene (the gene responsible for the fragile X syndrome). This syndrome is characterized by intellectual disability, developmental delay, tremor, ataxia, dementia, and POI [6, 7].
- *Galactosemia*: This somatic chromosomal defect may cause POI due to the toxic effects of increased galactose metabolites. This causes abnormalities in the carbohydrate composition of gonadotropins that reduce their bioactivity therefore impacting ovarian function [8].
- *Genes Associated with 46, XX Gonadal Dysgenesis*: In the last few years, new genes have been discovered using whole-exome sequencing. These mutations appear to be a rare cause of POI but have to be considered especially mainly in consanguineous families (STAG3, BRACA2, ESR2, SYCE1, MCM8, and MCM9).
- *Mutation in FOXL2 gene.*
- *Ataxia telangiectasia.*
- *Progressive external ophthalmoplegia*, a mitochondrial disorder with increased risk of POI.

- *Autoimmune Ovarian Failure:* Type I and type II syndromes of polyglandular autoimmune failure are associated with autoantibodies to multiple endocrine glands and other organs. In these disorders, the primordial follicles are spared, but there is strong histological evidence that POI occurs due to an intense lymphocytic infiltration of thecal cells. If effective immunosuppressive therapy is used early in the course of the disease, ovarian function might be preserved.

Iatrogenic Causes Chemotherapy, radiation therapy, surgery (bilateral oophorectomy).

Other Causes Viral infection, smoke cigarette, nulliparity.

Clinical Symptoms of POI

Most of the symptoms of POI are secondary to estrogen deficiency:

- **Vasomotor Symptoms**: Hot flushes and night sweats, sleep disorder, insomnia.
- **Vaginal dryness, dyspareunia, and decreased sexual desire.**
- **Irregular Menstrual Cycles** or **Amenorrhea with Infertility**: Women with POI should be informed that there is a small chance of spontaneous pregnancy and should be advised to use contraception if they wish to avoid pregnancy, although the probability of this happening is very low.

Risks and Health Complications of POI

- **Bone Loss**, Risk of Osteopenia, and Osteoporosis. A large number of studies have provided strong evidence that early age at menopause is associated with an increased risk of fracture (1.5- to 3-fold higher than the risk for women who experience menopause at the age of 50 years) [9, 10].

- The incidence of hip fracture in patients with POI diagnosed at 40 years of age is 9.4% compared with 3.3% in those women hitting menopause at age 50.
- **Cardiovascular morbidity** increases the mortality risk possibly related to endothelial dysfunction and increases the risk of type 2 diabetes mellitus (small increase in mortality due to ischemic heart disease and stroke) [10, 11].
- Untreated POI is associated with reduced life expectancy.
- **Infertility:** Any patient at risk for early menopause should consider fertility preservation because there are no interventions that have been shown to increase natural conception. Oocyte donation is an established option for fertility in POI patients [10, 12].
- **Sexual Disorders**: Reduction in sexual well-being and sexual function, vaginal discomfort, and dyspareunia.

- **Genito-Urinary Symptoms.**
- **Cognitive decline** and possible detrimental effect on cognition. This could reach more severe levels such as dementia.
- **Effects of Physical and Emotional Health** like Depression and Anxiety Disorders. This diagnosis destroys the patient's life plan with symptoms of grief and anger, negative self-image, and sadness. In these patients, psychological support should be offered [10].

Diagnosis of Premature Ovarian Failure

The diagnosis of POI is based on the following diagnostic criteria in women younger than 40 years of age:

- Oligo/amenorrhea for at least 4 months (amenorrhea is not required to make the diagnosis because POI patients frequently have an intermittent ovarian function).
- Elevated day 3 FSH level in the postmenopausal range (>25 IU/l on two occasions) and low serum estradiol.
- Transvaginal ultrasound.
- Chromosomal analysis and antibody testing should be performed in all women with POI without iatrogenic causes:
- Karyotyping.
- Test for Y-chromosomal material (if positive ovariectomy should be recommended) [13].
- Fragile X premutation testing.
- Screening in immune disorder should be considered in POI (21OH antibodies, TPO-Ab, adrenocortical antibodies (ACA)) [14].

    Most of the time the cause of POI is not identified, and these women are described as idiopathic POI.

    At the moment, there are no proven predictive tests to identify women that will develop POI and there are no established POI-preventing measures.

    Investigations to Exclude Other Disorders: pregnancy test, PRL serum concentration, and TSH-r.

Management of POI

The American College of Obstetrician and Gynecologist gives the following recommendations [15]:

- POI is a pathologic condition that should not be considered natural menopause.
- Common health risks of menopause are the same as POI but in the latter these risks may start as early as the age of 40 and the approach to health care in these women should be different.

- HRT is effective in treating the symptoms of hypoestrogenism and is able to control long-term health risks if not contraindicated. Climateric symptoms should be taken seriously by physicians because these can affect the quality of life and contribute to disease [16].
- HRT reduces the risk of osteoporosis, cardiovascular disease, and urogenital atrophy and improves the quality of life of women with POI [17].
- In POI patients, HRT manages osteoporosis more appropriately than bisphosphonates and should be the first-line therapy.
- HRT is able to control vasomotor symptoms and vaginal dryness. These symptoms may develop before menstrual cycle irregularity and amenorrhea occur.
- HRT is able to control emotional aspects of health like depression and anxiety, which mainly occur after an infertility diagnosis is made [18]. For many women with POI, infertility is the most devastating aspect of the diagnosis.
- The options for child-raising include egg donation using in vitro fertilization or adoption. Spontaneous pregnancies will occur in about 5% to 10% of women with 46, XX sPOI [19].
- Combined hormonal contraceptives prevent ovulation and pregnancy more than HRT and should be considered for those patients who wish for pregnancy prevention.
- The treatment with HRT should be continued until the age of natural menopause is reached (age 50–51 years).

Hormone Replacement Therapy Options

For young women with POI and estrogen deficiency, hormone therapy has to be considered a replacement and a completion of the correct hormonal asset, and it is up to the physician to clarify this point [20].

Estrogen Most of the studies showed that more than 50% of POI patients never took HRT or started HRT after many years from their primary diagnosis or discontinued it prior to age 45.

Ideally, any replacement therapy should mimic normal ovarian function. The transdermal routes of administration deliver hormones directly into the circulation avoiding complications due to the first passage effect on the liver when estrogen is given orally. Risks of venous thromboembolism are increased by oral estrogen [21] compared to transdermal estrogen use. In the ESTHER study on thromboembolism risk in estrogen users, the odds ratio for thromboembolism in women using oral estrogen was 4.2 (95% CI, 1.5–11.6) compared to 0.9 (95% CI, 0.4–2.1) in those using transdermal preparations [22].

In women with obesity or clotting disorders, the venous thromboembolism risk associated with oral estrogen is increased 5–8 times compared to transdermal users. There are three main types of estrogen formulation available, 17B-estradiol (E2), CEE, and ethinylestradiol (EE). E2 is typically esterified or micronized.

Recent trial encourages to use E2 therapy in younger women particularly for better improvement in BMD and for a better impact on long-term cardiovascular health [23].

Compared with oral contraceptive containing ethinylestradiol, 12 months of transdermal HRT resulted in significantly lower blood pressure, lower activation of renin–angiotensin–aldosterone system, and better renal function. This evidence strongly suggests that transdermal HRT is superior to combined oral contraceptives in promoting cardiovascular health in young women with POI [24].

There is no study that investigated the optimal estrogen dose for women with POI.

Progestins Estrogen and progestin should be prescribed in combination in any women with an intact uterus.

The NHI study provides the only long-term-controlled data published regarding HRT for young women with POI. The NHI study used transdermal estradiol with oral MAP (medroxyprogesterone acetate 10 mg). MAP is the only progestin for which we have evidence that demonstrates its ability to protect the endometrium from the risk of hyperplasia and endometrial cancer [25]. Progestin given less frequently than monthly is not recommended.

If oral micronized progestin is effective in inducing a full secretive endometrium in this context where higher dosages of estrogens are used (compared to postmenopausal women in HRT) remains an open question. Some young women with POI use HRT for decades. More supporting evidence regarding the effect of micronized progesterone on the endometrium in the context of a full replacement dose of estradiol is needed before recommending it as a first-line progestin in POI patients.

The North American Society of Menopause (NAMS) recommends systemic hormone therapy until age 50 to 51 years to all women with POI (without contraindications) to manage estrogen deficiency symptoms and prevent long-term health risks associated with POI [26].

Contraindications to estrogen therapy include a history of breast cancer, CHD, a previous venous thromboembolic event or stroke, active liver disease, unexplained vaginal bleeding, and high-risk endometrial cancer [27].

Testosterone Treatment with testosterone has been associated with improved sexual function in oophorectomized women but is not routinely recommended in the setting of POI because there are no adequate data regarding efficacy and long-term safety. Additional study is needed.

Sexuality and Quality of Life

Premature ovarian failure (POF) is a primary ovarian defect characterized by the absence of menarche (primary amenorrhea) or premature depletion of ovarian follicles before age 40 (secondary amenorrhea). It is a heterogeneous disorder affecting approximately 1% of women under the age of 40, 1:10,000 women under the age of 20, and 1:1000 women under the age of 30. The most severe forms present with absent pubertal development and primary amenorrhea (50% of these cases are at ovarian dysgenesis), while the forms with post-pubertal onset are characterized by the disappearance of menstrual cycles (secondary amenorrhea) associated with premature follicular depletion. As in the case of physiological menopause, POF presents with typical climacteric manifestations: infertility associated with palpitations, heat intolerance, hot flashes, anxiety, depression, and fatigue [28].

POF is biochemically characterized by low levels of gonadal hormones (estrogen and inhibins) and high levels of gonadotropins (LH and FSH) (hypergonadotropic amenorrhea). In addition to infertility, hormonal defects can cause serious neurological, metabolic, or cardiovascular consequences and lead to the early onset of osteoporosis. The heterogeneity of POF is also reflected in the variety of possible causes, including autoimmunity, toxic substances, drugs, and genetic defects. POF has a strong genetic component [29].

X chromosome abnormalities (e.g., Turner syndrome) represent the leading cause of primary amenorrhea associated with ovarian dysgenesis. Despite the description of several candidate genes, the cause of POF remains undetermined in the vast majority of cases. Management includes the replacement of the hormonal defect with estrogen/progestin preparations. The only solution currently available for fertility defect in women with absent follicular reserve is egg donation [30].

How important is family history? DW Cramer et al. [31] asked this question in a study conducted on a sample of 10,606 women between 45 and 54 years of age, selecting 344 cases with early menopause (mean age: 42.2 years) and 344 controls of the same age who were still menstruating or experienced menopause after the age of 46 years. Subjects were interviewed about their medical and family history, and blood samples were taken to identify women who were carriers of the classic or Duarte variant of galactosemia, a potential heritable factor for early menopause. Logistic regression analysis was used to estimate the risk of early menopause in women with and without a family history of early menopause.

Results: 1129 (37.5%) of early menopausal cases reported a family history of menopause before age 46 in a mother, sister, aunt, or grandmother compared with 31 (9.0%) of controls with an odds ratio (OR) of 6.1 (95% confidence interval [CI]: 3.9 to 9.4) after adjustment for smoking history, education, parity, and body mass index. The risk of early menopause associated with the same family history was higher: for family history in one sister, OR = 9.1 (95% CI: 3.1 to 26.5); multiple relatives, OR = 12.4 (95% CI: 4.4 to 34.2); and cases menopausal before age 40, OR = 8.4 (95% CI: 2.5 to 31.2). Cases with a family history of early menopause were no more likely to have galactose metabolism errors than cases without a family history or all controls, nor did they possess Turner's stigmata such as short stature, all of which suggests that in addition to the preferential recollection of family history by early menopausal women, a genetic factor including partial X chromosome deletions compatible with lack of male siblings may be intuited.

Premature menopause (POF) seldom occurs in adolescence as primary or secondary amenorrhea [32]. POF in youth is determined by genetic, autoimmune, or dysenzymatic causes. Over the past few decades, due to the high survival rate of childhood malignancies, the cause of POF has become ovarian failure secondary to chemo- and radiotherapy treatments (MIRF).

The fact remains that the relevance of this pathology has recently increased due to the progressive extension of life expectancy and the increasingly frequent postponement of conception beyond 30 years of age [33]. As female fertility already tends to decline 20 years before menopause, women with IOP generally have great difficulty conceiving. IOP presents with the typical manifestations of climacteric, particularly hot flashes and vaginal dryness, and a negative impact on glucose, lipid, and bone metabolism. These disorders predispose the woman with IOP to neuropsychological, cardiovascular, and osteoporosis repercussions. Thus, the premature onset of hypoestrogenism and infertility has a major impact on the well-being of the woman and her family.

This pathology then can induce in patients: [34].

1. Depression and anxiety related to loss of reproductive hormones and infertility.
2. Associated autoimmune adrenal insufficiency or hypothyroidism.
3. Reduced bone mineral density and increased risk of cardiovascular disease related to estrogen deficiency. Approximately 5–10% of women with primary ovarian insufficiency conceive and have a child.

In contrast to menopause proper (over age 50), premature ovarian failure is characterized by intermittent ovarian function in half of young women. These patients produce estrogen intermittently and sometimes even ovulate despite the presence of high gonadotropin levels.

On pelvic ultrasound examination, follicles are just as likely to be detected in patients more than 6 years after a diagnosis of premature ovarian failure as in patients less than 6 years after diagnosis. Therefore, the probability of follicle retrieval appears to remain stable during the normal reproductive life of these young women [35].

With regard to sexuality: This pathology involves hypoactive desire, vaginal dryness, disorders of orgasm and arousal, and dyspareunia. Sleep disorders can also affect the psychological sphere, negatively modifying the mood, the relationship with the partner, and the frequency of sexual intercourse.

Very often the partners of patients with premature ovarian failure put up with mood variations, impatience, and the neurological tension of their partners influencing in no small way conflict, misunderstanding, and emotional distance within the couple.

All of these factors have a dramatic effect on the lives of women and couples. In addition to the age of onset, ethnicity, lifestyle linked to sociocultural factors, the presence or absence of children, and single or cohabiting status, the sexual aspect can be experienced as humiliating, frustrating, painful, and tiring [36]. These patients do not rediscover the female "feeling" of sexuality due to depression, insomnia, decreased desire, difficulty in arousal, orgasm, dyspareunia, vaginal dryness, xerostomia, weight gain, and alteration of "body image." *"Feeling fat and not being able to lose weight," "not considering themselves desirable," and "feeling bloated, physically heavy" are often the expressions with which women suffering from premature ovarian failure describe themselves.*

Another difficult condition for these patients is the association with other diseases: dry eye syndrome [37], myasthenia gravis, rheumatoid arthritis, or systemic lupus erythematosus.

Smith et al. [37] conducted a study evaluating 65 patients with POF and 36 age-matched healthy control patients complaining of dry eye symptoms. Participants were administered the Ocular Surface Disease Index Questionnaire and the 25-item National Eye Institute Visual Function Questionnaire (NEI-VFQ 25). Assessments of ocular surface damage (Oxford and van Bijsterveld vital dye scores) and tear status (Schirmer test 1 [without anesthesia] and 2 [with anesthesia] and tear break-up time) were performed.

It was found that women with POF scored significantly worse than controls on all ocular surface damage parameters: Oxford score (3.2 vs 1.7; $P = 0.001$), conjunctival lissamine green (2.1 vs 1.3; $P = 0.02$), fluorescein corneal staining (1.2 vs 0.4; $P = 0.005$), and the van Bijsterveld score (2.1 vs 1.3; $P = 0.02$). In addition, the percentage of patients with POF who met the dry eye diagnostic criterion of a van Bijsterveld score greater than or equal to 4 was significantly higher among women with POF than among controls (20% vs 3%; $P = 0.02$). The POF group also tended to have worse scores than controls on self-reported symptoms, as measured by the overall ocular surface disease index (12.5 vs 2.1; $P < 0.001$) and the overall NEI-VFQ (94 vs 98; $P = 0.001$) after adjustment for age and race. Schirmer's test scores and tear break-up time did not differ. It was therefore concluded that women with POF were more likely to show ocular surface damage and dry eye symptoms than the age-matched control group.

Conclusion

The study by Groff et al. [38] at the National Institutes of Health Clinical Centre reports the lack of attention that clinicians often pay to patients' emotional responses immediately after being diagnosed with POF at an average age of 28 years. Following telephone interviews with a sample of 100 patients, 71% were dissatisfied with the way they had been informed by their doctor and 89% reported experiencing moderate-to-severe emotional distress at that time. The degree of emotional distress was positively correlated with the degree of dissatisfaction with the way women were informed of their diagnosis. Thorough and accurate medical information about POF, but little or no empathic and supportive approach by clinicians.

The diagnosis of POF can be emotionally traumatic and difficult for patients and partners to absorb. The results of the study suggest that the way in which patients are informed of this diagnosis can have a significant impact on their level of distress. They perceive a need for doctors to spend more time with them and provide more information about POF from a psycho-sexological and relational perspective [39].

References

1. Nelson LM. Clinical practice. Primary ovarian insufficiency. N Engl J Med. 2009;360:606.
2. Van Kasteren YM, Schoemaker J. Premature ovarian failure: a systematic review on therapeutic interventions to restore ovarian function and achieve pregnancy. Hum Reprod Update. 1999;5:483.
3. Sävendahl L, Davenport ML. Delayed diagnoses of Turner's syndrome: proposed guidelines for change. J Pediatr. 2000;137:455.
4. Sylvén L, Hagenfeldt K, Bröndum-Nielsen K, von Schoultz B. Middle-aged women with Turner's syndrome. Medical status, hormonal treatment and social life. Acta Endocrinol. 1991;125:359.
5. Schlessinger D, Herrera L, Crisponi L, et al. Genes and translocations involved in POF. Am J Med Genet. 2002;111:328.
6. Bodega B, Bione S, Dalprà L, et al. Influence of intermediate and uninterrupted FMR1 CGG expansions in premature ovarian failure manifestation. Hum Reprod. 2006;21:952.
7. Hagerman RJ, Leavitt BR, Farzin F, et al. Fragile-X-associated tremor/ataxia syndrome (FXTAS) in females with the FMR1 premutation. Am J Hum Genet. 2004;74:1051.
8. Kaufman FR, Reichardt JK, Ng WG, et al. Correlation of cognitive, neurologic, and ovarian outcome with the Q188R mutation of the galactose-1-phosphate uridyltransferase gene. J Pediatr. 1994;125:225.
9. De Vos M, Devroey P, Fauser BC. Primary ovarian insufficiency. Lancet. 2010;376:911.
10. The ESHRE Guideline Group on POI, Webber L, et al. ESHRE guideline: management of women with premature ovarian insufficiency. Hum Reprod. 2016;31(5):926–37.
11. Rocca WA, Grossardt BR, Miller VM, et al. Premature menopause or early menopause and risk of ischemic stroke. Menopause. 2012;19:272.
12. Oyesanya OA, Olufowoby O, Ross W, Sharif K, Afnan M. Prognosos of oocyte donation cycles. Fertil Steril. 2009;92:930–6.
13. Rocha VB, Guerra-junior G, Marquez de Faria AP, De Mello MP, Maciel Guerra AT. Complete gonadal dysgenesis in clinical practice: the 46 XY karyotype accounts for more than one third of cases. Fertil Steril. 2011;96:1431–4.
14. Husebye ES, Lovas K. Immunology of Addison's disease and premature ovarian failure. Endocrinol Metab Clin N Am. 2009;38:389–405.
15. Committee Opinion of American College of Obstetricians and Gynecologist. 2017:698.
16. Thurston RC. Are vasomotor symptoms associated with alterations in hemostatic and inflammatory markers? Study of Women's health Across the Nation. Menopause. 2011;18:1044–51.
17. Gallagher JC. Effect of early menopause on bone density and fracture. Menopause. 2007;14:567–71.
18. Schmidt PJ, Luff JA, Haq NA. Depression in women with spontaneous 46, XX primary ovarian insufficiency. J Clin Endocrinol Metab. 2011;96:278–87
19. Popat VB, Vanderhoof VH, Calis KA, Troendle JF, Nelson LM. Normalization of serum luteinizing hormone levels in women with 46, XX spontaneous primary ovarian insufficiency. Fertil Steril. 2008;89:429–33.
20. Sullivan SD, Sarrel PM, Nelson L. Hormone replacement therapy in young women with primary ovarian insufficiency and early menopause. Fert Steril. 2016;106:1588–99.
21. Smith NL, Blondon M, Wiggins KL, Harrington LB, et al. Lower risk of cardiovascular event in menopausal women taking oral estradiol compared with oral conjugated equine estrogens. JAMA Intern Med. 2014;174:25–31.
22. Canonico M, Oger E, Plu-Bureau G, Conard J, et al. Hormone replacement therapy and venous thromboembolism among postmenopausal women: impact of the route of estrogen administration and progestogens: the ESTHER study. Circulation. 2007;115:840–5.
23. Cartwright B, Robinson J, Seed PT, Fogelman I, Rymer L. Hormon replacement therapy versus the combined oral contraceptive pill in premature ovarian failure: a randomized controlled trial of effect on mineral density. J Clin Endocrinol Metab. 2016;101:3497–505.

24. Langrish JP, Mills NL, Bath LE, Warner P, Webb DJ, Kelnar, et al. Cardiovascular effects of physiological and standard sex steroid replacement regimens in premature ovarian failure. Hypertension. 2009;53:805–11.
25. Bjarnason K, Cerin A, Lindgren R, Weber T. Adverse endometrial effects during long cycle hormone replacement therapy. Scandinavian Long Cycle Study. Maturitas. 1999;32:161–70.
26. Position statement of NAMS. Menopause 2017;24(7):728–53.
27. Stuenkel CA, Davis SR, Gompel A, Lumsden MA, Murad MH, Pinkerton JV, Santen RJ. Treatment of symptoms of menopause. An Endocrine Society Clinical Practice Guideline. J Clin Endocrinol Metab. 2015;100(11):3975.
28. Beck-Peccoz P, Persani L. Insufficienza ovarica prematura. Orphanet J Rare Dis. 2006;1:9. https://doi.org/10.1186/1750-1172-1-9.
29. Chiauzzi VA, Bussmann L, Calvo JC, Sundblad V, Charreau EH. Circulating immunoglobulins that inhibit follicle-stimulating hormone receptor binding: a presumed diagnostic role in resistant ovary syndrome. Clin Endocrinol. 2004;61:46–54. https://doi.org/10.1111/j.1365-2265.2004.02054.x.
30. Achermann JC, Ozisik G, Meeks JJ, Jameson JL. Perspective: genetic causes of human reproductive diseases. J Clin Metab Endocrinol. 2002;87:2447–54. https://doi.org/10.1210/jc.87.6.2447.
31. Cramer DW, Xu H, Harlow BL. Family history as a predictor of early menopause. Fertil Steril. 1995;64(4):740–5. https://doi.org/10.1016/s0015-0282(16)57849-2. PMID: 7672145.
32. Garofalo P, De Sanctis V. Premature ovarian failure: menopause in the periadolescential period. Endocrinologist. 2003;4:19–28.
33. Persani L, Moretti C. Taking care of premature ovarian failure over time. Endocrinologist. 2016;17:111–3.
34. Martin LA, Porter AG, Pelligrini VA, Schnatz PF, Jiang X, Kleinstreuer N, Hall JE, Verbiest S, Olmstead J, Fair R, Falorni A, Persani L, Rajkovic A, Mehta K, Nelson LM, Rachel's Well Primary Ovarian Insufficiency Community of Practice Group. A design thinking approach to primary ovarian insufficiency. Panminerva Med. 2017;59(1):15–32. https://doi.org/10.23736/S0031-0808.16.03259-6. Epub 2016 Nov 9. PMID: 27827529.
35. Kalantaridou SN, Nelson LM. Premature ovarian failure is not premature menopause. Ann N Y Acad Sci. 2000;900:393–402. https://doi.org/10.1111/j.1749-6632.2000.tb06251.x. PMID: 10818427.
36. Persani L, Bonomi M, Rossetti R. Insufficienza ovarica primaria: elementi per una gestione up-to-date. L'Endocrinologo. 2015;16:45–50.
37. Smith JA, Vitale S, Reed GF, et al. Dry eye signs and symptoms in women with premature ovarian failure. Arco Ophthalmol. 2004;122:151–6.
38. Groff AA, Covington SN, Halverson LR, Fitzgerald OR, Vanderhoof V, Calis K, Nelson LM. Assessing the emotional needs of women with spontaneous premature ovarian failure. Fertil Steril. 2005;83(6):1734–41. https://doi.org/10.1016/j.fertnstert.2004.11.067. PMID: 15950644.
39. Hipp HS, Charen KH, Spencer JB, Allen EG, Sherman SL. Reproductive and gynecologic care of women with fragile X primary ovarian insufficiency. Menopause. 2016;23:993–9.

Endometriosis and Fertility

Chiara Bosisio, Francesco Maria Fusi, and Elena Vittoria Longhi

Endometriosis Definition

Endometriosis is a common gynecological condition affecting an estimated 2–10% of women of childbearing age. The name of this condition comes from the word "endometrium," which is the tissue that lines the uterus. It is unusual for endometrial tissue to spread beyond your pelvic region, but it is not impossible. During a woman's regular menstrual cycle, this tissue builds up and is shed if she does not become pregnant. Women with endometriosis develop tissue that looks and acts like endometrial tissue outside the uterus, usually on other reproductive organs inside the pelvis or in the whole abdominal cavity. Each month, this misplaced tissue responds to the hormonal changes of the menstrual cycle by building up and breaking down just as the endometrium inside the uterus does, resulting in small bleeding inside the pelvis. This means the tissue will grow, thicken, and break down. This leads to inflammation, swelling, and scarring of the normal tissue surrounding the endometriosis implants. Over time, the tissue that has broken down has nowhere to go and becomes trapped in pelvis. When the ovary is involved, blood can become embedded in the normal ovarian tissue, forming a "blood blister" surrounded by a fibrous cyst, called an endometrioma.

C. Bosisio
Maternal and Pediatric Department USSD Centro PMA, ASST Papa Giovanni XXIII, Bergamo, Italy

F. M. Fusi (✉)
Maternal and Pediatric Department USSD Centro PMA, ASST Papa Giovanni XXIII, Bergamo, Italy

School of Obstetrics University of Milano Bicocca, Milan, Italy
e-mail: ffusi@asst-pg23.it

E. V. Longhi
Department of Sexual Medical Center, San Raffaele Hospital, Milano, Italy

© Springer Nature Switzerland AG 2023

E. V. Longhi (ed.), *Managing Psychosexual Consequences in Chronic Diseases*,
https://doi.org/10.1007/978-3-031-31307-3_15

This tissue trapped in the pelvis or in the ovary can cause:

- irritation
- scar formation
- adhesions, in which tissue binds your pelvic organs together
- severe pain during your periods
- fertility problems

Endometriosis Symptoms

The symptoms of endometriosis vary. The following are the most common symptoms for endometriosis, but each woman may experience symptoms differently or some may not exhibit any symptoms at all. Pelvic pain is the most common symptom of endometriosis.

Symptoms of endometriosis may also include:

- Excessive menstrual cramps that may be felt in the abdomen or lower back
- Pain during intercourse
- Abnormal or heavy menstrual flow
- Infertility
- Painful urination during menstrual periods
- Painful bowel movements during menstrual periods
- Other gastrointestinal problems, such as diarrhea, constipation, and/or nausea

It is important to note that the amount of pain a woman experiences is not necessarily related to the severity of the disease. Some women with severe endometriosis may experience no pain, while others with a milder form of the disease may have severe pain or other symptoms.

A patient may also have no symptoms. It is important to get regular gynecological exams, which will allow the gynecologist to monitor any changes. This is particularly important if two or more symptoms are present.

Causes of Endometriosis

The exact cause of endometriosis is not known, and there are several theories regarding the cause, although no one theory has been scientifically proven. One of the oldest theories is that endometriosis occurs due to a process called retrograde menstruation. This happens when menstrual blood flows back through fallopian tubes into pelvic cavity instead of leaving the body through the vagina. One theory suggests that during menstruation, some of the tissue backs up through the fallopian tubes into the abdomen, a sort of "reverse menstruation," where it attaches and grows. Another theory is that hormones transform the cells outside the uterus into cells similar to those lining the inside of the uterus, known as endometrial cells. Another theory suggests that endometrial tissue may travel and implant via blood or lymphatic channels, similar to the way cancer cells spread. A third theory suggests that cells in any location may transform into endometrial cells. Endometriosis can also occur as a result of direct transplantation—in the abdominal wall after a cesarean section, for example. Additionally, it appears that certain families may have predisposing genetic factors to the disease. These displaced endometrial cells may be on pelvic walls and the surfaces of pelvic organs, such as bladder, ovaries, and rectum. They continue to grow, thicken, and bleed over the course of the menstrual cycle in response to the hormones of cycle. Some believe endometriosis might start in the fetal period with misplaced cell tissue that begins to respond to the hormones of puberty. This is often called the Mullerian theory. The development of endometriosis might also be linked to genetics or even environmental toxins.

Where Endometriosis Can Occur

The most common sites of endometriosis include:

- The ovaries
- The fallopian tubes
- Ligaments that support the uterus (uterosacral ligaments)
- The posterior cul-de-sac, i.e., the space between the uterus and rectum
- The anterior cul-de-sac, i.e., the space between the uterus and bladder
- The outer surface of the uterus
- The lining of the pelvic cavity

Occasionally, endometrial tissue is found in other places, such as:

- The intestines
- The rectum
- The bladder
- The vagina
- The cervix
- The vulva
- Abdominal surgery scars

Endometriosis Stages

A staging, or classification, system for endometriosis has been developed by the American Society of Reproductive Medicine. Endometriosis has four stages or types. It can be any of the following:

- Minimal
- Mild
- Moderate
- Severe

Different factors determine the stage of the disorder. These factors can include the location, number, size, and depth of endometrial implants. The stage of endometriosis is based on the location, amount, depth, and size of the endometrial tissue. Specific criteria include:

- The extent of the spread of the tissue
- The involvement of pelvic structures in the disease
- The extent of pelvic adhesions
- The blockage of the fallopian tubes

Stage 1—Minimal: In minimal endometriosis, there are small lesions or wounds and shallow endometrial implants on your ovary. There may also be inflammation in or around your pelvic cavity.

Stage 2—Mild: Mild endometriosis involves light lesions and shallow implants on an ovary and the pelvic lining.

Stage 3—Moderate: Moderate endometriosis involves deep implants on your ovary and pelvic lining. There can also be more lesions.

Stage 4—Severe: The most severe stage of endometriosis involves deep implants on your pelvic lining and ovaries. There may also be lesions on your fallopian tubes and bowels.

The stage of the endometriosis does not necessarily reflect the level of pain experienced, risk of infertility, or symptoms present. For example, it is possible for a woman in Stage 1 to be in tremendous pain, while a woman in Stage 4 may be asymptomatic.

Diagnosing Endometriosis

The symptoms of endometriosis can be similar to the symptoms of other conditions, such as ovarian cysts and pelvic inflammatory disease. Treating your pain requires an accurate diagnosis. For many women, simply having a diagnosis of endometriosis brings relief. Diagnosis begins with a gynecologist or other health care provider evaluating a patient's medical history and completing a physical examination, including a pelvic exam. A diagnosis of history and completing a physical examination, including a pelvic exam. A diagnosis of endometriosis can only be certain, though, when the doctor performs a laparoscopy, biopsies of any suspicious tissue, and the diagnosis is confirmed by examining the tissue beneath a microscope. Laparoscopy is a minor surgical procedure in which a laparoscope, a thin tube with a camera at the end, is inserted into the abdomen through a small incision. Laparoscopy is also used to determine the location, extent, and size of the endometrial growths.

Other examinations that may be used in the diagnosis of endometriosis include:

- **Ultrasound:** A diagnostic imaging technique that uses high-frequency sound waves to create an image of the internal organs transvaginal ultrasound or an abdominal ultrasound may be performed. Both types of ultrasound provide images of reproductive organs. They can help the gynecologist to identify cysts associated with endometriosis, but they are not effective in ruling out the disease.
- **CT scan:** A non-invasive diagnostic imaging procedure that uses a combination of X-rays and computer technology to produce horizontal, or axial, images— often called slices—of the body to detect any abnormalities that may not show up on an ordinary X-ray.
- **MRI scan:** A non-invasive procedure that produces a two-dimensional view of an internal organ or structure.
- **Laparoscopy:** The only certain method for identifying endometriosis is by viewing it directly. This is done by a minor surgical procedure known as a laparoscopy. Once diagnosed, the tissue can be removed in the same procedure.

Endometriosis Treatment Options

This condition can disrupt your life if it is left untreated. Endometriosis has no cure, but its symptoms can be managed.

Specific treatment for endometriosis will be determined by the health care provider based on:

- Overall health and medical history
- Current symptoms
- Extent of the disease
- Patient's tolerance for specific medications, procedures, or therapies
- Expectations for the course of the disease
- Patient's opinion or preference
- Patient's desire for pregnancy

If symptoms are mild, health care providers generally agree that no further treatment, other than pain medication, is necessary.

In general, treatment for endometriosis may include:

- "Watchful waiting" to observe the course of the disease
- Pain medication: non-steroidal anti-inflammatory drugs, such as ibuprofen or other over-the-counter analgesics
- Hormone therapy, including:

  - Oral contraceptives, with combined estrogen and progestin (a synthetic form of progesterone) hormones, to prevent ovulation and reduce menstrual flow
  - Progestins alone

– Gonadotropin-releasing hormone agonist, which stops ovarian hormone production, creating a sort of "medical menopause"
– Danazol, a synthetic derivative of testosterone (a male hormone)

Surgical techniques that may be used to treat endometriosis include:

• Laparoscopy (also used to help diagnose endometriosis): A minor surgical procedure in which a laparoscope, a thin tube with a lens and a light, is inserted into an incision in the abdominal wall; using the laparoscope to see into the pelvic area, the doctor can often remove the endometrial growths.
• Laparotomy: A more extensive surgery to remove as much of the displaced endometrium as possible without damaging healthy tissue
• Hysterectomy: Surgery to remove the uterus and possibly the ovaries

It may be frustrating to get diagnosis and treatment options early in the disease. Because of the fertility issues, pain, and fear that there is no relief, this disease can be difficult to handle mentally. Consider finding a support group or educating yourself more on the condition.

Relationship of Endometriosis to Infertility

Endometriosis is considered one of the three major causes of female infertility. According to the American Society for Reproductive Medicine, endometriosis can be found in 24–50% of women who experience infertility. Although 30–50% of infertile women have endometriosis, the reverse is also true, such that 30–50% of women with endometriosis have infertility [1]. Endometriosis may affect fertility by various mechanisms, including distortion of pelvic anatomy from adhesions, intraperitoneal inflammation, which can decrease oocyte quality and/or oocyte-sperm interactions, abnormal tubal transport, and implantation defects. Laparoscopic excision of endometriosis may have a beneficial effect on subsequent fertility; however, there is no role for the medical management of endometriosis in the setting of infertility with the exception of 3 to 6 months of pretreatment with GnRH analogue before IVF, which appears to increase live birth rates. Other forms of ovarian suppression before fertility treatments, such as CHC and Danazol, do not improve pregnancy or live birth outcomes. Intrauterine insemination (IUI) using clomiphene citrate (CC) for endometriosis is more likely to result in pregnancy than timed intercourse alone (9.5% vs 3.3%); however, CC is not as effective as gonadotropins. A large meta-analysis demonstrated that women with endometriosis have significantly decreased pregnancy rates following in vitro fertilization (IVF) compared with women with tubal factor infertility [2]; nevertheless, IVF remains the most effective fertility treatment for endometriosis, with a cumulative live birth rate greater than 60% after four cycles.

Because of age-related decreases in ovarian reserve and oocyte quality, the approach to the treatment of infertility in the setting of endometriosis should be based on age of the woman in addition to other coexisting infertility factors, if present. For example, if there is a surgically modifiable tubal factor, surgical intervention may be a good option, whereas with significant male factor, directly proceeding to IVF with intracytoplasmic sperm injection is the more reasonable approach. The stage of endometriosis also influences the choice of treatment for infertility.

Stage I/II Endometriosis and Infertility

For early-stage endometriosis, laparoscopic excision or ablation has a small, but significant positive effect on subsequent spontaneous fertility; however, the number needed to treat is 12, and if endometriosis is not found at every diagnostic laparoscopy for suspected early-stage disease, the number needed to treat may be as high as 40; that is, 40 laparoscopies to achieve one additional pregnancy. As a result, in asymptomatic women with possible early-stage endometriosis and normal ultrasound, laparoscopy is a low-yield intervention.

On the other hand, OI/IUI with gonadotropins has been shown to increase the pregnancy rate among women with known stage I/II endometriosis (15% vs 4.5% untreated), and although the success rate of OI/IUI among women with undiagnosed, early endometriosis is unknown, similar per-cycle pregnancy and cumulative live birth rates (about 20% and 65%, respectively) are seen following four cycles of OI/IUI among women with unexplained infertility and that due to minimal or mild endometriosis.

In asymptomatic women less than 35 years old, expectant management (EM) versus OI/IUI are reasonable initial treatment options. However, in symptomatic young women, laparoscopy for endometriosis will help with pain and increase fecundity; thus, surgery may be followed by EM or OI/IUI. If OI/IUI is not successful, IVF is the next step. In the older (>35 years old) woman with stage I/II endometriosis, pain should prompt laparoscopic intervention followed by OI/IUI or IVF; however, one of the latter two treatments can be pursued directly if pain is not present.

Stage III/IV Endometriosis

In advanced disease, pain regardless of age will also lead to surgical intervention as should large endometriomas (>4 cm), even if asymptomatic, for histopathologic confirmation, for easier access to ovaries for oocyte retrieval, and to prevent endometrioma rupture/leakage. Endometrioma resection also appears to have a beneficial effect on IVF success rates.

If pain or large endometriomas are not an issue in the older woman, a more aggressive approach with OI/IUI versus IVF without initial surgical intervention is recommended;

However, in the younger woman with no other infertility factors, initial surgery can be considered as an alternative to IVF. Repeated surgeries are not helpful for infertility, and, therefore, if initial surgical intervention fails to result in pregnancy, IVF should be pursued.

In conclusion, endometriosis is a chronic condition with no cure. We don't understand what causes it yet. But this doesn't mean the condition has to impact your daily life. Effective treatments are available to manage pain and fertility issues, such as medications, hormone therapy, and surgery. The symptoms of endometriosis usually improve after menopause.

Endometriosis and IVF

Endometriosis is one of the most challenging diseases for gynecologists helping infertile women to conceive. Many factors have been suggested to cause infertility in women with endometriosis, including pelvic adhesions, ovulatory dysfunction, disturbed folliculogenesis, and defective implantation. Using IVF, it is possible to bypass some disturbances of reproductive function. Several studies have shown that women with endometriosis have a lower ovarian response to gonadotrophins.

Although IVF has helped greatly to improve the chances of pregnancy for patients with endometriosis, however, outcomes of in vitro fertilization cycles in women with endometriosis are significantly worse than in patients without this condition.

Because of the use of IVF, information is available about embryo quality and rates of cell division, implantation, and pregnancy loss. Abnormalities in the nucleus and cytoplasm of embryos from women with endometriosis are six times more frequent than in women without endometriosis. These abnormalities include cytoplasmic fragmentation, darkened cytoplasm, reduced cell numbers, and increased frequency of arrested embryos leading to significantly fewer transferable embryos.

The impact of endometriosis on ovarian reserve and the quality of retrieved oocytes are evident. Lower implantation rates, however, raise the question whether this finding is purely the consequence of lower number and poorer quality of embryos, or whether it also reflects compromised endometrial receptivity [3].

Implantation problems are not limited to regular IVF. In oocyte donation cycles, a recipient's history of endometriosis might have a negative impact on implantation, pregnancy, and live birth rates. In a recent study, doctors split the eggs from the same donor in recipients with and without a history of endometriosis. The interesting thing about this study is that the women in this study had been in menopause for at least 1 year prior to attempting egg donation. The implantation and pregnancy rates were significantly lower in the endometriosis group compared with the control group (23.81% versus 31.48%, $P = 0.019$; 45.00% versus 58.33%, $P = 0.039$, respectively) [4].

In conclusion, although the mechanisms involved in endometriosis-related infertility are still not completely understood, some evidence suggests multiple factors that may potentially affect a patient's fertility. In addition to the pelvic anatomical alterations likely to compromise the gametic interaction and the altered steroidogenesis, ovulation and disrupted ovarian function, peritoneal changes seem to promote a harmful and pro-oxidative microenvironment, which may compromise the CC and the follicular microenvironment, affecting folliculogenesis and, possibly, the oocyte competence in women with endometriosis. Peritoneal alterations may also damage the spermatozoa and difficult gametes interaction. The role of compromised endometrial receptivity is still controversial; however, recent evidence points to a major role of the oocyte factor in impaired fertility of infertile women with endometriosis.

Sexuality and Quality of Life

Every patient suffering from endometriosis refers to an often conflicting relationship with their body. Femininity is often experienced as a threat, seduction as an intrusion into intimacy, and sensuality a drug only for men.

The study by Bellelis et al. [5] investigated the quality of life of patients diagnosed with endometriosis treated by laparoscopic technique.

A total of 892 post-laparoscopic patients with a histologically confirmed diagnosis of endometriosis were enrolled. The mean age was 33.2 ± 6.3 years and 78.7% of patients were Caucasian. 76.9% of the women in the sample had higher education. Most of the patients (56.5%) were nulliparous and 62.2% reported dysmenorrhea as their main complaint. Chronic pelvic pain was the most common symptom, followed by deep dyspareunia, reported by 56.8% and 54.7% of patients, respectively. Infertility was reported by 39.8% of the 892 patients in the sample. Endometriosis was most often diagnosed in the fourth decade of life. Patients with this condition presented with multiple symptoms for which a thorough history is necessary for a comprehensive diagnosis and monitoring of treatment results. In addition, parallel to psycho-sexological counseling of the patient and partner is highly suggested.

There is no doubt that women with endometriosis report higher chronic/cyclic pain and significantly more dyspareunia, dysmenorrhea, and dyschezia than women with other gynecological conditions (including uterine fibroids, pelvic adhesions, benign ovarian cysts, neoplasms, and congenital Mullerian anomalies) or a normal pelvis.

The study by Schliep et al. [6] investigated a group of 473 women, aged 18–44 years, who underwent diagnostic and/or therapeutic laparoscopy or laparotomy at one of 14 surgery centers located in Salt Lake City, UT and San Francisco, CA. Women with a history of surgically confirmed endometriosis were excluded. All women had completed a computer-assisted personal interview at baseline specifying 17 types of pain (rating severity using an 11-point visual analogue scale) and identifying any of 35 perineal, 60 anterior, and 60 posterior sites throughout the body for which they had experienced pain in the past 6 months.

Chronic pelvic pain was prevalent ($\geq 30\%$): women diagnosed with post-operative endometriosis, compared to women diagnosed with other gynecological disorders or a normal pelvis, reported more cyclic pelvic pain (49.5% vs. 31.0% and 33.1%, $P < 0.001$). In addition, women with endometriosis experienced more chronic pain (44.2 vs. 30.2%, $P = 0.04$) compared to women with a normal pelvis. *Deep pain with intercourse, cramping with menstruation, and pain with bowel evacuation were significantly more likely in women with endometriosis than those without (all $P < 0.002$).* A higher proportion of women diagnosed with endometriosis than women with normal pelvis reported vaginal pain (22.6 vs. 10.3%, $P < 0.01$), right labial (18.4 vs. 8.1%, $P < 0.05$), and left labial (15.3 vs. 3.7%, $P < 0.01$) pain along with pain in the right/left abdominopelvic hypogastric and umbilical regions for all.

This study seems to have shown that while women with endometriosis seem to experience more pelvic pain, particularly dyspareunia, dysmenorrhea, dyschezia, and pain in the vaginal and abdominopelvic area than women with other gynecological disorders or a normal pelvis, pelvic pain is commonly reported among women undergoing laparoscopy, even among women with no identified gynecological pathology.

But that is not all. The annual incidence of pelvic endometriosis among women aged 15–49 years and up to age 69 years was ascertained for the Icelandic population between 1981 and 2000 [7]. To identify cases, a centralized discharge-code registry was searched, as were all hospital databases and, for individual patients, all hospital records. Each visually diagnosed and histologically verified case of endometriosis was cross-checked against the national disease registry.

The revised classification system of the American Society for Reproductive Medicine was used for this purpose. The type of surgery at diagnosis and the presence of disease at five sites were recorded: deep pelvis, appendages, central pelvis, vesicouterine pouch, and ovaries.

In this study [7], 1383 women who had undergone surgical treatment were recruited and 811 (58.6%) had histological verification. 297 (36.9%) had minimal/light disease and 508 (63.1%) had moderate/severe disease. Crude annual incidence estimates were 0.1% for visually confirmed endometriosis and 0.06% for histologically verified endometriosis.

The annual age-standardized incidence was 0.1% and 0.05% for women aged 15–49 years. The most common site was the ovary, followed by the deep pelvis, central pelvis, appendages, and vesicouterine pouch. 1% had moderate/severe disease. *Crude annual incidence estimates were 0.1% for visually confirmed endometriosis and 0.06% for histologically verified endometriosis.*

It is not unheard of in the literature that endometriosis can begin as early as adolescence [8], with much anxiety on the part of young patients and parents.

Persistent pelvic pain, fear of infertility, and a painful and unrewarding sex life often affect patient compliance. The sexological approach can be educational for young women and can educate parents not to over-care and limit social contacts. The American Academy of Pediatrics guidelines on the assessment of the menstrual cycle recommend considering the menstrual cycle as an "additional vital sign" that helps to assess normal development and exclude pathological conditions [9].

Not excluding the psychological and relational aspect of the pathology, especially in young patients who are developing their body and sexual role and identity. Painful symptoms may thus alter the adolescents' state of mind, producing feelings of inadequacy, body dysmorphia, depression, emotional instability, irritability, impatience, hysteria, insomnia: symptoms that cannot be underestimated in a diagnosis and treatment of endometriosis.

Given the complexity of this pathology, scientific studies have also been applied to the possible consequences during pregnancy in patients diagnosed with endometriosis. One study [10] covered the period from January 2008 to October 2018 to test the hypothesis that endometriosis may increase the risk of preterm birth, miscarriage, preterm premature rupture of membranes, placenta previa, pre-eclampsia, pregnancy-induced hypertension (PIH), gestational diabetes cholestasis, small for gestational age (SGA) babies, antepartum hemorrhage, postpartum hemorrhage, placental abruption, placental retention, malpresentation, labor dystocia, caesarean section, stillbirth, neonatal death, and congenital malformations of the uterus, but the data are based on limited information. Be that as it may, the study by Kobayashi H et al. [10] confirmed this.

Lalani's study [11] also conducted a systematic review and meta-analysis of observational studies (1 January 1990–31 December 2017) that assessed the effect of endometriosis on maternal, fetal, and neonatal outcomes. Women over 20-week gestational age with endometriosis and a control group of pregnant women without endometriosis were examined.

The search strategy identified 33 studies (sample size, $n = 3{,}280{,}488$). Compared with women without endometriosis, women with endometriosis were more likely to have: pre-eclampsia (odds ratio [OR] = 1.18 [1.01–1.39]), gestational hypertension and/or pre-eclampsia (OR = 1.21 [1.05–1.39]), gestational diabetes (OR = 1.26 [1.03–1.55]), gestational cholestasis (OR = 4.87 [1.85–12.83]), placenta previa (OR = 3.31 [2.37–4.63]), antepartum hemorrhage (OR = 1.69 [1.38–2.07]), antepartum hospital admissions (OR = 3.18 [2.60–3.87]), miscarriage (OR = 1.71 [1.34–2.18]), labor dystocia (OR = 1.45 [1.04–2.01]), and caesarean section (OR = 1.86 [1.51–2. 29]). Fetuses and infants of women with endometriosis were also more likely to have premature rupture of membranes (OR = 2.33 [1.39–3.90]), preterm delivery (OR = 1.70 [1.40–2.06]), small for gestational age < 10% (OR = 1.28 [1.11–1.49]), admission to neonatal intensive care unit (OR = 1.39 [1.08–1.78]), stillbirth (OR = 1.29 [1.10, 1.52]), and neonatal death (MOR = 1.78 [1. 46–2.16]).

Conclusion

There is no doubt that patients diagnosed with endometriosis who conceive naturally have an increased risk of preterm delivery and neonatal admission to an intensive care unit. When severe adenomyosis is coexistent with endometriosis, women may be at increased risk of placenta previa and caesarean section. The study by

Berlanda et al. [12] included 355 pregnancies in the endometriosis group and 741 pregnancies in the control group. Women with endometriosis had a higher risk of preterm delivery <34 weeks (6.4% vs 2.8%, OR 2.42, CI 95% 1.22–4.82), preterm delivery <37 weeks (17.8% vs 9.7%, OR 1.98, CI 95% 1.23–3.19), and neonatal admission to the intensive care unit (14.1% vs 7.0%, OR 2.04, CI 95% 1.23–3.36). At post-hoc analysis, women with endometriosis and severe adenomyosis had a higher risk of placenta previa (23.1% vs 1.8%, OR 16.68, 95% CI 3.49–79.71), caesarean section (84.6% vs 38.9%, OR 8.03, 95% CI 1.69–38.25), and preterm delivery <34 weeks (23.1% vs 5.7%, OR 5.52, 95% CI 1.38–22.09).

Pregnancy aside, this pathology interferes with the patient's quality of life in every context of life: personal, professional, emotional, social, relational, and couple. Caregivers often complain of emotional distance from their partners, refusal of intimacy, hypersensitivity to touch, and discomfort even in the affective phases of foreplay. They may even completely and drastically reject any kind of physical complicity. To exclude, these aspects would be to overestimate the psychic qualities of the patient and the partner, fostering feelings of anger, exclusion, and inadequacy.

References

1. Pinar H, Kodaman MD. Current strategies for endometriosis management. Obstet Gynecol Clin North Am. 2015;42(1):87–101. Epub 2015 Jan 5.
2. Azem F, Lessing JB, Geva E, Shahar A, Lerner-Geva L, Yovel I, Amit A. Patients with stages III and IV endometriosis have a poorer outcome of in vitro fertilization–embryo transfer than patients with tubal infertility. Fertil Steril. 1999;72:1107–9.
3. Selam B, Arici A. Implantation defect in endometriosis: endometrium or peritoneal fluid. J Reprod Fertil Suppl. 2000;55:121–8.
4. Prapas Y, et al. History of endometriosis may adversely affect the outcome in menopausal recipients of sibling oocytes. Reprod Biomed Online. 2012;25:543–8.
5. Bellelis P, Dias JA Jr, Podgaec S, Gonzales M, Baracat EC, Abrão MS. Epidemiological and clinical aspects of pelvic endometriosis–a case series. Rev Assoc Med Bras. 2010;56(4):467–71. https://doi.org/10.1590/s0104-42302010000400022. English, Portuguese. PMID: 20835646.
6. Schliep KC, Mumford SL, Peterson CM, Chen Z, Johnstone EB, Sharp HT, Stanford JB, Hammoud AO, Sun L, Buck Louis GM. Pain typology and incident endometriosis. Hum Reprod. 2015;30(10):2427–38. https://doi.org/10.1093/humrep/dev147. Epub 2015 Aug 11. PMID: 26269529; PMCID: PMC4573450.
7. Gylfason JT, Kristjansson KA, Sverrisdottir G, Jonsdottir K, Rafnsson V, Geirsson RT. Pelvic endometriosis diagnosed in an entire nation over 20 years. Am J Epidemiol. 2010;172(3):237–43. https://doi.org/10.1093/aje/kwq143. Epub 2010 Jul 8. PMID: 20616202.
8. Dovey S, Sanfilippo J. Endometriosis and the adolescent. Clin Obstet Gynecol. 2010;53(2):420–8. https://doi.org/10.1097/GRF.0b013e3181dbdc61. PMID: 20436319.
9. American Academy of Pediatrics, Committee on Adolescence, American College of Obstetricians and Gynecologists, Committee on Adolescent Health Care. Menstruation in girls and adolescents: using the menstrual cycle as a vital sign. Pediatrics. 2006;118:2245–50.
10. Kobayashi H, Kawahara N, Ogawa K, Yoshimoto C. A relationship between endometriosis and obstetric complications. Reprod Sci. 2020;27(3):771–8. https://doi.org/10.1007/s43032-019-00118-0. Epub 2020 Jan 6. PMID: 32046459.

11. Lalani S, Choudhry AJ, Firth B, Bacal V, Walker M, Wen SW, Singh S, Amath A, Hodge M, Chen I. Endometriosis and adverse maternal, fetal and neonatal outcomes, a systematic review and meta-analysis. Hum Reprod. 2018;33(10):1854–65. https://doi.org/10.1093/humrep/dey269. PMID: 30239732; PMCID: PMC6145420.
12. Berlanda N, Alio W, Angioni S, Bergamini V, Bonin C, Boracchi P, Candiani M, Centini G, D'Alterio MN, Del Forno S, Donati A, Dridi D, Incandela D, Lazzeri L, Maiorana A, Mattei A, Ottolina J, Orenti A, Perandini A, Perelli F, Piacenti I, Pino I, Porpora MG, Scaramuzzino S, Seracchioli R, Solima E, Somigliana E, Venturella R, Vercellini P, Viganò P, Vignali M, Zullo F, Zupi E. Endometriosis Treatment Italian Club (ETIC). Impact of endometriosis on obstetric outcome after natural conception: a multicenter Italian study. Arch Gynecol Obstet. 2022;305(1):149–57. https://doi.org/10.1007/s00404-021-06243-z. Epub 2021 Oct 8. PMID: 34623489.

Polycystic Ovary Syndrome

Daniela Romualdi, Valeria Versace, Antonio Lanzone, and Elena Vittoria Longhi

Main Medical Characteristics

Polycystic ovary syndrome (PCOS) is a common endocrine–reproductive disorder affecting 8% to 13% of women of reproductive age worldwide. Although the exact aetiology of this syndrome still remains unknown, a complex physiopathologic setting including inappropriate gonadotrophin secretion, impaired glucose and insulin metabolism, hyperandrogenism and chronic anovulation is thought to produce the large spectrum of clinical and biochemical manifestations of PCOS [1].

Menstrual irregularities, anovulatory infertility, hirsutism and acne are variably combined in affected women and undergo fluctuations throughout the lifespan, from adolescence till menopause [2]. Besides hormonal and reproductive abnormalities, women with PCOS often show abnormal metabolic traits. Exaggerated insulin circulating levels, variably associated with reduced insulin sensitivity, constitute a frequent finding in PCOS women. Approximately 50% of affected women are obese and exhibit a proclivity to abdominal adiposity, which is considered the major determinant of insulin resistance and dyslipidaemia. In such patients, the imbalance in the insulin-mediated glucose metabolism seems only partially related to the degree of obesity: actually, although about 70% of obese women with PCOS

D. Romualdi
Department of Woman, Child Health and Public Health, Fondazione Policlinico Universitario Agostino Gemelli IRCCS, Università Cattolica del Sacro Cuore, Rome, Italy

Pia Fondazione di Culto e Religione, Azienda Ospedaliera Cardinale Panico, Tricase, Italy
e-mail: daniela.romualdi@policlinicogemelli.it

V. Versace · A. Lanzone (✉)
Department of Woman, Child Health and Public Health, Fondazione Policlinico Universitario Agostino Gemelli IRCCS, Università Cattolica del Sacro Cuore, Rome, Italy
e-mail: antonio.lanzone@policlinicogemelli.it

E. V. Longhi
Department of Sexual Medical Center, San Raffaele Hospital, Milano, Italy

© Springer Nature Switzerland AG 2023
E. V. Longhi (ed.), *Managing Psychosexual Consequences in Chronic Diseases*,
https://doi.org/10.1007/978-3-031-31307-3_16

exhibit an increased insulin secretion, the same feature is also found in 20–40% of normal-weight subjects [3]. Since women with PCOS often show more severe insulin resistance than weight-matched non-PCOS populations, it is theorized that women with PCOS have an intrinsic form of insulin resistance, which is mechanistically distinct from obesity-associated insulin resistance [4].

Hyperinsulinaemia is proposed as a key pathophysiological feature of PCOS contributing to both reproductive and metabolic disturbances. At the central level, hyperinsulinaemia seems to be involved in the dysregulation of LH secretion. At a peripheral level, insulin promotes ovarian androgen secretion by enhancing cytochrome P450c17α activity at the level of theca cells, in synergy with LH. This cogonadotropic effect is exerted both directly and indirectly, through the stimulation of insulin-like growth factor 1 (IGF-1) secretion and inhibition of IGF-1 binding protein production. Furthermore, PCOS thecal cells present an androgen hyperresponsiveness to the crosstalk between LH and insulin pathways. Insulin also decreases sex hormone-binding globulin (SHBG) synthesis in the liver, thus increasing the bioavailability of testosterone [5]. Therefore, hyperinsulinaemia could represent the key element of the interplay between systemic and intraovarian factors concurring to chronic anovulation in PCOS: it directly interferes with follicular development, it increases androgens synthesis, which in turn induces premature follicular atresia, and it seems to be directly correlated with anti-Müllerian hormone levels, which negatively regulates the early stage of follicular development [6].

Even if overall fecundity seems not to be severely impaired in PCOS, up to 30% of affected women are considered subfertile and may have increased time to pregnancy. When a pregnancy occurs spontaneously or after ovulation induction, several reports have documented a higher rate of obstetrical complications (early pregnancy loss, gestational diabetes, hypertensive disorders, preterm birth and perinatal mortality) compared with the general population. Insulin–glucose metabolism has a central role in determining pregnancy outcomes: it is commonly held that pregnancy itself represents a stressful clinical condition for glycaemic homeostasis by inducing physiologic insulin resistance. In PCOS women, the pancreatic function, which fulfils a compensatory adaptation before pregnancy, may fail to further overcome the insulin resistance induced by the gestational hormonal changes [7].

Insulin resistance may also contribute to increased cardiometabolic risk later in life. Actually, in PCOS patients, the prevalence of impaired glucose tolerance (IGT) and type 2 diabetes (DM) is 30–40% and 5–10%, respectively, which is a three- to sevenfold greater risk than an age-comparable population [8, 9]. Finally, PCOS women of all ages are at increased risk of endometrial cancer [10].

Due to the multitude of these clinical features, women with PCOS have a lower quality of life (QoL) compared to women without PCOS. Self-reported specific tools measuring this important health-related outcome in PCOS were developed, validated and applied in different countries across different ethnic groups. In particular, the PCOSQ scale includes domains to assess emotions, body hair, acne, weight, difficulties in conceiving and menstrual problems [11]. Several studies documented an increased prevalence of anxiety, poor body image, low self-esteem and depressive symptoms [12]. Furthermore, a large proportion of PCOS women suffer from delayed diagnosis and inadequate education and information provision by health professionals [13]. The key dimensions affecting QoL are a matter of controversy in different studies, likely due to variations across the lifespan, to different phenotypes and to cultural factors, but the major complaints are generally related to the presence of infertility, acne and hirsutism.

Main Tools for the Diagnosis of Polycystic Ovary Syndrome

In the last 30 years, the categorization of such a multifaceted condition has represented a challenge. Several criteria have been proposed for the diagnosis of PCOS. According to the 1990 National Institutes of Health (NIH) criteria, the diagnosis of PCOS required the presence of both oligo-anovulation and biochemical or clinical manifestations of hyperandrogenism [14]. The 2003 Rotterdam criteria by the European Society for Human Reproduction and Embryology (ESHRE) and the American Society for Reproductive Medicine (ASRM) introduced the ultrasonographic morphology of the ovaries (PCOM) as a further criterion for the diagnosis [15]. The threshold for PCOM should be revised regularly with advancing ultrasound technology, and age-specific cut-off values for PCOM should be defined. Using endovaginal ultrasound transducers with a frequency bandwidth that includes 8 MHz, the threshold for PCOM is a follicle number per ovary of ≥20 and/or an ovarian volume ≥10 ml on either ovary, ensuring no corpora lutea, cysts or dominant follicles are present. If using older technology, the threshold for PCOM could be an ovarian volume ≥10 ml on either ovary. This diagnostic approach was recently endorsed by the "International evidence-based guideline for the assessment and management of polycystic ovary syndrome" [16]. Accordingly, PCOS is diagnosed when at least two of the three key features of the syndrome are present (after the exclusion of related disorders), thus generating four main phenotypes based on their different combinations. There is increasing awareness that the four PCOS phenotypes may present different endocrine, reproductive and metabolic burdens.

Even if proposed by several authors, anti-Müllerian hormone levels should not be considered for the diagnosis of PCOS due to poor standardization of the assays and uncertain cut-off levels. Although insulin resistance is recognized as a key feature of PCOS, clinical measurement is not recommended at the current time for making diagnosis [16].

Main Treatments

The therapeutic approach is often complex and variable in relation to the primary symptom of the PCOS woman.

Lifestyle

Lifestyle modifications (preferably multicomponent including behavioural intervention, diet and exercise) represent the first step, irrespective of the goal to be achieved. In overweight-obese-PCOS women, a loss of 5% to 10% of body weight is able to provide significant clinical improvements and is to be considered successful weight reduction within 6 months [17]. Ongoing assessment and monitoring are important during weight loss and maintenance in all women with PCOS.

A variety of balanced dietary approaches could be recommended to reduce dietary energy intake and induce weight loss in women with PCOS with overweight and obesity. In these patients, there is no or limited evidence that any specific energy-equivalent diet type is better than another [18, 19].

Regular, moderate-intensity aerobic exercise over a short period should be encouraged in order to improve reproductive outcomes, in addition to reducing weight and insulin resistance, in young overweight women with PCOS. Outcomes are not dependent on the length of the exercise intervention nor the type and frequency of the exercise performed, as significant clinical benefits have been observed in sustainable programmes of 90 min of aerobic activity per week at moderate intensity [20].

Estro-Progestin (EP) Combinations

The estro-progestin (EP) combinations have been widely used for more than 30 years in women with PCOS: several studies have reported improvement in the main symptoms and signs of this syndrome, including hirsutism, acne and menstrual irregularities [21]. The beneficial effect of EP drugs is attributable to the suppression of LH secretion and to the reduction in ovarian androgen production; furthermore, these drugs are able to increase the hepatic discharge of sex hormone-binding globulin (SHBG), which in turn results in a reduction in the circulating levels of free, therefore bioavailable, testosterone [22]. However, especially in cases of long-term treatment, the EP formulations may be associated with a negative impact on the metabolic assessment. A recent meta-analysis reported that EP combinations are associated with the deterioration of some metabolic parameters in PCOS subjects [23]. This issue deserves particular attention in the light of the higher risk of cardiovascular disease due to the common presence of dyslipidaemia, hyperinsulinaemia and central body fat distribution in women with PCOS.

Insulin-Sensitizing Drugs

Insulin-sensitizing drugs may be prescribed to women with PCOS if non-pharmacological methods fail or as adjunctive therapy [16]. Out of the different classes of insulin-lowering drugs, metformin has been the most extensively studied in both short- and long-term treatment regimens. Metformin is a biguanide, which mainly acts by reducing hepatic glucose output. However, it also improves insulin sensitivity to some extent, independently of weight variations, and decreases intestinal absorption of glucose, gluconeogenesis, glycogenolysis and lipogenesis. In randomized trials, the administration of metformin induced an improvement in insulin sensitivity, BMI and menstrual pattern and a decrease in androgen levels in both normal-weight and obese-PCOS women [24]. This drug was also reported to ameliorate dyslipidaemia, endothelial function and measures of systemic inflammation, thus theoretically reducing the long-term risk of cardiovascular disease [25]. Administration of metformin during pregnancy in PCOS women seems to lower the risk of early pregnancy loss, but its putative role in the prevention of hypertensive disorders and gestational diabetes has not been confirmed [26]. The most common side effects related to metformin treatment are abdominal discomfort, nausea and diarrhoea [27].

The thiazolidinediones (troglitazone, rosiglitazone and pioglitazone) behave as a selective ligand for the PPAR-γ receptor, which is mainly expressed in adipocytes, pancreatic β-cells, vascular endothelium, macrophages and, in lower percentage, heart and skeletal muscle tissue. These compounds are able to enhance cellular insulin sensitivity with a post-receptor mechanism of action. In recent years, notwithstanding some discrepancies, several studies have reported a positive effect of these compounds on ovulatory dysfunction, ovarian and adrenal hyperandrogenism and insulin resistance in women with PCOS [28]. Data from a network meta-analysis comparing insulin-sensitizing drugs indicated that rosiglitazone had the most favourable effect on PCOS patients in terms of DHEAS, total testosterone, FSH and LH, while metformin performed better in terms of oestradiol, free testosterone and androstenedione [29]. Another meta-analysis of 11 RCTs showed no significant differences among the same two interventions in terms of fasting glucose, insulin or homeostasis model assessment of insulin resistance [30]. However, it cannot be disregarded that glitazones may be associated with relevant adverse effects: weight gain, fatigue, oedema, diarrhoea, anaemia, congestive heart failure and, particularly in the case of pioglitazone, increased risk of osteoporosis and bladder cancer. Thiazolidinediones are in category C of pregnancy medications.

Inositols (mainly MYO and/or d-Chiro) have been more recently proposed as a possible therapeutic approach in PCOS women. These molecules are found in some foods (mainly seeds and fruits) and can be synthetized endogenously by the adrenals. Inositols are also commercialized as oral supplements in different formulations and dosages. A recent Cochrane review [31] found evidence that D-chiro-inositol may improve the ovulation rate in the syndrome. By converse, there was no conclusive evidence that D-chiro-inositol may exert any effect on BMI, waist-to-hip ratio, blood pressure, hormonal parameters (except for serum sex hormone-binding globulin), fasting glucose, fasting insulin and plasma lipids (total cholesterol and triglycerides). Whereas there are insufficient data to evaluate the effect of myoinositol for the treatment of gestational diabetes, evidence from four trials of antenatal dietary supplementation with myoinositol during pregnancy shows a potential benefit for reducing the incidence of gestational diabetes [32].

A review of the literature suggests the availability of a plethora of alternative medical treatments to correct the metabolic dysfunction associated with PCOS (acarbose, naltrexone, alpha-lipoic acid, vitamin D). However, the data are not conclusive and there is an urgent need for large randomized controlled clinical trials to assess the real benefit/risk ratio of these therapeutic options.

Sexuality and Quality of Life

The effects of this pathology lead to various symptoms including hirsutism, infertility due to ovulation irregularities and obesity and diabetes [33]: acne and alopecia.

Rebecca Tzalazidis and Kirsten Oinonen of the University of Lakehead in Canada [34] assessed the relationship between polycystic ovary syndrome symptoms and the social and sexual habits of young women. In some subjects, symptoms of the syndrome were absent, while in others, they were present with varying severity. Previous research had shown that free social and sexual habits or an individual's orientation towards sexual activity without emotional involvement could be associated with an increased concentration of androgen hormones in the blood.

Based on this evidence, the study hypothesized that women with more severe PCOS symptoms were more likely to have hyperandrogenism associated with freer socio-sexual orientations. Subjects enrolled in the study completed questionnaires collecting information on polycystic ovary syndrome symptoms, socio-sexual orientations and sexual habits. Free socio-sexual orientations, free sexual desire, romantic interest in other women and frequency of masturbation were all found to be associated with symptoms of polycystic ovary syndrome, including the male-like distribution of hair. Sexuality scores were also higher in women in the group with more pronounced PCOS symptoms. Moreover, attraction to other women was more frequent in subjects with a confirmed diagnosis of polycystic ovary syndrome [35].

Many women with polycystic ovaries suffer from infertility, defined as follows:

- Inability of a woman under 30 years of age to become pregnant after 12 months of unprotected intercourse.
- Inability of a woman over 30 to become pregnant after 6 months of unprotected intercourse.
- Inability to carry a pregnancy to term.

As this condition affects obese women, lifestyle changes, such as weight loss, may improve the chances of pregnancy, but that is not all.

Women with polycystic ovaries have an increased risk of complications during pregnancy. As with patients with diabetes.

The following are the possible complications:

1. *Miscarriage: it apparently relates to obesity. Since many women who are obese are also insulin-resistant, researchers have endorsed insulin-sensitizing therapy that can significantly reduce the risk of miscarriage in pregnant women with PCOS.*

2. *Gestational Diabetes: pregnancy is usually associated with a certain degree of insulin resistance, but in gestational diabetes the body is unable to react correctly. In most cases, diabetes disappears after the baby is born. Women have had gestational diabetes and their children have a high risk of developing type 2 diabetes.*
3. *Preeclampsia: this syndrome is characterized by a sudden increase in blood pressure after the 20th week of gestation. Preeclampsia can cause damage to the mother's kidney, liver and brain. If left untreated, the disease can be fatal for the mother or the foetus. Preeclampsia can lead to eclampsia, a more severe form that can cause convulsions and coma in the mother.*

   If a patient contracts preeclampsia, the gynaecologist may devise a plan to try to prolong the pregnancy and give the foetus more time to grow and mature. Such a plan may include the mother taking medication to help prevent seizures and keep blood pressure levels within a normal range.
4. *Pregnancy-Induced Hypertension: in contrast to preeclampsia, in this case there is a general increase in blood pressure that can start before the 20th week of pregnancy. If left untreated, the condition may lead to preeclampsia.*
5. *Preterm Birth: it is a birth before 37 weeks of gestation. Many researchers believe that the increased risk of preterm birth is most evident among pregnant women with PCOS who have preeclampsia. Preterm infants are at risk of developing serious problems, including being underweight at birth or having underdeveloped lungs.*
6. *Caesarean Section: this type of birth may be more common among women with polycystic ovaries, who often have problems with obesity and high blood pressure. As it is a surgical procedure, the patient's psychophysical recovery may take a long time.*

As regards the aesthetic effects of the polycystic ovary, hirsutism appears to be one of the most annoying factors for patients with this diagnosis [36].

This is also because the abnormal growth of hair takes place in typically male areas of the body:

1. Upper lip
2. Chin
3. Abdomen
4. Chest
5. Back

Hirsutism affects around 10% of women and in most cases takes an idiopathic and benign form, with no particular cause; however, sometimes it can occur secondary to more serious conditions such as follows:

1. Polycystic ovary syndrome
2. Hypercortisolism (Cushing's syndrome)
3. Ovarian or adrenal tumours
4. Obesity
5. Medications

6. Acne
7. Male pattern baldness
8. Amenorrhoea (absence of menstruation)
9. Oligomenorrhoea (menstruation every 2–3 months)
10. Breast atrophy (shrinking of the breasts)
11. Muscular hypertrophy (enlargement of muscle masses)
12. Clitoral hypertrophy

It is therefore easy to deduce that polycystic ovary syndrome is associated with *anxiety, depression,* somatic symptoms, body dissatisfaction, *eating disorders* and reduced sexual satisfaction. A study by Yin and colleagues [37] summarized all the scores for mental disorders that were significantly more severe in women with PCOS than in healthy women. The scores for depressive symptoms, anxiety, emotional distress, eating disorders and somatization disorders were significantly higher in women diagnosed with PCOS than in the control group (no diagnosis of PCOS), whereas the scores for quality of life were significantly lower and those for sexual dysfunction much more severe.

These data are in line with other studies suggesting that women with polycystic ovary syndrome show a risk of up to four times higher of experiencing depressive symptoms and up to six times higher of displaying symptoms of anxiety, compared to women without PCOS [38, 39].

Conclusion

Polycystic ovary syndrome induces sufferers to undertake a clinical, physical, aesthetic, sexual and dietary revision with very high levels of conformity. The prevalence of physical, psychological and sexual disorders calls into question the sexual role and identity of women. Partners often overestimate the patients' psychological capacities and play down the mood disorders, apathy and sexual dysfunctions they report, sometimes with resignation and sometimes with generalized anxiety. With the participation of clinicians and sexologists, it would be possible to educate caregivers to more constructive relationship, sharing diet, physical exercises and aesthetic care as part of a two-person project. With regard to sexuality, it is possible to set up a rehabilitation process so that each couple can experience pleasant and above all exclusive intimacy.

References

1. Azziz R, Carmina E, Chen Z, Dunaif A, Laven JS, Legro RS, et al. Polycystic ovary syndrome. Nat Rev Dis Primers. 2016;2:16057. https://doi.org/10.1038/nrdp.2016.57.
2. Teede H, Deeks A, Moran L. Polycystic ovary syndrome: a complex condition with psychological, reproductive and metabolic manifestations that impacts on health across the lifespan. BMC Med. 2010;8:41. https://doi.org/10.1186/1741-7015-8-41.

3. Homburg R. Polycystic ovary syndrome. Best Pract Res Clin Obstet Gynaecol. 2008;22(2):261–74. https://doi.org/10.1016/j.bpobgyn.2007.07.009.
4. Corbould A, Kim YB, Youngren JF, Pender C, Kahn BB, Lee A, et al. Insulin resistance in the skeletal muscle of women with polycystic ovary syndrome involves both intrinsic and acquired defects in insulin signaling. Am J Physiol Endocrinol Metab. 2005;288(5):E1047–54. https://doi.org/10.1152/ajpendo.00361.2004.
5. Balen A. The pathophysiology of polycystic ovary syndrome: trying to understand PCOS and its endocrinology. Best Pract Res Clin Obstet Gynaecol. 2004;18:685–706. https://doi.org/10.1016/j.bpobgyn.2004.05.004.
6. Romualdi D, De Cicco S, Tagliaferri V, Proto C, Lanzone A, Guido M. The metabolic status modulates the effect of metformin on the antimullerian hormone-androgens-insulin interplay in obese women with polycystic ovary syndrome. J Clin Endocrinol Metab. 2011;96(5):E821–4. https://doi.org/10.1210/jc.2010-1725.
7. Boomsma CM, Eijkemans MJ, Hughes EG, Visser GH, Fauser BC, Macklon NS. A meta-analysis of pregnancy outcomes in women with polycystic ovary syndrome. Hum Reprod Update. 2006;12(6):673–83. https://doi.org/10.1093/humupd/dml036.
8. Apridonidze T, Essah PA, Iuorno MJ, Nestler JE. Prevalence and characteristics of the metabolic syndrome in women with polycystic ovary syndrome. J Clin Endocrinol Metab. 2005;90(4):1929–35. https://doi.org/10.1210/jc.2004-1045.
9. Rubin KH, Glintborg D, Nybo M, Abrahamsen B, Andersen M. Development and risk factors of type 2 diabetes in a nationwide population of women with polycystic ovary syndrome. J Clin Endocrinol Metab. 2017;102(10):3848–57. https://doi.org/10.1210/jc.2017-01354.
10. Barry JA, Azizia MM, Hardiman PJ. Risk of endometrial, ovarian and breast cancer in women with polycystic ovary syndrome: a systematic review and meta-analysis. Hum Reprod Update. 2014;20(5):748–58. https://doi.org/10.1093/humupd/dmu012.
11. Taghavi SA, Bazarganipour F, Montazeri A, Kazemnejad A, Chaman R, Khosravi A. Health-related quality of life in polycystic ovary syndrome patients: a systematic review. Iran J Reprod Med. 2015;13(8):473–82.
12. Dokras A, Stener-Victorin E, Yildiz BO, Li R, Ottey S, Shah D, et al. Androgen excess-polycystic ovary syndrome society position statement on depression, anxiety, quality of life and eating disorders in polycystic ovary syndrome. Fertil Steril. 2018;109(5):888–99. https://doi.org/10.1016/j.fertnstert.2018.01.038.
13. Deeks AA, Gibson-Helm ME, Paul E, Teede HJ. Is having polycystic ovary syndrome a predictor of poor psychological function including anxiety and depression? Hum Reprod. 2011;26(6):1399–407. https://doi.org/10.1093/humrep/der071.
14. Zawadski JK, Dunaif A. Diagnostic criteria for polycystic ovary syndrome: towards a rational approach. In: Dunaif A, Givens JR, Haseltine FP, Merriam GR, editors. Polycystic ovary syndrome. Boston: Blackwell Scientific Publications; 1992. p. 377–84.
15. Rotterdam ESHRE/ASRM-Sponsored PCOS consensus workshop group. Revised 2003 consensus on diagnostic criteria and long-term health risks related to polycystic ovary syndrome (PCOS). Hum Reprod. 2004;19(1):41–7. https://doi.org/10.1093/humrep/deh098.
16. Teede HJ, Misso ML, Costello MF, Dokras A, Laven J, Moran L, et al. Recommendations from the international evidence-based guideline for the assessment and management of polycystic ovary syndrome. Fertil Steril. 2018;110(3):364–79. https://doi.org/10.1016/j.fertnstert.2018.05.004.
17. Kiddy DS, Hamilton-Fairley D, Bush A, Short F, Anyaoku V, Reed MJ, et al. Improvement in endocrine and ovarian function during dietary treatment of obese women with polycystic ovary syndrome. Clin Endocrinol. 1992;36(1):105–11. https://doi.org/10.1111/j.1365-2265.1992.tb02909.x.
18. Toscani MK, Mario FM, Radavelli-Bagatini S, Wiltgen D, Matos MC, Spritzer PM. Effect of high-protein or normal-protein diet on weight loss, body composition, hormone, and metabolic profile in southern Brazilian women with polycystic ovary syndrome: a randomized study. Gynecol Endocrinol. 2011;27(11):925–30. https://doi.org/10.3109/09513590.2011.564686.

19. Stamets K, Taylor DS, Kunselman A, Demers LM, Pelkman CL, Legro RS. A randomized trial of the effects of two types of short-term hypocaloric diets on weight loss in women with polycystic ovary syndrome. Fertil Steril. 2004;81(3):630–7. https://doi.org/10.1016/j. fertnstert.2003.08.023.

20. Harrison CL, Lombard CB, Moran LJ, Teede HJ. Exercise therapy in polycystic ovary syndrome: a systematic review. Hum Reprod Update. 2011;17(2):171–83. https://doi.org/10.1093/humupd/dmq045.

21. Teede H, Tassone EC, Piltonen T, Malhotra J, Mol BW, Peña A. Effect of the combined oral contraceptive pill and/or metformin in the management of polycystic ovary syndrome: a systematic review with meta-analyses. Clin Endocrinol. 2019;91(4):479–89. https://doi.org/10.1111/cen.14013.

22. de Medeiros SF. Risks, benefits size and clinical implications of combined oral contraceptive use in women with polycystic ovary syndrome. Reprod Biol Endocrinol. 2017;15(1):93. https://doi.org/10.1186/s12958-017-0313-y.

23. Amiri M, Ramezani Tehrani F, Nahidi F, Kabir A, Azizi F, Carmina E. Effects of oral contraceptives on metabolic profile in women with polycystic ovary syndrome: a meta-analysis comparing products containing cyproterone acetate with third generation progestins. Metabolism. 2017;73:22–35. https://doi.org/10.1016/j.metabol.2017.05.001.

24. Nestler JE. Metformin for the treatment of the polycystic ovary syndrome. N Engl J Med. 2008;358(1):47–54. https://doi.org/10.1056/NEJMct0707092.

25. Sirmans SM, Weidman-Evans E, Everton V, Thompson D. Polycystic ovary syndrome and chronic inflammation: pharmacotherapeutic implications. Ann Pharmacother. 2012;46(3):403–18. https://doi.org/10.1345/aph.1Q514.

26. Romualdi D, De Cicco S, Gagliano D, Busacca M, Campagna G, Lanzone A, et al. How metformin acts in PCOS pregnant women: insights into insulin secretion and peripheral action at each trimester of gestation. Diabetes Care. 2013;36(6):1477–82. https://doi.org/10.2337/dc12-2071.

27. US FDA. Glucophage prescribing information for the US, 2008. Available at: http://www. accessdata.fda.gov/drugsatfda_docs/label/2008/020357s031,021202s016lbl.pdf.

28. Du Q, Yang S, Wang YJ, Wu B, Zhao YY, Fan B. Effects of thiazolidinediones on polycystic ovary syndrome: a meta-analysis of randomized placebo-controlled trials. Adv Ther. 2012;29(9):763–74. https://doi.org/10.1007/s12325-012-0044-6.

29. Huang R, Zhao PF, Xu JH, Liu DD, Luo FD, Dai YH. Effects of placebo-controlled insulin-sensitizing drugs on hormonal parameters in polycystic ovary syndrome patients: a network meta-analysis. J Cell Biochem. 2018;119(3):2501–11. https://doi.org/10.1002/jcb.26410.

30. Xu Y, Wu Y, Huang Q. Comparison of the effect between pioglitazone and metformin in treating patients with PCOS: a meta-analysis. Arch Gynecol Obstet. 2017;296(4):661–77. https://doi.org/10.1007/s00404-017-4480-z.

31. Morley LC, Tang T, Yasmin E, Norman RJ, Balen AH. Insulin-sensitising drugs (metformin, rosiglitazone, pioglitazone, D-chiro-inositol) for women with polycystic ovary syndrome, oligo amenorrhoea and subfertility. Cochrane Database Syst Rev. 2017;11:CD003053. https://doi.org/10.1002/14651858.CD003053.pub6.

32. Crawford TJ, Crowther CA, Alsweiler J, Brown J. Antenatal dietary supplementation with myo-inositol in women during pregnancy for preventing gestational diabetes. Cochrane Database Syst Rev. 2015;12:CD011507. https://doi.org/10.1002/14651858.CD011507.pub2.

33. Ferrazzi EM, Moghetti P, Fruzzetti F, Gambineri A, Fulghesu AM, Street ME, Rago R, Cetin I, Mandò C, Di Simone N, Genazzani AD, Apa R, De Leo V. Italian Advisory Board on ovary syndrome polycystic (PCOS): from observations to clinical experiences on the use of myoinositol (MYO) and alpha-lipoic acid (ALA) to improve the pictures of the syndrome. Minerva Ginecol. 2020;72(5):239–84.

34. Tzalazidis R, et al. Continuum of symptoms in polycystic ovary syndrome (PCOS): links with sexual behavior and unrestricted Sociosexuality. J Sex Res. 2021;58(4):532–44.

35. Néraud B, Jonard-Catteau S, Dewailly D. Polymicrocystic ovary syndrome. EMC - AKOS - Trattato di Medicina. 2007;9(2):1–7.

36. Harrison - Principles of internal medicine, vol. 1, 17th ed. McGraw Hill; 2009.
37. Yin X, Ji Y, Chan CLW, Chan CHY. The mental health of women with polycystic ovary syndrome: a systematic review and meta-analysis. Arch Women's Ment Health. 2021;24:11–27.
38. Berni TR, Morgan CL, Berni ER, Rees DA. Polycystic ovary syndrome is associated with adverse mental health and neurodevelopmental outcomes. J Clin Endocrinol Metabol. 2018;103(6):2116–25.
39. Brutocao C, Zaiem F, Alsawas M, Morrow AS, Murad MH, Javed A. Psychiatric disorders in women with polycystic ovary syndrome: a systematic review and meta-analysis. Endocrine. 2018;62(2):318–25.

Part X
Infertility

Male Infertility

**Fabrizio Ildefonso Scroppo, Anna Mercuriali, Zsolt Kopa,
and Elena Vittoria Longhi**

Introduction

Infertility is defined by the WHO as the inability of a non-contracepting, sexually active couple to achieve pregnancy in 1 year, and it affects 15% of the couples in Western industrialized European countries [1]. The prevalence of primary infertility, to conceive a first child, affects one in eight couples, and that of secondary infertility (to conceive a subsequent child) affects one in six. A male-associated factor can be found in ~50% of infertile relationships, mostly in the form of abnormal semen parameters. Recent advances allow to father a child for those men who previously had no chance of this [2].

Main Medical Characteristics

The intact testicular function is essential for male health: production of testosterone and sperm. Spermatogenesis is regulated by the hypothalamic–pituitary–gonadal (HPG) axis: Gonadotropin-releasing hormone (GnRH) controls the anterior

F. I. Scroppo (✉)
Andrology Service, Department of Urology, Istituto Clinico Villa Aprica, Como, Italy
e-mail: Fabrizio.Scroppo@grupposandonato.it

A. Mercuriali
Department of Endocrinology Unit, Ospedale di Circolo e Fondazione Macchi, Varese, Italy
e-mail: a.mercuriali@libero.it

Z. Kopa
Andrology Centre, Department of Urology, Semmelweis University, Budapest, Hungary

E. V. Longhi
Department of Sexual Medical Center, San Raffaele Hospital, Milano, Italy

© Springer Nature Switzerland AG 2023
E. V. Longhi (ed.), *Managing Psychosexual Consequences in Chronic Diseases*,
https://doi.org/10.1007/978-3-031-31307-3_17

pituitary gland by secreting the secretion of follicle-stimulating hormone (FSH) and luteinizing hormone (LH). LH regulates the function of testosterone production in the Leydig cells, while FSH regulates seminiferous tubule function, the spermatogenesis, which requires complex interactions between Sertoli cells, Leydig cells, and germ cells. The entire process to form elongated spermatids requires 74 days. After the spermatogenetic process, sperm mature and move toward collecting tubules to the storage and maturation area in the epididymis. The maturation process occurs in the epididymis and takes another 14 days. Vas deferens passes through the prostate gland where the sperm is mixed with additional fluid from the seminal vesicles. Sperm then enter the urethra by the ejaculation process. Obstructions or anatomical abnormalities along this pathway can also lead to male infertility.

A significant decreasing trend of the male fertility parameters can be observed in the last decades, theoretically due to gonadotoxic exposures; environmental conditions, toxins, and lifestyle factors (sedentary lifestyle, obesity, smoking, alcohol, etc.). In contrast, physical activity, reduced body weight, and reasonable diet will lead to the improvement of semen parameters and fertility. Quantitative and qualitative (globozoospermia and immotile cilia syndrome) spermatogenic impairment can have genetic, non-genetic, and presumed genetic causes. Genetic alterations [3] (Y chromosome microdeletions, sex chromosome anomalies: e.g., 47,XXY and 46,XX syndromes, partial androgen insensitivity, chromosomal structural anomalies: translocations and inversions) may result in male infertility. Congenital abnormalities can predict later sub/infertility and can enhance the risk of testicular malignancies (testicular dysgenesis syndrome). Endocrine disturbances (e.g., hypogonadisms and delayed puberty) and immunological factors (antisperm antibodies) are also well-known factors of male infertility. Anabolic and androgenic steroid abuse is an increasingly prominent cause of male factor infertility. Reduced male fertility can also be the result of acquired urogenital abnormalities (e.g., previous testicular torsion and previous surgery), infections of the urogenital tract, and increased scrotal temperature (e.g., as a consequence of varicocele). Malignancies (e.g., testicular tumors and hematological malignancies) can cause a major decrease in fertility. Sexual and ejaculatory dysfunctions are also relevant factors. Although a revolutionary improvement has been made in the past decade in both diagnostics and surgical treatment, ~25–30% of the male infertility cases remained idiopathic [4]. The effect of aging on male fertility is not completely clear [5]. Young men have spermatids present in 90% of seminiferous tubules, which decreases to 50% by the age of 50–70 and to 10% by the age of 80. Additionally, 50% of Sertoli cells are lost by the age of 50. In aging men, pregnancy rates are significantly lower, conception often takes longer, and the prevalence of congenital and genetic abnormalities in newborns is even higher (see Table 1).

Table 1 Male conditions, mechanism, and effects on male health

Medical condition	Mechanism	Effect
Environmental conditions, toxins, and lifestyle factors	Toxins, less physical activity, recreational drugs	Spermatogenic and/or sperm function defect
Genetic alterations	Sex chromosomal or autosomal diseases	Spermatogenic failure
Endocrine disturbances	Altered hormonal regulation	Central stimulatory problems, peripheral spermatogenic defect
Testicular maldescent	Testicular dysgenesis, Sertoli and Leydig cell dysfunction	Sub/infertility, hypogonadism, testicular cancer
Malignancies	Oncotherapies	Spermatogenic defect, DNA fragmentation
Acquired urogenital abnormalities	Testicular torsion, prostate surgery	Spermatogenic defect, ejaculatory problems
Infections	Oxidative stress	Sperm membrane damage, DNA fragmentation, sperm function problems
Immune infertility	Autoantibodies	Affected sperm motility, penetration defect
Anabolic and androgenic steroid use	Negative feedback	Spermatogenic impairment, endogenous testosterone production stop
Sexual and ejaculatory dysfunctions	Intercourse problems	Fertilization defect
Aging	Affected sperm function	Less pregnancy rates, higher rate of miscarriages, higher incidence of genetic problems in the offspring

Diagnosis

Medical Examination

First of all, an accurate **medical history** is essential, focusing in particular on lifestyle, any risky work activities, concomitant pathologies, interfering therapies on spermatogenesis, sexual development (if cryptorchidism, puberty disorders), erectile dysfunction, and if there are ejaculate changes in the last period; it is also important to investigate age and pathologies of the partner in order to establish the successive iter for the couple.

The **physical examination** consists of evaluation of BMI, scrotal palpation (testicular volume and consistency, epididymis, vas deferens, possible neoformations, and varicocele), and exclusion of penile malformations [6].

Semen Analysis

- **Spermiogram** is the diagnostic gold standard; it must be interpreted according to WHO 2010 reference values [7] (Table 2) and must be performed at least twice after 3 months, as the seminal parameters are subjected to variability over time.
- **Biological and Functional Tests**: They are second-level tests; the most used are the separation by gradients (to recover the most mobile spermatozoa, also in foresight of assisted fertilization techniques), the DNA fragmentation test (as a possible cause of fertility in the absence of other alterations of the seminal parameters or in case of repeated abortions) [8], the MAR test (to evaluate the presence of antibodies on the surface of the spermatozoon), and the eosin test (in case of immobility or severe asthenozoospermia, it evaluates vitality).
- **Other Examinations**: Based on the diagnostic question, culture tests of spermatic fluid or prostate secretion [9], serological tests, and search for spermatozoa in the urine may be required.

Hormone Levels

The study of hormonal profile is fundamental to assess the extent of testicular damage and if there are endocrine dysfunctions at the base [10].

- **FSH, LH, and total testosterone** are the first-level tests. FSH is the hormone that directly stimulates spermatogenesis, while LH mainly regulates the production of testosterone by the testicle. In the case of testicular insufficiency,

Table 2 Parameters for spermiogram

Parameter	Normal values	Meaning
Volume	>1.5 ml	If reduced (hypoplasia), there may be obstruction, retrograde ejaculation, or hypogonadism
Aspect	Grey-opalescent	If altered, there may be an infection or blood
pH	>7.2	It becomes acidic in case of obstruction of ejaculatory ducts
Viscosity	Normal	Increased if there is infection of the accessory glands
Agglutination	Absent	It is present if inflammation or antisperm antibodies
Leukocytes	$<1 \times 10^6$/ml	Increased if inflammation
Concentration	$>15 \times 10^6$/ml	Oligozoospermia is reduced sperm count per ml; in cryptozoospermia, spermatozoa are present only after centrifugation; azoospermia is the total absence of spermatozoa
Progressive motility	>32%	Asthenozoospermia is reduced sperm motility; akinesia is the complete immobility
Morphology	>4%	Teratozoospermia are the structural changes in the head, central part, or tail

there is often a profile of hypergonadotropic hypogonadism (increased LH and FSH, with reduced or still normal testosterone). Instead, in pre-testicular forms, there are reduced levels of both FSH, LH, and testosterone (hypogonadotropic hypogonadism).

- The assay of **free testosterone** is not currently a reliable method; however, it can be calculated using an equation between total testosterone, albumin, and SHBG.
- As second level, based on particular clinical or anamnestic data, it may be required the study of **metabolic profile** (diabetes mellitus), **thyroid function** (dysthyroidism), **PRL** (hyperprolactinemia), **estradiol** (estrogen-secreting tumors), or **other pituitary hormones** (in case of hypogonadotropic hypogonadism, it is indicated to differentiate isolated forms from multiple pituitary deficits).

Imaging Diagnostics

- **Scrotal ultrasound** [11] is helpful in identifying the main pathological patterns most frequently associated with male infertility: reduced testicular volume or hypoechoic structure (in case of hypogonadism, congenital, or acquired), inhomogeneous ecopattern (testicular tumors, ectasia of rete testis, and microlithiasis), cryptorchidism, enlarged or cystic epididymis (e.g., for epididymitis, traumatic outcomes or obstructive causes), agenesis, or dilation of the vas deferens. The visualization of the spermatic plexus in B mode also allows us to identify the presence of varicocele and the evaluation of the diameter of the intrafunicular sperm veins.

  Usually, the ultrasound study continues with the **color Doppler** investigation in search of spermatic venous refluxes of pathological significance, represented by the presence of basal spermatic venous reflux in orthostatism and/or prolonged response to the Valsalva maneuver [12]. Furthermore, the study of vascularization of the testicular pulp and epididymis is useful for the diagnosis of orchiepididymitis and testicular torsion.
- **Trans-rectal ultrasound (TRUS)** allows the study of the prostate and distal seminal pathways. In addition to excluding mono- or bilateral agenesis of the seminal vesicles, it serves to assess the presence of prostate–vesicular inflammations and to document any ectasias of the seminal vesicles and/or ejaculatory ducts, secondary to functional obstructive pathology, or conditioned by the presence of intraprostatic cysts (originated by Mullerian or Wolffian ducts). TRUS is not performed routinely, but only in case of hypoplasia or suspected inflammatory pathology.

Genetic Analysis

Genetic investigations are indicated in case of azoospermia or severe oligo-asthenoteratozoospermia [13].

- **Karyotype** can be already requested in case of sperm concentration less than ten million per ml, and it allows to highlight alterations of sex chromosomes (the most frequent is correlated with Klinefelter syndrome) or autosomal ones (translocations, etc.)
- Search for **microdeletions of the Y chromosome** is indicated in case of sperm concentration less than five million per ml; in particular, in the AZF region there are several genes involved in spermatogenesis.
- **Mutations of CFTR gene** (cystic fibrosis) are responsible for a condition of agenesis of the vas deferens or ejaculatory ducts (not detectable on physical examination); suspicion criteria may be also a seminal volume less than 1.5 ml and pH less than 7.

Finally, in the presence of documented alterations, adequate genetic counseling is important, also aimed at calculating any risk of transmission to the fetus.

Main Nonsurgical Treatments

Lifestyle

First of all, a healthy lifestyle should be observed [14]. Indeed, overweight, smoking, alcohol, use of anabolics or drugs, stressful conditions, and exposure to high temperatures (sauna, Turkish bath, and some jobs) can cause a significant decrease in fertility potential, which is reversible.

Nutraceutical

Supplements are often used in idiopathic infertility, after a complete diagnostic process, in the presence of documented alterations of seminal parameters and fragmentation of sperm DNA, and repeated failures with assisted reproduction techniques [15]. Their function is to reduce oxidative stress, which leads to a reduction in sperm quality, to supply the amino acids necessary for spermatogenesis, to regulate the mitochondrial energy metabolism or to improve viscosity. However, the evidence is low due to the lack of comparative studies between the individual molecules, their combinations, doses, and optimal duration of treatment. Furthermore, the potential side effects in case of overdose should not be ignored and the physiological oxidative stress necessary for the fertilization of the oocyte by the spermatozoa must not be completely inhibited [16].

The most commonly used active ingredients are listed as follows:

1. **Folic acid**—necessary for the integrity of sperm DNA.
2. **Arginine**—precursor of spermine and spermidic synthesis, antioxidant.
3. **Astaxanthin**—carotenoid that acts as membrane stabilizing, antioxidant.
4. **Carnitine**—essential for mitochondrial beta-oxidation, improves motility and concentration.

5. **Coenzyme Q10**—antioxidant and cofactor for mitochondrial transport chain, improves all parameters.
6. **Glutathione**—antioxidant, improves all parameters.
7. **Myo-Inositol**—FSH second messenger, regulates spermatogenesis and osmotic balance.
8. **N-Acetylcysteine**—mucolytic action, improves viscosity and motility, increases sperm volume.
9. **Selenium**—antioxidant, improves concentration and motility.
10. **Vitamin C**—antioxidant, improves concentration and motility.
11. **Vitamin E**—antioxidant, increases motility.
12. **Zinc**—antioxidant, stabilizes sperm chromatin.

Hormonal Therapy

An effective spermatogenesis requires the action of both follicle-stimulating hormone (FSH) and luteinizing hormone (LH).

Idiopathic Male Infertility

- **FSH therapy** (human or recombinant) can also be considered when there are normal levels of gonadotropins, as numerous data are in favor of an improvement of the seminal parameters in case of oligozoospermia, oligoasthenozoospermia, or high spermatic DNA fragmentation index [17]; on the other hand, a lack of response to treatment occurs when there are already high FSH levels. The most commonly used dosages are 150 IU subcutaneously or intramuscularly three times a week for 3 months.
- **Antiestrogens** (SERMs) increase the endogenous secretion of LH, FSH, and testosterone, as they block the negative feedback of estrogens on the hypothalamic–pituitary axis. Clomiphene 50 mg per day or tamoxifen 10 mg has been proven effective in increasing the pregnancy rate in case of idiopathic infertility; however, they are off-label in men, so they need the signature of the informed consent and their cost is total load of the patient.
- **Aromatase inhibitors** (letrozole, anastrozole) have a mechanism similar to SERMs, but their use is not currently recommended for a possible loss of bone mass [18].

Infertility Due to Hypogonadotropic Hypogonadism

- **Human chorionic gonadotropin** (hCG) has an action similar to LH. The dosage is 1500–2000 IU subcutaneously or intramuscularly three times a week for at least 6 months (dose and duration should be finalized to normalize testosterone levels). If after 6–9 months of therapy the patient still remains azoospermic or severely oligozoospermic, FSH therapy should be added at a dose of 75–150 IU three times a week.

- **Pulsatile GnRH** can be considered in case of hypothalamic pathology. It is a subcutaneous hormone infusion pump that stimulates the release of gonadotropins (GnRh) every 2 h; the initial dose of 25 ng/kg can be increased up to 600 ng/kg, until normal testosterone levels are reached. This therapeutic option is severely limited by poor compliance and high costs.
- **Testosterone replacement therapy**, instead, is contraindicated in case of desire of paternity because it inhibits the release of FSH and LH.

Other Therapies

The following treatments are aimed at resolving specific causes [19].

Infertility Due to Post-Testicular Causes

- **Antibiotic therapy** is used in case of didymal, epididymal, or accessory glands infections; the choice is guided by semen culture or by cultural examination of expressed prostatic secretion when chronic bacterial prostatitis is suspected. Main antimicrobial agents usually include fluoroquinolones, macrolides, or tetracyclines [20].
- **Anti-inflammatory therapy** can be considered alone or in combination with antibiotics, in order to reduce symptoms of inflammation and oxidative stress, in case of the persistence of leukospermia or autoimmune forms. Belonging to this category, there are NSAIDs, cortisone, and phytotherapy with fibrinolytic and anti-edema action, such as escin or bromelain.

Infertility Due to Extra-Gonadic Hormonal Causes

- Hyperprolactinemias, dysthyroidisms, and diabetes mellitus require the specific pharmacological treatment prescribed by an endocrinologist or diabetologist.

Sexual Dysfunctions

The most commonly used drugs do not seem to interfere negatively on the seminal parameters [21].

- In the case of premature ejaculation, dapoxetine 30–60 mg on demand should be considered.
- For erectile dysfunction, PDE5 inhibitors are indicated in the oral form (sildenafil, tadalafil, vardenafil, and avanafil) or through intra-cavernous administration (alprostadil).

Surgical Treatments

Most important conditions in male infertility with surgical therapeutic consequences are schematized in Table 3.

Varicocele

Surgical correction (**varicocelectomy**) results in semen analysis improvement in ~75% of patients when indicated correctly; that is in the case of long infertile relation (minimally 1, but even 2 years), palpable varicoceles with oligozoospermia in younger male patients (age of the partner is also a significant influencing factor in order to optimize the cost/benefit ratio in infertility setting!). The microsurgical subinguinal approach is the gold standard treatment option to preserve the testicular artery and lymphatics. Then, laparoscopy or open surgical techniques using subinguinal or inguinal incisions are employed. In more countries, radiological interventions are also used for varicocele treatment [22].

Azoospermia

Obstructive Azoospermia

Absence of spermatozoa in the ejaculate despite normal spermatogenesis. Prevalence of OA accounts for ~10% of patients presenting for fertility evaluation. Testicular volume is usually normal with normal gonadotropin levels.

Table 3 Male infertility conditions and related effects on fertility

Disease	Definition	Effects on fertility
Varicocele	Dilated, tortuous veins of the pampiniform plexus in the spermatic cord, reported in about 15% of the fertile male population and ~40% of infertile males	Decreased testicular arterial blood flow, increased level of vasoconstrictor agents, temperature elevation. Decreased Leydig cell function may cause spermatogenetic defect and decreased sperm function
Azoospermia	Total absence of sperm in the ejaculate	Infertility
Obstructive azoospermia (OA)	Absence of spermatozoa in the ejaculate despite normal spermatogenesis—Testis volume is usually normal with normal gonadotropin levels	Reversible infertility
Non-obstructive azoospermia (NOA)	Spermatogenic failure due to either a lack of appropriate stimulation by gonadotropins or a testicular impairment (primary testicular failure), usually presents with low testicular volume and elevated FSH (except of hypogonadotropic hypogonadism)	Irreversible infertility, 50% chance of focal spermatogenesis

Table 4 Sites of obstructions and related treatment

Site of obstruction	Definition	Treatment
Rete testis	Sperms cannot enter the epididymis, loss of the maturation process	TESE
Epididymis	Due to infectious etiology	Tubulo-vasectomy, MESA, TESE
Vas deferens	Congenital uni/bilateral absence	MESA, TESE
Ejaculatory duct	Due to infectious etiology	TURED

Surgical treatment of obstructive azoospermia [23] (see also Table 4):

- Vasectomy reversal (vasovasostomy); after a vasectomy operation (mostly performed for birth control), microsurgical reconstruction of the vas deferens for fertility potential restoration.
- Tubulo-vasectomy; modern microsurgical reconstruction of congenital or post-inflammatory occlusions at the epididymal level. New anastomosis between one dilated epididymal tubule and the vas deferens to bypass the obstructed part of the seminal ways.
- Microsurgical epididymal sperm aspiration (MESA); in the case when microsurgical reconstruction is not possible or failed. Sperms from the epididymis can be used for in vitro fertilization with a higher success rate compared to testicular sperms.
- Testicular sperm extraction (TESE or testicular biopsy) [24]; in obstructive azoospermia TESE is applied to retrieve testicular sperm for assisted reproductive technique (intracytoplasmic sperm injection—ICSI). Indicated when reconstruction or MESA cannot be used or failed and can be performed also less invasively with percutan methods.
- Transurethral Resection of the Ejaculatory Duct (TURED) [25]; for the treatment of ejaculatory duct obstruction.

Non-obstructive Azoospermia (NOA)

A failure of spermatogenesis is caused by either a lack of appropriate stimulation by gonadotropins (usually primary or secondary hypogonadism) or a testicular impairment (primary testicular failure). Possible etiologies show a wide palette from genetic disorders or local testicular insults resulting in dysfunction of the hypothalamic–pituitary–testis axis. NOA is usually present with low testicular volume and elevated FSH (except of hypogonadotropic hypogonadism).

At about 50% of non-obstructive azoospermia cases, spermatogenesis may be focal; spermatozoa (or elongated spermatids) can be surgically found and used for assisted reproduction, intracytoplasmic sperm injection (ICSI). This is the only option in NOA to father a child. Multiple random bilateral testicular sperm extraction (TESE) is the method of choice. Microsurgical TESE increases retrieval rates

[26]. ICSI results are significantly weaker in NOA compared to obstructive azoospermia (18% vs. 28%).

Non-Palpable Testicular Masses: Organ-Sparing Surgery

With the widespread use of scrotal ultrasound for male infertility, a greater number of incidental testicular lesions are being identified. Recently, there has been an increasing trend toward organ-sparing microsurgery to prevent fertility and androgen substitution and improve health-related quality of life. The majority (~80%) of small non-palpable testicular masses are benign lesions.

Semen Cryopreservation

It allows sperm storage at temperatures below 0 °C for an indefinite time, although current techniques may still cause damage and deterioration over time. It is recommended in the case of [27]:

- Any kind of surgical sperm retrieval (MESA, TESE, microTESE), in order to avoid further sperm-finding procedures for assisted reproduction.
- Neoplastic or autoimmune diseases that must be treated with therapies capable of altering the reproductive function (e.g., chemo/radiotherapy).
- Progressive diseases that can affect fertility.
- Progressive and serious deterioration of the quality of the seminal fluid over time.
- Spinal cord injured men.
- Surgical interventions that may alter the mechanisms of ejaculation (e.g., prostatectomy, vasectomy) or fertility.
- Sperm donation.

Sexuality and Quality of Life

Male infertility appears to be a pathology that causes much suffering to both patients and their partners. The initial astonishment at the diagnosis of infertility soon gives way to anxiety and feelings of inadequacy: a sense of guilt toward the partner and obsessive behavior while waiting for the result of treatment, such as daily exercise (morning run) and diet (weight loss) [28].

A study by Irisawa et al. [29] evaluated the sexual behavior of 156 infertile patients by interview. It was found that the intensity of sexual desire of infertile patients was weaker than that of fertile males in the corresponding age groups, especially between 34 and 40 years of age. The frequency of morning erection in infertile patients was highest between the ages of 24 and 30 and decreased with age. On the other hand, there was no significant reduction in the intensity of erection during sexual intercourse. While 6% of infertile patients reported disturbance of arousal and ejaculation, 16% of partners expressed dissatisfaction with their sex life. This was often accompanied by anxiety and mood disorders.

Erectile dysfunction is often associated with male infertility [30]: a 2013 study evaluating 22,682 interviews with men and women aged 15–44 years reported that, in the United States, up to 12% of men have fertility problems [31]. It seems that sexual dysfunction in men is often present in the general population, with 20–30% of adult men worldwide reporting at least one sexual disorder, with prevalence increasing with age. The estimated prevalence of erectile dysfunction and premature ejaculation in men of reproductive age ranges from 12% to 19% and 8% to 31%, respectively [32–35].

The types of sexual dysfunction that lead to male infertility include erectile dysfunction and ejaculation disorders, such as anejaculation, retrograde ejaculation, and severe premature ejaculation, with organic, iatrogenic, relational, and/or psychogenic causes. It should be noted that male fertility may be impaired by sexual dysfunction per se, as in the case of psychogenic erectile dysfunction, or, more often, infertility may be caused by the negative effect exerted on sperm parameters by a systemic disease or the drug used to treat such diseases, which may also lead to sexual dysfunction [36].

In particular, ejaculation disorders affecting male fertility are mainly those that lead to aspermia (dry ejaculation), which can occur [37] either due to the inability to transport sperm (anejaculation) or the inability to ejaculate in an anterograde direction (retrograde ejaculation).

The simultaneous presence of sexual dysfunction in the female partner of an infertile couple may contribute to the deterioration of erectile function.

Women with secondary infertility had lower female sexual function index scores in orgasm, satisfaction, arousal, and desire than women with primary infertility [38–40].

Hassanzadeh et al. [41] found that in 300 infertile Iranian men, 129 suffered from premature ejaculation, of which 74% had the permanent form and 26% had acquired premature ejaculation. These results are similar to those reported by Serefoglu et al. [42] in a study of 261 Turkish men attending an outpatient urology clinic with a self-reported complaint of premature ejaculation (62.5% with the permanent form and 16.1% with the acquired form). By contrast, in an Italian study [43] Lotti et al. reported that of 244 men seen consecutively, with couple infertility, 38 had premature ejaculation, of which 38.5% had the permanent form and 61.5% had the acquired form. These data were similar to those reported by Basile Fasolo et al. [44] in 2658 Italian men with premature ejaculation admitted to outpatient clinics for free andrological examination (21.4% with permanent premature ejaculation and 69.8% with acquired premature ejaculation).

The study by Ramezanzadeh et al. [45] showed that sexual desire was negatively associated with the duration of infertility and positively associated with the frequency of coitus. Furthermore, no significant difference in sexual desire was observed between subjects with a recent (<3 months) or long-term (3–180 months) diagnosis of infertility ($P = 0.075$).

Similar results have been reported by others using the validated IIEF-15 instrument [46].

Reduced sexual desire in infertile couples has been related to the fact that sexual activity is focused on procreation rather than on the playful aspects and that intrusive medical requirements affect intimacy [47].

But What of the Couple: How Do They Experience This Pathological Situation?

Most publications have also analyzed the relationship between male infertility and marital instability. Some studies report low sexual satisfaction following the diagnosis of infertility. Drosdzol and Skrzypulec [48] found that male infertility became more intolerable for the couple depending on the duration of infertility (3–6 years). Andrews et al. [49] found a weak association between male fertility-related stress and sexual dissatisfaction in 157 infertile couples (but the duration of infertility was not indicated).

Smith et al. [50] investigated sexual satisfaction among 357 men in infertile couples (duration of infertility: 1.4–2.3 years) and found a low-to-medium value.

Monga et al. [51] suggested that perceived male infertility leads to feelings of inadequacy, decreased self-esteem, and increased stress levels, which affect sexual satisfaction. A 2014 study investigating sexuality, self-esteem, and partnership quality [52] in 153 males from infertile couples showed that infertility is associated with reduced sexual and general relationship satisfaction, self-esteem, and confidence, using the Self-Esteem and Relationship Questionnaire (SEAR).

With regard to orgasmic function: Jain et al. [53] reported male orgasm failure in 8% of a sample of 175 infertile men (using a questionnaire not validated according to ICD-103), while Saleh et al. found [54] that 11% of 405 men undergoing infertility evaluation revealed problems with orgasm (using the IIEF-15). In particular, these patients failed to collect sperm for a second analysis, by masturbation or during sexual intercourse at home, after abnormalities in one or more sperm parameters were detected. They also reported severe anxiety.

Rabo et al. [55] reported that the average sexual activity of 110 men with Klinefelter's syndrome examined for infertility was significantly lower than that of 325 normozoospermic and functional men.

Yoshida et al. [56] found a prevalence of sexual dysfunction in 67.5% of 40 men with Klinefelter syndrome who complained of infertility (39 with azoospermia and one with severe oligoasthenospermia). However, men with Klinefelter syndrome showed no significant difference in the frequency of sexual dysfunction compared with a control group of 55 infertile non-azoospermic men. The average monthly frequency of sexual intercourse in patients with Klinefelter syndrome was significantly higher than in the control group, probably because they wanted to continue to have sexual relations after the diagnosis of azoospermia. Corona et al. [57] found severe erectile dysfunction in 22.7% of 23 men with Klinefelter syndrome, while 60.9% had hypoactive sexual desire, 9.5% suffered premature ejaculation, and 9.5% delayed ejaculation.

It is now clear that couples' infertility involves significant psychological stress: the European Society of Human Reproduction and Embryology (ESHRE) has developed guidelines for clinical practice. These guidelines provide recommendations to improve the quality of psychosocial care for couples with infertility and during ART. ESHRE guidelines [58] report that patients starting first-line infertility treatment or ART do not have worse marital and sexual relationships than the general population and that patients receiving fertility treatment do not have higher prevalence rates of sexual dysfunction than the general population.

Everyday clinical evidence also shows that, in infertile men, erectile dysfunction is associated with mood disorders and generalized anxiety (assessed by questionnaires: IIEF-15-EFD—the MHQ), especially in patients with azoospermia compared to other categories of infertile men. In addition, men with azoospermia show higher rates of premature ejaculation and sexual desire with reduced orgasmic function (due to depressive and somatized anxiety) than fertile men.

Conclusion

Erectile dysfunction and male infertility are considered early indicators of poor general health. Men with azoospermia show the highest rates of psychological and general health disorders associated with a higher prevalence of sexual dysfunction. Finally, drugs commonly used for general health problems can lead to sperm abnormalities and sexual dysfunction, and therefore, adequate information must be provided to patients. There is no doubt, in all of this, that knowing the sexual history of the couple and of individuals would offer clinicians and the sexologist better references to understand: the patient's and partner's compliance, the couple's relationship, the obsessiveness regarding the parental project, the conditioning of social networks (friends who have already had children), and families (families of origin pressing for a grandchild).

References

1. Jungwirth A, Diemer T, Kopa Z, Krausz C, Minhas S, Tournaye H. European Association of Urology guidelines on male infertility. EAU Annual Congress Barcelona; 2019.
2. Pan MM, Hockenberry MS, Kirby EW, Lipshultz LI. Male infertility diagnosis and treatment in the era of in vitro fertilization and intracytoplasmic sperm injection. Med Clin North Am. 2018;102(2):337–47.
3. Krausz C, Riera-Escamilla A. Genetics of male infertility. Nat Rev Urol. 2018;15(6):369–84.
4. Tournaye H, Krausz C, Oates RD. Novel concepts in the aetiology of male reproductive impairment. Lancet Diabetes Endocrinol. 2017;5(7):544–53.

5. Pino V, Sanz A, Valdés N, Crosby J, Mackenna A. The effects of aging on semen parameters and sperm DNA fragmentation. JBRA Assist Reprod. 2020;24(1):82–6.
6. Nieschlag E, Lenzi A. The conventional management of male infertility. Int J Gynaecol Obstet. 2013;123(Suppl 2):S31–5.
7. World Health Organization. Department of Reproductive Health and Research. WHO laboratory manual for the examination and processing of human semen. 5th ed. New York: Cambridge University Press; 2010.
8. Muratori M, Marchiani S, Tamburrino L, Cambi M, Lotti F, Natali I, Filimberti E, Noci I, Forti G, Maggi M, Baldi E. DNA fragmentation in brighter sperm predicts male fertility independently from age and semen parameters. Fertil Steril. 2015;104(3):582–90.e4.
9. La Vignera S, Condorelli RA, Vicari E, Salmeri M, Morgia G, Favilla V, Cimino S, Calogero AE. Microbiological investigation in male infertility: a practical overview. J Med Microbiol. 2014;63(Pt 1):1–14.
10. Kathrins M, Niederberger C. Diagnosis and treatment of infertility-related male hormonal dysfunction. Nat Rev Urol. 2016;13(6):309–23.
11. Lotti F, Maggi M. Ultrasound of the male genital tract in relation to male reproductive health. Hum Reprod Update. 2015;21(1):56–83.
12. Cavallini G, Scroppo FI, Colpi GM. The clinical usefulness of a novel grading system for varicocoeles using duplex Doppler ultrasound examination based on postsurgical modifications of seminal parameters. Andrology. 2019;7(1):62–8.
13. Krausz C, Escamilla AR, Chianese C. Genetics of male infertility: from research to clinic. Reproduction. 2015;150(5):R159–74.
14. National Institute for Health and Clinical Excellence. Fertility problems: assessment and treatment. London: Royal College of Obstetricians & Gynaecologists; 2013.
15. Calogero AE, Aversa A, La Vignera S, Corona G, Ferlin A. The use of nutraceuticals in male sexual and reproductive disturbances: position statement from the Italian Society of Andrology and Sexual Medicine (SIAMS). J Endocrinol Investig. 2017;40(12):1389–97.
16. Agarwal A, Parekh N, Panner Selvam MK, et al. Male oxidative stress infertility (MOSI): proposed terminology and clinical practice guidelines for management of idiopathic male infertility. World J Mens Health. 2019;37(3):296–312.
17. Barbonetti A, Calogero AE, Balercia G, Garolla A, Krausz C, La Vignera S, Lombardo F, Jannini EA, Maggi M, Lenzi A, Foresta C, Ferlina A. The use of follicle stimulating hormone (FSH) for the treatment of the infertile man: position statement from the Italian Society of Andrology and Sexual Medicine (SIAMS). J Endocrinol Investig. 2018;41(9):1107–22.
18. Chehab M, Madala A, Trussell JC. On-label and off-label drugs used in the treatment of male infertility. Fertil Steril. 2015;103(3):595–604.
19. Calogero AE, Condorelli RA, Russo GI, et al. Conservative nonhormonal options for the treatment of male infertility: antibiotics, anti-inflammatory drugs, and antioxidants. Biomed Res Int. 2017;2017:4650182.
20. Wagenlehner FME, Pilatz A, Weidner W, et al. Prostatitis, epididymitis and orchitis. In: Cohen J, Powderly WJ, Opal SM, editors. Infectious diseases. 4th ed. Elsevier; 2017. p. 532–8.
21. Yang Y, Ma Y, Yang H, et al. Effect of acute tadalafil on sperm motility and acrosome reaction: in vitro and in vivo studies. Andrologia. 2014;46(4):417–22.
22. Maheshwari A, Muneer A, Lucky M, Mathur R, McEleny K, British Association of Urological Surgeons and the British Fertility Society. A review of varicocele treatment and fertility outcomes. Hum Fertil (Camb). 2020;7:1–8.
23. Brannigan RE. Introduction: Surgical treatment of male infertility: a state-of-the-art overview. Fertil Steril. 2019;111(3):413–4.
24. Akerman JP, Hayon S, Coward RM. Sperm extraction in obstructive azoospermia: what's next? Urol Clin North Am. 2020;47(2):147–55.
25. Avellino GJ, Lipshultz LI, Sigman M, Hwang K. Transurethral resection of the ejaculatory ducts: etiology of obstruction and surgical treatment options. Fertil Steril. 2019;111(3):427–43.
26. Flannigan RK, Schlegel PN. Microdissection testicular sperm extraction: preoperative patient optimization, surgical technique, and tissue processing. Fertil Steril. 2019;111(3):420–6.

27. Gupta S, Sekhon LH, Agarwal A. Sperm banking: when, why, and how? In: Sabanegh ES, editor. Male infertility problems and solutions. Humana Press: Totowa; 2011. p. 107–18.
28. Rantala ML, Koskimies AI. Sexual behavior of infertile couples. Int Fertil J. 1988;33(1):26–30. PMID: 2896169.
29. Irisawa S, Shirai M, Matsushita S, Kagayama M, Iehijo S. Sexual behavior in Japanese males. Tohoku J Exp Med. 1966;90:125–32.
30. Boivin J, Bunting L, Collins JA, Nygren KG. International estimates of the prevalence of infertility and seeking treatment: potential need and demand for medical treatment for infertility. Hum Reprod. 2007;22:1506–12.
31. Chandra A, Copen CE, Stephen EH. Infertility and impaired fertility in the United States, 1982–2010: National Survey of Family Growth data. Natl Health Stat Report. 2013;67:1–18.
32. Parazzini F, et al. Frequency and determinants of erectile dysfunction in Italy. Eur Urol. 2000;37:43–9.
33. Mirone V, Ricci E, Gentile V, Basile Fasolo C, Parazzini F. Determinants of the risk of erectile dysfunction in a wide range of Italian men attending andrology clinics. Eur Urol. 2004;45:87–91.
34. Moreira ED Jr, Hartmann U, Glasser DB, Gingell C, GSSAB Investigators Group. A population survey of sexual activity, sexual dysfunction and behaviors associated with seeking help in middle-aged adults and the elderly in Germany. Eur J Med Res. 2005;10:434–43.
35. Moreira ED Jr, Glasser DB, Gingell C, GSSAB Investigators Group. Sexual activity, sexual dysfunction and associated behaviors of seeking help in middle-aged and older adults in Spain: a population survey. J Urol World. 2005;23:422–9.
36. World Health Organization. International statistical classification of diseases and related health problems - 10th revision. WHO; 2016. http://www.who.int/classifications/icd/en/
37. Mehta A, Sigman M. Management of dry ejaculate: a systematic review of aspermia and retrograde ejaculation. Fertil Steril. 2015;104:1074–81.
38. Lara LA, et al. Effect of infertility on the sexual function of couples: state of the art. Endocr Metab Immune Drug Discov. 2015;9:46–53.
39. Keskin U, et al. Differences in the prevalence of sexual dysfunction between primary and secondary infertile women. Fertil Steril. 2011;96:1213–7.
40. Davari Tanha F, Mohseni M, Ghajarzadeh M. Sexual function in women with primary and secondary infertility compared with controls. Int J Impot Res. 2014;26:132–4.
41. Hassanzadeh K, Yavari-kia P, Ahmadi-Asrbadr Y, Nematzadeh-Pakdel A, Alikhah H. Characteristics of premature ejaculation in infertile men. Pak J Biol Sci. 2010;13:911–5.
42. Serefoglu EC, Cimen HI, Atmaca AF, Balbay MD. The distribution of patients seeking treatment for premature ejaculation disorder according to the four premature ejaculation syndromes. J Sex Med. 2010;7:810–5.
43. Lotti F, et al. Impaired sperm quality is associated with sexual dysfunction based on its severity. Hum Reprod. 2016;31:2668–80.
44. Basile Fasolo C, Mirone V, Gentile V, Parazzini F, Ricci E. Premature ejaculation: prevalence and associated conditions in a sample of 12,558 men who participated in Andrology Prevention Week 2001 - a study by Italian Society of Andrology (SIA). J Sex Med. 2005;2:376–82.
45. Ramezanzadeh F, Aghssa MM, Jafarabadi M, Zayeri F. Alterations of sexual desire and satisfaction in male partners of infertile couples. Fertil Steril. 2006;85:139–43.
46. Marci R, et al. Procreative sex in infertile couples: the decay of pleasure? Qual Health Result Life. 2012;10:140.
47. Reder F, Fernandez A, Ohl J. Does sexuality still have a place for couples treated with assisted reproductive techniques? J Gynecol Ostetus Biol Reprod. 2009;38:377–88.
48. Drosdzol A, Skrzypulec V. Evaluation of marital and sexual interactions of polish infertile couples. J Sex Med. 2009;6:3335–46.
49. Andrews FM, Abbey A, Halman LJ. Infertility stress, marriage factors, and subjective Well-being of wives and husbands. J Health Soc Behav. 1991;32:238–53.
50. Smith JF, et al. Sexual, marital and social impact of a man's perceived infertility diagnosis. J Sex Med. 2009;6:2505–15.

51. Monga M, Alexandrescu B, Katz SE, Stein M, Ganiats T. Impact of infertility on quality of life, marital adjustment, and sexual function. Urology. 2004;63:126–30.
52. Wischmann T, et al. Sessualità, autostima e qualità del partenariato nelle donne e negli uomini sterili. Geburtshilfe Frauenheilkd. 2014;74:759–63.
53. Jain K, Radhakrishnan G, Agrawal P. Infertility and psychosexual disorders: relationship in infertile couples. Indian J Med Sci. 2000;54:1–7.
54. Saleh RA, Ranga GM, Raina R, Nelson DR, Agarwal A. Sexual dysfunction in men undergoing infertility assessment: an observational cohort study. Fertil Steril. 2003;79:909–12.
55. Raboch J, Mellan J, Stárka L. Klinefelter syndrome: development and sexual activity. Arch Sex Behav. 1979;8:333–9.
56. Yoshida A, et al. Sexual function and clinical features of patients with Klinefelter syndrome with the main male infertility disorder. Int J Androl. 1997;20:80–5.
57. Corona G, et al. Sexual dysfunction in subjects with Klinefelter's syndrome. Int. J Androl. 2010;33:574–80.
58. Gameiro S, et al. ESHRE guideline: routine psychosocial care in infertility and medically assisted reproduction: a guide for fertility staff. Hum Reprod. 2015;30:2476–85.

The Klinefelter Syndrome

Silvani Mauro and Elena Vittoria Longhi

The Klinefelter syndrome (KS) is a syndrome characterized by the presence of at least one extra X chromosome in the chromosome set. In 85% of cases, the karyotype is 47XXY, while the remaining 15% of cases have different aneuploidies, for example 48XXXY, 48XXYY or 49XXXXY. In 18% of cases, mosaicisms are present. The first clinical observation of this syndrome dates back to 1942 by Harry Klinefelter, who described a case of azoospermia, gynaecomastia and small testicles [1]. The cause of this pathology may be attributed to the non-disjunction of the original paternal or maternal gametes, during the first or second meiotic division; with less frequency, it can also be generated by a non-meiotic disjunction of the sex chromosomes of the zygote, which, in this case, would be responsible for the mosaicisms observed. The incidence of the syndrome increases with the age of the mother and, instead, does not correlate with the age of the father [2]. Azoospermia is attributed to the extra X chromosome, which reduces the viability of the germ cells present in the foetal testicles and which, thus, undergo degenerative phenomena during childhood until they disappear during adolescence. The mechanism by which Leydig cells would no longer produce testosterone is not yet fully clarified [3, 4]. The presence at birth of infants with the 47XXY karyotype is estimated at 1–4/1000 births. The actual prevalence is greater if we think that the cases diagnosed at birth and in adulthood are greater, so as to constitute the more common form of male hypogonadism.

S. Mauro (✉)
Urologist and Oncosurgery, Biella, Italy

E. V. Longhi
Department of Sexual Medical Center, San Raffaele Hospital, Milano, Italy

© Springer Nature Switzerland AG 2023

227

E. V. Longhi (ed.), *Managing Psychosexual Consequences in Chronic Diseases*,
https://doi.org/10.1007/978-3-031-31307-3_18

Clinical Manifestations

There are two clinical categories, the classic form and the variants; sometimes, the syndrome expresses mosaicism, i.e. with cell lines that can present chromosome alterations or not.

In the classic form, the clinical manifestations are represented by testicles of reduced volume (with a volume of less than 10 cm^3) and of increased consistency and gynaecomastia is present in 85% of cases. The expression of hypogonadism can vary from mild forms of reduction in secondary sexual characteristics to forms of fully blown eunuchoidism [1, 3, 5]. Severe azoospermia or oligozoospermia is present. Recently, spermatozoa have been found in the seminal fluid of a number of patients affected by the Klinefelter syndrome and pregnancies have occurred without the use of MART (Medically Assisted Reproductive Technologies). At puberty, the testicles become small and hard, while prior to this period they have a regular consistency. This aspect is related to the action of the gonadotropin FSH, which determines hyalinosis and fibrosis of the seminiferous tubules. The apparently hyperplastic Leydig cells, compared to the volume of the didymus, actually present structural alterations, such as mitochondria anomalies where the Reinke crystals are absent, leading to a decreased synthesis of testosterone even in the presence of high levels of LH and also under stimulation with hCG. All this translates into blocking the synthesis of testosterone and in increasing the production of oestradiol, which is responsible for the appearance of gynaecomastia. These patients are taller than normal (>75th percentile), which is not only linked to androgen deficiency but also to osteopenia related to the chromosomal abnormality. The excessive growth of long bones begins before puberty, and the bone age is the registry age. The ratio between the measurement of the opening of the arms and the height is equal to or less than 1, unlike patients with eunuchoid appearance due to androgenic deficit in which the excessive growth of the lower and upper limbs is identical [6, 7]. The intellectual quotient is lower than normal in 15–25% of the patients, while the remaining patients have personality and learning disorders, difficulty in verbal expression and easy fatigue, difficulty in concentrating and memory loss related to androgen deficiency. In this category of patients, the incidence of diabetes for insulin resistance, breast cancer and varicosity of the lower limbs is higher. In the classical forms, diagnosed in adulthood, the reduction in androgens can lead to loss of libido, a decrease in volume and muscle tone propensity towards the development of thromboembolisms and an increased risk of mortality from diabetes and cardiovascular diseases.

In the variant forms are included all patients with extra X chromosomes; the anomalies of the classic form being all the more accentuated the more X chromosomes are present. Some have severe mental retardation, scrotum hypoplasia, cryptorchidism and growth retardation. There is a very rare form (1/10,000 births) in which the Y chromosome is missing altogether. These patients have the same anomalies as the more accentuated classic Klinefelter with associated hypospadias of various degrees.

Mosaicisms

These patients have multiple stem cell lines of which at least 5% have a normal karyotype. In these patients, the clinical picture is much more undefined and graded than the classic form. If the karyotype of the testicular cell line is normal, the gonadal function can be maintained and in some cases fertility has also been documented [1–10].

Diagnosis

The diagnosis of Klinefelter syndrome in pre-pubertal age is difficult, with the clinical signs being mild, difficult to detect or completely absent. Sexual development can be regular, sometimes delayed or incomplete. During post-puberty, instead, the following are manifested: reduced testicular volume, altered skeletal proportions, high plasma levels of FSH and LH and low levels of testosterone. Gynaecomastia is sometimes expressed and diagnosed on the occasion of the screening of the male-factor in the context, for example, of couple infertility. The diagnosis is cytogenetic with presence in all cell lines or only in part of the 47XXY kit [9–11].

Klinefelter Syndrome and Fertility

The Klinefelter syndrome is the main cause of infertility due to a chromosomal impairment, affecting 1 in 1000 males at birth. The incidence is 3–4% of infertile and 10–12% of azoospermic individuals. This trisomy originates in 90% of cases from a non-disjunction of the X chromosome during maternal meiosis, while only 10% of cases are due to errors that occur during paternal meiosis [1–5, 8]. Twenty per cent (20%) of subjects affected by KS also present mosaicisms (46XY-47XXY). The development of KS seems to be highly correlated with the age of the mother (>40 years old). Recent studies have also shown deletions of the AZF a-b-c region of the Y chromosome in individuals affected by KS. In view of the scarcity of symptoms, only 10% of the individuals affected receive a pre-pubertal diagnosis. In adulthood, the spectrum of symptoms can range from a normal condition to one of severe hypogonadism, which explains why a large part of KS patients does not receive an adequate diagnosis. The diagnosis is almost always confirmed following an assessment for couple infertility, where there is azoospermia, cryptozoospermia and very severe oligoasthenoteratospermia. Sometimes, the hormonal picture expresses normal or low testosterone values as opposed to high LH values, in the context of a compensated hypogonadism. No medical therapy is possible for the treatment of infertility. With testicle biopsy, spermatozoa are found in 50% of KS patients. Spermatozoa in the ejaculate of non-mosaic KS patients are found in

7.7–8.4% of cases; spontaneous pregnancies have been recorded in these cases. The percentage of microtese pregnancies is in the order of 55% compared to techniques with episodic sampling in which it goes down to 42%. The risk of transmission of aneuploidy in non-mosaic KS patients, in the case of offspring born by adopting the TESE ISCSI technique, is one in 100 cases [1, 3–6, 8]. As regards the treatment of KS patients for infertility, an important concept to be underlined is that the seminiferous tubule of spermatogonial stem cells and of the interstitial compartment of Leydig in these patients presents a normal histological picture from childhood until puberty. In pre-pubertal age, the testosterone levels and other markers of Leydig function (insulin-like 3) and sertoli function (inhibin B and anti-Mullerian factor) are normal. At puberty, and sometimes also in the pre-pubertal phase, the spermatogonia and the populations of the Leydig/Sertoli cells are reduced until the end of puberty; therefore, in adults, a hyalinisation of the seminiferous tubule is observed with the disappearance of the spermatogonia and hyperplasia of the Leydig cells in a framework of fibrosis/atrophy of the testicles [10, 11]. For this reason, a number of authors recommend the TESE (testicular sperm extraction) technique in KS patients during pre-puberty, at around 12 years old or during phase 3, i.e. during the phase of pubertal development with cryopreservation of spermatogonia. To carry out this fertility prevention programme, it is obviously necessary to perform: a double prenatal and noninvasive neonatal test to diagnose KS. Prenatal screening can be performed on the DNA of foetal cells circulating with the PCR technique or through an analysis of the gene map of the X chromosome, e.g. AR (Xp) and SHOX (Xp/Xy) or the autosomal gene GAPDH (12p), and allows to diagnose any chromosome aneuploidies including KS. This allows us to identify the patients with KS, who will be able to be subjected to the ISCI/TESE programme. An increasing number of patients with KS are making requests for paternity and to have the right to participate in the ISCSI/TESE programme. In vitro SSCs increase their number by 18 times after 64 days. Lue and collaborators have shown that, in mice, cells with an euploid kit in contact with XXY cells are able to restore spermatogenesis. The TESE technique applied to young people affected by KS brings different results in relation to age. Wikstrom and co-workers report the results of their study related to testicular biopsy, which was conducted on 14 adolescents; the research revealed that spermatogonia A of p and d types were present in seven subjects, aged 10–12.5 years, while they were completely absent in the other seven adolescents, aged 11.7–14 years [1–7–9]. Thus, TESE with pre-adolescent/adolescent cryopreservation offers better results than the same procedure in adulthood. An 8% share of non-mosaic KS patients can present sperm in the seminal fluid. Up to 50% of non-mosaic KS patients have sperm in the testis collected with TESE or micro-TESE.

Sexuality and Quality of Life

The sexuality of Klinefelter patients is often overlooked by specialists, because they are not always prepared to answer questions from patients, parents and adolescents.

In the 1960s and 1970s, systematic screening in psychiatric hospitals detected 1.3% KS among hospitalized boys, which is ten times more than in the general population, and between 0.6% and 1% KS among hospitalized patients.

The study by Raboch et al. [12] evaluated plasma testosterone levels in 105 patients with Klinefelter syndrome aged 16 to 45 years: it was found that at each 5-year interval, male hormone values were lower than in a control group of 25 healthy adolescents and 85 fertile, able-bodied men. Analysis of heterosexual development using the HTDM Questionnaire in 110 patients with Klinefelter syndrome aged 21 to 40 years, who were examined primarily for infertility and signs of imperfect somatosexual development, revealed a marked delay in sociosexual development compared with that in 325 normozoospermic men from infertile marriages. For 8 of the 12 items on the HTDM questionnaire, the differences were statistically significant. Examination using the SAM questionnaire in these two groups revealed that the sexual activity of subjects with Klinefelter syndrome was significantly weaker than that of fertile, able-bodied men. For 15 of the 18 items on the SAM questionnaire, the differences were statistically significant.

Interest in Klinefelter patients has also been studied with extensive research by psychiatrists. Ad esempio, la ricerca di Keber et al. [13].

Interest in Klinefelter patients has also included extensive psychiatric and scientific studies, for example, the research by Keber et al. [13]

Here, a wide variety of psychiatric disorders and related studies are described, noting that KS boys are described as mostly shy, with little energy and initiative and few friends: they cry more often than their peers. Neuropsychological studies show a significantly lower verbal IQ than controls, while performance IQ is generally normal and global IQ is in the normal range with large individual variations. Language acquisition is consistently delayed. However, there is no increase in aggression. Several hypotheses have been proposed to explain the psychological aspects of KS such as low androgen levels during foetal and infantile development, personality disorder related to hypogonadism and delayed mitosis of cells with an extra X chromosome, but none of these can explain the specificity of psychological problems associated with KS. As to therapeutic aspects, specialists are inclined to androgen replacement therapy in the case of testosterone blood levels being too low, from the time of FSH increase (around the age of 11–15 years). This prevents osteoporosis, back pain and excessive fatigue often seen in males with KS; testosterone also improves social drive, mood, concentration and work capacity. Where the diagnosis of KS is made in adulthood, androgen therapy has also shown some efficacy, although less than when started earlier. Because of the oral and written language problems of KS boys between the ages of 5 and 12, Graham et al. recommend preventative guidance for these boys. In addition, they insist on the importance of parental instruction, speech therapy, reducing the duration of instruction given by teachers and, particularly, stimulating and stable childhood conditions. Although androgens are generally thought to increase aggression, no consistent data in the literature demonstrating that restoring physiological blood levels of androgens increases crime or aggression have been found.

Keber's systematic study concludes that Klinefelter syndrome is common and, if undiagnosed (which seems most commonly to be the case), these patients have increased risks of developing psychiatric disorders. Therefore, psychiatrists and child psychiatrists should bear that diagnosis in mind when examining boys or men who exhibit physical traits typical of KS (height, underdeveloped testes) associated with school problems and/or psychiatric disorders. In fact, if the diagnosis is confirmed by endocrinology and genetic testing, psychological follow-up and treatment with testosterone undecanoate (in the case of abnormal blood levels of testosterone) should be initiated. This therapy would generally improve physical well-being, mood, concentration and work capacity. There are no consistent data in the literature showing that restoring physiological blood levels of testosterone would be dangerous for KS men with severe psychiatric problems.

That said through the HTDM and SAM Questionnaires, heterosexual development and sexual activity were studied in the following groups of males: [14]

1. A control group of 345 married men with infertile marriages (adequately somato-sexually developed) showed normozoospermia in the ejaculate and good potency.
2. A group of 48 unilateral and 57 bilateral adult cryptorchids.
3. 101 married patients with distinct testicular hypoplasia (with the axis of both sex glands less than 30 mm).
4. 110 patients with Klinefelter's syndrome.
5. 14 patients with hypogonadotropic hypogonadism.

Delayed heterosexual development was found only in two groups (groups 4 and 5), and in all four pathological specimens, markedly reduced activity in sexual life was ascertained.

The study by Otonicar et al. [15] investigated the psychological and behavioural characteristics of Klinefelter patients and their partners (group 1-$n = 17$) to see if they differed from couples with idiopathic infertility (group 2; $n = 16$) and fertile couples (group 3 $n = 17$). They investigated the attitudes of the three groups towards pregnancy, labour and sexuality to find potential differences among the three groups.

In addition, they tested the hypotheses of below-average intelligence and quality of social life of patients with Klinefelter syndrome compared with patients in the control group. Data were collected using the history interview, the questionnaire on attitudes towards pregnancy, labour and sexuality (SSG) and the MMPI-2 personality questionnaire.

The results showed that patients with Klinefelter syndrome and their partners did not differ significantly from couples with idiopathic infertility (group 2), having some schizoid traits in the personality structure and mostly negative attitudes towards pregnancy, labour and sexuality. However, a significant difference appeared between the Klinefelter syndrome group and the group of fertile couples. The hypothesis of lower-than-average intelligence was not confirmed, but the quality of social life of men with Klinefelter syndrome was found to be much lower. It could be concluded at the end of the study that in the management of infertile couples in which the man has Klinefelter syndrome, the personality structure should be taken into account, as this has an important impact on the outcome of treatment, by identifying schizoid traits in personality structure and negative attitudes towards pregnancy, labour and sexuality.

Conclusion

Klinefelter syndrome encompasses a significant number of symptoms, personality traits, and affective–sexual interactions. Among other things, an increased risk of autistic traits has been reported in Klinefelter syndrome (KS). Some studies have shown an increased incidence of gender dysphoria (GD) and paraphilia in autism spectrum disorder. One particular study by Fisher [16] assessed the presence of (1) paraphilic fantasies and behaviours and (2) GD symptomatology in KS. A sample of 46 KS patients and 43 healthy males in the control group (HC) was examined. Subjects were studied by several psychometric tests, such as Autism Spectrum Quotient (AQ) and Reading the Mind in the Eyes Revised (RME) to measure autistic traits, Gender Identity/GD questionnaire (GIDYQ-AA) and Sexual Addiction Screening Test (SAST). Psychopathological symptoms of bodily distress were assessed using the Symptom Checklist 90 Revised (SCL-90-R). The presence and frequency of any paraphilic fantasies and behaviours were assessed using a clinical interview based on criteria from the Diagnostic and Statistical Manual of Mental Disorders, Fifth Edition. Finally, all included individuals were assessed by Wechsler Adult Intelligence Scale-Revised to assess intelligence quotient (IQ). Results: KS patients reported significantly lower total, verbal and performance IQ scores and obsessive–compulsive symptoms. KS also showed higher autistic traits according to the RME and AQ tests. Regarding sexuality, KS showed a significantly higher frequency of voyeuristic fantasies during masturbation (52.2% versus 25.6%) and higher SAST scores ($P = 0.012$). Obsessive symptoms were confirmed in the relationship between Klinefelter and significantly higher gender dysphoric symptoms mediated by the presence of autistic traits.

References

1. Aksklaed L, Juul A. Testicular function and fertility in men with Klinefelter syndrome a review. Eur J Endocrinol. 2013;168:R67–76.
2. Wikstrom AM, Dunkel L. Klinefelter Syndrome. Best Pract Trs Clin End. 2011;25:239–50.
3. Herlihy M, Lachlan M. Screening for Klinefelter Syndrome. Curr Opin END DIAB OBES. 2015;22:224–9.
4. Anderson AM, Nuller J, Skakkebaek NE. Different role of prepubertal and post pubertal germ cells and Sertoli cells in the regulation of serum inhibin B levels. J Clin End Metab. 1998;83:4451–8.
5. Potton I, Brosse A, Groupe Fertipreserve. Infertility treatment in Klinefelter syndrome. Gynec Obst Fert. 2011;39:529–32.
6. Malbur M, Repping S, Gyltay J. The genetic origin of Klynefelter syndrome and its effect on spermatogenesis. Fert Ster. 2012;98:253–60.
7. Murphy TF. Parents choice in banking boys testicular tissue. J Med Ethics. 2010;36:806–9.
8. Norton ME, Jelliffe LL, Currier LJ. Chromosome abnormalities detected by current prenatal screening and non invasive prenatal testing. Obest Gynecol. 2012;207:314.
9. Butler G. Klinefelter's syndrome does not cause delayed puberty. BMU. 2013;346:1518.
10. River N, Milazzo JP, Perdrix A, Castanet M, Sibert L, et al. The feasibility of fertility preservation in adolescents with Klinefelter syndrome. Hum Reprod. 2013;28:1468–79.

11. Ramasamy R, Ricci JA, Palermo GD, Godstein LV. Successful fertility treatment for Klinefelter's syndrome. J Urol. 2009;182:1108–13.
12. Raboch J, Mellan J, Stárka L. Klinefelter's syndrome: sexual development and activity. Arch Sex Behav. 1979;8(4):333–9. https://doi.org/10.1007/BF01541877. PMID: 475580.
13. Kebers F, Janvier S, Colin A, Legros JJ, Ansseau M. En quoi le syndrome de Klinefelter peut-il intéresser le psychiatre et le pédopsychiatre? [What is the interest of Klinefelter's syndrome for (child) psychiatrists?]. Encephale. 2002;28(3 Pt 1):260–5. French. PMID: 12091788.
14. Raboch J, Mellan J. Sexual development and activity of men with disturbances of somatic development. Andrologia. 1979;11(4):263–71. https://doi.org/10.1111/j.1439-0272.1979. tb02202.x. PMID: 40461.
15. Otonicar B, Velikonja V, Zorn B. Traits de personnalité des hommes atteints de syndrome de Klinefelter et de leurs partenaires [Personality traits of men with Klinefelter syndrome and their partners]. Gynecol Obstet Fertil. 2001;29(2):123–8.
16. Fisher AD, Castellini G, Casale H, Fanni E, Bandini E, Campone B, Ferruccio N, Maseroli E, Boddi V, Dèttore D, Pizzocaro A, Balercia G, Oppo A, Ricca V, Maggi M. Hypersexuality, paraphilic behaviors, and gender dysphoria in individuals with Klinefelter's syndrome. J Sex Med. 2015;12(12):2413–24.

Part XI
Inflammatory Bowel Diseases

Crohn's Disease

Giulia Roda and Elena Vittoria Longhi

Introduction

Crohn's disease (CD) is a chronic inflammatory bowel disease with a progressive and destructive course over time [1]. CD is one of the two subtypes of inflammatory bowel diseases (IBD), which include CD and ulcerative colitis (UC). Its prevalence and incidence are increasing worldwide [2]. The global prevalence of IBD has been increasing since the year 2000 and now affects up to one in 200 individuals in Western countries [2]. Higher rates of incidence with a peak between the second and fourth decades of life have been described in Ashkenazi Jews, urban populations and population in the northern latitudes [2]. However, many epidemiologic studies have revealed an increased incidence in the elderly. In Western countries, no sex-related prevalence has been determined, while a male prevalence has been associated with the risk to develop CD in Asia [2]. Moreover, recent studies have shown an increase in the incidence of CD in Asia [3].

Several factors contribute to the pathogenesis of CD such as a dysregulated immune system, an altered microbiome, genetic susceptibility and environmental factors [4]. More than 200 loci associated with CD risk have been discovered with genome-wide association studies (GWAS) in addition to the intracellular pattern recognition receptor gene *NOD2* (*CARD15*) discovered in 2001 [5–8].

Clinically, CD affects mostly young patients and symptoms are typically abdominal pain, chronic diarrhoea, urgency, weight loss and fatigue [1].

Familial inheritance of CD has been shown with concordance rates amongst monozygotic twins around ~50% [1, 9].

G. Roda (✉)
IBD Center, Humanitas Research Hospital, Milan, Italy
e-mail: giulia.roda@humanitas.it

E. V. Longhi
Department of Sexual Medical Center, San Raffaele Hospital, Milano, Italy

© Springer Nature Switzerland AG 2023
E. V. Longhi (ed.), *Managing Psychosexual Consequences in Chronic Diseases*,
https://doi.org/10.1007/978-3-031-31307-3_19

Diagnosis still relies on endoscopy and histological assessment of biopsy specimens.

Given its progressive nature, the management of this chronic disease is based on a prompt assessment of disease extent and severity and of prognostic factors able to predict complications such as stenosis or perianal disease. Therapeutic interventions aim to induce deep and long-lasting remission and to avoid surgery and other complications in the long term. Achieving mucosal healing, defined as restitution of the mucosal epithelium as absence of ulcers, represents nowadays the target of the treatment as it leads to outcome improvement, including decreased risk of surgery, frequency of relapse rates and quality of life (QOL) [10].

Therefore, treatment with biological therapies and/or immunosuppressant drugs or novel small molecules in combination with tight control and adjustment of the therapy (treat-to-target approach) based on a specific target could impact the natural history of the disease and determine disease modification with improvement of clinical outcomes, a decrease in complications and need for hospitalization and surgery [11–13].

Main Medical Characteristics

CD symptoms are heterogeneous and depend on disease location (ileo vs colon vs upper digestive tract), severity of inflammation and disease behaviour (including complications).

Natural History

CD is characterized by skip intestinal lesions that can affect the entire gastrointestinal (GI) tract and involves chronic, relapsing transmural inflammation. CD has different phenotypes: 'stricturing disease' due to fibrosis; 'penetrating disease' due to fistulas between the gut and other structures (intestinal tract, bladder, vagina, etc.); disease lacking these features, which is termed 'inflammatory' or 'non-stricturing, non-penetrating disease'; and 'stricturing, penetrating disease'. During CD natural history, disease phenotype can evolve from inflammatory disease to structuring and/or penetrating disease. Studies investigating what patients will evolve towards a complicated disease are still lacking. However, data have shown that early treatment can modify the natural history of the disease. Moreover, repeated cycles of inflammation can lead to bowel damage that could be irreversible [14]. Disease location remains stable over time. A third of patients with CD present with large bowel disease, 30% with ileocolonic disease and a 30% with small bowel disease. 30% to 75% of patients have upper GI tract involvement [15, 16]. CD is characterized by periods of remission and flares, which occur randomly. Up to 50% of patients require intestinal resection within 10 years of a CD diagnosis. The major complications given the progressive nature of the disease are strictures and perianal involvement, which are present in 50% of all patients with CD within 10 years of a diagnosis. Population-based cohort studies have demonstrated that up to 30% of patients with CD have bowel damage at diagnosis, and half of these patients need surgery in the 20 years following a CD diagnosis [17, 18]. Forty per cent of patients have bowel damage within 1 year of diagnosis and present worse outcomes, including high rates of surgery and hospitalization. Around a third of CD patients have perianal disease at diagnosis [19].

Symptoms

In clinical practice, the typical CD patient is a young patient with right lower quadrant abdominal pain, chronic diarrhoea without blood in the majority of cases (ileal localization) and weight loss. When the colon is affected, rectal bleeding is the major symptom. Fever is related to a septic complication such as abscesses. In the stricturing phenotype, bowel obstruction leads to hyperactive bowel sounds, nausea and vomiting. In the penetrating phenotype, fistulas or abscesses cause the major symptoms [20].

In 50% of patients with CD, extraintestinal manifestations (EIMs) including skin, joint or eye can be present before intestinal disease diagnosis. Axial arthropathy (including ankylosing spondylitis and sacroiliitis) and erythema nodosum parallel intestinal activity. Peripheral arthropathy (type 2 polyarticular) and pyoderma gangrenosum are usually independent of disease activity (except for type 1—pauciarticular arthropathy) and can persist when CD is in remission [21].

Patients with CD have an increased risk of developing colorectal cancer and small bowel cancers compared with the general population [22]. Moreover, a three-fold increased risk of deep venous thrombosis and pulmonary embolism compared with the general population has been determined by several studies [23].

Among the *risk factors*, smoking has been identified as the only modifiable risk factor associated with early disease onset, need for immunosuppression, increased need for surgical interventions and higher rates of post-operative disease recurrence [1]. Family history of IBD is another well-known risk factor for CD.

Physical examination should assess abdominal signs of inflammation and or the presence of abscesses and signs of malnutrition, dehydration, anaemia or malabsorption. Perianal region examination should be given to all the patients with suspected or established diagnosis of CD to exclude a perianal involvement such as skin lesions (ulcerations and skin tags), anal canal lesions (stenosis, fissures and ulcers) and fistulas in the presence or absence of abscesses.

Main Tools for Diagnosis of CD

Diagnosis of CD can be challenging. Indeed, a combination of assessments is needed such as assessment based on clinical history, physical examination and diagnostic tests (serological and faecal biomarkers), cross-sectional imaging and endoscopy and histological evaluation of biopsy specimens [23, 24].

The diagnosis of CD is often delayed by 5–9 months due to the variability of the disease. This window of 5–9 months highly impacts the quality of life and the natural history of the disease with complications and ileocolic resection. The early identification of early symptoms and signs is pivotal to reduce the diagnostic delay and manage the patient within the therapeutic window of opportunities. Recently, a Red Flags Index has been developed to enable early and timely diagnosis of CD. It includes eight items (non-healing or complex perianal fistula or abscess or perianal lesions, first-degree relative with confirmed inflammatory bowel disease, weight loss (5% of usual body weight) in the last 3 months, chronic abdominal pain, nocturnal diarrhoea, mild fever in the last 3 months, no abdominal pain 30–45 min after meals, predominantly after vegetables and no rectal urgency) to help to discriminate functional gut disorders from CD. This index has been developed to help clinicians in primary or secondary care for an early diagnosis of IBD because it is highly predictive of CD [25] (Fig. 1).

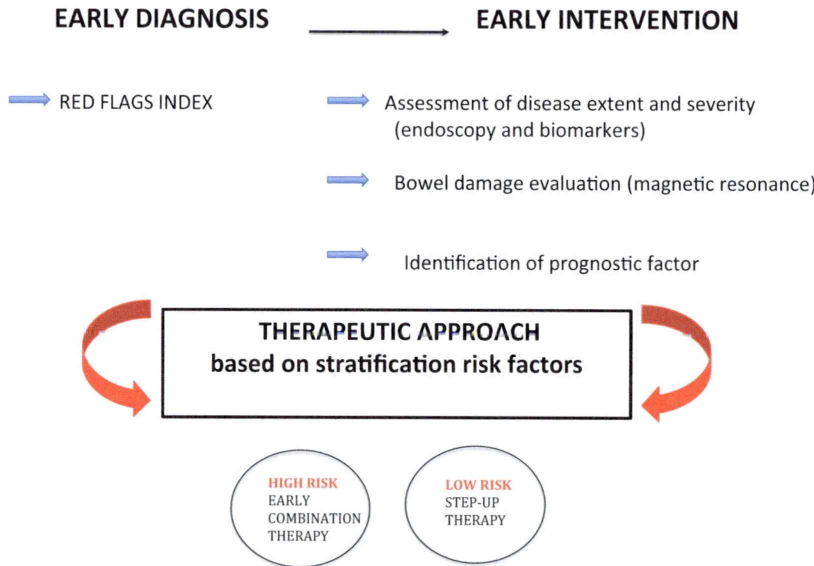

Fig. 1 From early diagnosis to early intervention in CD

The main clinical score to assess response to treatment is the Crohn's disease activity Index (CDAI), which is used in clinical trials. A simplified version of the CDAI is the Harvey Bradshaw index (HBI), which includes only clinical parameters without laboratory analysis, and it is easier to use also in clinical practice.

Typically, routinary blood test in active CD shows thrombocytosis, increased C-reactive protein (CRP) and anaemia. Hypoalbuminaemia and vitamin deficiencies might be present, especially in extensive small bowel disease. C-reactive protein is a serological biomarker used in clinical practice to monitor disease activity. CRP is not a diagnostic marker, and around one-third of patients have normal CRP levels despite active disease and one-third have increased CRP levels despite clinically inactive disease [26].

Sixty per cent of CD patients are positive for antimicrobial antibodies, such as anti-*Saccharomyces cerevisiae* antibodies (ASCA), 10% to 15% for auto-antibodies, such as perinuclear anti-neutrophil cytoplasmic antibodies (pANCA).

To assess disease activity, faecal calprotectin, a stool biomarker, is used in clinical practice. Its concentrations correlate with neutrophil infiltrates in the gut. This marker is mostly used in clinical practice to screen patients for endoscopy as patients with a concentration of less than 40 μg/g with associated symptoms typical of irritable bowel syndrome have been shown to be associated with a low risk of IBD (1%) [27]. Thus, faecal calprotectin is a useful biomarker to monitor disease activity, assess response to therapy and predict clinical relapse and postoperative recurrence [28].

Endoscopy remains the gold standard for diagnosis. Endoscopic findings for a diagnosis of CD include a patchy distribution of inflammation and skip lesions. Typically, intestinal lesions are aphthoid erosions defined as ulcer with a diameter lower than 5 mm or ulcers that tend to be longitudinal with a cobble-stone appearance and with a diameter greater than 5 mm. Ulcers can be superficial or deep, based on the muscularis propria involvement. The Simplified Endoscopic Score for Crohn's disease (SES-CD) is an endoscopic score important to compare assessments and to define response to treatment by evaluating mucosal healing as therapeutic goal. Endoscopy is also crucial to screen for colorectal cancer, and a surveillance programme is recommended for patients affected by IBD. In patients with clinical suspicion of CD but negative findings by ileocolonoscopy and radiological examinations, small-bowel capsule endoscopy (SBCE) is recommended [29].

To confirm CD diagnosis, histological examination of endoscopic biopsies is the gold standard. Typical microscopic features of CD are as follows: focal (discontinuous) chronic inflammation, focal crypt irregularity, granulomas and irregular villous architecture in the terminal ileum [30].

Assessment of disease extent and complications (such as stenosis, fistulas and abscesses) with cross-sectional imaging is important in CD. Bowel ultrasonography (BUS), CTE and MRI enterography (MRE) have comparable accuracy for both diagnosis of CD and the detection of complications [31, 32].

Main Surgical Treatments

In the past decade, treatment goals have changed from treating symptoms to treating beyond symptoms to modify the natural history of the disease and improved outcomes such as reduction in the risk of relapse, decrease in hospitalization rates, achievement of steroid-free remission and resection-free intervals. In the past, patients were started on aminosalicylates, steroids or thiopurine, and when they failed these therapies, a step-up approach was initiated with dose escalation. However, data have shown that this strategy fails to change the course of disease.

Endoscopic healing, usually defined as the absence of ulcerations, is the major therapeutic target in IBD because it correlates with better outcomes.

In patients with severe Crohn's or complicated disease, a top-down approach might be considered.

The treatment of CD includes an induction phase and a maintenance phase. The most widely used drugs in CD are corticosteroids, immunosuppressants, biologicals (anti-TNFs), anti-adhesion molecules (vedolizumab) and anti-IL-12/IL-23 molecules (ustekinumab). 5-aminosalicylates have not shown efficacy in CD and antibiotics that are used in complicated CD.

According to guidelines, mild-to-moderately active disease should be treated with steroids (budesonide or prednisone) [29, 33]. Although budesonide and prednisolone are not effective for maintaining remission, steroid discharge with a steroid-sparing agent should be a major therapeutic goal because of the side effects associated with prolonged exposure. Nutritional therapy is pivotal in the presence of weight loss and in the pre-operative window.

Thiopurines and methotrexate should be considered for maintenance therapy, and they are associated with a reduced need for surgery [34]. However, an increased risk of cancer such as lymphoma, non-melanoma skin cancers, myeloid disorders and urinary tract cancers is associated with these drugs [35].

Biological agents (anti-TNFs agents, vedolizumab and ustekinumab) can be used for induction and/or maintenance therapy of CD.

According to drug labelling, anti-TNF agents (infliximab, adalimumab and certolizumab pegol) effective to induce and maintain remission are restricted to patients not responsive to steroids or thiopurine. Certolizumab is only available in North America, Switzerland and a few other countries.

Infliximab is the first anti-TNFs, and it has shown efficacy to treat perianal disease.

Moreover, infliximab as monotherapy or combined with azathioprine was significantly more effective than azathioprine alone when steroid-free remission and mucosal healing rates at 6 months were evaluated [36].

Immunogenicity is a major issue with all monoclonal antibodies; it is reduced by the combination with an immunosuppressant drug.

Vedolizumab is a gut-selective intravenously administered monoclonal antibody blocking $\alpha 4\beta 7$ integrin, with efficacy in induction and maintenance of clinical remission in refractory and luminal CD. Vedolizumab is used in patients with multiple comorbidities or in the elderly patients due to infection risk from other biologics.

Ustekinumab is a monoclonal antibody directed against interleukin-12 and interleukin-23. After an intravenous infusion for induction, it is administered subcutaneously every 8 weeks for maintenance therapy. Ustekinumab has shown superiority to placebo in anti-TNF naïve and refractory patients with moderate-to-severe CD.

In clinical practice, biological therapies, such as anti-TNF agents, ustekinumab and vedolizumab, are preferred drugs compared to thiopurines in high-risk patients and showed superiority on several clinical trials.

In patients who fail to respond to or stop responding to biological agents, switching between different non-anti-TNFs (different mechanisms of action) and switching to another anti-TNF biological drug are options.

CD patients usually undergo surgery when the disease is refractory to medical treatment, in the presence of complications (stenosis, fistula, abscesses or cancer) and intolerance to medical therapy. Surgery is not curative in CD. A multidisciplinary team should be responsible for surgery decision.

The exact surgical procedure depends on the underlying reason for the surgery. In the presence of multiple strictures, removal of the most prominent stricture with an anastomosis and intraoperatively dilatation or strictureplasty of the remaining ones is the ideal treatment option to preserve the intestine. Bowel resection and fistulotomy are indicated in fistulizing CD in case of fistula communicating with the intestinal tract such as enterovesicular fistulae, enterovaginal fistulae or enterocutaneous fistulae. Surgical drainage of the abscess may be required depending on the size and presence of septic symptoms. Perianal fistula and abscess often require surgical intervention with drainage and placement of a seton.

Sexuality and Quality of Life

Psychological disorders are common in patients with Crohn's disease (CD). The study by Cozaru et al. [21] aimed to determine the frequency with which depression and anxiety occur in patients with CD by tracking some socio-demographic and medical variables and checking the relationship between depression and age, stage of evolution and duration of the disease.

Two groups of patients were followed (sex ratio F:M—1/1): a group of 45 patients diagnosed with CD and a control group of 45 patients with enterocolitis (EC). The Beck Depression Inventory (BDI) was used to assess depression and the State-Trait Anxiety Inventory (Spielberger) to assess anxiety.

The results showed that 62.34% of patients with Crohn's disease had moderate and severe depression, in contrast to the control group, where only 16.46% had moderate or severe depression.

Higher than average levels of anxiety were found in both groups, suggesting that this is associated with a greater extent with MICI.

The anxiety and depression levels of patients with active disease were higher than those of EC, but not of patients in remission. The depression score of the CD sample was higher than that of the EC sample ($P < 0.001$). There was no significant difference in trait anxiety between the groups. Based on these results, it is clear that screening for depression and anxiety should be performed routinely as part of improving the quality of care in individuals with this condition.

In particular, if the patients are children, certain precautions need to be considered. Children with diagnosed inflammatory bowel diseases such as Crohn's disease face the daunting prospect of living with a chronic condition. In addition to psychological stress, children suffer from the side effects of therapy; in particular, corticosteroid therapies are problematic in the growth phase. This highlights the need for less aggressive alternative therapies for children and adolescents living with such a chronic condition. Elemental diets are widely used and accepted treatment options. Several paediatric patients with Crohn's disease also use complementary, alternative and integrative therapies to reduce or avoid drug therapies.

The study by Schwermer et al. [22] investigated elemental diets (Flexical, Elemental 028), semi-elemental diets (Pregomin), polymeric diets (Modulen IBD), whole protein formulas and ω-3 fatty acid supplementation. The data indicated that dietary therapies were equal to or more effective than corticosteroid therapies when used for the treatment of Crohn's disease.

However, it should be considered that the psychic part of children, strongly influenced by the symptoms of Crohn's disease, is reflected in their parents' anxiety and guilt throughout the course of their lives. In addition to diet, children and parents need to be supported to avoid making pathology the only yardstick for adherence to sociality, integration with the peer group and normal pre- and post-puberty growth processes.

Many of these children show depression, anxiety and sleep and behavioural disorders because they feel alienated and inadequate in the world around them [23].

In this connection, the study by Badarnee et al. [24] investigated not only external stress factors but also personal psychological characteristics that increase patients' vulnerability to stress.

The psychological characteristics of 49 patients diagnosed with Crohn's disease and 56 patients in the control group were compared. The psychological characteristics were defined by four types of assessment: assessment of oneself, general assessment of the future, assessment of the therapy and assessment of the difficulties to be overcome.

The types of assessments differed between the two groups and patients were characterized by six items:

- How to get over the routine
- Strive for the love of others
- Take care of your body and health
- Do things only at your own pace
- Express negative emotions without rules
- Feeling too identified with others

Children with MICI are characterized by chronic stress (e.g. over-identification with others) and interpersonal conflicts (e.g. doing things only at one's own pace) as well as an unequal quality of life in relation to the peer group.

That is not all. Although there have been significant advances in medical therapies for the treatment of Crohn's disease, it is estimated that 50% of patients will require surgery within the first decade of the disease's duration [25]. Of these patients, a considerable number will develop recurrent symptoms within the first postoperative year. To prevent disease recurrence, many clinicians use postoperative prophylactic therapy. Randomized controlled trials, although limited in number, have shown that a prophylactic postoperative strategy is effective in reducing recurrences (both clinical and endoscopic) in high-risk patients [26].

Among the factors affecting the frequency of postoperative recurrence, the study by Yamamoto et al. [27] reviewed the literature in focusing on the following factors: age at disease onset, sex, family history of Crohn's disease, smoking, duration of Crohn's disease before surgery, prophylactic medical treatment (corticosteroids, 5-aminosalicylic acid (5-ASA) and immunosuppressants), anatomical site of involvement, indication for surgery (perforating or non-perforating disease), length of the resected bowel, anastomotic technique, presence of granuloma in the specimen, disease involvement at the resection margin, blood transfusions and postoperative complications.

Smoking significantly increases the risk of recurrence (the risk is approximately twice as high), especially in women and heavy smokers. Quitting smoking reduces the rate of postoperative recurrence. Several studies have shown a higher risk when the duration of the disease before surgery was short. There were, however, different definitions of 'short' among the studies.

In addition, different clinical studies have shown a higher recurrence rate in patients with perforating disease than in those with non-perforating disease. However, the evidence of different recurrence rates in perforating and non-perforating disease is not conclusive. The result of Yamamoto's research showed that the factors examined (age at disease onset, gender, family history of Crohn's disease, anatomical site of disease, length of resected bowel, presence of granuloma in the specimen, blood transfusions and post-operative complications) were not predictive of post-operative recurrence.

The most significant factor influencing postoperative recurrence of Crohn's disease remains smoking.

A more recent study with regard to this, by Ozgur et al. [28], revisited the medical records of patients with CD, treated surgically between January 2003 and January 2015. Data including demographic and clinical characteristics of the patients were recorded. Recurrence was assessed on the basis of the Crohn's Disease Activity Index or endoscopic findings. The majority of the 112 patients were male ($n = 64$, 57.1%), and 61 (54.4%) of them were active smokers. The median follow-up was 113 (range: 61–197) months. Disease recurrence occurred in 16 (14.3%) patients at a median of 13.5 months. The endoscopic recurrence rate was 8% ($n = 9$) at 1 year, 12.5% ($n = 14$) at 5 years and 13.4% ($n = 15$) at 10 years.

The results of the study suggest that patients' age at diagnosis, penetrating disease, intra-abdominal abscess and concomitant fistula and abscess are the risk factors for CD recurrence after surgery. Only 0.9% of patients underwent colonoscopic balloon dilatation at 1 year, and 8 (7.1%) patients required resection at a median of 36 months. Patient age at diagnosis ($P = 0.033$), penetrating disease behaviour ($P = 0.011$), intra-abdominal abscess ($P = 0.040$) and concomitant fistula and intra-abdominal abscess ($P = 0.017$) were associated with disease recurrence.

But let us ask ourselves: How do patients experience Crohn's disease? How do they cope with anxiety, depression and sexual activity?

There is no doubt that sexual function is more affected by active disease than by disease in remission in both women and men. The partial sexual function score in women and men with active disease is significantly lower than in patients with disease in remission and/or under control, indicating a worse sexual function during the period when the disease is active [29, 30]. In the study by Timmer et al. [31], an alteration in sexual function was shown in women regardless of disease activity compared with the control group: low sexual activity (63%), 17% no sexual activity and 20% moderate or high activity.

Another study by Timmer et al. [32] also shows that increasing disease duration improves all outcomes, suggesting that over time the patient develops effective coping strategies.

It is easy to deduce that *body image and sex role are also questioned by patients diagnosed with Crohn's disease, irrespective of gender.*

Studies seem to show that there are no major differences in the perception of body image between patients with Crohn's disease (73.2%) and patients with rectal ulcerative colitis (60%). In the two diseases [33], reciprocal influences between body image and intimacy, libido, body perception and sexual activity [29] of patients emerged, particularly in women. 66.8% of the patients in the study (56) reported an impairment of body image. A decrease in the frequency of sexual activity was found in the majority of women with Crohn's disease and in all those patients with such severity of active disease that sexual intercourse was impaired. Half of the women and between one-third and one-half of the men reported a decrease in sexual desire or libido after diagnosis and with active disease [34].

The occurrence of sexual dysfunction in people with Crohn's disease is between 10% and 60% in men and 52% to 60% in women.

The main sexual dysfunctions found in patients are decreased frequency of sexual activity, decreased libido and impaired body image. Erectile dysfunction and arousal disturbance are more likely to be found in male patients, while altered body image, vaginal dryness, hypoactive desire and arousal disturbance are found in female patients.

Intimacy, which is already much compromised, also leads to states of anxiety, depression, mood disorders, compulsiveness or food restriction and sleep disorders. So much so that 88.5% of patients indicate a severe impairment of their quality of life.

The role of specialists and sexologists in these cases becomes fundamental: 61% of women and 46% of men affected by Crohn's disease have requested information on the impact of the disease on intimacy and sexuality, identifying their specialist as the appropriate interlocutor to clarify their doubts. In particular, female patients are more likely to seek information, even if this does not result in an actual conversation with the health professional, especially if the treating professional is of the opposite sex [35].

Although issues related to sexual disorders are considered very important by the patient, they are rarely discussed with the care team. The likelihood that the patient will address these issues elsewhere is minimal. It has been found that women are less likely to disclose such information to a general practitioner or gastroenterologist (especially if the doctor is of the opposite sex), but to a sexologist, seen as the clinician who cannot judge, it would be easier, especially if he or she is part of the clinical team [36].

It goes without saying, in relation to this picture of the psychological and relational repercussions in patients diagnosed with Crohn's disease, that the progression of the disease and the medical treatments condition the relationship with the caregivers: partners and family members.

In fact, 50.2% of 347 patients suffering from Crohn's disease (208 patients) and rectal ulcerative colitis (124 patients) and indeterminate colitis (15 patients) declared a negative effect of the disease in the sphere of affective, but also professional and social relationships [36].

Last but not least, caregivers, who are often attributed by the medical team with an overestimation of their psychic and relational abilities with the patient and healthcare professionals, if involved, show helplessness, frustration, anger, repressed aggressiveness, anhedonia, chronic fatigue and mood disorders.

Conclusion

What can be said? The complexity of Crohn's disease alongside the chronicity and variance of the clinical process induces the patient and caregivers to compromise on life. The therapeutic and follow-up agenda conditions every long- and short-term plan. The relationship with the clinicians often appears to be the only social and therapeutic contact. It is difficult to meet friends because of the unpredictability of the symptoms and the loneliness often induced by the pathology. The clinicians, while observing these aspects, try to encourage and support, but there is still a lack of preparation in these matters.

Moreover, even looking at the Crohn's disease activity index (CDAI), there is no mention of aspects arising from the disease. The assumption that the multidisciplinary team can be a useful reference point not only for patients but also for the clinicians themselves is confirmed. The psychosexologist could be a figure of facilitation and conveyance in the communication with the patient and the caregiver, as an element of support in the compliance of the therapeutic process.

References

1. Torres J, Mehandru S, Colombel J-F, Peyrin-Biroulet L. Crohn's disease. Lancet. 2017;389:1741–55.
2. Ng SC, et al. Worldwide incidence and prevalence of inflammatory bowel disease in the twenty-first century: a systematic review of population-based studies. Lancet. 2017;390:2769–78.
3. Ng SC, et al. Incidence and phenotype of inflammatory bowel disease based on results from the Asia-pacific Crohn's and colitis epidemiology study. Gastroenterology. 2013;145(1):158–65.
4. Ananthakrishnan AN, et al. Environmental triggers in IBD: a review of progress and evidence. Nat Rev Gastroenterol Hepatol. 2017;15:39–49.
5. Ogura Y, et al. A frameshift mutation in NOD2 associated with susceptibility to Crohn's disease. Nature. 2001;411:603–6.
6. Yamazaki K, et al. Single nucleotide polymorphisms in TNFSF15 confer susceptibility to Crohn's disease. Hum Mol Genet. 2005;14:3499–506.
7. Huang H, et al. Fine-mapping inflammatory bowel disease loci to single-variant resolution. Nature. 2017;547:173–8.
8. The International IBD Genetics Consortium (IIBDGC), et al. Analysis of five chronic inflammatory diseases identifies 27 new associations and highlights disease-specific patterns at shared loci. Nat Genet. 2016;48:510–8.
9. Halfvarson J, Bodin L, Tysk C, Lindberg E, Järnerot G. Inflammatory bowel disease in a Swedish twin cohort: a long-term follow-up of concordance and clinical characteristics. Gastroenterology. 2003;124:1767–73.
10. Bernstein CN, et al. Increased burden of psychiatric disorders in inflammatory bowel disease. Inflamm Bowel Dis. 2019;25:360–8.
11. Reinink AR, Lee TC, Higgins PDR. Endoscopic mucosal healing predicts favorable clinical outcomes in inflammatory bowel disease: a meta-analysis. Inflamm Bowel Dis. 2016;22:1859–69.
12. Shah SC, Colombel J-F, Sands BE, Narula N. Systematic review with meta-analysis: mucosal healing is associated with improved long-term outcomes in Crohn's disease. Aliment Pharmacol Ther. 2016;43:317–33.
13. Peyrin-Biroulet L, et al. Selecting therapeutic targets in inflammatory bowel disease (STRIDE): determining therapeutic goals for treat-to-target. Am J Gastroenterol. 2015;110:1324–38.
14. Peyrin-Biroulet L, Loftus EV, Colombel J-F, Sandborn WJ. The natural history of adult Crohn's disease in population-based cohorts. Am J Gastroenterol. 2010;105:289–97.
15. Kuriyama M, Kato J, Morimoto N, Fujimoto T, Okada H, Yamamoto K. Specific gastroduodenoscopic findings in Crohn's disease: comparison with findings in patients with ulcerative colitis and gastroesophageal reflux disease. Dig Liver Dis. 2008;40:468–75.
16. Sawczenko A, Sandhu BK. Presenting features of inflammatory bowel disease in Great Britain and Ireland. Arch Dis Child. 2003;88:995–1000.
17. Thia KT, Sandborn WJ, Harmsen WS, Zinsmeister AR, Loftus EV. Risk factors associated with progression to intestinal complications of Crohn's disease in a population-based cohort. Gastroenterology. 2010;139:1147–55.
18. Fiorino G, Bonifacio C, Peyrin-Biroulet L, Danese S. Preventing collateral damage in Crohn's disease: the Lémann index. J Crohns Colitis. 2016;10:495–500.
19. Fiorino G, et al. Prevalence of bowel damage assessed by cross-sectional imaging in early Crohn's disease and its impact on disease outcome. J Crohns Colitis. 2017;11(3):274–80.
20. Peyrin-Biroulet L, et al. Perianal Crohn's disease findings other than fistulas in a population-based cohort: inflamm. Bowel Dis. 2012;18:43–8.
21. Cozaru GC, Papari AC, Sava N, Papari A. P-1363 - Assessment of anxiety and depression in patients with Chron disease. Eur Psychiatry. 2012;27(Suppl 1):1–10.
22. Schwermer M, Fetz K, Längler A, Ostermann T, Zuzak TJ. Complementary, alternative, integrative and dietary therapies for children with Crohn's disease – A systematic review. Complement Ther Med. 2020;52:102493.

23. Paiva AS, Faria A, Loureiro H. Diet impact perception in inflammatory bowel disease patients. Clin Nutr ESPEN. 2021;46:S663.
24. Badarnee M, Weiss B, Shouval D, Kreitler S. Motivational disposition towards psychological characteristics of Israeli children with inflammatory bowel diseases: a case-control study. J Pediatr Nurs. 2022;62:e131–8.
25. Rice HE, Chuang E. Current management of pediatric inflammatory bowel disease. Semin Pediatr Surg. 1999;8(4):221–8.
26. Cohen-Mekelburg S, Schneider Y, Gold S, Scherl E, Steinlauf A. Risk stratification for prevention of recurrence of postoperative Crohn's disease. Gastroenterol Hepatol (N Y). 2017;13(11):651–8. PMID: 29230144; PMCID: PMC5717880.
27. Yamamoto T. Factors affecting recurrence after surgery for Crohn's disease. World J Gastroenterol. 2005;11(26):3971–9. https://doi.org/10.3748/wjg.v11.i26.3971. PMID: 15996018; PMCID: PMC4502089.
28. Ozgur I, Kulle CB, Buyuk M, Ormeci A, Akyuz F, Balik E, Bulut T, Keskin M. What are the predictors for recurrence of Crohn's disease after surgery? Medicine (Baltimore). 2021;100(14):e25340.
29. Knowles SR, et al. Illness perceptions in IBD influence psychological status, sexual health and satisfaction, body image and relational functioning: a preliminary exploration using Structural Equation Modeling. J Crohn's Colitis. 2013;7:e344–50.
30. O'Connor M, Bager P, Duncan J, Gaarenstroom J, Younge L, Detre. N-ECCO Consensus statements on the European nursing roles in caring for patients with Crohn's disease or ulcerative colitis. J Crohn's Colitis. 2013;7(9):744–64.
31. Timmer A, Kemptner D, Bauer A, Takses A, Ott C, Furst A. Determinants of female sexual function in inflammatory bowel disease: a survey based cross-sectional analysis. BMC Gastroenterol. 2008;8(1):45.
32. Timmer A, Bauer A, Kemptner D, Furst A, Rogler G. Determinants of male sexual function in inflammatory bowel disease: a survey-based cross-sectional analysis in 280 men. Inflamm Bowel Dis. 2007;13(10):1236–43.
33. Muller KR, Prosser R, Bampton P, Mountifield R, Andrews JM. Female gender and surgery impair relationships, body image, and sexuality in inflammatory bowel disease: patient perceptions. Inflamm Bowel Dis. 2010;16(4):657–63.
34. O'Toole A, Winter D, Friedman S. Review article: the psychosexual impact of inflammatory bowel disease in male patients. Aliment Pharmacol Ther. 2014;39(10):1085–94.
35. Dolak F, et al. The reflection of the quality of life of people with Crohn's disease in nursing. Neuroendocrinol Lett. 2014;35(Suppl 1):19–25.
36. Borum ML, Igiehon E, Shafa S. Physicians may inadequately address sexuality in women with inflammatory bowel disease. Inflamm Bowel Dis. 2010;16(2):181.

Part XII
Hypogonadism

Hypogonadism

Mariano Galdiero and Elena Vittoria Longhi

Introduction

Male hypogonadism (HG) is a clinical syndrome that results from impaired testicular functions, steroidogenesis and gametogenesis and is consequently associated with low testosterone (T) concentration (T deficiency) and/or altered semen quality. In clinical practice, the term 'hypogonadism' is commonly used to identify the clinical syndrome related to low T concentration more than the altered spermatogenesis. HG can be classified as congenital or acquired and also as primary or secondary in relation to the type of alteration of the hypothalamic–pituitary–testicular axis [1]. Abnormalities of the testicular function itself cause primary (hypergonadotropic) HG, whereas defects of the hypothalamus or the pituitary cause secondary (central, hypogonadotropic) HG (Table 1). In some cases, both central and testis functions can be affected resulting in a mixed form of HG. Furthermore, HG-like syndrome can also be caused by an impairment in androgen activity for example through reduced levels of free T in case of increased levels of the sex hormone-binding globulin (SHBG) by which T is bound [2]. Causes of hypogonadism may be organic or functional. Organic HG is only a curable disease, frequently permanent, while functional HG is caused by conditions that disrupt gonadotropins and T concentrations, but it is potentially reversible by treating the underlying aetiology [3]. T actions are related not only to direct genomic and non-genomic effects, but also to indirect estrogenic-induced effects. T production by the foetal testis induces the differentiation of internal genitalia and the correct testis descent. During puberty, T is the main regulator of secondary sexual characteristics development, male fertility

M. Galdiero (✉)
Department of Internal Medicine, Endocrinology and Andrology Section, A. Rizzoli Hospital, Ischia Island, Naples, Italy
e-mail: mariano.galdiero@aslnapoli2nord.it

E. V. Longhi
Sexual Medical Center, San Raffaele Hospital, Milano, Italy

© Springer Nature Switzerland AG 2023
E. V. Longhi (ed.), *Managing Psychosexual Consequences in Chronic Diseases*,
https://doi.org/10.1007/978-3-031-31307-3_20

Table 1 Classification of the major causes of hypogonadism

Primary hypogonadism	Secondary hypogonadism
Organic	*Organic*
Klinefelter syndrome (47,XXY and variants)	Hypothalamic/pituitary tumour
Cryptorchidism, anorchia	Iron overload syndromes
Chemotherapy/radiotherapy	Infiltrative/infection disease of the hypothalamus/pituitary
Orchidectomy	Congenital hypogonadotropic hypogonadism
Orchitis	• *Kallmann syndrome (isolated)*
Torsion/trauma	• *Idiopathic (isolated)*
Noonan syndrome	• *Combined (+ other hormonal deficiency)*
HIV infection	
Functional	*Functional*
Ageing	Hyperprolactinaemia
Drugs	Opioids, steroids, GnRH analogues
Pollutants	Alcohol and marijuana abuse
Chronic kidney disease	Systemic illness
	Nutritional deficiency/strenuous physical exercise
	Severe obesity, metabolic syndrome, type II diabetes
	Organ failure (liver, heart and lung)
	Traumatic brain injury

Modified by Refs. [2] and [3]. GnRH: gonadotropin-releasing hormone

and growth pubertal spurt. During adulthood, T is involved in sexual function and behaviour, maintenance of bone health, regulation of body composition (muscle mass and fat distribution) and glucose or lipid metabolism while is still unclear the possible effects on mood and cognitive functions. The so wide spectrum of T effects explains the necessity of a correct HG diagnosis and the comprehension of T deficiency sign, symptoms and related pathology [1].

Main Medical Characteristics of Hypogonadism

Clinical manifestations of HG are related to the time of onset (prepubertal or postpubertal), to the severity and duration of T deficiency and individual variation in androgen sensitivity. Patients diagnosed with prepubertal onset of HG can manifest eunuchoid body habitus with disproportionately long arm and legs, lack of development of secondary sex characteristics (scant pubic and axillary hair, and high-pitched voice, reduced muscle mass, reduced penis length, hypospadias or ambiguous genitalia), small testis or cryptorchidism and gynaecomastia and can result in delayed puberty [4]. On the other hand, postpubertal HG can present with a wide spectrum of sign and symptoms not always pathognomonic of T deficiency, but often suggestive of T deficiency or only associated with T deficiency [2]. From adult age to elderly, many signs and symptoms can overlap with clinical characteristics of concomitant diseases (i.e. cardiovascular, neurological, kidney, bone and metabolic) or to the age itself. The link between these diseases and T deficiency is so strong that to date is not clear if T deficiency could be a causative factor or a consequence of the above-mentioned diseases so represents a marker of poor general health.

Main Diagnostic Tool for Hypogonadism

Anamnesis and physical examination can induce suspicion of HG by identifying one or more signs and symptoms as shown in Fig. 1 but, according to current guidelines, the diagnosis of HG in adulthood requires the presence of low total T and/or free testosterone levels in a patient with at least one symptom/sign of androgen deficiency [2, 5]. The first step of the diagnostic process is to identify if T levels are below normal levels. The last Endocrine Society guidelines established only a lower limit of the normal total T levels (9.2 nmol/L) to perform diagnosis of HG [2], while the previous guideline considered a 'grey' zone between 8 and 12 nmol/L of suspected HG with values below 8 nmol/l as diagnostic for HG [5]. This 'borderline range' is very recently considered also by the European Academy of Andrology guidelines [6]. In case of borderline, T levels or 'grey zone' is suggested to repeat morning fasting total T with free T levels by an equilibrium dialysis method or by calculating it by a specific Vermeulen formula including SHBG levels and albumin concentration. Although normal free T levels have not been established, the lower limit established by the laboratory should be used to diagnose HG. This precaution results useful in case of a condition associated with altered SHBG concentration. For example, diabetes, obesity, glucocorticoids and anabolic steroids,

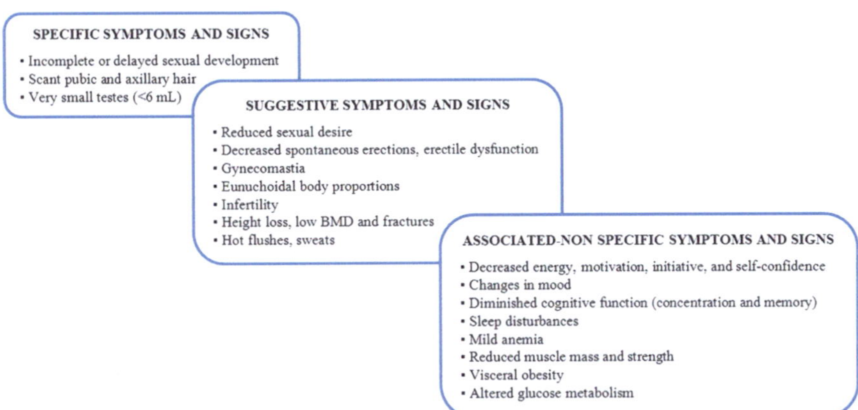

Fig. 1 Characteristics specific, suggestive or associated with hypogonadism. (Modified by Ref. [2])

hypothyroidism and nephritic syndrome are associated with decreased SHBG levels, while ageing, hyperthyroidism and liver diseases exert increased SHBG levels. Once HG has been confirmed, the second step is to measure gonadotropins (LH and FSH) levels in order to distinguish between primary and secondary HG. In the first case, LH and FSH are elevated, while, in case of secondary HG, gonadotropins are low or inappropriately normal in relation to an expected compensatory response to low T levels. In order to identify the aetiology of hypothalamic, pituitary and/or testicular dysfunction further biochemical (i.e. prolactin or other pituitary tropins), genetic (karyotype or specific gene mutation) or radiological (ultrasound scan or pituitary MRI) is required. In men of couples with a desire for offspring, semen analyses should be performed [2, 4–6].

Treatment

Correct classification of HG and the identification of HG aetiology are fundamental to ensure the patient a correct therapeutic approach. The milestone of HG treatment is T replacement therapy (TRT), but some clinical considerations need to be done before starting TRT. In case of secondary hypogonadism, when the desire for fatherhood is present, the correct approach is represented by gonadotropin treatment as human chorionic gonadotropin (hCG), exerting LH-like effects, plus FSH in order to induce spermatogenesis together with normalization of T levels [7].

Furthermore, the identification of reversible organic or functional condition requires specific treatment. Between organic causes of HG functional pituitary adenomas are for example reversible conditions by dedicated management. Furthermore, HG can reverse by lifestyle intervention in the case of obesity, type II diabetes, inadequate nutrition or scant/intensive exercise, or by discontinuing the use or abuse of alcohol and some drugs [8]. The goal of TRT is to induce and/or maintain secondary sex characteristics and to correct symptoms of testosterone deficiency. The treatment should be personalized according to the age of patient, patient's preference, estimated compliance, concomitant diseases, different pharmacokinetics of drugs and also cost. Many T formulations were proposed among years with different types of administration, pharmacokinetic profile, dosage and clinical advantages or disadvantages. Native T is nowadays available only as transdermal preparation, while chemical modifications (alkylation or esterification), by decreasing liver catabolism, allow a better T bioavailability and pharmacokinetics of injectable or oral T preparation. T undecanoate is the most used formulation of oral T. It is absorbed by the lymphatic system so bypassing the liver. The disadvantage of this T type is the irregularity of T levels in relation to lipid content assumed by diet and the necessity of administration two to three times a day. A variety of transdermal T types, such as native T, has been proposed. Both patches (standard dosage 5–10 mg/day) and gel (40–80 mg/day) allow a single-daily administration and provide uniform T serum levels during the day, similar to circadian T rhythm with a good safety profile. Injectable T preparation is esters in oily depot for i.m. injection. T enanthate and cypionate are available for clinical use at 200–250 mg every 2–4 weeks. T propionate is available in as dose of 100 mg to administer every 2–4 days. A formulation of T undecanoate for i.m. administration is also available and allows a single administration every 10–14 weeks. Injectable T preparations, although less expensive than transdermal ones, induce a supraphysiological increase in T concentration during the first days after administration followed by a constant decline until the subsequent injection with an increase in side effects, especially irritability, polycythaemia and fluctuation of symptoms with patient discomfort. Other preparations proposed during the years are transbuccal (gingival) T and subcutaneous implantation but were both of non-relevant clinical success. TRT is contraindicated in patients planning fertility, in patient with known or suspect prostate (PSA level > 4 ng/mL) or breast cancer, elevated haematocrit (>48–50%) or thrombophilia/venous thromboembolism, severe obstructive sleep apnoea syndrome, severe lower urinary tract symptoms, severe heart failure (class III or IV New York Hearth Association—NYHA) and myocardial infarction or stroke within the last 6 months [2, 4–6]. Relevant outcomes of TRT treatment are secondary sexual characteristics, sexuality, body composition, metabolism, bone health and mood. In men who have not undergone complete pubertal development, TRT therapy induces the development of secondary sex characteristics, including facial and body hair growth, deepening of the voice, muscle and bone accretion, penile enlargement, and pigmentation of the scrotum and their maintenance during life [9]. Regarding sexuality, observational studies and meta-analyses demonstrated TRT-positive effect on erectile function, libido, morning erections, orgasmic function and sexual satisfaction [10] and a recent randomized placebo-controlled trial on 788 clearly hypogonadism men, TRT compared to placebo, was documented to modestly increase sexual interest and sexual activity from flirting to sexual intercourse. The size of these effects was inversely related to the baseline T concentrations and proportional to the increase in T concentrations during TRT. Greater effects on libido and sexual activity than on erectile function were observed [11]. The effect of TRT on erectile has been recently investigated in a meta-analysis on men with functional HG, in which a modest improvement of erectile function was obtained only in subject diagnosed with moderate erectile dysfunction and not in more severe conditions [12]. Furthermore, TRT does not significantly improve sexual function and activity in men who do not have low T concentrations [13]. A further outcome is body composition. TRT consistently improves body composition (similar reduction in fat mass and increase in lean mass) in HG men, without changing in total body weight or body mass index (BMI) when compared with placebo or diet alone [14, 15].The metabolic effects of TRT are far from fully comprehension, and the data nowadays available are conflicting. Although some studies reported an amelioration of HbA1c and glycaemia on TRT, more consistent data on the amelioration of body composition and insulin resistance are available [16, 17]. Regarding the TRT outcome of bone health, TRT was shown to improve bone quality in HG men with low or moderate fracture risk [11], to improve bone mineral density, both in the spine and in the hip [18], but no data are available regarding a possible reduction in fracture risk in HG. Finally, TRT slightly improves the positive and reduces the negative aspects of mood [19]. Although epidemiological studies have reported an association between lower T concentrations and late-onset, low-grade, persistent depressive disorder [20], limited evidence of TRT benefits on this condition is available [21].

Sexuality and Quality of Life

According to Masters and Johnson's linear model, the male sexual response is based on four stages defined as the human sexual response cycle.

The *arousal phase* represents the first stage of the sexual response and is a consequence of physical or mental erotic stimuli leading to sexual arousal.

The next stage is the *plateau phase,* which precedes sexual orgasm. In this phase, the erect penis reaches maximum rigidity and the male urethral sphincter contracts to prevent retrograde ejaculation and urospermia. The plateau phase usually ends with orgasm, which is often characterized by antegrade ejaculation.

The *resolution phase* allows the baseline condition to be reached and the penis to return to a flaccid state. In 1979, Kaplan added the concept of desire and the sexual response model was condensed into three phases: desire, arousal and orgasm [22].

In the last decade, the validity of linear models has been questioned. In particular, Basson has proposed a nonlinear model of sexual response emphasizing that desire can come before or after arousal and that orgasm can contribute to, but is not necessary, satisfaction and resolution [23].

Consequently, a reduction in ejaculatory/orgasmic reactions may reflect a lack of sexual motivation; hyperexcitability in subjects with delayed ejaculation or reduced ejaculate volume may result from a disjunction between genital and subjective arousal, generating a vicious circle [23, 24].

Clinical studies have clearly shown that the *endocrine system* plays a key role in regulating all the steps involved in sexual activity. The *adrenal pathway and growth hormones* are involved in the mechanisms that support the arousal phase, contributing to increased heart and respiratory rates and increased blood pressure, which is essential for penile tumescence and pelvic vasocongestion. Thyroid hormones are involved in the *regulation of sexual desire and contribute to the control of ejaculation.* Finally, androgens and testosterone (T) in particular are involved in regulating all phases of the sexual response cycle [25–27].

A singular study by Martínez-Riera et al. [28] investigated the response of androgens, weak androgens, oestrogen and gonadotropins to clomiphene in alcoholics.

The study determined the levels of serum testosterone, sex hormone-binding protein (SHBG), dehydroepiandrosterone, androstenedione, LH, FSH, prolactin and oestradiol, on day 1 and day 6 after admission and after an 8-day course of clomiphene 200 mg/day, in a sample of 63 male patients (25 with and 38 without liver cirrhosis).

The same test was performed on 15 healthy volunteers.

Cirrhotic patients showed a decrease in basal testosterone levels and a loss of circadian rhythm with recovery after clomiphene. Although basal testosterone levels in non-cirrhotic alcoholics did not differ from those of controls, there was a significant improvement after discontinuation. SHBG levels were higher in both groups of alcoholics than in controls, indicating a worse degree of hypogonadism, as only the free hormone is active. Before clomiphene testing, serum LH and FSH levels were not significantly higher in either the alcoholic group compared to the control group. After clomiphene, both LH and FSH increased. Androstenedione and oestradiol showed similar behaviour (parallelism) in the alcoholic and cirrhotic groups, showing in both cases higher levels than in the control group, and an increase after clomiphene, possibly reflecting the peripheral conversion of androgens to oestrogen. Since clomiphene has no effect on the adrenal cortex, the increase in androstenedione after clomiphene indicates its testicular (directly or after testosterone conversion) rather than adrenal origin. Higher serum oestradiol levels have been observed in cirrhosis with ascites or gynaecomastia.

The male adolescent may present with various endocrinological problems, the most frequent of which is the *delay or absence of puberty due to constitutional retardation of growth and development.* This form does not require therapy and must be distinguished from other forms of *hypogonadism (primary or secondary)* by endocrine tests (LHRH test, secretion of LH nightly pulses, basal plasma testosterone level and after HCG and brain NMR). Treatment of hypogonadism consists of replacement therapy with testosterone or testicular stimulation with HCG or LHRH.

Another frequently occurring disease is gynaecomastia, which is usually caused by the physiological enlargement of the mammary gland during pubertal development, and may sometimes be secondary to *hypogonadism, tumours and liver function abnormalities.* Severe or psychologically disturbing gynaecomastia can be corrected by reduction mammaplasty. Very often adolescents can present with diseases related to poor eating habits. Obesity is common, and anorexia is also becoming a major problem in the male population.

As for females [29], delayed puberty is defined in girls by the absence of breast development beyond 13 years and in boys by the absence of testicular enlargement (<4 ml) beyond 14 years. Simple investigations lead to the diagnosis of central or peripheral hypogonadism and constitutional delay of puberty.

In girls, delayed puberty is rare (2% of cases), and often, organic, ergo Turner's syndrome should be systematically suspected. In boys, delayed puberty is often constitutional and functional. Treatment options are: remove the etiological conditions of hypogonadism when possible, hormone replacement therapy (oestrogen in girls and testosterone in boys) and psychological management.

But There Is More.

A large body of scientific literature indicates that sexual dysfunction, and in particular erectile dysfunction (ED), may be an early surrogate marker of several disease states such as *diabetes mellitus, hypertension, metabolic syndrome (MetS) and depression.* Furthermore, it has been suggested that ED could also be considered the first sign of impending coronary heart disease (CHD) and an efficient predictor of silent CHD in a diabetic population, independent of glyco-metabolic control and ED severity.

Hypogonadism is frequently associated with MetS both in subjects with and without ED, with insulin resistance being the presumed pathogenetic link. In subjects with erectile dysfunction, hypogonadism may exacerbate sexual dysfunction due to its typical symptoms, such as decreased sexual desire and mood disorders. However, hypogonadism itself has been associated with an increased risk of cardiovascular and overall mortality.

On the subject of pubertal delays, Kallmann syndrome (SK) is a congenital form of *idiopathic hypogonadotropic hypogonadism* in which hypogonadism is associated with olfactory deficit (hypo/anosmia) and other non-reproductive defects (renal agenesis, synkinesis, cleft palate and syndactyly).

SK can be sporadic or familial, with X-linked, autosomal (dominant or recessive) or hereditary inheritance. A mutation in genes regulating GnRH neuron migration and/or olfactory bulb morphogenesis (KAL1, FGFR1, FGF8, PROKR2, PROK2 and CHD7) has been found in 30% of cases.

SK manifests itself as delayed or absent puberty after 18 years of age in males and 16 years of age in females, together with olfactory deficit and, inconsistently, somatic abnormalities. Low gonadotropin and testosterone (T) or oestradiol (E2) levels are diagnostic of hypogonadism only after the age of 18 (in males) and 16 (in females) and between the second week and the third month of life in children with micropenis and/or cryptorchidism [30].

The odour test and magnetic resonance imaging are useful tools to assess the sensory deficit and morphology of the olfactory bulbs.

To induce puberty, increasing doses of intramuscular (im) or transdermal (td) T in men or E2 (oral, td) in women are administered. After puberty, therapy can be continued with T undecanoate im (every 10–12 weeks) in the male and with oestrogen–progestin combinations in the female. A period of discontinuation should be scheduled after the completion of puberty in order to define reversible forms.

Conclusion

Hypogonadism appears to be a complex pathology starting in adolescence. Patients of various ages undergo clinical examinations and therapies that may facilitate and induce pubertal growth or adequate sex life in young adults and patients over 50. However, the physical and human demands to which these patients are subjected may affect therapeutic compliance over time. Changes in sexual function and the aesthetic aspects of prolonged hormone therapies should be evaluated with individual patients and their partners. Sexologically, it is useful to share the therapeutic pathway in order to offer individuals the possibility of 'choosing' the best quality of life and 'supporting' psychic motivation over time, which is too often disrupted by the results of drug therapy.

References

1. Matsumoto AM, Bremner WJ. Testicular disorders. In: Melmed S, Polansky KS, Larsen PR, Kronenberg HM, editors. Williams textbook of endocrinology. 13th ed. New York, NY: Elsevier; 2016. p. 688–777.
2. Bhasin S, Brito JP, Cunningham GR, Hayes FJ, Hodis HN, Matsumoto AM, Snyder PJ, Swerdloff RS, Wu FC, Yialamas MA. Testosterone therapy in men with hypogonadism: an endocrine society clinical practice guideline. J Clin Endocrinol Metab. 2018;103(5):1715–44.
3. Lenzi A, Balercia G, Bellastella A, Colao A, Fabbri A, Foresta C, Galdiero M, Gandini L, Krausz C, Lombardi G, Lombardo F, Maggi M, Radicioni A, Selice R, Sinisi AA, Forti G. Epidemiology, diagnosis, and treatment of male hypogonadotropic hypogonadism. J Endocrinol Investig. 2009;32(11):934–8.
4. Dohle GR, Arver S, Bettocchi C, Jones TH, Kliesch S. EAU guidelines on male hypogonadism. 2018. https://uroweb.org/guideline/male-hypogonadism/.
5. Wang C, Nieschlag E, Swerdlo R, Behre HM, Hellstrom WJ, Gooren LJ, Kaufman JM, Legros J-J, Lunenfeld B, Morales A, Morley JE, Schulman C, Thompson IM, Weidner W, Wu FCW. Investigation, treatment, and monitoring of late-onset hypogonadism in males: ISA, ISSAM, EAU, EAA, and ASA recommendations. Eur Urol. 2009;55:121–30.
6. Corona G, Goulis DG, Huhtaniemi I, Zitzmann M, Toppari J, Forti G, Vanderschueren D, Wu FC. European Academy of Andrology (EAA) guidelines on investigation, treatment and monitoring of functional hypogonadism in males. Andrology. 2020;8:970.
7. Finkel DM, Phillips JL, Snyder PJ. Stimulation of spermatogenesis by gonadotropins in men with hypogonadotropic hypogonadism. N Engl J Med. 1985;313(11):651–5.
8. Corona G, Rastrelli G, Morelli A, et al. Treatment of functional hypogonadism besides pharmacological substitution. World J Mens Health. 2019;38:256.
9. Giagulli VA, Triggiani V, Carbone MD, Corona G, Tafaro E, Licchelli B, Guastamacchia E. The role of long-acting parenteral testosterone undecanoate compound in the induction of secondary sexual characteristics in males with hypogonadotropic hypogonadism. J Sex Med. 2011;8(12):3471–8.
10. Rastrelli G, Guaraldi F, Reismann Y, Sforza A, Isidori AM, Maggi M, Corona G. Testosterone replacement therapy for sexual symptoms. Sex Med Rev. 2019;7(3):464–75.
11. Snyder PJ, Bhasin S, Cunningham GR, et al. Lessons from the testosterone trials. Endocr Rev. 2018;39:369–86.
12. Corona G, Rastrelli G, Morgentaler A, Sforza A, Mannucci E, Maggi M. Meta-analysis of results of testosterone therapy on sexual function based on international index of erectile function scores. Eur Urol. 2017;72:1000–11.
13. Basaria S, Harman SM, Travison TG, Hodis H, Tsitouras P, Budoff M, Pencina KM, Vita J, Dzekov C, Mazer NA, Coviello AD, Knapp PE, Hally K, Pinjic E, Yan M, Storer TW, Bhasin S. Effects of testosterone administration for 3 years on subclinical atherosclerosis progression in older men with low or low-normal testosterone levels: a randomized clinical trial. JAMA. 2015;314(6):570–81.
14. Corona G, Giagulli VA, Maseroli E, et al. Therapy of endocrine disease: testosterone supplementation and body composition: results from a meta-analysis study. Eur J Endocrinol. 2016;174:R99–116.

15. NgTang Fui M, Hoermann R, Zajac JD, Grossmann M. The effects of testosterone on body composition in obese men are not sustained after cessation of testosterone treatment. Clin Endocrinol. 2017;87:336–43.
16. Jones TH, Arver S, Behre HM, et al. Testosterone replacement in hypogonadal men with type 2 diabetes and/or metabolic syndrome (the TIMES2 study). Diabetes Care. 2011;34:828–37.
17. Hackett G, Cole N, Bhartia M, Kennedy D, Raju J, Wilkinson P, BLAST Study Group. Testosterone replacement therapy improves metabolic parameters in hypogonadal men with type 2 diabetes but not in men with coexisting depression: the BLAST study. J Sex Med. 2014;11:840–56.
18. Rochira V, Antonio L, Vanderschueren D. EAA clinical guideline on management of bone health in the andrological outpatient clinic. Andrology. 2018;6:272–85.
19. Wang C, Alexander G, Berman N, Salehian B, Davidson T, McDonald V, Steiner B, Hull L, Callegari C, Swerdloff RS. Testosterone replacement therapy improves mood in hypogonadal men—a clinical research center study. J Clin Endocrinol Metab. 1996;81(10):3578–83.
20. Shores MM, Sloan KL, Matsumoto AM, Moceri VM, Felker B, Kivlahan DR. Increased incidence of diagnosed depressive illness in hypogonadal older men. Arch Gen Psychiatry. 2004;61(2):162–7.
21. Shores MM, Kivlahan DR, Sadak TI, Li EJ, Matsumoto AMA. A randomized, double-blind, placebo-controlled study of testosterone treatment in hypogonadal older men with subthreshold depression (dysthymia or minor depression). J Clin Psychiatry. 2009;70(7):1009–16.
22. Corona G, Forti G, Maggi M. Hypoactive sexual desire in man: the role of the andrologist. Italian J Obstet Gynecol. 2006;28(6):269–76. ISSN 1971-1433.
23. Corona G, Boddi V, Gacci M, et al. Perceived reduction in ejaculate volume in patients with erectile dysfunction: psychological correlates. J Androl. 2011;32:333–9.
24. Rowland DL. Psychophysiology of ejaculatory function and dysfunction, Mondo. J Urol. 2005;23:82–8.
25. Corona G, Isidori AM, Aversa A, et al. Endocrinological control of sexual desire and arousal/erection of men. J Sex Med. 2016;13:317–37.
26. Corona G, Jannini EA, Vignozzi L, et al. Hormonal control of ejaculation. Nat Rev Urol. 2012;9:508–19.
27. Gabrielson AT, Sartor RA, Hellstrom WJG. The impact of thyroid disease on sexual dysfunction in men and women. Sex Med Rev. 2019;7(1):57–70.
28. Martínez-Riera A, Santolaria-Fernández F, González Reimers E, Milena A, Gómez-Sirvent JL, Rodríguez-Moreno F, González-Martín I, Rodríguez-Rodríguez E. Alcoholic hypogonadism: hormonal response to clomiphene. Alcohol. 1995;12(6):581–7. https://doi.org/10.1016/0741-8329(95)02006-3. PMID: 8590623.
29. Edouard T, Tauber M. Retard pubertaire [Delayed puberty]. Arch Pediatr. 2010;17(2):195–200. https://doi.org/10.1016/j.arcped.2009.09.017. Epub 2009 Nov 4. PMID: 19892534.
30. Sinisi AA, Maione L, Bellastella G, et al. Diagnosis and therapy of hypogonadism in Kallmann's syndrome. Endocrinologist. 2011;12:8 19.

Part XIII
Neurology

Chronic Migraine

Bruno Colombo and Elena Vittoria Longhi

Migraine and Chronic Migraine: Characteristics and Diagnosis

Migraine is a very frequent neurological disorder. It is estimated that more than one billion people worldwide have been diagnosed with migraine, which means that approximately 12% of the adult population meet the criteria for migraine. Migraine is most prevalent between the ages of 25 and 55 years [1]. According to the International Classification of Headache Disorders (ICHD-3), the disease is a condition in which headaches recur at irregular intervals, attacks lasting from 4 to 72 h, with total freedom from symptoms between attacks [2]. Several hours before the headache begins, there may be prodromal symptoms, which can involve altered mood or behavior. The most common premonitory symptoms are impaired concentration, irritability, fatigue, yawning, and food cravings. Migraine aura, immediately preceding the onset of headache, occurs in approximately 15% of sufferers. The most common form is a visual disturbance (in 90% of patients suffering from aura), a blind spot that increases in minutes, and/or a distinct pattern of scintillating lights (unformed flashes or fortification phenomena). These symptoms commonly resolve before the headache. Symptoms such as one-sided numbness or dysphasia can precede or follow visual aura. The migraine headache usually develops gradually, frequently on one side of the head (60% of patients), although bilateral, deep-seated headaches are common. The throbbing pain (in 50% of cases) is felt deeply behind one or both eyes. The pain intensity is at least moderate or severe during attacks.

B. Colombo (✉)
Neurological Department, Headache and Pain Unit, San Raffaele Hospital, Vita-Salute University, Milan, Italy
e-mail: colombo.bruno@hsr.it

E. V. Longhi
Department of Sexual Medical Center, San Raffaele Hospital, Milano, Italy

© Springer Nature Switzerland AG 2023
E. V. Longhi (ed.), *Managing Psychosexual Consequences in Chronic Diseases*,
https://doi.org/10.1007/978-3-031-31307-3_21

Nausea frequently accompanies the headache, and in some cases, vomiting occurs. Light, even normal levels, can increase the patient's distress (photophobia, in 94% of cases) as can noise (phonophobia in 91% of cases) and movements. Migraine pain is aggravated by physical activity (90% of cases) or head movement. Sufferers often just want to retire to a darkened room. Feelings of depression and hopelessness may accompany the attack, making it more difficult to continue normal activities. Patients under migraine attack may wish to sleep to escape the pain and related symptoms, but the headache may keep them awake. After the attack, the sufferer is usually tired and washed out for some hours [3].

Several factors are suggested as being associated with migraine: 60–70% of people who suffer from migraine have parents or other close relatives who suffer from it. There is also evidence of an association between migraine and depression and of higher levels of psychological distress among those with migraine, particularly females, as compared to subjects without migraine. It emphasized the relationship between stress and migraine attacks: In some cases, the relief of stress ("the weekend migraine") is reported as a precipitating factor. Hormonal factors and a relationship with the menstrual cycle have also been frequently observed ("menstrual migraine") [4].

Migraine can be divided into episodic migraine (EM) with the criterion of <15 headache days per month and chronic migraine (CM) with >15 days headache days per month in the last 3 months. According to ICHD-3 criteria, in CM 8 more days per month are characterized by migraine attacks [2].

It is estimated that 1–4% of the population meet the criteria for CM. However, the true prevalence of CM is not so easy to estimate: In particular, difficulties in epidemiological research are due to patient recall bias, heterogeneous data collection instruments, and the potential for patients to overestimate headache frequency. CM frequently develops from EM: This process has been named as "progression," "transformation," or "chronification." The annual progression rate from EM to CM is about 3%. Patients with CM often overuse symptomatic drugs (triptans or nonsteroidal anti-inflammatory drugs). This situation may lead to a complication of migraine, the so-called medication overuse headache. This entity is defined as intake of analgesics on >15 days per month or triptans and combination analgesics on >10 per month. The 1-year population prevalence of CM and medication overuse is approximately 1–3%. The greatest risk of progression from EM to CM is associated with butalbital-containing medication and opioids [5].

CM is almost three times more common in women than in men, with a first peak in younger age (18–29 years) and a second peak in adult age (40–49 years).

In 25% of patients affected by CM headache, the disability related to pain is defined as very severe according to Migraine Disability Assessment Scale (MIDAS). In fact, the Global Burden of Diseases (GBD) has classified migraine as the second-world cause of years lived with disability and the first cause in under 50 s in both genders. A recent Italian study reported that CM has a high economic burden, with annual direct cost 4.8-fold higher than that of EM (Euro 2037 vs Euro 427) due to more visits, diagnostic tests, and drug use. Costs were significantly higher for women than for men and increased with age [6].

CM is a dynamic state, with patients moving in and out of the chronic state. The possibility to remit from CM to EM is 26% within 2 years [7].

Several modifiable risk factors increase the risk of developing CM, in particular, high baseline migraine attack frequency (one or more per week), obesity, snoring, caffeine consumption, and inadequate treatment of attacks. Other important risk factors are low socioeconomic status, anxiety, bipolar disorders, comorbid pain disorders, asthma and allergies, previous head injury, allodynia (normal non-noxious tactile stimuli to the skin is experienced as painful), and female sex. In one study, the increased severity of depression is reported to worsen the risk to transform EM to CM. Moreover, the presence of depression preceded migraine progression, suggesting a possible causal link [8]. The strongest data about risk factors for the transformation of EM to CM demonstrate that increased headache day frequency, overuse of acute migraine drugs, and depression are the most important factors. People with CM are more likely to experience specific comorbidities.

Pathophysiological dysfunctions responsible for migraine chronification are not completely understood. Patients affected by CM might have a lower sensory threshold and eventually an increased susceptibility to the neurological mechanisms contributing to migraine attacks. Central and peripheral sensitization processes can have a pivotal role in determining CM state. Admittedly, compared to EM patients, CM subjects have higher interictal plasma levels of certain vasoactive neuropeptides (biomarkers of functions of trigeminal and autonomic system) such as calcitonin gene-related peptide (CGRP) and vasoactive intestinal peptide (VIP), thus confirming an altered interictal activity both of the trigeminal and cranial autonomic system [9–11]. Of note, dysfunction of cortical and subcortical brain areas involved in pain control and processing, such as cingulate cortex (somatosensory and anterior), thalamus, and hypothalamus, might also have a crucial role in migraine chronification. A possible hypothesis (although not completely supported by definite experimental evidence) is that increased continuous nociceptive processing may lead to an overactivation of the descending pain-modulating network (projections from frontal lobe, hypothalamus, and amygdala on periaqueductal gray), resulting in higher oxidative stress and consequent dysregulation of pain modulation [12]. This process may further lower the pain threshold for developing new attacks, leading to a possible conversion on CM [9]. Particularly, according to neuroimaging studies, CM patients have a more distinct dysfunction of the pain inhibitory network and an increased sensitization of the central pain pathways. It is still questionable if these brain alterations are specific biomarkers that predispose EM patients to convert on CM state or just a reflection of maladaptive and/or adaptive responses to the increasing migraine frequency [13].

CM and Quality of Life

CM is not life-threatening, but it is quality of life-threatening. For many patients, the persistence of pain and the recurrence of attacks are the things that make it so difficult to live with. CM can greatly disrupt and restrict a sufferer's working and social life and has a pervasive effect on daily activities and also on workplace activities. It is small wonder that many CM sufferers feel that they are discriminated against at work. They may fail to achieve promotion, or in extreme cases, may risk losing their job because of their migraine. From the point of view of the employer, one of the most disturbing aspects of CM is the persistence of attacks and duration of pain. With many illnesses, an employer may be able to plan ahead, for example, if a staff member is going to be off for a certain period due to a scheduled operation. In contrast, someone affected by CM may be perceived as an unreliable employee due to both the number of days that a person is ineffective and the number of days he actually loses due to the continuous and intractable pain. The reduction in work productivity may be assessed in terms of presenteeism (hours or days in which patients affected by CM worked less productively due to migraine. Patients stay on the workplace but work at a lower level due to headaches) and absenteeism (loss of paid work days, in this situation patients affected by migraine avoid a full day of work due to headaches). The negative effect on paid work gives the reason on the high indirect cost of CM: 70% of the total cost per individual per year is represented by productivity loss [14]. The Headwork questionnaire is a specific tool developed to measure work-related disability in patients with EM and CM without regard to the use of medications. This questionnaire takes into account migraineurs work-related disability on different levels, considering not only the specific tasks that could be reduced by migraine pain, but also on peculiar features of the workplace environment that contribute to disability at work [15].

Treatment of Chronic Migraine

The aim of treatment of CM is the prevention of migraine attacks. The standard first-line pharmacological treatments include both neuromodulant (such as topiramate and sodium valproate) and botulinum—neurotoxin A. Nonpharmacological therapies such as occipital nerve stimulation and electric supraorbital stimulation have also been used in small clinical trials. Recently, a new class of drugs (anti-CGRP/R antibodies) is proving very promising for CM prophylaxis in several clinical trials [16].

Topiramate

According to Italian treatment guidelines, topiramate has the highest level of recommendation for the prophylactic treatment of CM patients [17]. The putative activity is possibly due to an inhibition of neuronal hyperexcitability. In two large randomized controlled trials, topiramate reduced headache days versus placebo in CM patients. Furthermore, topiramate is cost-effective and noninvasive. Topiramate is relatively well-tolerated: Adverse events commonly associated include fatigue, nausea, paresthesia, concentration, and memory disturbances [12]. In rare cases, severe psychological adverse events were reported, such as aggravation of depressive symptoms. Given this specific peculiarity, considering the significant comorbidity rates of depression and CM, it might not be the first-line drug in CM patients with comorbid mood disturbances [5].

Onabotulinum Toxin/A (OBT-A)

Up to now, OBT-A (formulation of botulin toxin A administered to at least 31 injection sites across seven head and neck muscles, every 12 weeks) is the only treatment specifically approved for the treatment of CM [18]. The putative pharmacological activity is due to the prevention of central sensitization, inhibiting the release of CGRP from peripheral nociceptive neuron, interfering with TRP channels. OBT-A has been shown to reduce total headache days in CM patients, with or without MOE, according to a standardized scheme (PREEMPT-scheme). Treatment efficacy was observed at 24 and 56 weeks. Therapy was generally well-tolerated: The only adverse events were pain, swelling, and bruising in the site of injection [16].

Anti-CGRP/R Monoclonal Antibodies

Anti-CGRP/R monoclonal antibodies are macromolecules that bind to the CGRP ligand or its receptor neutralizing the effects of excessive CGRP released in the trigeminal sensory nerve fibers during migraine attacks [19]. CGRP is a member of the calcitonin family of peptides (37-amino acids neuropeptide), which in humans exists in two forms, alpha and beta. CGRP is a pro-inflammatory vasodilating molecule involved in central and peripheral pathophysiological events in migraine. Seminal studies showed that CGRP levels increase in jugular venous blood during migraine attacks and are elevated interictally in the peripheral circulation in patients with both EM and CM [11]. Monoclonal antibodies are made from living cells or organisms, have high molecular weight, have long half-life, and are catabolized bypassing liver metabolism (degraded to peptides or amino acids). Studies of monoclonal antibodies as prophylaxis therapy for CM have shown efficacy in randomized controlled trials. Three anti-CGRP antibodies are approved in the USA and Europe for the prophylactic treatment of CM: erenumab, which targets the CGRP receptor, and fremanezumab and galcanezumab, which targets the CGRP ligand. They are all administered once a month subcutaneously, or once every three months for fremanezumab. The results of clinical trials showed the efficacy and safety (mild-to-moderate injection site reactions) of anti-CGRP/R monoclonal antibodies as prophylactic therapy in patients with CM, with an observed treatment effect within 4 weeks after the initial dose [16].

Last but not least, we have to consider that there is an aspect of CM that is almost impossible to quantify: It is the fear, the guilt, and the despair that is frequently admitted by migraineurs when at least they feel able to talk about it. For this reason, we should rediscover the value of empathy and re-establish therapeutic alliances, but more importantly we should enhance doctors who know how not only to employ technical devices or drugs but also to approach human beings, both the patients, and who look after them, through a highly emotional process of integration. In this respect, the humanistic education of the doctor needs to surface as a key value in a kind of medicine where the psychological approach has a creative and active role, both in practice and culturally.

Comorbidities of Chronic Migraine

1. Psychiatric comorbidities

    (a) Depression
    (b) Bipolar disorders
    (c) Anxiety
    (d) Chronic pain and fibromyalgia

2. General comorbidities (somatic)

    (e) Hypertension
    (f) Stroke and cerebrovascular events
    (g) Asthma
    (h) Allergies
    (i) Sinusitis and bronchitis.

Sexuality and Quality of Life

It is known that migraine, as a chronic condition observed mainly in women, negatively affects the quality of life [20] and sexual function [21]. Several studies have investigated the relationship between migraine and sexual function.

On the other hand, however, some authors have suggested that migraine sufferers report higher levels of sexual desire than those with tension-type headache.

Depression and anxiety would appear to be heightened in migraine sufferers [22] while also causing handicap in many areas of life [23].

A sample of 50 women were referred to the migraine center of the Department of Neurology, School of Medicine, Acibadem University, between May 2011 and May 2012. Only female patients were selected, due to their predominant demand for outpatient consultation. The diagnosis of migraine with or without aura was confirmed by two specialists in neurology, in accordance with the second edition of the International Headache Society (IHS) International Classification of Headache Disorders (ICHD-II) of 2004 [24]. To be eligible for the study, patients had to be between 18 and 50 years old, with a history of migraine for at least 6 months, and be in a sexual relationship during the previous 6 months.

Patients with tension-type headache, diabetes mellitus, or hypertension and patients who were pregnant, lactating, or postmenopausal were excluded.

The socio-demographic data request questionnaires, Migraine Disability Rating Scale (MIDAS) [25], Female Sexual Function Index (FSFI) [26], Beck Depression Inventory (BDI) [27], and Beck Anxiety Inventory (BAI) [28] were used for self-assessment.

The Results?

The mean age of the patients at the time of the study visit was 31.9 (6.5) years, 90% of the participants had been married for approximately 8.1 (6.3) years, and 50% of them had a child. The majority of patients (90%) had a diagnosis of migraine without aura with a mean duration of 7.2 (4.8) years. The mean Migraine Disability Rating Scale (MIDAS) score was 19.3 (12.8), and in 40%, the disability was severe.

Sixty percent of patients had mild, moderate, or severe depression; the mean score was 16.3.

Furthermore, 45 women reported low sexual function. The other scores were as follows: desire 3.4 (1.0), arousal 4.0 (1.3), orgasm 4.2 (1.4), satisfaction 4.5 (1.5), and pain 4.9 (1.6) on a low mean score [28].

From these results, there appears to be no clear correlation between migraine and sexual dysfunction. However, in a recent study by Bestepe et al. [29] using the Arizona Sexual Experiences Scale (ASEX), patients with migraine reported higher rates of sexual dysfunction than healthy patients but lower rates than patients with tension-type headache. No relationship between sexuality and migraine frequency, severity, or duration was reported.

However, a well-established relationship between migraine, depression, and anxiety has been confirmed [30].

Randolph et al. [31] conducted an interesting study on the quality of questions to ask migraine patients: 85 patients, 71 females (83.5%), and 14 males (16.5%). Using the 2004 International Headache Society criteria for migraine, the following questions were asked, "Does light bother you during a headache?" If the answer was "no," subjects were then asked, "during a headache, would you prefer to be in sunlight or in a dark room?" "Does noise bother you during a headache?" If the answer was "no," subjects were then asked, "during a headache, would you rather be in a room with loud music or a quiet room?"

Strangely enough, most of those concerned initially denied there and then any photophobia and phonophobia, whereas following further questions 93% of patients responded in the affirmative. This led scholars to recommend detailed diagnoses and multiple questions on the same topics.

There is more.

Reviewing the literature, we notice the study by Kucukdurmaz et al. [32], which aimed to determine the incidence of risk factors associated with sexual function and distress in premenopausal women with migraine. Sixty-nine women diagnosed with migraine were included. Sexual function and distress were assessed by the Female Sexual Function Index (FSFI) and the revised Female Sexual Distress Scale (FSDS-R), respectively. Depression and anxiety were studied using the Hospital Depression and Anxiety Scale (HADS). Migraine-related disability was assessed by the Migraine Disability Rating Scale (MIDAS), and mean pain severity was determined by the visual analog scale (VAS). Fifty-five women reported sexual dysfunction. Underlying this was found to be a very high index of depression.

Therefore, the diagnosis of migraine should be conducted jointly by a team: neurologist, sexologist, psychiatrist, and physiatrists, especially with respect to the practice of breathing and relaxation.

Relaxation and Yoga in the Treatment of Migraine.

What Then of the Dizziness Associated with Migraine? Teggi et al. [33] evaluated the prevalence of vertigo in a population of 2672 patients diagnosed with headaches, which were hemicranial, pulsatile, phonophobia, and photophobia-associated and worsened on exertion. Patients were asked to respond to a questionnaire; demographic data and previous dizziness and/or vertigo were addressed in the first part. The mean age of the sample was 48.3 ± 15 years, and 46.7% were male.

A total of 1077 (40.3%) subjects reported vertigo/dizziness during their lifetime, and the mean age of the first vertigo attack was 39.2 ± 15.4 years. In the second part, they were asked about the characteristics of vertigo (age of the first episode, rotational vertigo, recurrent episodes, positional exacerbation, presence of cochlear symptoms) and lifetime presence of migraines. An effect regarding age and sex was demonstrated, with symptoms 4.4-fold higher in females and 1.8-fold higher in persons older than 50 years. In the total sample of 2672 responders, 13.7% reported a spinning sensation, 26.3% relapsing episodes, 12.9% positional exacerbation, and 4.8% cochlear symptoms; 34.8% reported headaches during their lifetime. Subjects who suffered from migraine had an increased rate of relapsing episodes, positional exacerbation, cochlear symptoms, and a lower age of onset of the first episode of dizziness/vertigo.

In contrast, Pacor et al. [34] conducted a study on the frequency of migraine and an adverse reaction to foods. Migraine was present in 41 of 300 patients (13.6%). 38 of these 41 subjects were treated with an elimination diet; 25 (65.7%) achieved significant improvement. In a further study on the same subject, 24 patients were affected by food intolerance and only one by food allergy. The remaining 13 subjects with migraine were subsequently subjected to pharmacological treatment.

Conclusion

Wanting to extend clinical research, it emerges that migraine and multiple sclerosis (MS) are two neurological disorders that affect different aspects of women. Sexual function is one of the comorbidities that are not well considered in these cases. Some recent studies have evaluated sexual function in women suffering from migraine or MS. Eighty-six married migraine patients and 86 married MS cases of the same age were asked to complete valid and reliable Beck Depression Inventory (BDI) and FSFI (Female Sexual Function Index) questionnaires. The BDI score was higher in women with migraine than in MS cases, and BDI scores in both groups were high in cases with sexual dysfunction. The BDI score was significantly correlated with the total FSFI and its subscales in both groups. Multiple linear regression analysis between FSFI as dependent variable and age, BDI, and education level as independent variables showed that age and BDI were independent predictors of FSFI in both groups. Sexual dysfunction should be considered in women with MS or migraine.

References

1. Colombo B. Migraine: pathophysiology and classification. In: Colombo B, Teggi R, editors. Vestibular migraine and related syndromes. Springer; 2014. p. 1–15.
2. International Headache Society. The international classification of headache disorders, 3rd edition. Cephalalgia. 2018;38:1–211.
3. Dodick WD. Migraine. Lancet. 2018;391:1315–30.
4. Maasumi K, Tepper SJ, Kriegler JS. Menstrual migraine and treatment options: review. Headache. 2016;2017(57):194–208.
5. May A, Schulte LH. Chronic migraine: risk factors, mechanisms and treatment. Nat Rev. 2016;12:455–64.
6. GBD 2016 Disease and injury incidence and prevalence collaborators. Global, regional and national incidence, prevalence and years lived with disability for 328 diseases and injuries for 195 countries, 1990-2016: a systematic analysis for the Global Burrden of Disease Study 2016. Lancet. 2017;390(10100):1211–59.
7. Serrano D, Lipton RB, Scher AI, et al. Fluctuations in episodic and chronic migraine status over the course of 1 year: implication for diagnosis, treatment and clinical trial design. J Headache Pain. 2017;18(1):101.
8. Ashina S. Depression and risk of transformation of episodic to chronic migraine. J Headache Pain. 2012;13:615–24.
9. Bigal ME, Lipton RB. Clinical course in migraine: conceptualizing migraine transformation. Neurology. 2008;71:848–55.
10. Cernuda Morollon E. Increased VIP levels in peripheral blood outside migraine attacks as a potential biomarker of cranial parasympathetic activation in chronic migraine. Cephalalgia. 2015;35:310–6.
11. Cernuda Morollon E. Interictal increase of CGRP levels in peripheral blood as a biomarker for chronic migraine. Neurology. 2013;81:1191–6.
12. Aurora SK, Brin MF. Chronic migraine: an update on physiology, imaging, and the mechanism of action of two available pharmacologic therapies. Headache. 2017;57:109–25.
13. Colombo B, Messina R, Rocca MA, et al. Imaging the migrainous brain: the present and the future. Neurol Sci. 2019;S1:49–54.
14. Munakata J, Hazard E, Serrano D, et al. Economic burden of transformed migraine: results from the American Migraine Prevalence and Prevention study. Headache. 2009;49:498–508.
15. D'Amico D, Grazzi L, Grignani E, et al. HEADWORK questionnaire: why do we need a new tool to assess work-related disability in patients with migraine? Headache. 2020;60(2):497–504.
16. Agostoni EC, Barbanti P, Calabresi P, Colombo B, et al. Current and emerging evidence-based treatment options in chronic migraine: a narrative review. J Headache Pain. 2019;20:92–101.
17. Sarchielli P, Granella F, Prudenzano MP, et al. Italian guidelines for primary headaches: 2012 revised version. J Headache Pain. 2012;13(S2):31–70.
18. Frampton JE, Silberstein S. OnabotulinumtoxinA: a review in the prevention of chronic migraine. Drugs. 2018;78(5):589–600.
19. Tso AR, Goasby PJ. Anti-CGRP monoclonal antibodies: the next era of migraine prevention? Curr Treat Options Neurol. 2017;19(8):27.

20. Bigal ME, Lipton RB, Stewart WF. The epidemiology and impact of migraine. Curr Neurol Neurosci Rep. 2004;4:98–104. https://doi.org/10.1007/s11910-004-0022-8.
21. Houle TT, Dhingra LK, Remble TA, Rokicki LA, Penzien DB. Not tonight, do I have a headache? Headache. 2006;46:983–90. https://doi.org/10.1111/j.1526-4610.2006.00470.
22. Burri A, Spector T, Rahman Q. The etiological relationship between anxiety sensitivity, sexual distress, and female sexual dysfunction is in part genetically moderate. J Sex Med. 2012;9:1887–96. https://doi.org/10.1111/j.1743-6109.2012.02710.
23. Antonaci F, Nappi G, Galli F, Manzoni GC, Calabresi P, Costa A. Migraine and psychiatric comorbidity: a review of clinical findings. J Headache. 2011;12:115–25. https://doi.org/10.1007/s10194-010-0282-4.
24. Stewart WF, Lipton RB, Dowson AJ, Sawyer J. Development and testing of MIDAS (Migraine Disability Assessment) questionnaire to assess headache-related disability. Neurology. 2001;56:20–8. https://doi.org/10.1212/WNL.56.suppl_1.S20.
25. Ertas M, Siva A, Dalkara T, Uzuner N, Dora B, Inan L, Idiman F, Sarica Y, Selcuki D, Sirin H, Oguzhanoglu A, Irkec C, Ozmenoglu M, Ozbenli T, Ozturk M, Saip S, Neyal M, Zarifoglu M. Turkish MIDAS Group: the validity and reliability of the Turkish Migraine Disability Assessment Questionnaire (MIDAS). Headache. 2004;44:786–93. https://doi.org/10.1111/j.1526-4610.2004.04146.
26. Rosen R, Brown C, Heiman J, Leiblum S, Meston C, Shabsigh R, Ferguson D, D'Agostino R Jr. The Female Sexual Function Index (FSFI): a multidimensional self-assessment tool for assessing female sexual function. J Marital Sex Ther. 2000;26:191–208. https://doi.org/10.1080/009262300278597.
27. Hisli N. Reliability and validity of Beck's depression inventory among college students [in Turkish]. Psikoloji Dergisi. 1989;7:3–13.
28. Wiegel M, Meston C, Rosen R. The female sexual function index (FSFI): cross-validation and development of clinical cutoff scores. J Marital Sex Ther. 2005;31:1–20.
29. Bestepe E, Cabalar M, Kucukgoncu S, Calıkusu C, Ornek F, Yayla V, Erkoc S. Sexual dysfunction in women with migraine versus tension-type headache: a comparative study. Int J Impot Res. 2011;23:122–7. https://doi.org/10.1038/ijir.2011.16.
30. Yalug I, Selekler M, Erdogan A, Kutlu A, Dundar G, Ankarali H, Aker T. Correlations between alexithymia and pain severity, depression and anxiety among chronic and episodic migraine patients. Psychiatry Clin Neurosci. 2010;64:231–8. https://doi.org/10.1111/j.1440-1819.2010.02093.x.
31. Randolph W, et al. Headache: the diary of pain in the head and face presentation of the research. The use of questions to determine the presence of photophobia and phonophobia during migraine. J Head Face Pain. 2007;48(3):395–7. https://doi.org/10.1111/j.1526-4610.2007.00920.x.
32. Kucukdurmaz F, Inanc Y, Inanc Y, et al. Disfunzione sessuale e disagio nelle donne in premenopausa con emicrania: associazione con depressione, ansia e disabilità correlata all'emicrania. Int J Impot Res. 2018;30:265–71. https://doi.org/10.1038/s41443-018-0049-z.
33. Teggi R, Manfrin M, Balzanelli C, Gatti O, Mura F, Quaglieri S, Pilolli F, Redaelli de Zinis LO, Benazzo M, Bussi M. Point prevalence of vertigo and vertigo in a sample of 2672 subjects and correlation with headaches. Acta Otorinolaringoiatria Ital. 2016;36(3):215–9. https://doi.org/10.14639/0392-100X-847.
34. Pacor ML, Nicolis F, Cortina P, Peroli P, Venturini G, Andri L, Corrocher R, Lunardi C. Emicrania e alimenti [Migraine and food]. Recenti Prog Med. 1989;80(2):53–5. Italian. PMID: 2711014.

Sleep Disorders

Luigi Ferini-Strambi, Maria Salsone, and Elena Vittoria Longhi

Introduction

Sleep is a complex and fascinating phenomenon occurring in all known animal species. It is critical to health, especially for memory consolidation [1]. Two different sleep states are known, rapid eye movement (REM) sleep and non-REM sleep, which in turn is divided into three stages (so-called N1–N3). Briefly, brain waves become slower and more synchronized in the progression from the NREM stages: N1 is considered the stage of transition between wake and sleep in which it is possible to experience "hypnic jerks," signals of muscle relax; N2 is the stage in which we spend most of our sleep and is characterized by a specific pattern of electroencephalogram (EEG) including sleep spindles and K-complexes; and finally, N3 referred to as "deep" or "slow-wave" sleep differs mainly from the other two stages for the presence of delta waves on EEG recording. N3 is needed for an individual feeling of well-being and refreshment. During a typical night, sleep is characterized by the cyclic occurrence of REM and NREM forth at least four to five times [1]. Finally, several sleep characteristics should be considered in order to better define sleep health: (1) sleep duration, the total amount of sleep obtained per 24 h; (2) sleep continuity or efficiency, the ease of falling asleep and returning to sleep; (3)

L. Ferini-Strambi (✉)
Department of Clinical Neurosciences, Vita-Salute San Raffaele University, Milan, Italy

Department of Clinical Neurosciences, Neurology-Sleep Disorder Center, IRCCS San Raffaele Scientific Institute, Milan, Italy
e-mail: ferinistrambi.luigi@hsr.it

M. Salsone
Institute of Molecular Bioimaging and Physiology, National Research Council, Milan, Italy
e-mail: salsone.maria@hsr.it

E. V. Longhi
Department of Sexual Medical Center, San Raffaele Hospital, Milano, Italy

© Springer Nature Switzerland AG 2023

E. V. Longhi (ed.), *Managing Psychosexual Consequences in Chronic Diseases*,
https://doi.org/10.1007/978-3-031-31307-3_22

timing, the placement of sleep within the 24-h day; (4) alertness/sleepiness, the ability to maintain attentive wakefulness; and (5) satisfaction/quality, the subjective assessment of "good" or "poor" sleep [2].

Sleep and urological medicine are two related entities and are not completely surprising for some reasons. First, sleep is an age-related phenomenon becoming more fragmented and with more night-time awakenings over time, and thus, disturbed sleep may occur in subjects with other age-related diseases such as urological disorders. Most middle-aged and older subjects frequently experience changes in their sexual health as a consequence of the natural aging process and those changes can lead to manifest dysfunctions including erectile dysfunction (ED), decreased libido, loss of pubic and body hair, and impaired orgasmic and ejaculatory function. Second, sleep is crucial for the circadian rhythm of testosterone secretion, being strongly dependent on REM sleep. Indeed, nocturnal testosterone starts to rise at sleep onset reaching a peak during the first REM sleep cycle. Thus, it is possible to speculate that insufficient/fragmented sleep or sleep disruption could influence testosterone secretion. In line with this, accumulating pieces of evidence have demonstrated that sleep is disrupted in ED populations. In this context, sleep disorders may be also considered potential risk factors for the development of sexual or urological dysfunctions.

This chapter opens with a brief presentation of the most frequent sleep disorders such as obstructive sleep apnea, insomnia disorder, and restless legs syndrome, including clinical presentation followed by a focus on the main sexual dysfunctions occurring in these disorders. This approach could be of clinical relevance, since sleep disorders negatively affect the quality of life of patients with sexual dysfunctions, and they are usually associated with a greater risk of developing cognitive decline. Thus, early detection of sleep disorders in these patients could offer several advantages. Pharmacological and non-pharmacological treatments might have benefits for urological patients with sleep disturbances by reducing the impact of sleep disturbances not only on the pathology but also by improving the quality of life for both patients and their carers.

Sleep Disorders and Sexual Dysfunction

Obstructive Sleep Apnea

Obstructive sleep apnea (OSA) is the most common sleep-related breathing disorder. It is a chronic disorder characterized by repetitive collapse of the upper airway during sleep resulting in increased arousals, sleep fragmentation, and decreased oxygenation [3]. The prevalence of OSA is strictly dependent on its gravity, ranging from 6% to 17% in the general population at ≥ 15 events/h apnea–hypopnea index (AHI) and shows a higher rate in men and increases with age [4]. Clinically, the most frequent symptoms reported by OSA patients are excessive daytime sleepiness (EDS), fatigue, and mood problems [5, 6]. In addition, these patients may exhibit cognitive dysfunction with impairment in attention, memory, and executive functions [7]. Thus, OSA has been associated with an increased risk for mild cognitive impairment and dementia in both cross-sectional and prospective observational studies [8]. Most studies have observed higher risk among those with more severe OSA, supporting the hypothesis that nocturnal hypoxia may be responsible for brain vascular changes [7, 9], while the presence of EDS may also contribute to neurocognitive impairment in OSA patients [10]. Finally, robust neuroimaging evidence suggests that OSA may accelerate amyloid deposition in the brain over time [11, 12]. Considering the higher prevalence of the disease and the clinical relevance of the symptoms, many researchers tried to develop simple and noninvasive tools for OSA screening. Indeed, screening and early diagnosis of OSA might be relevant because untreated OSA often presents severe consequences and complications of the disease. Full-night polysomnography (PSG) remains the gold standard procedure for OSA diagnosis [13] although it may present several limitations as the high expense and the inconvenience of an overnight sleep study. Continuous positive airway pressure (CPAP) remains still now the most efficacious treatment for the complete resolution of sleep apnea [14].

Sexual Dysfunction in OSA

There is evidence that OSA and ED, a common disorder characterized by a consistent inability to attain or maintain a penile erection, or both, sufficient for adequate sexual relations [15], are strictly related. Indeed, these two disorders often coexist, with about half of the male OSA population having ED and vice versa. This association has been supported by epidemiological and clinical studies. Guilleminault et al., among the first, reported an increased prevalence of ED among a population of patients with OSA [16]. Moreover, studies conducted in sleep clinic populations described similar findings with an ED prevalence ranging between 41% and 80% [17]. In line with these findings, Chen et al. in a recent cross-sectional study found that ED incidence in OSA patients was 9.44-fold higher compared with non-OSA patients [18]. In addition, the severity of OSA could play a role to predict the development of ED in these patients. In a Korean study, Shin et al. [19] investigated the correlation between OSA and ED, or disease-specific quality of life. They also analyzed specific PSG parameters in predicting ED in OSA patients. They found that ED was not associated with AHI, but it significantly correlated with decreased minimum oxygen saturation. Moreover, when the cutoff values for the desaturation were set at 77%, the positive predictive ED in OSA value was equal to 89.9% [19].

The association between OSA and ED, however, remains until debatable since conflicting results have been also reported. Some authors [20], in a study on 70 healthy married men aged 45–75 years and others [21] in a community study dwelling men aged 67 years, found no association between these two disorders. Their results did not support the notion that sleep disorders may be involved in the increased prevalence of erectile impotence in healthy older individuals [20]. On the other hand, a recent systematic review and meta-analysis aimed to answer this enigma [17]. Twenty-eight observational studies, 19 cross-sectional design studies, seven case–control studies, and two cohort studies were included. Interestingly, their results indicate that in patients without OSA, the risk of ED was significantly lower compared with patients with OSA [17]. Taken together, these findings indicate that OSA may be associated with a higher risk of ED.

The underlying mechanism of interaction between OSA and ED remains until unknown. In the last years, three main theories have been proposed including (1) hormonal effect of testosterone (Fig. 1); (2) peripheral neuropathy due to hypoxemia; and (3) vascular endothelial dysfunction [22]. Although the relationship between testosterone and OSA is really complicated, it has been reported that testosterone plays a crucial role in the pathogenesis of OSA. Indeed, many studies found that OSA patients had lower serum testosterone, and there was a negative correlation between sleep parameters such as AHI, oxygen desaturation index, and testosterone level [22]. On the other hand, some authors [23] demonstrated that androgen treatment significantly increased the number of apneas in hypogonadal patients and others [24] that Marfan's syndrome patients may have a worsened OSA after testosterone injection. Concerning the second hypothesis, some authors evaluated the bulbocavernosus reflex and the somatosensory-evoked potentials of the pudendal nerve, the most widely established method of documenting pudendal neuropathies as cause of impotence in OSA [25]. The bulbocavernosus reflex was altered in almost all OSA patients and those with altered reflex presented more severe condition characterized by a higher AHI, a higher percentage of sleep time spent with SaO_2 <90%, and a lower daytime PaO_2. In OSA, ED seems to be related to a peripheral nerve dysfunction probably due to nocturnal hypoxia [25]. Finally,

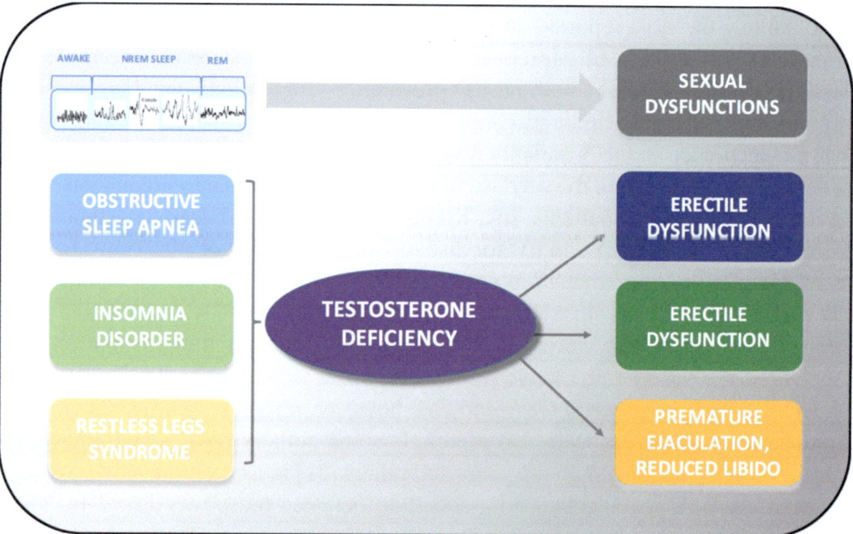

Fig. 1 Hypothetical mechanisms linking sleep disorders to sexual dysfunctions. Schematic representation of main sleep disorders causing a decrease in testosterone levels

vascular endothelial dysfunction may be involved in the pathogenesis of ED in OSA, as demonstrated by the elevation of inflammatory markers such as interleukin (IL)-6 and IL-8 found in these patients [26]. These and other pieces of evidence support the hypothesis that endothelial dysfunction may be the common pathophysiological mechanism linking OSA with both ED and cardiovascular complications [27].

Several longitudinal and cross-sectional studies investigated in OSA the effect of CPAP treatment on ED, although this remains until controversial. Among longitudinal investigations, Budweiser et al. [28] evaluated whether CPAP therapy may have a long-term effect on sexual function including ED in OSA males. CPAP users experienced an improvement in overall sexual function and in low mean nocturnal oxygen saturation compared with CPAP non-user. Interestingly, results from a study assessing the sexual functioning in male and female partners before and after CPAP therapy in OSA did not report the beneficial effect of CPAP on the patients but improved sexual function in women after their male partner underwent nasal CPAP also had psychological benefits [29]. Finally, a trial assessing the effect of 3 months of CPAP on cardiovascular risk in OSA patients with type 2 diabetes demonstrated that CPAP therapy improves somnolence and promotes exercise but that there is no direct benefit for sexual function, in particular for total or free testosterone serum [30]. In a randomized trial of CPAP and vardenafil, the first-line therapy for ED, moderate-to-severe OSA, and ED were randomized to 12 weeks of CPAP or sham CPAP and 10 mg daily vardenafil or placebo in a two-by-two factorial design [31]. Their main results demonstrated that (1) CPAP increased the frequency of sleep-related erections and overall sexual satisfaction, but did not change erectile function or treatment or relationship satisfaction; (2) vardenafil did not alter erectile function or sleep-disordered breathing, but did improve overall self-esteem and relationship satisfaction; (3) adherent CPAP improved erectile function, sexual desire, overall sexual, self-esteem, relationship, and treatment satisfaction, as well as sleepiness, and quality of life; and (4) adherent vardenafil use did not consistently change nocturnal erection quality. On this basis, the authors suggest that adherent CPAP or vardenafil use improves ED and quality of life [31]. Finally, a recent systematic review and meta-analysis clarified the anti-ED effect of CPAP and further compare the efficacy between CPAP, phosphodiesterase type 5 inhibitors, and combination therapy on erectile function in OSA concurrent ED. Results showed that CPAP significantly ameliorated, especially total erectile events, moreover international index of erectile function score, and nocturnal penile rigidity, whereas no significant improvements have been reported in nocturnal penile tumescence circumference. These findings provided promising insights about CPAP-based ED treatment for OSA patients [32].

Finally, convergent evidence links OSA to nocturia, a common urological disorder in middle-aged and older patients defined as the need to wake up one or more times to void urine during sleep [33–36]. The biological mechanism underlying the pathogenesis of nocturia in OSA patients is related to an increase in circulating levels (both urine and plasma) of natriuretic peptide (ANP). Indeed, total urine output, plasma ANP, and urine ANP excretion have been reported significantly higher among OSA subjects with higher AHI levels [37]. The increase in ANP levels might lead to the suppression of arginine vasopressin in these patients [22].

In conclusion, other pieces of evidence support the close association between OSA and ED. In particular, OSA is associated with a higher risk of ED. Although crucial is the role of testosterone in the pathogenesis of ED in these patients, endothelial dysfunction as a common mechanism to explain cardiovascular complications in both disorders is emerging. Preliminary longitudinal investigations suggest a beneficial effect of CPAP treatment on ED and quality of life. Further well-designed controlled clinical trials and longitudinal prospective studies are needed.

Insomnia Disorder

Insomnia disorder (ID) is the most highly prevalent sleep disorder having a prevalence of about 7% in the European population [38]. Epidemiologic studies also suggest that overall about 30% to 35% of the population has at least one of the insomnia symptoms occasionally, and 9% to 10% of the population meets the diagnostic criteria for insomnia disorder [22, 39, 40]. ID is defined as a disorder of sleep initiation or maintenance, followed by a feeling of non-restorative sleep and several diurnal consequences ranging from occupational and social difficulties to cognitive impairment [3]. The diagnosis is based on the clinical evaluation of subjective symptoms in accordance with the fifth edition of the Diagnostic and Statistical Manual of Mental Disorders (DSM-5) and the third version of the International Classification of Sleep Disorder (ICSD-3) published criteria [3, 41], while PSG evaluation provides to exclude the presence of another sleep disorders. Notably, ID is also one of the most common mental disorders. It is also well documented that ID patients have an increased risk to develop depression and dementia, especially Alzheimer's disease [42, 43]. It is emerging the hypothesis that ID is an umbrella of different clinical subtypes, each with its own specific multivariate profile of characteristics, rather than a single clinical entity. A combination of indices of sleep quality and quantity associated with mental and physical health, childhood trauma, life events, fatigue, sleepiness, hyperarousal, hyperactivity, other sleep disorders, lifetime sleep history, chronotype, depression, anxiety, mood, quality of life, personality, happiness, worry, rumination, and others should be considered [44]. Since the clinical relevance of ID, a timely treatment is due. Cognitive-behavioral therapy for insomnia is recommended as the first-line treatment for this disorder in adults of any, whereas a pharmacological intervention can be offered if cognitive-behavioral therapy is not sufficiently effective or not available [45].

Sexual Dysfunction in Insomnia Disorder

Sexual dysfunction is more common among older men, and insomnia has been reported as an independent risk factor related to sexual dysfunction, along with cardiovascular disease, diabetes, and depression [22]. A possible explanation for this phenomenon is that insomnia and insufficient sleep are strictly related to a decrease in the level of testosterone levels [19, 46–48] (Fig. 1). This is not surprising, since as abovementioned, the nocturnal testosterone levels are strictly related to the REM sleep stage. Thus, it is possible to speculate that diurnal testosterone rhythm might be also a sleep-related phenomenon. In this context, some authors have reported that during fragmented sleep, nocturnal testosterone rise was observed only in subjects who showed REM episodes indicating that sleep-related rise in serum testosterone levels was linked with the appearance of first REM sleep [49]. Moreover, it has been also demonstrated that while sleep loss in the early part of the night does not affect testosterone levels, early awakening and wakefulness during the second part of the night reduce its morning circulating concentrations [50]. In line with this, Leproult R et al. investigated the effect of 1 week of sleep restriction on testosterone levels in young healthy men [51]. They found that daytime testosterone levels were decreased by 10% to 15% in a group of 10 healthy young men whose sleep was restricted to 5 h per night for eight nights [51]. Another study performed on 24 healthy young men with acute sleep loss found lowered salivary testosterone level (but not cortisol) reactive aggression [52]. By contrast, results from recent randomized controlled studies of short sleeper vs habitual sleep suggest that sleep restriction does not adversely affect plasma testosterone levels in healthy young men [53]. Contrasting results may be probably due to the methodological differences used to investigate the duration and timing of sleep.

In conclusion, insomnia could adversely affect the circadian level of serum testosterone causing sexual dysfunction. Confirmatory longitudinal studies should be performed in order to evaluate the influence of sleep duration and quality on testosterone concentrations over time.

Restless Legs Syndrome

Restless legs syndrome (RLS) is a common sleep-related movement disorder characterized by an urge to move the limbs frequently accompanied by uncomfortable and unpleasant sensations that are difficult to describe. Patients define their symptoms as burning, twitching, or pain in their lower limbs. However, in the most severe cases the symptomatology can be perceived also in the upper limbs [54]. It is commonly considered a disorder with a clear prevalence in females, but although lower in men, it affects approximately 4.1% to 7.6% of men [22]. The clinical onset of the disease has a circadian trend with a peak in the evening or at night and starts during period of rest or inactivity. Indeed, an exacerbation of unpleasant sensations is reported in those situations where immobility is forced such as driving, flying long distance, watching movies in theater, and attending business meetings. Patients may employ different strategies to alleviate the discomfort [54, 55]. Despite sleep macrostructure and microstructure are significantly altered by the presence of periodic limb movement sleepiness is not universally reported by all patients [54, 56]. Although the exact pathogenesis remains until debated, two forms of RLS have been proposed: idiopathic or secondary occurs in comorbidity with other medical conditions such as polyneuropathy, iron deficiency anemia, multiple sclerosis, hypertension, and cardiovascular diseases. As a chronic condition, RLS requires treatment in the long term. Different drugs in particular dopamine agonists have shown to have a good efficacy in reducing patients' symptomatology and are considered first-line treatment, while alpha-2-delta agonists are recognized as a valid alternative [54, 57].

Sexual Dysfunction in Restless Legs Syndrome

RLS and sexual dysfunction have similar pathophysiological features including autonomic dysfunction and dopamine deficiency. Thus, it is not surprising that these two conditions may coexist. Gao et al. examined whether men with RLS have a higher prevalence of ED. They found that men with RLS had a higher likelihood of concurrent ED, and the magnitude of the observed association was increased with a higher frequency of RLS symptoms. On this basis, they suggest that ED and RLS share common determinants [58]. In addition, a prospective study has been conducted by Li Y et al., for examining whether RLS was associated with a higher risk of developing ED based on 6 years of follow-up. Results demonstrated that after adjustment for potential confounders, such as age, body mass index, smoking, physical activity, other sleep disorders, and snoring status, men with RLS were more likely to develop ED than those without the syndrome [59]. Not only ED, however, occurs in RLS patients. Kurt et al. found that premature ejaculation was more prevalent in RLS than in control patients while the rate of ED did not differ between the groups [60]. Sleepiness, anxiety, and sexual dysfunction have been reported in men hemodialysis patients with RLS [61]. Finally, men with RLS may exhibit also reduced libido and depression mood more often than controls [62] (Fig. 1). To date, there is no evidence about the efficacy of dopaminergic agents on ED or sexual dysfunction in men with RLS.

In conclusion, although there are only a few studies about RLS and sexual dysfunction, there is a convergence that RLS may be associated with these conditions, especially within ED. Future research should be focused on the efficacy of RLS treatments on sexual dysfunctions in these patients.

Conclusions and Future Directions

In conclusion, there is convergence supporting the relationship between sleep disorders and sexual dysfunctions since disturbed sleep is frequently reported in these patients. Of note, it appears that some sleep disorders, in particular OSA, may be more likely associated with some specific sexual dysfunctions such as ED. Considering the clinical relevance of this research topic, we suggest that in addition to receiving a neurological evaluation, patients with sleep disorders must be also evaluated for sexual function. On the other hand, urologists should investigate the impact and the contribution of sleep disorders on male sexual function and dysfunction in their patients. Finally, the research agenda should include further studies in a longitudinal prospective cohort for better characterizing the direction and the nature of the relationship between sleep disorders and sexual dysfunctions and the establishment of new biomarkers. Additional research is also needed to elucidate the mechanisms underlying the pathogenesis of sexual dysfunction linked to sleep disorders and evaluate the efficacy of treatments for sleep disorders in urological patients.

Quality of Life and Sexuality

Pieces of evidence support the association between sleep disorders and sexual dysfunctions. The main biological link between these two conditions is related to the circadian secretion of testosterone. Indeed, nocturnal testosterone secretion is modulated by the sleep stages, starting to rise at sleep onset with a peak during the first REM sleep cycle. Thus, it is possible to speculate that sleep disorders could adversely affect serum testosterone levels. There is a convergence that sleep loss, especially during the second part of the night, in the early awakening, and wakefulness, reduces its morning circulating concentrations. Considering the clinical relevance of the association between sleep disorders and sexual dysfunctions, the objective of this chapter is to summarize and discuss the cross-sectional and longitudinal studies on the main sleep disorders occurring in the most common urological and sexual disorders. Obstructive sleep apnea is more likely associated with the development of erectile dysfunction (ED) and nocturia, insomnia disorder is frequently concurrent with ED, and restless legs syndrome may often exhibit premature ejaculation and reduced libido. Emphasis is placed on the early detection of sleep disorders in urological patients in order to provide them with timely treatment for overall health. Although a beneficial effect of continuous positive airway pressure treatment on sexual dysfunctions and quality of life has been also reported, confirmatory studies should be performed for evaluating the influence of sleep on testosterone concentrations over time and the efficacy of treatments. Conversely, caution should be considered in treating patients affected by sleep disorders with testosterone.

Among studies on sleep disorders, patients with sexsomnia are often mentioned.

These patients fill out the Paris Arousal Disorder Severity Scale (PADSS) and are monitored for 1–2 nights with video-polysomnography.

The most striking findings include seventeen patients (70.6% male, aged 17–76 years) with sexsomnia and showed amnestic caressing of bedmate ($n = 11$), full sexual intercourse ($n = 8$), masturbation ($n = 8$), and spontaneous orgasm ($n = 1$). Sexual behaviors are more directed during sleep than during wakefulness ($n = 12$), leading to six sexual assaults, including intramarital rape ($n = 3$), assault of a family member ($n = 2$), rape of a friend ($n = 1$), and forensic consequences ($n = 2$). In 47% of patients with sexsomnia, there was a history or current occurrences of sleepwalking/night terrors. Patients with sexsomnia had more N3 awakenings than matched healthy controls and the same amount as normal sleepwalkers. Half of them presented evidence of cortico-cortical dissociation, including concomitant slow (mainly frontal) and fast (mainly temporal and occipital) electroencephalography (EEG) rhythms, with concomitant N3 penile erection in one case. Of 89 sleepwalkers, 10% had previous episodes of amnestic sexual behaviors, with a higher PADSS-A score and a trend of higher total PADSS score than the 80 sleepwalkers without sexsomnia.

The male predominance of sexsomnia and the serious clinical and forensic consequences are generally confirmed in these studies. The results suggest a continuum of regular sleepwalking, sleepwalking with occasional sexsomnia, and near-exclusive sexsomnia.Conflict of InterestsThe authors declare not to have commercial or financial relationships that could represent as a potential conflicts of interest.

References

1. Ferini-Strambi L, Galbiati A, Marelli S. Sleep microstructure and memory function. Front Neurol. 2013;4:159.
2. Buysse DJ. Sleep health: can we define it? Does it matter? Sleep. 2014;37:9–17.
3. American Academy of Sleep Medicine. International classification of sleep disorders. 3rd ed. Darien, IL: American Academy of Sleep Medicine.
4. Ferini-Strambi L, Lombardi GE, Marelli S, Galbiati A. Neurological deficits in obstructive sleep apnea. Curr Treat Options Neurol. 2017;19(4):16.
5. Gottlieb DJ, Whitney C, Bonekat WH, Iber C, James GD, Lebowitz M, et al. Relation of sleepiness to respiratory disturbance index: the Sleep Heart Health Study. Am J Respir Crit Care Med. 1999;159:502e7.
6. Aloia MS, Arnedt JT, Davis JD, Riggs RL, Byrd D. Neuropsychological sequelae of obstructive sleep apnea-hypopnea syndrome: a critical review. J Int Neuropsycologichol Soc. 2004;10:772–85.
7. Gagnon K, Baril AA, Gagnon JF, Fortin M, Decary A, Lafond C, Desautels A, Montplaisir J, Gosselin N. Cognitive impairment in obstructive sleep apnea. Pathol Biol. 2014;62(5):233–40.
8. Leng Y, McEvoy CT, Allen IE, Yaffe K. Association of sleep-disordered breathing with cognitive function and risk of cognitive impairment: a systematic review and meta-analysis. JAMA Neurol. 2017;74:1237.
9. Bucks RS, Olaithe M, Rosenzweig I, Morrell MJ. Reviewing the relationship between OSA and cognition: where do we go from here? Respirology. 2017;22(7):1253–61.
10. Steiropoulos P, Galbiati A, Ferini-Strambi L. Detection of mild cognitive impairment in middle-aged and older adults with obstructive sleep apnoea: does excessive daytime sleepiness play a role? Eur Respir J. 2019;53:1801917.
11. Liguori C, Mercuri NB, Izzi F, et al. Obstructive sleep apnea is associated with early but possibly modifiable Alzheimer's disease biomarkers changes. Sleep. 2017;40(5)
12. Yun CH, Lee HY, Lee SK, et al. Amyloid burden in obstructive sleep apnea. J Alzheimers Dis. 2017;59:21.
13. Kapur V, Auckley D, Chowdhuri S, Kuhlmann DC, Mehra R, Ramar K, et al. Clinical practice guideline for diagnostic testing for adult obstructive sleep apnea: an American academy of sleep medicine clinical practice guideline. J Clin Sleep Med. 2017;13(3):479–504.
14. Ftikhar IH, Bittencourt L, Youngstedt SD, Ayas N, Cistulli P, Schwab R, et al. Comparative efficacy of CPAP, MADs, exercise-training, and dietary weight loss for sleep apnea: a network meta-analysis. Sleep Med. 2017;30:7–14.

15. NIH Consensus Conference. Impotence. NIH consensus development panel on impotence. JAMA. 1993;270:83–90.
16. Guilleminault C, Eldridge FL, Tilkian A, Simmons FB, Dement WC. Sleep apnea syndrome due to upper airway obstruction: a review of 25 cases. Arch Intern Med. 1977;137:296–300.
17. Kellesarian SV, Malignaggi VR, Feng C, Javed F. Association between obstructive sleep apnea and erectile dysfunction: a systematic review and meta-analysis. Sex Med J. 2018;30:129–40.
18. Chen KF, Liang SJ, Lin CL, Liao WC, Kao CH. Sleep disorders increase risk of subsequent erectile dysfunction in individuals without sleep apnea: a nationwide population-base cohort study. Sleep Med. 2016;17:64–8.
19. Shin HW, Rha YC, Han DH, Chung S, Yoon IY, Rhee CS, et al. Erectile dysfunction and disease-specific quality of life in patients with obstructive sleep apnea. Int J Impot Res. 2008;20:549–53.
20. Schiavi RC, Mandeli J, Schreiner-Engel P, Chambers A. Aging, sleep disorders, and male sexual function. Biol Psychiatry. 1991;30:15–24.
21. Bozorgmehri S, Fink HA, Parimi N, Canales B, Ensrud KE, Ancoli-Israel S, et al. Association of sleep-disordered breathing with erectile dysfunction in community dwelling older men. J Urol. 2017;197:776–82.
22. Wook Cho J, Duffy JF. Sleep, sleep disorders, and sexual dysfunction. World J Mens Health. 2019;37(3):261–75.
23. Schneider BK, Pickett CK, Zwillich CW, Weil JV, McDermott MT, Santen RJ, et al. Influence of testosterone on breathing during sleep. J Appl Physiol. 1985;1986(61):618–23.
24. Cistulli PA, Grunstein RR, Sullivan CE. Effect of testosterone administration on upper airway collapsibility during sleep. Am J Respir Crit Care Med. 1994;149:530–2.
25. Fanfulla F, Malaguti S, Montagna T, Salvini S, Bruschi C, Crotti P, et al. Erectile dysfunction in men with obstructive sleep apnea: an early sign of nerve involvement. Sleep. 2000;23:775–81.
26. Bouloukaki I, Papadimitriou V, Sofras F, Mermigkis C, Moniaki V, Siafakas NM, et al. Abnormal cytokine profile in patients with obstructive sleep apnea-hypopnea syndrome and erectile dysfunction. Mediat Inflamm. 2014;2014:568951.
27. Hoyos CM, Melehan KL, Phillips CL, Grunstein RR, Liu PY. To ED or not to ED e Is erectile dysfunction in obstructive sleep apnea related to endothelial dysfunction? Sleep Medicine Reviews. 2015;20:5–14.
28. Budweiser S, Luigart R, Jörres RA, Kollert F, Kleemann Y, Wieland WF, et al. Long-term changes of sexual function in men with obstructive sleep apnea after initiation of continuous positive airway pressure. J Sex Med. 2013;10:524–31.
29. Acar M, Kaya C, Catli T, Hancı D, Bolluk O, Aydin Y. Effects of nasal continuous positive airway pressure therapy on partners' sexual lives. Eur Arch Otorhinolaryngol. 2016;273:133–7.
30. Knapp A, Myhill PC, Davis WA, Peters KE, Hillman D, Hamilton EJ, et al. Effect of continuous positive airway pressure therapy on sexual function and serum testosterone in males with type 2 diabetes and obstructive sleep apnoea. Clin Endocrinol. 2014;81:254–8.
31. Melehan KL, Hoyos CM, Hamilton GS, Wong KK, Yee B, McLachlan RI, et al. Randomized trial of CPAP and vardenafil on erectile and arterial function in men with obstructive sleep apnea and erectile dysfunction. J Clin Endocrinol Metab. 2018;103(4):1601–11.
32. Li Z, Fang Z, Xing N, Zhu S, Fan Y. The effect of CPAP and PDE5i on erectile function in men with obstructive sleep apnea and erectile dysfunction: a systematic review and meta-analysis. Sleep Med Rev. 2019;48:101217.
33. van Kerrebroeck P, Abrams P, Chaikin D, Donovan J, Fonda D, Jackson S, et al. The standardisation of terminology in nocturia: report from the Standardisation Sub-committee of the International Continence Society. Neurourol Urodyn. 2002;21:179–83.
34. Middelkoop HA, Smilde-van den Doel DA, Neven AK, Kamphuisen HA, Springer CP. Subjective sleep characteristics of 1,485 males and females aged 50-93: effects of sex and age, and factors related to self-evaluated quality of sleep. J Gerontol A Biol Sci Med Sci. 1996;51:M108–15.
35. Burgio KL, Johnson TM 2nd, Goode PS, Markland AD, Richter HE, Roth DL, et al. Prevalence and correlates of nocturia in community-dwelling older adults. J Am Geriatr Soc. 2010;58:861–6.

36. Bliwise DL, Foley DJ, Vitiello MV, Ansari FP, Ancoli-Israel S, Walsh JK. Nocturia and disturbed sleep in the elderly. Sleep Med. 2009;10:540–8.
37. Umlauf MG, Chasens ER, Greevy RA, Arnold J, Burgio KL, Pillion DJ. Obstructive sleep apnea, nocturia and polyuria in older adults. Sleep. 2004;27:139–44.
38. Wittchen HU, Jacobi F, Rehm J, et al. The size and burden of mental disorders and other disorders of the brain in Europe 2010. Eur Neuropsychopharmacol. 2011;21:655–79.
39. Morin CM, LeBlanc M, Daley M, Gregoire JP, Mérette C. Epidemiology of insomnia: prevalence, self-help treatments, consultations, and determinants of help-seeking behaviors. Sleep Med. 2006;7:123–30.
40. Ohayon MM, Reynolds CF 3rd. Epidemiological and clinical relevance of insomnia diagnosis algorithms according to the DSM-IV and the International Classification of Sleep Disorders (ICSD). Sleep Med. 2009;10:952–60.
41. American Psychiatric Association. Diagnostic and Statistical Manual of Mental Disorders (DSM-5). 5th ed. Washington, DC: American Psychiatric Press; 2013.
42. Baglioni C, Battagliese G, Feige B, et al. Insomnia as a predictor of depression: a meta-analytic evaluation of longitudinal epidemiological studies. J Affect Disord. 2011;135:10–9.
43. Ju YS, Ooms SJ, Sutphen C, Macauley SL, Zangrilli MA, Jerome G, et al. Slow wave sleep disruption increases cerebrospinal fluid amyloid-β levels. Brain. 2017;140(8):2104–11.
44. Benjamins JS, Migliorati F, Dekker K, et al. Insomnia heterogeneity: characteristics to consider for data-driven multivariate subtyping. Sleep Med Rev. 2017;36:71–81.
45. Riemann D, Baglioni C, Bassetti C, et al. European guideline for the diagnosis and treatment of insomnia. Sleep Res. 2017;26(6):675–700.
46. Wu JL, Wu RS, Yang JG, Huang CC, Chen KB, Fang KH, et al. Effects of sleep deprivation on serum testosterone concentrations in the rat. Neurosci Lett. 2011;494:124–9.
47. Carter JR, Durocher JJ, Larson RA, DellaValla JP, Yang H. Sympathetic neural responses to 24-hour sleep deprivation in humans: sex differences. Am J Physiol Heart Circ Physiol. 2012;302:H1991–7.
48. Auyeung TW, Kwok T, Leung J, Lee JS, Ohlsson C, Vandenput L, et al. Sleep duration and disturbances were associated with testosterone level, muscle mass, and muscle strength: a cross-sectional study in 1274 older men. J Am Med Dir Assoc. 2015;16(630):e1–6.
49. Luboshitzky R, Zabari Z, Shen-Orr Z, Herer P, Lavie P. Disruption of the nocturnal testosterone rhythm by sleep fragmentation in normal men. J Clin Endocrinol Metab. 2001;86:1134–9.
50. Schmid SM, Hallschmid M, Jauch-Chara K, Lehnert H, Schultes B. Sleep timing may modulate the effect of sleep loss on testosterone. Clin Endocrinol. 2012;77:749–54.
51. Leproult R, Van Cauter E. Effect of 1 week of sleep restriction on testosterone levels in young healthy men. JAMA. 2011;305:2173–4.
52. Cote KA, McCormick CM, Geniole SN, Renn RP, MacAulay SD. Sleep deprivation lowers reactive aggression and testosterone in men. Biol Psychol. 2013;92:249–56.
53. Smith I, Salazar I, RoyChoudhury A, St-Onge MP. Sleep restriction and testosterone concentrations in young healthy males: randomized controlled studies of acute and chronic short sleep. Sleep Health. 2019;5(6):580–6.
54. Ferini-Strambi L, Carli G, Casoni F, Galbiati A. Restless legs syndrome and Parkinson disease: a causal relationship between the two disorders? Front Neurol. 2018;9:551.
55. Allen RP, Picchietti DL, Garcia-Borreguero D, Ondo WG, Walters AS, Winkelman JW, et al. International Restless Legs Syndrome Study Group., Restless legs syndrome/Willis-Ekbom disease diagnostic criteria: updated International Restless Legs Syndrome Study Group (IRLSSG) consensus criteria–history, rationale, description, and significance. Sleep Med. 2014;15:860–73. https://doi.org/10.1016/j.sleep.2014.03.025.
56. Kallweit U, Siccoli MM, Poryazova R, Werth E, Bassetti CL. Excessive daytime sleepiness in idiopathic restless legs syndrome: characteristics and evolution under dopaminergic treatment. Eur Neurol. 2009;62:176–9. https://doi.org/10.1159/000228261.

57. Rinaldi F, Galbiati A, Marelli S, Ferini Strambi L, Zucconi M. Treatment options in intractable restless legs syndrome/Willis-Ekbom disease (RLS/WED). Curr Treat Options Neurol. 2016;18(7):7. https://doi.org/10.1007/s11940-015-0390-1.
58. Gao X, Schwarzschild MA, O'Reilly EJ, Wang H, Ascherio A. Restless legs syndrome and erectile dysfunction. Sleep. 2010;33:75–9.
59. Li Y, Batool-Anwar S, Kim S, Rimm EB, Ascherio A, Gao X. Prospective study of restless legs syndrome and risk of erectile dysfunction. Am J Epidemiol. 2013;177:1097–105.
60. Kurt O, Yazici CM, Alp R, Sancak EB, Topcu B. Is it only a sleeping disorder or more? Restless legs syndrome and erectile function. Scand J Urol. 2016;50:392–5.
61. Dikici S, Bahadir A, Baltaci D, Ankarali H, Eroglu M, Ercan N, et al. Association of anxiety, sleepiness, and sexual dysfunction with restless legs syndrome in hemodialysis patients. Hemodial Int. 2014;18:809–18.
62. Ulfberg J, Nyström B, Carter N, Edling C. Prevalence of restless legs syndrome among men aged 18 to 64 years: an association with somatic disease and neuropsychiatric symptoms. Mov Disord. 2001;16:1159–63.

Multiple Sclerosis

Maria Chiara Buscarinu, Giulia Pellicciari, Silvia Romano, Marco Salvetti, and Elena Vittoria Longhi

Epidemiology and Pathogenesis

Multiple sclerosis (MS) is an immune-mediated inflammatory demyelinating disorder of the central nervous system (CNS) characterized by myelin and axonal damage, which can affect both white and gray matters. The main pathologic hallmark of MS is the demyelinating plaque characterized by an immunologic response mediated by CD8+ and CD4+ T cells and B cells, all contributing to the pathogenesis of MS [1].

The course of MS is highly variable and unpredictable. In most patients, the disease is initially characterized by episodes of reversible or partially reversible neurological deficits, often followed by progressive neurological impairment.

The prevalence of MS has increased progressively over time, particularly in women; to date, the number of subjects affected by MS is about 2.3 million worldwide [2].

The reasons for this increase, similarly to its causes, remain unclear. Probably, we are dealing with changes in environmental exposures since the increase seems to be too fast to be attributable to heritable factors [3]. Some possible explanations are the availability of more advanced imaging techniques [4] or changes in lifestyle, such as lack of vitamin D [5], obesity, and increased smoking [6].

Prevalence studies have shown a different geographic distribution characterized by distinct areas of disease frequency related to latitude (high-, medium-, and low-risk areas) [7], and it is generally accepted that the prevalence of MS tends to increase with increasing distance from the equator (Northern Europe is more

M. C. Buscarinu · G. Pellicciari · S. Romano · M. Salvetti (✉)
Department of Neuroscience, Mental Health and Sense Organs (NESMOS), Sapienza University of Rome, Rome, Italy
e-mail: silvia.romano@uniroma1.it

E. V. Longhi
Department of Sexual Medical Center, San Raffaele Hospital, Milano, Italy

E. V. Longhi (ed.), *Managing Psychosexual Consequences in Chronic Diseases*,
https://doi.org/10.1007/978-3-031-31307-3_23

affected than the Eastern countries). Italy is considered among the high-risk countries for MS, with the primacy of Sardinia, which has a prevalence of 299 cases per 100,000 inhabitants, against the figure referring to the rest of the peninsula significantly lower (179 cases per 100,000) [8].

MS is commonly diagnosed between 20 years and 40 years of age although it can affect younger and older individuals. Pediatric MS typically presents a favorable short-term prognosis but a higher probability (more than 50%) of developing a secondary progressive form after the age of 30 years [9].

Similar to other autoimmune diseases, MS is more prevalent in women than in men with a prevalence ratio increasing from 2.3 to 3.5:1 in the last decades [10, 11].

Many studies have attempted to analyze the genetic aspects of this disease. MS is characterized by some degree of familiarity; the risk in second-degree relatives with 25% genetic similarity is 1–2%, whereas in third-degree relatives with 12.5% genetic similarity, this risk is less than 1% [12]. Studies on monozygotic twins have confirmed concordance values from 10% to 31%, which are about six times the concordance rate in dizygotic twins (2.5–5%) [13, 14].

The role of MHC alleles is well known [15, 16], and a susceptibility linked to the DR15 and DQ6 haplotypes and the corresponding DRB1 * 1501, DRB5 * 0101, DQA1 * 0102 and * 0602, and DQB2 genotypes has been reported [17].

Through genome-wide association studies (GWAS), several new MS susceptibility loci have been identified related to the immune response and microglia biology [18]. However, genes alone are not sufficient to determine pathology.

Chronic infections due to herpes viruses, the neurotrophic human herpes virus 6 (HHV6) [19] and lymphotropic Epstein–Barr virus (EBV) [20], or autoimmune processes due to infection [21] have long been studied among the most important environmental factors.

EBV infection, which affects about 95% of the population [22], seems to be a risk factor when contracted in old age and in typical adolescent age, associated with mononucleosis as a clinical manifestation. Moreover, an anatomopathological study has shown the presence of EBV-infected B cells in lymphoid follicle-like structures in the cerebral meninges of some MS patients suggesting a correlation among the reactivation of the virus in the follicles, acute inflammation, and relapses [23].

Recently, using a "candidate interactome" approach, an interaction between disease-associated genetic variants and EBV proteins with a potential role in MS etiology has been highlighted. EBV infection can be considered a necessary condition, but in itself not sufficient to cause the disease. Multiple exogenous and endogenous viral factors are been described as potentially able to affect the etiopathogenesis of MS as genes coding for immune system components, related to antiviral response, or allelic variants of genes that encode a viral protein known as EBNA2 [24].

Among the environmental factors, smoking, vitamin D deficiency, diet, and exposure to UV radiations have been described as factors involved in MS onset and/or progression [25].

Vitamin D deficiency has been correlated with a greater risk for MS. Cholecalciferol performs multiple functions on our body such as maintaining calcium homeostasis, regenerating myelin, and regulating the immune system [26].

Cigarette smoking has been demonstrated to increase the risk of MS approximately 50% [27]. Over the past 10 years, also obesity has been highly emphasized as a modifiable risk factor for MS. Adolescent patients with a BMI greater than 27 present an increased risk of two to three times that of their normal-weight peers. Not only is obesity taken into account, but also being overweight. There is, however, an important difference: Obesity is associated with an increased probability of onset of MS in children [28].

In conclusion, researchers agree that gene–environment interactions, together with stochastic events, play the most important role in MS etiology [29, 30].

Clinical Presentation

Clinical features both in terms of onset of disease and in terms of short-and long-term evolution are highly variable across patients. Due to the random and wide spatial distribution of lesions, MS can result in symptoms and signs of CNS involvement in all functional systems, although some symptoms are common and others are rare. Typical symptoms include optic neuritis, brainstem syndromes such as internuclear ophthalmoplegia, diplopia and dysarthria, cerebellar syndromes, and transverse myelitis.

Pyramidal impairment, with paresis or plegia, and sensory involvement with paraesthesia, pallesthesia, sensory ataxia, and Lhermitte signs are very common. Autonomic functions (urinary dysfunction and sexual and gastrointestinal disorders) can also be impaired in about 90% of patients significantly affecting the quality of life. The most frequent and most disabling symptom is fatigue, which can be defined as an overwhelming sense of tiredness, lack of strength, and energy compared to the level of activity exercised. Cognitive and *psychological disorders are frequently reported.* Some mood disorders occur more often in people with MS than in the general population, and this predisposition might be due to a complex interaction of factors, which include the disease course, genetic predisposition, and life events leading to a sense of loss and grief. Cognitive impairment occurs in 40–65% of MS patients, typically involving complex attention, information processing speed, (episodic) memory, and executive functions, and often emerges early in disease, but impairment is more prevalent and may differ qualitatively among persons with progressive forms.

Other less frequent symptoms are paroxysmal disorders, epileptic manifestations, and trigeminal neuralgia.

There are no specific tests for MS, and the diagnosis often relies on a careful medical history, a neurologic examination, and various tests including magnetic resonance imaging (MRI) of the brain and spinal cord and cerebrospinal fluid (CSF) analysis for ruling out other conditions that might produce similar signs and symptoms.

The specific changes in CSF are the detection of oligoclonal bands (OCB), which occur in the vast majority of MS patients. A lack of OCB can represent a red flag leading to consider possible alternative diagnoses [31].

On the MRI, there could be an involvement of a single anatomical region, as presented by a monofocal attack, or the involvement may consist of more than one anatomical CNS region as described in multifocal attacks. MRI is used not only as a diagnosis tool, but it is also fundamental to estimate lesion load, disease activity (scans with gadolinium), atrophy, and axonal loss, as well as to follow their progression.

However, the Revised McDonald Criteria published in 2018 include specific guidelines for using MRI and CSF analysis to speed the diagnostic process (Table 1) [32], and clinical experience is often necessary for approaching MS diagnosis, for example, when distinguishing a noninflammatory optic neuropathy or myelopathy from optic neuritis or myelitis may be challenging.

Based on the clinical course, it is possible to identify four subtypes [33]:

1. *Relapsing–Remitting MS (RRMS):* It is the most common form, affecting more than 50% of MS patients. It is characterized by relapses followed by full or partial recovery of impaired functions, with a stable course and lack of progression during periods between relapses.
2. *Secondary Progressive MS (SPMS):* It may develop in some patients with relapsing–remitting disease. The disease course continues to worsen with or without periods of remission or leveling off of symptom severity (plateaus). For many patients, treatment with disease-modifying agents helps delay such progression.
3. *Primary Progressive MS (PPMS):* It affects approximately 10% of MS patients. Symptoms worsen gradually from the beginning. There are no relapses or remis-

Table 1 Revised McDonald criteria for the diagnosis of multiple sclerosis

Clinical presentation	Additional data needed for diagnosis
≥2 clinical attacks and objective evidence of ≥2 lesions	None
≥2 clinical attacks and objective evidence of 1 lesion	DIS: An additional attack implicating a different CNS site OR by MRI[a]
1 clinical attack and objective clinical evidence of ≥2 lesions	DIT: An additional clinical attack OR by MRI[b] OR CSF-specific oligoclonal bands
1 clinical attack and objective evidence of 1 lesion	DIS: An additional clinical attack implicating a different CNS site OR by MRI[a] OR DIT: An additional clinical attack OR by MRI[b] OR CSF-specific oligoclonal bands

Adapted from Thompson et al. [32]

CNS central nervous system, *CSF* cerebrospinal fluid, *DIS* disseminated in space, *DIT* disseminated in time, *MRI* magnetic resonance imaging

[a]DIS by MRI: new lesions on follow-up imaging or both gadolinium-enhancing and non-enhancing lesions on single MRI

[b]DIS by MRI: ≥1 symptomatic or asymptomatic lesion in ≥2 areas including cortical/juxtacortical, periventricular, infratentorial, or spinal

sions, but there may be occasional plateaus. This form of MS shows a poor or no response to the drugs typically used to treat the disease.

4. *Progressive-Relapsing MS:* It is a rare form, affecting fewer than 5% of patients. It is progressive from the onset, with intermittent flare-ups of worsening symptoms along the way. There are no periods of remission.

Other rare phenotypes are the clinically isolated syndrome (CIS) and the radiologically isolated syndrome (RIS). CIS is defined as the first clinical manifestation of a demyelinating inflammatory disease, which could be MS, but still does not meet the diagnostic criteria of temporal dissemination. More complex is RIS, which is defined as the occasional finding, during an imaging examination performed for another purpose, of a finding suggestive of demyelination on an inflammatory basis in the absence of signs or symptoms of any kind [34]. RIS has never been considered a subtype of MS since it does not meet the clinical criteria for diagnosis. However, diagnostic suspicion can reasonably arise when the lesions found have morphology and localization strongly suggestive of disease.

Therapy

Currently, there is no cure that can achieve a complete recovery for MS.
Clinical management should take into account three different aims:

- To treat acute exacerbations.
- To decrease the number and severity of relapses, to decrease progression, and to prevent/minimize neuronal damage (disease-modifying therapies, DMTs).
- To prevent and/or treat complications due to MS and to preserve quality of life (QoL) (symptomatic treatment).

Treatment of acute relapses is based on the use of high-dose corticosteroids (methylprednisolone 1 g/day IV from 3 to 5 days). This treatment has few side effects and is effective in promoting the recovery of neurological deficits if promptly initiated. If the treatment with glucocorticoids does not have the expected efficacy, plasmapheresis can be used (off-label), the benefits of which would derive from the elimination of humoral factors and pathogenic plasma factors such as antibodies, complement factors, and cytokines.

In the last years, due to a greater understanding of MS physiopathology, the therapeutic scenario of DMT has changed quite radically, impacting disease severity [35] (Table 2).

DMTs are able to reduce the frequency and severity of relapses and consequently long-term disability. There are currently several drugs approved by the Food and Drug Administration (FDA):

- Injective therapies (interferons or glatiramer acetate) for RRMS patient with mild/moderate disease activity.
- Infusion therapies (*natalizumab*, *ocrelizumab*, and *alemtuzumab*) for patients with more active disease or aggressive form.

Table 2 MS treatment

Generic name/brand name	Recommended dose	Indication
Injectable drugs		
Interferon beta-1b/Betaseron or Extavia	250 mcg SC every other day	RR MS (including CIS)
Interferon beta-1a/AVONEX	30 mcg IM once weekly	RR MS (including CIS)
Interferon beta-1a/Rebif	22–44 mcg SC TIW	RR MS
Interferon beta-1b/Extavia	250 mcg SC every other day	RR MS (including CIS)
Peg-INF beta-1b/PLEGRIDY	125 mcg SC every other day	RR MS
Glatiramer acetate/Copaxone or Copemyl	20 mg SC once daily 40 mg SC TIW	RR MS
Orally administered drugs		
Fingolimod/Gilenya	0.5 mg once	RR MS
Dimethyl fumarate/TECFIDERA	120 mg BID for 1 week; then 240 mg BID	RR MS
Teriflunomide/AUBAGIO	7 mg or 14 mg once daily	RR MS
Cladribine/Mavenclad	3.5 mg/kg body weight over 2 years, administered as 1 treatment course of 1.75 mg/kg per year. Each treatment course consists of 2 treatment weeks, one at the beginning of the first month and one at the beginning of the second month of the respective treatment year	RR MS
Siponimod/MAYZENT	2 mg once	RR and SPMS
Injectable drugs		
Natalizumab/TYSABRI	300 mg IV infusion every 4 weeks	RR MS
Alemtuzumab/Lemtrada	First year: 12 mg IV infusion on 5 consecutive days Second year: 12 mg IV infusion for 3 consecutive days	RR MS in patients with poor response to ≥ 2 previous DMTs
Ocrelizumab/OCREVUS	Start dose: 300 mg IV infusion, followed by a second 300 mg IV infusion 2 weeks latersubsequent dose: 600 mg IV infusion every 6 months	RR or PP MS

BID twice daily, *CIS* clinically isolated syndrome, *MT* disease-modifying therapy, *IM* intramuscular, *IV* intravenous, *MS* multiple sclerosis, *SC* subcutaneous, *TIW* three times weekly

- Oral therapies for mild–moderate MS forms (dimethyl fumarate and teriflunomide) and for subjects with more aggressive forms (fingolimod, siponimod, and cladribine).

The choice of a specific agent should be individualized considering disease activity, comorbidities, risk factors, and patient preferences.

Considering non-pharmacological treatment, physical therapy and occupational therapy have been shown useful to decrease complications that arise from fatigue, weakness, and spasticity [36, 37]. Several studies have demonstrated that exercise has many positive benefits in MS patients including improved quality of life and sense of well-being and decreased depression [38, 39].

Various approaches to cognitive rehabilitation have been attempted in MS subjects using both a traditional rehabilitation program performed by speech therapists and psychologists [40] and a computerized program of rehabilitation [41]. This system is more interactive and seems to seriously help patients in the rehabilitation process [41, 42].

Sexuality and Quality of Life

Patients with multiple sclerosis (MS) not only suffer from the consequences of acute attacks of the disease and its progression but also from residual symptoms associated with lesions in different areas of the brain and spinal cord. These patients can develop a wide range of problems including depression, tremors, sensory disturbances, visual disturbances, cognitive impairments, and depression. Sexual dysfunction (DS) is also one of the destructive manifestations of the disease that negatively affects the quality of life, mood regulation, and interpersonal relationships; unfortunately, DS is often underreported. The prevalence of DS in MS patients is substantial, with reported rates modified from 50% to 73% in male patients and 45% to 70% in female patients [43–45].

Notably, the study by McCabe et al. [45] assessed the impact of symptom exacerbation among men and women with multiple sclerosis (MS) on sexuality and relationship satisfaction. A total of 321 individuals with MS (120 men, M age = 48.10 years; 201 women, M age = 45.78 years) and 239 individuals in the general population (79 men, M age = 53.93 years; 160 women, M age = 45.89 years) completed measures of relationship satisfaction and sexuality and then completed them again 18 months later. Results showed that both men and women with MS reported significantly higher levels of sexual dysfunction than the general population. Women in all groups reported significantly higher levels of sexual dysfunction but also higher levels of sexual activity than men in each time period. They also reported significantly higher levels of sexual satisfaction at the 18-month follow-up. These results showed that men and women respond similarly to MS and that MS patients do not necessarily experience lower levels of sexual interaction or relationship quality when they suffer an increase in their physical symptoms.

In addition, a study by Miller et al. [46] conducted at the Multiple Sclerosis Center, Carmel Medical Center, Technion–Israel Institute of Technology, Haifa, Israel, assessed the HRQOL of 215 outpatients with MS in their clinic using the MSQOL-54 and Fatigue Severity Scale (FSS) and that of 172 healthy controls using the SF-36 (a subset of the MSQOL-54). They then compared QOLs among MS subgroups defined by disability, gender, and occupation and calculated linear and nonlinear relationships between the level of disability as measured by the Expanded Disability Status Scale (EDSS) and MSQOL-54 dimensions.

The result was that the QOL of MS patients measured by SF-36 is lower than that of controls, especially with regard to the physical aspects of the disease. The relationship between physical disability, as measured by EDSS, and all 14 MSQOL-54 and FSS dimensions appeared negative. Women would appear to be better able to "cope psychologically" with the debilitating aspects of MS.

In general, bladder, bowel, and sexual dysfunction are often neglected symptoms in patients with multiple sclerosis (MS) and may be associated with lower health-related quality of life (HRQoL). The objective of the study by Vitkova et al. [47] was to explore the association of bladder, bowel, and sexual dysfunction with HRQoL in patients with MS stratified by disease duration ($\leq$5 and >5 years) and controlled for clinical and socio-demographic variables.

The study included 223 MS patients (mean age 38.9 $\pm$ 10.8 years, 67% female, mean EDSS 3.0 $\pm$ 1.5) who completed the Short-Form-36 Health Survey, the Bladder Control Scale, and the Bowel Control Scale. The Physical Component Summary (PCS) and the Mental Component Summary (MCS) of the SF36 were also used as dependent variables. It was found that bladder and sexual dysfunction were associated with lower HRQoL in MS patients even when MS had been diagnosed for a relatively short time.

The Bladder, Urological Disease, and Sexual Dysfunction

Genitourinary dysfunction is also common in women with multiple sclerosis (MS), but few studies have evaluated the association between bladder and sexual dysfunction in these patients. Borello-France et al. [48] recruited 133 women with MS who completed questionnaires regarding general health status, bladder function, and sexual function. Results: 61% of the sample indicated that they had a problem with bladder control and 47% that their neurological problems interfered with their sex life. Over 70% of the sample reported becoming aroused and experiencing orgasm during sexual activity. Lack of a sexual partner and indication of bothersome neurological problems were the best predictors of sexual dysfunction. There was one unexpected result: Incontinent patients reported higher levels of orgasm than non-incontinent women.

A study by Borello-Francia et al. [48] recruited 133 women with MS who completed questionnaires regarding general health status, bladder function, and sexual function. Results: 61% of the sample indicated that they had a problem with bladder control. 47% that their neurological problems interfered with their sex life. Over 70% of the sample reported becoming aroused and experiencing orgasm during sexual activity. Lack of a sexual partner and indication of bothersome neurological problems were the best predictors of sexual dysfunction. There was one unexpected result: Incontinent patients reported higher levels of orgasm than non-incontinent women.

An additional finding emerged from the research of Lew-Starowicz et al. [49] studying differences and similarities in male and female sexual response in a sample of 204 patients with MS. The questionnaires used included the International Index of Erectile Function, the Female Sexual Function Questionnaire, the Quality of Sexual Life Questionnaire, the Beck Depression Inventory, and the Expanded Disability Status Scale.

It was found that disease course and duration did not predict patients' SF. Negative correlations were found for brainstem symptoms with orgasmic function and overall satisfaction in men and between cognitive functioning and the partner domain in women sufferers compared with their partners.

Interestingly, brainstem symptoms were proponents of arousal in women. More than half (52.1%) of patients reported depression. Mood disorders and depression negatively affected desire, erectile function, and overall satisfaction with sex life in men and with orgasm and sexual pleasure in women.

The main gender difference appeared to be decreased desire on SQoL in women with no such correlation in men. The negative evaluation of the relationship with the partner significantly influenced the domains of SF and SQoL in women and desire in men with MS.

How do partners of MS patients respond? Rosen's [50] study started from clinical experience: Patients with MS reported female sexual interest/excitement disorder (FSIAD) as well as depression and lower sexual and relationship satisfaction than healthy control subjects. Ninety-seven women and their partners ($n = 97$) and 108 control couples were recruited. Both groups completed questionnaires on sexual desire, sexual distress, sexual function, sexual satisfaction, sexual communication, relationship satisfaction, depression, and anxiety.

Partners of patients with MS and FSIAD reported sexual dysfunction (erectile dysfunction, premature ejaculation), hypoactive desire, and increased sexual distress [51].

That is not all. In these chronic diseases, partner relationships and affectivity can also be therapeutic or iatrogenic tools. In this sense, O'Connor et al. [52] studied the impact of neurological disease on marital relationship satisfaction.

Participants included 423 patients and 335 caregivers with motor neuron disease (MND), Huntington's disease (HD), Parkinson's disease, and multiple sclerosis (MS).

Results showed that patients and caregivers with MH had significantly lower levels of relationship satisfaction and sex life satisfaction than the other three disease groups. In addition, patients with MH indicated a significantly higher level of relational satisfaction than their caregivers. For patients with MS and MND, social support fueled relationship satisfaction, whereas for patients with Parkinson's disease, social support and sex life satisfaction fueled marital relationship satisfaction.

Conclusion

Living with a multiple sclerosis (MS) patient challenges your relationship and the role of your partner. To this end, Relationship Matters (RM) is a relationship enrichment program that integrates information and resources from the National Multiple Sclerosis Society with marriage counseling. The neurologist and the psychosexologist should interact to improve communication within the couple. The MS patient is of course the focus of attention in the course of treatment and in overcoming consequent dysfunction. However, the partner is alone and the medical culture often overestimates the psychological and relational capacity. Often, the moments of crisis of the partner are also a cue to understanding feelings of inadequacy, failure, and anger. Supporting the couple and individuals is often a condition for increasing therapeutic compliance of the patient and complicity between the two [53].

References

1. Wu GF, Alvarez E. The immunopathophysiology of multiple sclerosis. Neurol Clin. 2011;29(2):257–78.
2. Multiple Sclerosis International Federation. What is MS? 2019. https://www.msif.org/about-ms/what-is-ms/.
3. Koch-Henriksen N, Sørensen PS. The changing demographic pattern of multiple sclerosis epidemiology. Lancet Neurol. 2010;9(5):520–32.
4. Gajofatto A, Stefani A, Turatti M. Prevalence of multiple sclerosis in Verona, Italy: an epidemiological and genetic study. Eur J Neurol. 2013;20(4):697–703.
5. Pierrot-Deseilligny C, Souberbielle JC. Vitamin D and multiple sclerosis: an update. Mult Scler Relat Disord. 2017 May;14:35–45.
6. Zhang P, Wang R, Li Z, Wang Y, Gao C, Lv X, Song Y, Li B. The risk of smoking on multiple sclerosis: a meta-analysis based on 20,626 cases from case-control and cohort studies. PeerJ. 2016;15(4):e1797.
7. Atlas of MS. Mapping multiple sclerosis around the world. London: Multiple Sclerosis International Federation; 2013. Available at: http://www.msif.org/about-ms/publications-and-resources.
8. Battaglia MA, Bezzini D. Estimated prevalence of multiple sclerosis in Italy in 2015. Neurol Sci. 2017;38(3):473–9.
9. Banwell B, Ghezzi A, Bar-Or A, Mikaeloff Y, Tardieu M. Multiple sclerosis in children: clinical diagnosis, therapeutic strategies, and future directions. Lancet Neurol. 2007;6(10):887–902.
10. Ahlgren C, Oden A, Lycke J. High nationwide prevalence of multiple sclerosis in Sweden. Mult Scler. 2011;17:901–8.
11. Compston A, Coles A. Multiple sclerosis. Lancet. 2002;359:1221–123.
12. Goodin DS. The genetic basis of multiple sclerosis: a model for MS susceptibility. BMC Neurol. 2010;10:101.
13. Dyment DA, Ebers GC, Sadovnick AD. Genetics of multiple sclerosis. Lancet Neurol. 2004;3:104–10.
14. Ristori G, Cannoni S, Stazi MA, et al. Multiple sclerosis in twins from continental Italy and Sardinia: a nationwide study. Ann Neurol. 2006;59(1):27–34.
15. Compston DA, Batchelor JR, McMonald WI. B-lymphocyte alloantigens associated with multiple sclerosis. Lancet. 1976;308:1261–5.

16. Terasaki PI, Park MS, Olpez G, Ting A. Multiple sclerosis and high incidence of a B lymphocyte antigen. Science. 1976;193:1245–7.
17. Olerup O, Hillert J. HLA class I-associated genetic susceptibility in multiple sclerosis: a critical evaluation. Tissue Antigens. 1991;38:1–15.
18. International Multiple Sclerosis Genetics Consortium. Multiple sclerosis genomic map implicates peripheral immune cells and microglia in susceptibility. Science. 2019;365(6460):eaav7188.
19. Engdahl E, Gustafsson R, Huang J, et al. Increased serological response against human herpesvirus 6a is associated with risk for multiple sclerosis. Front Immunol. 2019;10:2715.
20. Ascherio A, Munger KL. Epstein-Barr virus infection and multiple sclerosis: a review. J Neuroimmune Pharmacol. 2010;5(3):271–7.
21. Ascherio A, Munger KL. Environmental risk factors for multiple sclerosis. Part the role of infection. Ann Neurol. 2007;61(4):288–99.
22. Wingerchuk DM. Environmental factors in multiple sclerosis: Epstein-Barr virus, vitamin D, and cigarette smoking. Mt Sinai J Med. 2011;78(2):221–30.
23. Serafini B, Rosicarelli B, Franciotta D, et al. Dysregulated Epstein-Barr virus infection in the multiple sclerosis brain. J Exp Med. 2007;204:2899–912.
24. Mechelli R, Manzari C, Policano C, et al. Epstein-Barr virus genetic variants are associated with multiple sclerosis. Neurology. 2015;84:1362–8.
25. Ascherio A. Environmental factors in multiple sclerosis. Expert Rev Neurother. 2013;13(12 Suppl):3–9.
26. Antico A, Tampoia M, Tozzoli R, Bizzaro N. Can supplementation with vitamin D reduce the risk or modify the course of autoimmune diseases? A systematic review of the literature. Autoimmun Rev. 2012;12:127–36.
27. Rosso M, Chitnis T. Association between cigarette smoking and multiple sclerosis: a review. JAMA Neurol. 2019;77:245.
28. Munger KL, Bentzen J, Laursen B, et al. Childhood body mass index and multiple sclerosis risk: a long-term cohort study. Mult Scler. 2013;19:1323–9.
29. Olsson T, Barcellos LF, Alfredsson L. Interactions between genetic, lifestyle and environmental risk factors for multiple sclerosis. Nat Rev Neurol. 2017;13:25–36.
30. Bordi I, Ricigliano VA, Umeton R, et al. Noise in multiple sclerosis: unwanted and necessary. Ann Clin Transl Neurol. 2014;1(7):502–11.
31. Calabrese M, Gasperini C, Tortorella C, et al. "Better explanations" in multiple sclerosis diagnostic workup: a 3-year longitudinal study. Neurology. 2019;92:e2527.
32. Thompson AJ, Banwell BL, Barkhof F, et al. Diagnosis of multiple sclerosis: 2017 revisions of the McDonald criteria. Lancet Neurol. 2018;17(2):162–73.
33. Lublin FD, Reingold SC, Cohen JA, et al. Defining the clinical course of multiple sclerosis: the 2013 revisions. Neurology. 2014;83:278–86.
34. Lebrun C, Bensa C, Debouverie M, et al. Association between clinical conversion to multiple sclerosis in radiologically isolated syndrome and magnetic resonance imaging, cerebrospinal fluid, and visual evoked potential: follow-up of 70 patients. Arch Neurol. 2009;66:841–6.
35. Tintorè M, Vidal-Jordana A, Sastre-Garriga J. Treatment of multiple sclerosis - success from bench to bedside. Nat Rev Neurol. 2019;15(1):53–8.
36. Buzaid A, Dodge MP, Handmacher L, Kiltz PJ. Activities of daily living: evaluation and treatment in persons with multiple sclerosis. Phys Med Rehabil Clin N Am. 2013;24:629–38.
37. Motl RW, Sandroff BM, Kwakkel G, et al. Exercise in patients with multiple sclerosis. Lancet Neurol. 2017;16:848–56.
38. Woldańska-Okońska M. Rehabilitation in multiple sclerosis. Adv Clin Exp Med. 2017;26:709–15.
39. Amatya B, Khan F, Galea M. Rehabilitation for people with multiple sclerosis: an overview of Cochrane reviews. Cochrane Database Syst Rev. 2019;1:CD012732.
40. Goverover Y, Chiaravalloti ND, O'Brien AR, DeLuca J. Evidenced-based cognitive rehabilitation for persons with multiple sclerosis: an updated review of the literature from 2007 to 2016. Arch Phys Med Rehabil. 2018;99:390–407.

41. Dana A, Rafiee S, Gholami A. Motor reaction time and accuracy in patients with multiple sclerosis: effects of an active computerized training program. Neurol Sci. 2019;40:1849–54.
42. Harand C, Daniel F, Mondou A, Chevanne D, Creveuil C, Defer G. Neuropsychological management of multiple sclerosis: evaluation of a supervised and customized cognitive rehabilitation program for self-used at home (SEPIA): protocol for a randomized controlled trial. Trials. 2019;20:614.
43. Zorzon M, Zivadinov R, Bosco A, et al. Sexual dysfunction in multiple sclerosis: a case-control study. I. Attendance and comparison of groups. Mult Scler. 1999;5:418–27.
44. Demirkiran M, Sarica Y, Uguz S, et al. Multiple sclerosis patients with and without sexual dysfunction: are there differences? Mult Scler. 2006;12:209–14.
45. McCabe MP. Exacerbation of symptoms among people with multiple sclerosis: impact on sexuality and relationships over time. Arch Sex Behav. 2004;33:593–601.
46. Miller A, et al. Health-related quality of life in multiple sclerosis: the impact of disability, gender and employment status. What Life Ris. 2006;15(2):259–71. https://doi.org/10.1007/s11136-005-0891-6.
47. Vitkova M. Health-related quality of life in multiple sclerosis patients with bladder, bowel and sexual dysfunction. Disabil Rehabil. 2014;36(12):987–92. https://doi.org/10.3109/0963828 8.2013.825332.
48. Borello-France D, Leng W, O'Leary M, Xavier M, Erickson J, Chancellor MB, et al. Bladder and sexual function in women with multiple sclerosis. Mult Scler. 2004;10(4):455–61. https://doi.org/10.1191/1352458504ms1060oa.
49. Lew-Starowicz M, et al. Correlations of sexual function in male and female patients with multiple sclerosis. Sex Med. 2014;11(9):2172–80. https://doi.org/10.1111/jsm.12622.
50. Rosen NO, et al. Partners also experience the consequences: a comparison of sexual, relational and psychological adjustment of women with sexual interest/arousal disorder and their partners to control couples. Sex Med. 2019;16(1):83–95. https://doi.org/10.1016/j.jsxm.2018.10.018.
51. Rosen NO, Dubé JP, Corsini-Munt S, et al. Partners also experience the consequences: a confrontation between the sexual, relational and psychological adjustment of women with sexual interest/arousal disorder and their partners to control couples. J Sex Med. 2019;16:83–95.
52. O'Connor EJ, McCabe MP, Firth L. The impact of neurological disease on marital relationships. J Sex Marital Ther. 2008;34(2):115–32. https://doi.org/10.1080/00926230701636189.
53. Tompkins SA, Roeder JA, Thomas JJ, Koch KK. Effectiveness of a relationship enrichment program for couples living with multiple sclerosis. Int J MS Care. 2013;15(1):27–34. https://doi.org/10.7224/1537-2073.2012-002. PMID: 24453760; PMCID: PMC3883030.

Alzheimer's Disease

Lorenzo Pinessi and Elena Vittoria Longhi

Alzheimer's disease is a dramatic pathological occurrence for the patient, his family, caregivers and doctors.

It is worsening, practically unstoppable, and it is poorly responsive to the drugs available today; it seriously worsens the quality of life and reduces its duration.

It is not the only form of dementia, but the most common (about 40–50% of all dementias). Relatively infrequent (<1%) in 60-year-olds, it shows an exponential increase with age, reaching 25–30% in elderly subjects over 85 years old. The female sex is most affected and constitutes the greatest risk factor with age. Other risk factors are family history, head injuries, low folate and vitamin B12 levels, hyperhomocysteinaemia, arterial hypertension, diabetes and dyslipidaemia. Good education, physical and mental activity, moderate wine consumption and abundant quantities of fish in the diet are protective factors.

Diagnosis

Early clinical and neuroradiological diagnosis is important for a correct therapeutic approach, especially useful in the initial stages of the disease in order to slow down its progression. In the late pre-terminal stages, Alzheimer's disease is not clinically distinguishable from other dementias.

Often, these are mixed forms: Alzheimer's disease (AD) associated with vascular dementia (VD) or frontotemporal dementia (FTD).

L. Pinessi (✉)
Neurological Clinic and Specialization School in Neurology, University of Turin, Turin, Italy

Department of Neuroscience and Mental Health, Molinette-Città della Salute, Turin, Italy
e-mail: lorenzo.pinessi@unito.it

E. V. Longhi
Department of Sexual Medical Center, San Raffaele Hospital, Milano, Italy

© Springer Nature Switzerland AG 2023
E. V. Longhi (ed.), *Managing Psychosexual Consequences in Chronic Diseases*,
https://doi.org/10.1007/978-3-031-31307-3_24

Clinically, these three important and frequent forms of dementia are generally well differentiated in their initial stages, as already mentioned.

Brain magnetic resonance imaging (MRI) and the measurement of CSF biomarkers (tau protein, phospho-tau and beta-amyloid) are an important diagnostic aid.

The neurological clinical characteristics of the appearance of the first symptoms, their severity and course, the presence of vascular risk factors, any familiarity, the patient's behaviour (minimizes or does not memory deficits and behavioural alterations), the presence of depressive psychiatric pathology (depressive pseudo-dementia), etc., almost always allow us, together with the anamnesis, to make a diagnosis of correct probability.

With the progressive increase in the population in old age due to the increase in life expectancy, Alzheimer's disease (and other forms of dementia) constitutes one of the main social and health problems today and in the future.

The chances of presenting this pathology increase, as mentioned, with the passing of the years (70–80 years, late-onset form), even if there are cases of onset at an earlier age (50–60 years, early-onset form). We have to remember that the age of the first patient with dementia described by Alois Alzheimer was 51 years (Frau Auguste). Alzheimer and Italian Gaetano Perusini neuropathologists first described (1906, 1910) both the symptomatological characteristics and the neuropathological alterations present in the brain. Today, we know that several alterations are associated with Alzheimer's disease: cerebral-cortical atrophy, amyloid senile plaques (however present in smaller numbers in senile brains), which accumulate diffusely outside the neurons, altering their functioning, being made up of extracellular fibrils of the Aβ42 protein and neurofibrillary tangles made up of intracellular aggregates of abnormal forms of the tau protein.

Treatment

The brain areas most affected by the degenerative process are the hippocampus, the amygdala, the cingulate cortex, the frontal lobes and the cortical associative area.

Since the 1970s, studies in neurochemistry, neuropharmacology, neurogenetics and neuroimaging have greatly improved and deepened our knowledge on the pathogenesis, diagnostics and therapy of Alzheimer's disease.

An "enormous" number of scientific publications on this subject have been produced and continued to be produced.

In 1976, a selective loss of cholinergic neurons in the brain was highlighted, which led to a reduction in cholinergic transmission with the consequent appearance of cognitive and memory disorders typical of the disease. This discovery allows in fact the only therapeutic possibility used today, which consists precisely in enhancing the cholinergic transmission and increasing the availability of acetylcholine (ACh) in the synaptic space due to the effect of the inhibitory drugs of the enzyme acetylcholinesterase (AChEIs).

However, the effectiveness of these drugs (donepezil, rivastigmine and galantamine) is modest, although therapy started early is always recommended in order to obtain some results. They are generally well tolerated; undesirable side effects are represented by gastrointestinal and dysautonomic disorders; contraindications to use are cardiological (complete block of the left branch, sinus node disease) and pneumological (bronchial asthma).

Subsequently, the involvement of other neurotransmitters such as dopamine and serotonin was shown as glutamic acid. In particular, the excitotoxic glutamatergic dysregulation seems to be inhibited by memantine, with the indication for the latter in the moderate–severe phases of AD.

Clinically, Alzheimer's disease begins in a subtle and insidious way, often scotomized or denied by the patient. These are initial mnesic and modest cognitive deficits (mild cognitive impairment, MCI) and mild behavioural and personality alterations.

Short-term memory is impaired with remote and autobiographical memory retention for at least a few years.

There are temporal–spatial abnormalities and disorientation, and praxis disorders that were modest at first and then worsened. Autonomous life and speech are progressively reduced, as well as understanding, writing, reading and attention.

Delusions and hallucinations (atypical neuroleptics are useful), anxiety and depression, especially in the initial stages of the disease (SSRI drugs are useful) and alterations in the sleep-wake rhythm (night is mistaken for day and vice versa).

Finally, the patient becomes completely dependent on washing, dressing, eating, etc. The clinical picture worsens within a few years until the exitus (after 8–10 years from onset).

In addition to the aforementioned pharmacological interventions, unfortunately still not decisive today, there are some types of non-pharmacological interventions, summarized here as follows:

- Physical activity and motor rehabilitation. Rehabilitation and cognitive stimulation.
- Occupational therapy with interventions on daily activities.
- Information and psychological support aimed in particular at caregivers (relatives and assistance staff, carers).
- Additional complementary interventions such as music therapy and aroma therapy [1–11].

Sexuality and Quality of Life

Hartmans et al. [12] reviewed the clinical studies published to date on the sexuality of patients diagnosed with Alzheimer's disease. In particular, with regard to the association between sexual behaviour and cognitive functioning the results appeared discordant.

Derouesné et al. [13] showed that changes in sexual behaviour were not related to general cognitive functioning and duration of dementia, but to the severity of behavioural changes and limitations in daily activities perceived by the spouse. Ballard et al. [14] on the other hand found a trend towards an association between better general cognitive functioning and an ongoing sexual relationship.

Abnormal sexual behaviour such as hypersexuality is often reported by caregivers. However, this behaviour seems rare in patients with dementia [15]. One study compared sexual changes in patients with Alzheimer's disease and those with frontotemporal dementia (FTD) and found the same frequency of increased sexual desire in both conditions (8%) [16]. Other research on caregiver perceptions of the influence of dementia on sexuality in marriage showed that increased demand for sex was found in 5% of couples [17]. Reported inappropriate sexual behaviours are often the result of a failure to take into account spouses' feelings and background sexual education (inhibited, influenced by religion, family backgrounds, etc.).

A single study on dementia on erectile functioning showed impaired cognitive sequencing, forgetfulness and decline in decision-making ability to negatively influence sexual behaviour [18]. This negative influence on sexual behaviour could be explained by reduced frontal lobe activity.

Miller et al. [19] then evaluated weight gain, cravings for sweets/carbohydrates, hyposexuality and compulsions in frontal lobe dementia (FLD) compared to Alzheimer's disease (AD). FLD is progressive dementia with a high rate of misdiagnosis, and therefore, better diagnostic criteria are needed for FLD. Fourteen patients who met the research criteria for AD were compared with 14 with suspected FLD.

Hypersexuality

Caregivers were questioned about weight gain, sweet or carbohydrate preference, sexual desire and patient compulsions. Differences were compared with Fisher's exact test.

Comparative Results Showed

FLD versus AD: weight gain in patients with FLD was 64% (AD 7%), carbohydrate craving was 79% (versus 0%) and compulsive behaviour was 64% (versus 14%). In FLD, the first symptoms were often changes in diet or hyposexuality. Compulsions were more bizarre and severely disabling in FLD than in AD. Changes in diet, hyposexuality and disabling compulsions were described as prominent early symptoms in FLD but not in AD.

Craving for Sweets

More recently, the study by De Giorgi et al. [20] has shown that in elderly patients with dementia, a combination of cognitive impairment, impaired judgement and personality changes is likely to contribute to changes in sexual attitude and behaviour. The most common alteration reported in people with dementia is apathy and indifference to sex [21]. However, inappropriate sexual behaviour (ISB), also known as sexually disinhibited behaviour or hypersexuality, has been consistently described in most dementia syndromes.

What Do Scholars Mean by ISB?

The concept of ISB has developed over time, and one of the latest definitions appears in the study by De Medeiros et al. [22]: "ISB is specific sexual behavior character-ized by an apparent loss of control or a search for intimacy that is out of place in the social context or directed toward the wrong goal; the behavior may not be sexual in its form, but rather in its suggestion".

That is, ISB can be divided into conventional and nonparaphilic (sexual interest arises within socially and culturally accepted boundaries), versus unconventional and paraphilic (sexual arousal that deviates, involving, for example, children, animals and non-consenting persons) [23].

The study by Lyketsos et al. [24] shows that the overall prevalence of behavioural and psychiatric symptoms of dementia is 50–80%; therefore, most people with dementia may manifest some of these symptoms. Reportedly, the occurrence of ISB in individuals with dementia ranges from 7% to 25%, with a higher prevalence in residents of skilled nursing facilities and in patients with more severe cognitive impairment. [25] Physical manifestations appear to be more frequent in males, [26] whereas in women they appear to be more verbal.

In the light of all this, there is no doubt that ISB can be a threat to patients' mental and physical health; for example, repeated masturbation can cause genital trauma [27] or cause anxiety, distress and embarrassment in caregivers, often disrupting the continuity of care at home and leading to home confinement or institutionalization. [28].

Conclusion

The treatment of Alzheimer's disease requires a systemic approach. It is not only the patient who suffers from the progression of the disease but the whole family: partners and children. The aspect of care and protection of the person is only the beginning of a daily relationship where it is difficult to decipher the behaviour of the patient without giving an emotional (as well as clinical) meaning. Many partners feel overwhelmed by their partner's IBS, disowning the man they had always known before the disease. In this case, the psychosexologist can be a valuable translator of the feelings of both the caregiver and the patient. There is no doubt that clinicians should be interested in these sometimes neglected issues, given that they are consequent to the disease. In fact, each patient experiences the disease beyond the symptoms: sensitivity, character, personality and the life of the couple are additional filters to help understand the treatment and the individual.

References

1. Braak H, Braak E. Demonstration of amyloid deposits and neurofibrillary changes in the whole brain sections. Brain Pathol. 1991;1(3):213–6.
2. Gosche KM, et al. Hippocampal volume as an index of Alzheimer neuropathology findings from the nun study. Neurology. 2004;58:1476–82.
3. Snider BJ, et al. Cerebrospinal fluid biomarkers and rate of cognitive decline in very mild dementia of the Alzheimer type. Arch Neurol. 2009;66:638–45.
4. Deardorff WJ, et al. Behavioral and psychological symptoms in Alzheimer's dementia and vascular dementia. Handb Clin Neurol. 2019;165:5–32.
5. Loureiro JC, et al. Passive antiamyloid immunotherapy for Alzheimer's disease. Curr Opin Psychiatry. 2020;33:284–91.
6. Cummings J, et al. Alzheimer's disease drug development pipeline: 2020. Alzheimers Dement. 2020;6:1–29.
7. Hoenig MC, et al. Alzheimer's disease neuroimaging initiative. assessment of tau tangles and amyloid-β plaques among super agers using PET imaging. JAMA Netw Open. 2020;3:e2028337.
8. Iadecola C. Revisiting atherosclerosis and dementia. Nat Neurosci. 2020;23(6):691–2.
9. Breijyeh Z, et al. Comprehensive review on Alzheimer's disease: causes and treatment. Molecules. 2020;25:5789.
10. Yiannopoulou KG, et al. Current and future treatments in Alzheimer disease: an update. J Cent Nerv Syst Dis. 2020;12:1–12.
11. Cummings J. Drug development for psychotropic, cognitive-enhancing, and disease-modifying treatments for Alzheimer's disease. J Neuropsychiatry Clin Neurosci. 2021;33:3–13.
12. Hartmans C, Comijs H, Jonker C. Cognitive functioning and its influence on sexual behavior in normal aging and dementia. Int J Geriatr Psychiatry. 2014;29:441–6. https://doi.org/10.1002/gps.4025.
13. Derouesné C, Guigot J, Chermat V, et al. Changes in sexual behavior in Alzheimer's disease. Alz Dis Assoc Disord. 1996;10(2):86–92.
14. Ballard CG, Solis M, Gahir M, et al. Sexual intercourse in people with marital dementia. Int J Geriatr Psychiatry. 1997;12:447–51.
15. Burns A, Jacoby R, Levy R. Psychiatric phenomena in Alzheimer's disease. IV: behavioral disorders. Br J Psychiatry. 1990;157:86–94.
16. Miller BL, Darby AL, Swartz JR, et al. Dietary changes: sexual compulsions and behaviors in frontotemporal degeneration. Dementia. 1995;6:195–9.
17. Eloniemi-Sulkava U, Notkola IL, Hämäläinen K, et al. Perceptions of the spouse's caregiver on the influence of dementia on marriage. Int Psychogeriatr. 2002;14:47–58.
18. Davies HD, Zeiss AM, Shea EA, et al. Sessualità e intimità nei malati di Alzheimer e nei loro partner. Disabilità sessuale. 1998;16(3):193–203.

19. Miller BL, et al. Dietary changes, compulsions and sexual behavior in frontotemporal degeneration. Dement Geriatr Cogn Disord. 1995;6:195–9. https://doi.org/10.1159/000106946.
20. De Giorgi R, Series H. Treatment of inappropriate sexual behavior in dementia. Curr Treat Options Neurol. 2016;18:41. https://doi.org/10.1007/s11940-016-0425-2.
21. Tsai SJ, Hwang JP, Yang CH, Liu KM, Lirng JF. Inappropriate sexual behavior in dementia: a foreplay. Alzheimer's Disorder Assoc. 1999;13(1):60–2.
22. De Medeiros K, Rosenberg PB, Baker AS, Onyike CU. Comportamenti sessuali impropri negli anziani con demenza che vivono in strutture residenziali. Dement Geriatr Cogn Disord. 2008;26(4):370–7.
23. Kafka MP, Prentky R. A comparative study of non-paraphilic sexual addictions and paraphilias in men. J Clin Psychol. 1992;53(10):345–50.
24. Lyketsos CG, Lopez O, Jones B, Fitzpatrick AL, Breitner J, DeKosky S. Prevalence of neuropsychiatric symptoms in dementia and mild cognitive impairment: results from the cardiovascular health study. JAMA. 2002;288(12):1475–83.
25. Burns A, Jacoby R, Levy R. Psychiatric phenomena in Alzheimer's disease. IV: behavioral disorders. Brit. J Psychol. 1990;157:86–94.
26. Onishi J, Suzuki Y, Umegaki H, Endo H, Kawamura T, Imaizumi M, et al. Behavioral, psychological and physical symptoms in group homes for the elderly with dementia. Int Psicogeriatr. 2006;18(1):75–86.
27. Haddad PM, Benbow SM. Sexual problems associated with dementia: part 2. Etiology, evaluation and treatment. Int J Geriatr Psychopharmacol. 1993;8(8):631–7.
28. Wallace M, Safer M. Hypersexuality among older adults with cognitive problems. Geriatr Nurs. 2009;30(4):230–7.

Sexuality and Traumatic Brain Injury

Anna Mazzucchi, Alessandra Redolfi, and Elena Vittoria Longhi

Introduction

Traumatic brain injury (TBI) can lead to motor, cognitive and behavioural disorders that can affect psychological functioning not only for the patient [1, 2] but also for all families' members [3–5]. For this reason and its epidemiological incidence, TBI is recognized as an international public health problem and it is defined as a silent epidemic [6].

Deficits resulting from head injury can also invalidate the possibility of establishing and maintaining interpersonal relationships, including those related to the affective sexual dimension. It is known that sexuality is a basic need of the human being and part of one's personal identity. Sexuality influences thoughts and feelings, actions and interaction and, in sum, people's mental and physical health [7]. Despite this, in a study by Moreno and colleagues [8], 72% of patients with TBI (n = 38) declared they almost never talked about sexuality with a health professional. Patients express the need for greater openness in dealing with the topic of sexuality on the clinical and relational level. A recent clinical guideline for patients with moderate and severe brain injury recommends the need to promote discussions on sexuality by medical health personnel [9]: less than 0.01% of all TBI studies evaluate sexuality specifically [10].

To describe changes that can occur in patients' affective and sexual life following a traumatic brain injury, it is necessary to understand the aspects that commonly

A. Mazzucchi (✉)
Department for Acquired Brain Injury Rehabilitation, Don Carlo Gnocchi Foundation, Milan, Italy

A. Redolfi
Spalenza Rehabilitation Centre, Don Carlo Gnocchi Foundation, Rovato, Italy
e-mail: aredolfi@dongnocchi.it

E. V. Longhi
Department of Sexual Medical Center, San Raffaele Hospital, Milano, Italy

© Springer Nature Switzerland AG 2023
E. V. Longhi (ed.), *Managing Psychosexual Consequences in Chronic Diseases*,
https://doi.org/10.1007/978-3-031-31307-3_25

affect the different components of the correlated neurophysiological functions [11–13]. Primary effects are directly related to the damages or dysfunctions of the central nervous system produced by the trauma. These consequences may depend on the alterations of cortical and subcortical structures but also on the dysfunction of neurochemical system and the interference with hypothalamic and brainstem structures. Other effects are related to physical and neuropsychological changes that affect the expressions of sexual activity: i.e. the physical limitations to perform movements emblematic of lovemaking and/or the behavioural and cognitive involvement in sexuality manifestations. So, post-traumatic subjects could manifest a decrease in interest in sex activity, in sex drive, in sex appeal, in controlling impulses, in the quality of interactive behaviour with partner, etc. Lastly, other adverse effects could be consequence of psychosocial influences, such as changes in body image, loss of sexual identity, low self-confidence, depression and/or anxiety.

Studies involving TBI patients have shown the presence of sexual problems like decrease in sex drive [14–16], decrease in frequency of intercourse [15], erectile dysfunction [15, 17–20], low self-confidence [15, 16], declines in sex appeal [15] and deficits in the ability to form sexual images [16]. Ponsford and colleagues [21] asked a group of 208 moderate-to-severe TBI patients about the reason for changes in their sexual behaviour. TBI patients referred fatigue, decreased mobility, low confidence, diminished sex appeal and decreased ability to communicate, confirming how different effects of head trauma are actually interconnected. It is also well known that the significant changes occurring after a traumatic brain injury may also compromise a couple's relationship [22, 23], leading to a decrease in the display of affection and cohesion [24], reduced communication [25] and less relational satisfaction [24]. Bivona and colleagues [26] showed a reduction in desire and frequency of sexual activity in both TBI patients and partners and highlighted the possibility that these data reflect relational dysfunctions.

Neuroanatomical, Neurophysiological and Neurochemical Structures Correlated with Sexual Activity

From the neuroanatomical point of view, sexual behaviour is regulated in the brain by several cortical areas, such as the orbitofrontal and the prefrontal cortex, many subcortical structures, such as thalamus and the hypothalamus, amygdala, the caudate nucleus, the insula, the anterior cingulate cortex, several nuclei of the brainstem and by the spinal cord. So, the finely adjusting and acting of this multifaceted and flexible complex behaviour require the contribution and the appropriate interfaced and sequencing of many components [11, 12, 27–29]. From the neurophysiological point of view, the prefrontal cortex and the orbitofrontal cortex are involved in planning complex cognitive behaviours, personality expression, decision-making, behavioural adaptation and moderating correct social behaviour [29]. From the neurochemical point of view, several studies pointed out that dopamine is the main neurotransmitter that could generate sexual motivation, suggesting that the increase in dopamine levels would lead the behavioural shift towards hypersexuality and, on the contrary, the decrease in dopamine, like in consequence of traumatic brain injury, would induce hypo-sexuality. Also, serotonin, norepinephrine, acetylcholine, histamine and many endocrine factors would be integrated to guarantee the correct functioning of sexuality in all the interconnected mechanisms and components [27–29].

The Assessment of Sexuality After TBI

As functioning in one domain can affect functioning in other domains, literature underlines the importance of adopting a bio-psychosocial approach for the assessment of sexuality after a traumatic brain injury [30]. In a study involving professional who work with TBI's patients [31], only 24% of 267 clinicians declared to speak about sexuality issues with patients and partner as an aspect of their usual practice. The assessment of sexuality after TBI has not yet become a clinical practice, and probably also for this reason, the literature concerning specific tools for the assessment of sexuality is still limited. Among these, the first tools specific for the TBI's population were the Psychosexual Assessment Questionnaire (PAQ) [15], the Sexual Interest and Satisfaction Scale (SISS) [17] and the Sexual Adjustment Questionnaire (SAQ) [17]. These tools can only be administered to patients and not to partners, and limited psychometric information is available.

In 2003, Ponsford and colleagues have created the Sexual Questionnaire (SQ) [21] as an adaptation of the previous tools described above. It compares post-injury aspects of sexuality with pre-injury status on a five-point Likert scale and can be administered to males' and females' patient, singles and engaged. There are, however, some limits, such as it measures quantitative changes only and not qualitative changes, and it is only for patients and displays limited psychometric information. Recently, to overcome these psychometric limitations, Stolwyk and colleagues performed a factorial analysis of answers to the Sexual Questionnaire, administered to 865 TBI's patients [32]. Based on the analysis, items from the original SQ have been organized into subscales named Sexual Functioning, Relationship Quality and Self-Esteem and Mood subscales. The authors renamed this new toll Brain Injury Questionnaire of Sexuality (BISQ). The BISQ is actually the most validated measure of sexual functioning for TBI patient. However, the tool does not allow to deepen partners' appraisal about sexuality and to obtain information about the quality of the sentimental relationship, in terms of feeling, affection and complicity.

Verschuren's conceptual models of sexual health following chronic diseases [33] emphasize the importance not only of sexual functioning, but also of sexual well-being, that is the personal emotional experience and how it is evaluated in terms of one's personal life and relation with the partner. While studying sexual health in people with chronic disease, the author also underlines how it is essential to pay attention to the relationship with partner because it plays an important role in adaptation to the disease and to sexual life.

In line with this theoretical framework, our research group formed a new Italian questionnaire, named Brain Injury Sexual Relational Questionnaire (BISRQ), whose psychometric properties have been considered in a recent study (D'Amato et al., submitted, [34]). The questionnaire's structure allows evaluating sexual functioning, sexual well-being, sentimental life and appraisal of the impact of ABI on sexual and sentimental lives, for both patient and partners. Appraisal about sexuality for single patients is therefore possible, answering only questions in the patient section. The questionnaire was administered to 146 patients with severe acquired brain injury and 80 partners; the study was approved by the Ethics Committee of Don Carlo Gnocchi Foundation. For the purposes of this chapter, we report limited related findings. Partners obtain significantly lower scores on all subscales, except for the Sexual Importance Subscale. For example, 60% of patients reported satisfaction in relation to sexual life, differently from 35% of partners. Regardless of the different reasons that can explain the evaluations of partners and patients [34–39], the discrepancy that emerged leads us to the interpretation of a couple dynamic in which poor communication and poor internal sharing prevail. BISRQ scores allow the clinician to construct a representation of different perceptions of patients and partners about sexuality and could be used as a starting point to explore intimacy aspects and to take care also about that. During the research's data collection, we finally recruited 37 caregivers (77% of them parent of single patients; 23% other relatives) with the aim of investigating their opinions regarding the sexuality of single patients: 80% of them reported that sexuality played an important or very important role for the patient before the brain injury. Only 49% of caregivers declared the same importance for the patient after brain injury. Furthermore, half of the caregivers consider patients' sexual desire intensity as absent or low. Patients' parents seem not to know much about the sexual life of their relative and consider this topic a secondary aspect, in line with literature describing individuals with disabilities perceived as asexual [40].

International guidelines largely emphasize the need for the family's involvement in the patient's rehabilitation process [41, 42]. Family represents in fact a central nucleus of responsibility for the well-being, safety and coordination of patient care [43]. For this reason, and considering the multifactorial aetiology of sexuality difficult after TBI, it is necessary for clinicians to promote the deepening and treatment of this matter.

Treatment of Sexuality as an Interdisciplinary Intervention

Arango Lasprilla and colleagues [31] investigated the reasons why professionals who work with TBI patients do not talk about sexuality as a clinical practice: 43% of 324 professionals declare patients do not ask for information on this topic and 34% that patients do not report having problem related to sexuality. Cultural and personal variables can obstruct requesting help. As proposed by Moreno and colleagues [8], if rehabilitation team accepts the need for an interdisciplinary approach to sexuality and recognizes this topic as a fundamental role of a holistic intervention, then a collaborative approach can help to meet patient's needs. The authors suggested to use the PLISSIT model [44], largely used in the field of sexology since the 70 s. PLISSIT is an acronym to describe four levels of evaluation and intervention: Permission, Limited Information, Specific Suggestion and Therapeutic Intervention.

According to the author who proposed this model [44], people with sexual problems can solve them if they have permission to discuss sexuality, if they receive concrete, relevant and limited information on specific sexual issues and if they receive suggestions on ways to deal with sexual problems. The model provides the possibility of a counselling intervention gradual that allows clinicians to take care of the aspects of sexuality according to their own level of competence and attitude.

More recently, Taylor and Davis proposed the extended PLISSIT model [45], specific for addressing the sexual well-being of individuals with an acquired disability or chronic illness.

All team's members can play a role in addressing a different aspect of sexuality [8]; for example, if there are motor limitations, a physiotherapist may suggest compensation systems; if there are neurocognitive impairments, a neuropsychologist can provide adaptations; and if there are side effects of the drugs, a neurologist may decide to modify the therapy.

Therapeutic intervention level involved referral for specialist intervention, such as psychosexual therapy or relationship counselling. The literature does not identify evidence-based intervention models specific to brain injury population, which is characterized by a specific set of motors, cognitive and emotional disorders. Only recently, Backhaus and colleagues developed a new 16-week couple group intervention for individuals with brain injury [46, 47]. It is the first couple's therapy specifically created for people with a brain injury that was empirically investigated in a prospective study. Intervention's objectives are dyadic adjustment and communication; there is no form, however, dedicated specifically to sexuality.

Other treatments are proposed for couple intimacy, such as narrative therapy approach [48] or emotionally focused therapy [49]. This approach considers the couple as the focus of intervention, in line with the literature mentioned, which underlines the need for a bio-psychosocial approach to sexuality. However, there is a need to develop intervention models that take into account the complexity of the topic and that allow to help the rehabilitation team in the management of sexual difficulties.

In 2019, Moreno's research group [50] finally published a review reporting operational aspects of rehabilitation professionals' discussion of sexuality, providing guidance about prerequisites for discussing sexuality, tools supporting dialog, time to start and type of professional to engage. This review should be the first step towards the integration of sexuality as a necessary component in the rehabilitation of individuals with TBI, as it is for other aspects widely considered in the literature.

References

1. Carroll E, Coetzer R. Identity, grief and self-awareness after traumatic brain injury. Neuropsychol Rehabil [Internet]. 2011;21(3):289–305.
2. Malec JF, Brown AW, Moessner AM, Stump TE, Monahan P. A preliminary model for post-traumatic brain injury depression. Arch Phys Med Rehabil [Internet]. 2010;91(7):1087–97.
3. Tramonti F, Bonfiglio L, Bongiovanni P, Belviso C, Fanciullacci C, Rossi B, Chisari C, Carboncini MC. Caregiver burden and family functioning in different neurological diseases. Psychol Health Med [Internet]. 2019;24(1):27–34.
4. Whiffin CJ, Ellis-Hill C, Bailey C, Jarrett N, Hutchinson PJ. We are not the same people we used to be: an exploration of family biographical narratives and identity change following traumatic brain injury. Neuropsychol Rehabil [Internet]. 2019;29(8):1256–72.
5. Lond BJ, Williamson IR. Stuck in a loop of fear: a phenomenological exploration of careers' experiences supporting a spouse with acquired brain injury. Disabil Rehabil [Internet]. 2018;40(24):2907–15.
6. Zitnay GA. Lessons from national and international TBI societies and funds like NBIRTT. Acta Neurochir Suppl [Internet]. 2005;93:131.
7. Edwards WM, Coleman E. Defining sexual health: a descriptive overview. Arch Sex Behav [Internet]. 2004;33(3):189–95.
8. Moreno A, Gan C, Zasler N, McKerral M. Experiences, attitudes, and needs related to sexuality and service delivery in individuals with traumatic brain injury. NeuroRehabilitation [Internet]. 2015;37(1):99–116.
9. Truchon C, Kagan C, Bayley M, Swaine B, Lamontagne ME, Marshall S, Gargaro J. INESSS-ONF clinical practice guidelines for the rehabilitation of adults having sustained a moderate-to-severe TBI. Brain Injury [Internet]. 2017;31(6–7):741.
10. Turner D, Schöttle D, Krueger R, Briken P. Sexual behavior and its correlates after traumatic brain injury. Curr Opin Psychiatry [Internet]. 2015;28(2):180–7.
11. Mesulam MM. Behavioral neuroanatomy: large scale networks, association cortex, frontal syndromes, the limbic system, and hemispheric specialization. In: Mesulam MM, editor. Principles of behavioral and cognitive neurology. 2nd ed. New York: Oxford University Press; 2000. p. 1–120.
12. Baird AD, Wilson SJ, Bladin PF, Saling MM, Reutens DC. Neurological control of human sexual behaviour: insights from lesion studies. J Neurol Neurosurg Psychiatry [Internet]. 2007;78(10):1042–9.
13. Ahmad TG, Yeates G. Sex and sexuality after brain injury. Nottingham: Headway–The Brain Injury Association; 2017.
14. Sandel ME, Williams KS, Dellapietra L, Derogatis LR. Sexual functioning following traumatic brain injury. Brain Inj [Internet]. 1996;10(10):719–28.
15. Kreutzer JS, Zasler ND. Psychosexual consequences of traumatic brain injury: methodology and preliminary findings. Brain Inj [Internet]. 1989;3(2):177–86.
16. Simon FC, Ponsford J. The role of imagery in sexual arousal disturbances in the male traumatically brain injured individual. Brain Inj [Internet]. 1999;13(5):347–54.
17. Kreuter M, Dahllöf AG, Gudjonsson G, Sullivan M, Siösteen A. Sexual adjustment and its predictors after traumatic brain injury. Brain Inj [Internet]. 1998;12(5):349–68.
18. Moreno JA, Gan C, Zasler N. Neurosexuality a transdisciplinary approach to sexuality in neurorehabilitation. NeuroRehabil [Internet]. 2017;41(2):255–9.
19. Sander AM, Maestas KL, Pappadis MR, Sherer M, Hammond FM, Hanks R. NIDRR traumatic brain injury model systems module project on sexuality after TBI. Sexual functioning 1 year after traumatic brain injury: findings from a prospective traumatic brain injury model systems collaborative study. Arch Phys Med Rehabil [Internet]. 2012;93(8):1331–7.
20. Stolwyk RJ, Downing MG, Taffe J, Kreutzer JS, Zasler ND, Ponsford JL. Assessment of sexuality following traumatic brain injury: validation of the brain injury questionnaire of sexuality. J Head Trauma Rehabil [Internet]. 2013;28(3):164–70.

21. Ponsford J. Sexual changes associated with traumatic brain injury. Neuropsychol Rehabil [Internet]. 2003;13(1–2):275–89.
22. Godwin EE, Kreutzer JS, Arango-Lasprilla JC, Lehan TJ. Marriage after brain injury: review, analysis, and research recommendations. J Head Trauma Rehabil [Internet]. 2011;26(1):43–55.
23. Williams C, Wood RL. The impact of alexithymia on relationship quality and satisfaction following traumatic brain injury. J Head Trauma Rehabil [Internet]. 2013;28(5):E21–30.
24. Peters LC, Stambrook M, Moore AD, Zubek E, Dubo H, Blumenschein S. Differential effects of spinal cord injury and head injury on marital adjustment. Brain Inj [Internet]. 1992;6(5):461–7.
25. Ponsford J, Olver J, Ponsford M, Nelms R. Long-term adjustment of families following traumatic brain injury where comprehensive rehabilitation has been provided. Brain Inj [Internet]. 2003;17(6):453–68.
26. Bivona U, Antonucci G, Contrada M, Rizza F, Leoni F, Zasler ND, Formisano R. A biopsychosocial analysis of sexuality in adult males and their partners after severe traumatic brain injury. Brain Inj [Internet]. 2016;30(9):1082–95.
27. Calabrò RS, Bramanti P. Neuroanatomy and physiology of human sexuality. In: Calabrò RS, editor. Male sexual dysfunction in neurological diseases: from pathophysiology to rehabilitation. New York: Nova Science Publisher; 2011. p. 1–24.
28. Georgiadis JR. Functional neuroanatomy of human cortex in relation to wanting sex and having it. Clin Anat [Internet]. 2015;28(3):314–23.
29. Calabrò RS, Cacciola A, Bruschetta D, Milardi D, Quattrini F, Sciarrone F, la Rosa G, Bramanti P, Anastasi G. Neuroanatomy and function of human sexual behavior: a neglected or unknown issue? Brain Behav [Internet]. 2019;9:e01389.
30. Moreno JA, Arango Lasprilla JC, Gan C, McKerral M. Sexuality after traumatic brain injury: a critical review. NeuroRehabilitation [Internet]. 2013;32(1):69–85.
31. Arango-Lasprilla JC, Olabarrieta-Landa L, Ertl MM, Stevens LF, Morlett-Paredes A, Andelic N, Zasler N. Provider perceptions of the assessment and rehabilitation of sexual functioning after traumatic brain injury. Brain Inj [Internet]. 2017;31(12):1605–11.
32. Stolwyk RJ, Downing MG, Taffe J, Kreutzer JS, Zasler ND, Ponsford JL. Assessment of sexuality following traumatic brain injury: validation of the Brain Injury Questionnaire of Sexuality. J Head Trauma Rehabil. 2013;28(3):164–70.
33. Verschuren JE, Enzlin P, Dijkstra PU, Geertzen JH, Dekker R. Chronic disease and sexuality: a generic conceptual framework. J Sex Res [Internet]. 2010;47(2–3):153–70.
34. D'Amato A, Gugliotta M, Redolfi A, Maietti A, Sapienza S, Mazzucchi A. Sexual and relational life after severe acquired brain injury: evaluation in an Italian population and treatment's implications. 2015 (poster presented to 3rd European Congress of NeuroRehabilitation, Vienna, 1-4 Dicembre 2015).
35. Bibby H, McDonald S. Theory of mind after traumatic brain injury. Neuropsychologia [Internet]. 2005;43(1):99–114.
36. Ubukata S, Tanemura R, Yoshizumi M, Sugihara G, Murai T, Ueda K. Social cognition and its relationship to functional outcomes in patients with sustained acquired brain injury. Neuropsychiatr Dis Treatm [Internet]. 2014;10:2061–8.
37. Bivona U, Formisano R, De Laurentiis S, Accetta N, Di Cosimo MR, Massicci R, Ciurli P, Azicnuda E, Silvestro D, Sabatini U, et al. Theory of mind impairment after severe traumatic brain injury and its relationship with caregivers' quality of life. Restor Neurol Neurosci [Internet]. 2015;33(3):335–45.
38. Klonoff PS. Psychotherapy after brain injury: principles and techniques. Guilford Press; 2010. p. 45–69.
39. Perlesz A, Kinsella G, Crowe S. Psychological distress and family satisfaction following traumatic brain injury: injured individuals and their primary, secondary, and tertiary careers. J Head Trauma Rehab [Internet]. 2000;15(3):909–29.
40. Esmail S, Darry K, Walter A, Knupp H. Attitudes and perceptions towards disability and sexuality. Disabil Rehabil [Internet]. 2010;32(14):1148–55.

41. Marshall S, Bayley M, McCullagh S, Velikonja D, Berrigan L. Clinical practice guidelines for mild traumatic brain injury and persistent symptoms. Can Fam Physician [Internet]. 2012;58(3):257–67.
42. Carney N, Totten AM, O'Reilly C, Ullman JS, Hawryluk GW, Bell MJ, Rubiano AM. Guidelines for the management of severe traumatic brain injury. Neurosurg [Internet]. 2017;80(1):6–15.
43. De Goumoëns V, Didier A, Mabire C, Shaha M, Diserens K. Families' needs of patients with acquired brain injury: acute phase and rehabilitation. Rehabil Nurs [Internet]. 2019;44(6):319–27.
44. Annon JS. The PLISSIT model: a proposed conceptual scheme for the behavioral treatment of sexual problems. J Sex Educ Ther [Internet]. 1976;2:1–15.
45. Taylor B, Davis S. The extended PLISSIT model for addressing the sexual wellbeing of individuals with an acquired disability or chronic illness. Sex Disabil [Internet]. 2007;25(3):135–9.
46. Backhaus S, Neumann D, Parrot D, Hammond FM, Brownson C, Malec J. Examination of an intervention to enhance relationship satisfaction after brain injury: a feasibility study. Brain Inj [Internet]. 2016;30(8):975–85.
47. Backhaus S, Neumann D, Parrot D, Hammond FM, Brownson C, Malec J. Investigation of a new couples intervention for individuals with brain injury: a randomized controlled trial. Arch Phys Med Rehabil [Internet]. 2019;100(2):195–204.
48. Hawkins LG, Eggleston D, Brown CC. Utilizing a narrative therapy approach with couples who have experienced a traumatic brain injury to increase intimacy. Contemp Fam Ther [Internet]. 2019;41(3):304–15.
49. Kowal J, Johnson SM, Lee A. Chronic illness in couples: a case for emotionally focused therapy. J Marital Fam Ther [Internet]. 2003;29(3):299–310.
50. Deschênes PM, Lamontagne ME, Gagnon MP, Moreno JA. Talking about sexuality in the context of rehabilitation following traumatic brain injury: an integrative review of operational aspects. Sex Disabil [Internet]. 2019:1–18.

Parkinson's Disease

Mario G. Rizzone, Leonardo Lopiano, and Elena Vittoria Longhi

Introduction

Parkinson's disease (PD) is a neurodegenerative disorder characterized by progressive loss of dopaminergic neurons of the substantia nigra pars compacta (SNpc), which is anatomically located in the mesencephalon, and formation of intraneuronal alpha-synuclein inclusions defined as Lewy bodies.

PD is the second most common neurodegenerative disorder after Alzheimer's disease, with an incidence rate of about 14/100.000 people from the general population. This incidence grows up to 160/100.000 when considering individuals older than 65 years [1]. The prevalence of PD is about 150/100.000 individuals in the general population, while it is higher than 400/100.000 in the elderly. PD is slightly prevalent in males than in females (M/F incidence ratio 1.3).

Aetiopathogenesis

Although the aetiology of PD still remains controversial, it is largely accepted that its pathophysiology is multifactorial, resulting from the interaction between genetic and environmental factors [2].

The role of genetics has been demonstrated by the identification of several PD-related gene mutations with either an autosomal dominant or recessive inheritance [3]. The SNCA gene codifies for α-synuclein, and the LRRK2 gene deserves

M. G. Rizzone (✉) · L. Lopiano
Department of Neuroscience, 'Rita Levi Montalcini'—University of Turin, Turin, Italy
e-mail: mariogiorgio.rizzone@unito.it; leonardo.lopiano@unito.it

E. V. Longhi
Department of Sexual Medical Center, San Raffaele Hospital, Milano, Italy

E. V. Longhi (ed.), *Managing Psychosexual Consequences in Chronic Diseases*,
https://doi.org/10.1007/978-3-031-31307-3_26

to be mentioned as the most common loci for autosomal dominant PD mutations with variable penetrance among family members. On the other hand, PARK2 gene is regarded as the most frequently affected locus for autosomal recessive PD mutations, which are responsible for about 50% of cases of early-onset PD. Despite being less frequently involved, PINK1 and DJ1 are also genes carriers of recessive mutations associated with PD. Finally, mutations in the GBA gene, which is responsible for Gaucher's disease, have been recently demonstrated to play an important role as a risk factor for PD.

With respect to possible environmental causes of PD, several risk factors have been reported, such as exposure to pesticides or heavy metals, rural life, agricultural occupation and traumatic head injury [4].

Several pathophysiological mechanisms have been suggested to account for the progressive neuronal loss observed in PD brains, which include α-synuclein misfolding and aggregation, neuroinflammation, impairment of the ubiquitin–proteasome system, mitochondrial dysfunction and oxidative stress [2]. Neurodegeneration in PD brains typically affects the dopaminergic neurons located in the mesencephalic SNpc, whose damage/loss determines the clinical onset of motor symptoms observed in patients with PD. However, neuronal loss is not only confined to this brain structure. It has been suggested that the earliest pathological changes may involve neurons from the spinal cord and the autonomic nervous system, to progressively spread to the medulla oblongata, olfactory bulb, substantia nigra and midbrain and eventually to cortical areas (Braak's hypothesis) [5]. The involvement of non-dopaminergic pathways accounts for the presence of several non-motor symptoms of PD.

Clinical Features

Motor Symptoms

PD is characterized by the presence of three cardinal motor symptoms: bradykinesia, rigidity and rest tremor. According to the diagnostic criteria of the Movement Disorders Society, bradykinesia is defined as slowness of movement and decrement in amplitude or speed when movements are continued; rigidity refers to velocity-independent resistance of major joints to passive movements; rest tremor is defined as a 4- to 6-Hz tremor in fully resting limbs, which is suppressed during movement initiation [6]. Typically, the clinical onset of PD is characterized by asymmetric bradykinesia associated with hand rest tremor and/or rigidity. Patients may present with facial hypomimia and hypophonic speech. Micrography is also a common feature that is observed in patients who are affected in their dominant hemisphere. In early disease stages, the only detectable walking abnormality may be a reduction in pendular synkinesis on the affected body side. With the progression of the disease, bradykinesia, rigidity and rest tremor can worsen to progressively involve both sides of the body. Patient gait may become shuffled, with short steps, sometimes freezing when turning or passing an open door. Postural abnormalities with flexed trunk and limbs may also appear. Balance often worsens with disease progression and increases the risk of falls. The motor symptoms of PD typically show an excellent response to symptomatic therapy with dopaminergic drugs. However, in patients at more advanced PD stages, motor fluctuations and drug-induced involuntary movements (dyskinesias) may appear, which often represent one of the major causes of disability [7]. Motor fluctuations, which typically appear after the introduction of levodopa therapy, are characterized by a quick transition from good control of motor symptoms (on condition) to their acute reappearance (off condition). Conversely, when patients are in the on condition, dyskinesias may appear, which consists of involuntary choreiform and/or dystonic movements of the neck, trunk and limbs. Dyskinesias may be highly disabling with a significant impact on patients' quality of life.

Non-motor Symptoms

PD does not only affect the motor system. There are many non-motor symptoms belonging to the clinical picture of PD, whose appearance may precede many years of the clinical onset of motor symptoms, in the so-called prodromal phase of PD [8]. Non-motor manifestations of PD include hyposmia, constipation, rapid eye movement sleep behaviour disorder (RBD), excessive daily sleepiness, anxiety and depression. Autonomic symptoms, such as urinary urgency or incontinence and symptomatic postural hypotension, are most common in the intermediate–advanced stages of the disease. At later stages of PD, cognitive impairment often occurs, whose progression leads to the development of dementia in a very high percentage of patients. Hallucinations and paranoid ideation are also seen in PD patients, although they are most frequently related to dopaminergic treatment [7, 8].

Diagnosis

The diagnosis of PD is clinical and is based on the presence of the characteristic motor symptoms associated with suggestive non-motor features. A good and persistent response to dopaminergic therapy and the absence of symptoms suggestive of other neurological conditions support a correct diagnosis of PD [6]. As part of the diagnostic process, it is always recommended that patients receive a brain MRI or CT scan to exclude secondary parkinsonisms (vascular, hydrocephalus, tumours, etc.). Conversely, more specific assessments, such as positron emission tomography (PET) or single photon emission computed tomography (SPECT) to detect abnormalities in the SNpc dopaminergic nerve terminals projecting to the striatum, are indicated in selected cases only [8].

Therapy

Currently, the treatment of PD remains symptomatic, in the absence of any available disease-modifying treatment to slow down the progression of the disease. Therapy options include both pharmacological and surgical interventions.

The dopaminergic drugs that are currently available allow to obtain excellent control of motor symptoms in patients at early disease stages. At later disease stages, although the response to dopaminergic drugs remains satisfactory, a high percentage of patients develop drug-induced complications, i.e. motor fluctuations and dyskinesias [2, 8, 9]. At most advanced stages of the disease, motor symptoms tend to become increasingly resistant to dopamine therapy, and worsening in non-motor symptoms may represent an additional source of disability.

Levodopa still represents the 'gold standard' for the pharmacological treatment of PD, being the most effective drug for motor symptoms. Levodopa has a plasmatic half-life of 1–2 h, is absorbed at the jejunoileal level and transformed to dopamine, which acts as replacement therapy at the level of the surviving nigral dopaminergic terminals.

Levodopa has a high tolerability and causes infrequent side effects (common to all dopaminergic drugs) such as nausea, vomiting, postural hypotension and hallucinations.

The main issue related to levodopa therapy is the occurrence of motor complications (motor fluctuations and dyskinesias) in a high percentage of patients who have been on treatment for 3–5 years.

Levodopa dosages vary, depending on the stage of the disease, between 300 and 1500 mg daily, which are usually fractioned into 3–8 doses.

Other therapy options for PD include dopamine agonists, monoamine oxidase-B inhibitors (i-MAO-B), catechol-O-methyltransferase inhibitors (i-COMT) and amantadine. Anticholinergic drugs are currently considered a second-choice treatment due to their unfavourable side-effect profile [9].

Dopamine agonists act directly on the striatal dopaminergic receptors. Compared to levodopa, they have lower efficacy on motor symptoms with a higher incidence of dopaminergic side effects (nausea, vomiting, orthostatic hypotension, impulse control disorder and daily sleepiness). In contrast, they cause motor complications very infrequently, which is the major advantage of their clinical use. Nowadays, the most commonly used dopamine agonists are the long-acting–non-ergot derivatives, such as pramipexole extended release, ropinirole extended release and rotigotine (the latter in transdermal patch formulation). These drugs are either used as monotherapy in patients at early PD stages, or in association with levodopa. Apomorphine is a dopamine agonist with a very short half-life, which is administered by single-dose subcutaneous injections for the treatment of sudden motor blocks, or by continuing subcutaneous infusion for the management of patients at advanced disease stages.

The i-MAO-B (selegiline, rasagiline, safinamide and zonisamide) and i-COMT (entacapone, tolcapone and opicapone) are enzyme inhibitors, which increase or prolong the duration of levodopa effect.

Amantadine is currently used for the treatment of dyskinesias.

In patients with advanced PD, whose motor fluctuations and dyskinesias become poorly responsive to oral therapy, treatment strategies may include continuous infusion of subcutaneous apomorphine or intraduodenal levodopa gel via PEG-J. In these patients, surgical treatment is also a suitable therapeutic option. The bilateral continued electrical stimulation of specific brain targets (i.e., subthalamic nucleus and internal globus pallidus) through implantable pulse generators (deep brain stimulation—DBS) has proven efficacious in determining significant improvements of PD motor symptoms, with a reduction in drug-induced complications [9].

Sexuality and Quality of Life

A number of impulse control disorders, including compulsive sexual behaviour, have been described in Parkinson's disease. The excessive sexual demands of Parkinsonian men can lead to significant tension within the couple.

In-depth sexual interviews reveal that these cases may reflect various types of sexual dysfunction that present as hypersexuality.

A study by Bronner et al. [10] aimed to analyse cases of presumed and true male compulsive sexual behaviour and to propose a practical tool for clinicians, to assist them in the diagnosis and management of compulsive sexual behaviour and other sexual dysfunctions in Parkinsonian patients.

The sexual assessment revealed that only one in three patients were experiencing true hypersexuality caused by compulsive sexual behaviour.

The majority of patients diagnosed with Parkinson's disease had erectile dysfunction, difficulty reaching orgasm (delayed ejaculation) and a gap in desire within the couple.

Another study by Bronner et al. [11] identified four types of sexual preoccupation:

1. Sexual behaviour with underlying sexual dysfunction
2. Discrepancy in sexual desire with a partner after the restoration of desire
3. Hypersexuality and compulsive sexual behaviour
4. Sexual behaviour with the underlying restless genital syndrome

Understanding of these types of behaviour can only come through the psychosexual counselling of the caregiver and, if possible, the couple.

This has led the clinic not to limit itself to the treatment of motor symptoms of Parkinson's disease (PD), but also of non-motor symptoms, in particular cognitive and neurobehavioural complications, which affect the quality of life of the caregiver who lives in constant distress.

Impulse control disorders constitute a group of psychiatric disorders in the Diagnostic and Statistical Manual of Mental Disorders (DSM-IV-TR) [12] and are characterized by the inability to resist an impulse, drive or temptation to perform a typically pleasurable activity that is ultimately harmful to the person or others due to its excessive nature.

Pathological gambling (PG) is the most common ICD, and other ICDs without formal DSM-IV-TR diagnostic criteria include compulsive sexual behaviour and compulsive buying [13].

Uncontrolled eating disorder, classified as eating disorder in the DSM-IV-TR, shares many of the clinical features of ICDs. Recent observational studies suggest that a number of ICDs may occur with greater frequency in PD than in the general population and may be associated with the use of dopamine agonists (DA).

Other related disorders reported to occur in PD and characterized by repetitive or compulsive behaviours include the following:

1. Dopamine dysregulation syndrome (DDS) or hedonic homeostatic dysregulation [14], an addiction-like state characterized by excessive use of dopaminergic medications, particularly levodopa and short-acting DAs (e.g. subcutaneous apomorphine)

2. Punding, an intense fascination with meaningless movements or activities (e.g. picking up, arranging or disassembling objects) [15]

3. Walkabout, defined as excessive and aimless wandering [14]

In one epidemiological study of 3090 patients with PD, in 46 movement disorder centres in the United States and Canada, an ICD has to date been identified in 13.6% of patients (gambling = 5.0%, sexual behaviour = 3.5%, buying = 5.7% and uncontrolled eating disorder = 4.3%) and 4.9% had two or more ICDs [16].

A total of 15 cases of DDS were reported in the original description of this dopamine dysregulation syndrome and other related disorders in patients with PD, but a cross-sectional or cumulative prevalence rate was not reported.

With regard to punding, in one series that examined PD patients with higher levodopa equivalent daily dosages (LEDDs), 14% met the criteria for punding, but another larger study of unselected PD patients reported a prevalence rate of 1.4% [17].

There is more. Sexuality in these patients often discomfits caregivers.

A study by Bronner et al. [11] identifies four common types of sexual preoccupation behaviours in people with PD:

1. Sexual behaviour with underlying sexual dysfunction

2. Discrepancy in sexual desire with a partner after restoration of desire

3. Hypersexuality and compulsive sexual behaviour

4. Sexual behaviour with the underlying restless genital syndrome

---

Understanding these four behavioural types can help healthcare providers explain to and educate PD sufferers and their partners, help reduce stress and tension between them and help them manage these sexual problems.

Not least because the caregiver has an important therapeutic role. While emotionally, physically and psychologically demanding, the role of the PD patient's partner is also costly and time-consuming. The cost of caregiving is typically borne by the family, and one survey estimated that the average caregiver spends an average of 22 h per week performing the role.

The caregiver has a unique and privileged view of the patient's condition, and often, due to symptoms of apathy, cognitive impairment and depression, they can provide a more accurate assessment of symptoms and the effect of treatment. It is therefore critical that the caregiver be involved in clinical appointments and treatment decisions whenever possible [18].

In this regard, in a clinical trial [19] of caregivers in an outpatient Palliative Care Service for PDRD, data became available on PD patient aggression through interviews, punctuated every 3 months for 12 months.

Measures of illness severity, quality of life, mood and caregiver burden were included in the correlation and relative risk models, adjusting for age, sex and diagnosis.

Of 170 caregivers, 31 (18.2%) reported physical assault and 18 (10.6%) reported sexual assault. The 12-month cumulative incidence of physical and sexual assault was 21.1% (23/109) and 16.0% (19/119), respectively. The cumulative incidence of physical aggression was associated with patient depression ($r = 0.37$), patient-perceived quality of life ($r = -0.26$), caregiver burden ($r = 0.26$), caregiver-perceived quality of life ($r = -0.26$) and caregiver anxiety ($r = 0.20$). Age, gender, cognitive impairment and dementia were not associated with cumulative sexual aggression.

Furthermore, sexual problems are commonly reported in PD (68% of men and 36% of women). [20] Gender differences in SD patterns have been demonstrated. In men, the predominant SD was found to be erectile dysfunction (ED), difficulty achieving orgasm and premature ejaculation (EP), whereas the predominant symptoms for women with PD were low sexual desire and difficulty with arousal and with orgasm. [21].

Female patients were less dissatisfied with their sex lives than males. [22] In a recent study of 89 patients with PD, although men reported significantly higher sexual desire, women were more satisfied with their sex lives [23]; the explanation offered was that male SD interfered with the traditional active role, creating a devastating effect on men's self-esteem and overall sexual experience; this idea has also been suggested by others. [24].

There is also a difference between caregivers: Which is better? A woman or a man?

A cross-sectional, longitudinal study [25] among participants with PD enrolled in the National Parkinson's Foundation Parkinson's Outcomes Project from 2009 to 2014 at 21 international sites studied 7209 participants (63% men and 37% women) with PD.

Men had a mean age of 66.0 (SD: 9.8) years, and women had a mean age of 66.9 (SD: 9.7) years. More men than women had a caregiver (88.4% vs 79.4%, $p < 0.0001$).

Caregiver burden was measured by the Multidimensional Caregiver Strain Index (MCSI).

Male caregivers reported greater strain than female caregivers (MCSI score 19.9 vs 16.4, $p < 0.0001$). These differences persisted after controlling for age, stage of illness, number of comorbidities, cognitive and mobility measures and health-related quality of life. In addition, the odds of accompanying a caregiver to the baseline visit were lower for women than men (odds ratio: 0.76, 95% confidence interval [CI]: 0.67–0.86) and women had a faster rate of using a paid caregiver than men (hazard ratio: 1.76, 95% CI: 1.35–2.28) after controlling for potential confusion.

Thus, it is shown that caregivers show greater perseverance in caring for their partners, but also a very high distress index is often underestimated by doctors and nurses.

It also follows that their disappointment concerning their own future and their ability to plan seems strongly compromised. [26].

In this regard, a qualitative study using semi-structured interviews of female caregivers of PD patients presenting with delusions was conducted. Thematic analysis was employed using MAXQDA 2018.

Twelve participating spouses (SPs) were interviewed.

Four themes emerged as follows:

Managing disbelief: trying to make sense of the delusional content
Hypervigilance: constant attention to bizarre and threatening speech and behaviour
Defensive strategy: anticipating delusions and potential consequences
Hiding and exposing: ambivalence about revealing the effect of delusions but wanting support

Conclusion

Education about potential neurobehavioural changes should be forthcoming for both patients and caregivers.

Clinicians should be aware that the impact of delusions on caregivers is often greater than revealed in clinical interviews. Interdisciplinary teams liaising separately with spousal caregivers can improve the disclosure and delivery of appropriate psychological and educational support.

Teamwork would give the psychosexologist the opportunity to validate the caregiver's needs, desires and motivation to go on, even as the partner's illness progresses. Moreover, the caregiver could be taught to separate 'the person (partner)' from the disease. In this sense, delusions and physical and sexual aggressiveness would be easier to accept if reported to the disease and not to the chosen affective partner and likewise for all the other progressive symptoms of PD.

References

1. Hirtz D, Thurman DJ, Gwinn-Hardy K, Mohamed M, Chaudhuri AR, Zalutsky R. How common are the "common" neurologic disorders? Neurology. 2007;68(5):326–37.
2. Jankovic J, Tan EK. Parkinson's disease: etiopathogenesis and treatment. J Neurol Neurosurg Psychiatry. 2020;91(8):795–808.

3. Karimi-Moghadam A, Charsouei S, Bell B, Jabalameli MR. Parkinson disease from mendelian forms to genetic susceptibility: new molecular insights into the neurodegeneration process. Cell Mol Neurobiol. 2018;38(6):1153–78.

4. Ascherio A, Schwarzschild MA. The epidemiology of Parkinson's disease: risk factors and prevention. Lancet Neurol. 2016;15(12):1257–72.

5. Braak H, Del Tredici K, Rub U, de Vos RA, Jansen Steur EN, Braak E. Staging of brain pathology related to sporadic Parkinson's disease. Neurobiol Aging. 2003;24(2):197–211.

6. Postuma RB, Berg D, Stern M, Poewe W, Olanow CW, Oertel W, Obeso J, Marek K, Litvan I, Lang AE, et al. MDS clinical diagnostic criteria for Parkinson's disease. Mov Disord. 2015;30(12):1591–601.

7. Hayes MT. Parkinson's disease and parkinsonism. Am J Med. 2019;132(7):802–7.

8. Kalia LV, Lang AE. Parkinson's disease. Lancet. 2015;386(9996):896–912.

9. Armstrong MJ, Okun MS. Diagnosis and treatment of Parkinson disease: a review. JAMA. 2020;323(6):548–60.

10. Bronner G, Hassin-Baer S. Exploring hypersexual behavior in men with Parkinson's disease: is it compulsive sexual behavior? J Parkinsons Dis. 2012;2(3):225–34.

11. Bronner G, Hassin-Baer S, Gurevich T. Sexual concern behavior in Parkinson's disease. J Parkinsons Dis. 2017;7(1):175–82.

12. American Psychiatric Association. Diagnostic and statistical manual of mental disorders, 5th ed., text revision. Washington, DC; American Psychiatric Association; 2000.

13. Grant JE, Levine L, Kim D, et al. Impulse control disorders in inpatient adult psychiatric patients. Am J Psychiatry. 2005;162:2184–8.

14. Giovannoni G, O'Sullivan JD, Turner K, et al. Hedonistic homeostatic dysregulation in patients with Parkinson's disease on dopamine replacement therapy. J Neurol Neurosurg Psychiatry. 2000;68:423–8.

15. Evans AH, Katzenschlager R, Paviour D, et al. Punding in Parkinson's disease: its relationship to dopamine dysregulation syndrome. Mov Disord. 2004;19:397–405.

16. Weintraub D, Koester J, Potenza MN, et al. Dopaminergic therapy and impulse control disorders in Parkinson's disease: the leading results of a cross-sectional study of over 3,000 patients movement disorders. 2008.

17. Miyasaki J, Hassan KL, Lang AE, et al. Punding prevalence in Parkinson's disease. Mov Disord. 2007;22:1179–81.

18. Hiseman P, et al. The burden of the caregiver and the non-motor symptoms of Parkinson's disease, author links open the Jon P. Hiseman1 overlay panel. Int Rev Neurobiol. 2017;133:479–97.

19. Macchi ZA, Miyasaki J, Katz M, Galifianakis N, Sillau S, Kluger BM. Prevalence and cumulative incidence of caregiver-reported aggression in advanced Parkinson's disease and related disorders. Neurol Clin Pract. 2021;11(6):e826–33. https://doi.org/10.1212/CPJ.0000000000001110.

20. Brown RG, Jahanshahi M, Quinn N, et al. Sexual function in Parkinson's disease patients and their partners. J Neurol Neurosurg Psychiatry. 1990;53(6):480–6.

21. Koller WC, Vetere-Overfield B, Williamson A, et al. Sexual dysfunction in Parkinson's disease. Clin Neuropharmacol. 1990;13(5):461–3.

22. Bronner G, Cohen OS, Yahalom G, et al. Correlations of the quality of sexual life in male and female patients with Parkinson's disease and their partners. Parkinsonism Relat Disord. 2014;20:1085–8.

23. Celikel E, Ozel-Kizil ET, Akbostanci MC, et al. Assessment of sexual dysfunction in patients with Parkinson's disease: a case-control study. Eur J Neurol. 2008;15(11):1168–72.

24. Connolly BS, Lang AE. Drug treatment of Parkinson's disease: a review. JAMA. 2014;311(16):1670–83.

25. Dahodwala N, Shah K, He Y, Wu SS, Schmidt P, Cubillos F, Willis AW. Sexual inequalities in access to caregiving in Parkinson's disease. Neurology. 2018;90(1):e48–54. https://doi.org/10.1212/WNL.0000000000004764.

26. Deutsch CJ, Robertson N, Miyasaki JM. Psychological impact of Parkinson disease disappointments on spouse's caregivers: a qualitative study. Brain Sci. 2021;11(7):871. https://doi.org/10.3390/brainsci11070871.

Part XIV
Odontoiatry

Periodontal Disease

Mauro Belluz and Elena Vittoria Longhi

Gingivitis and periodontitis are inflammatory conditions caused by the formation and persistence of microbial biofilms on the hard, non-shedding surfaces of teeth.

Etiopathogenesis and Clinical Expression

Gingivitis is the first manifestation of the inflammatory response to the biofilm. It is reversible (i.e., if the biofilm is disrupted gingivitis resolves), but if biofilms persist gingivitis becomes chronic. In some subjects, chronic gingivitis progresses to periodontitis.

Besides the presence of a disease-associated biofilm, these subjects are exposed to additional risk factors including smoking and systemic comorbidities.

Periodontitis is characterized by non-reversible tissue destruction resulting in progressive loss of attachment eventually leading to tooth loss.

Severe periodontitis is the sixth most prevalent disease of mankind [1]; it is associated with reduced quality of life and masticatory dysfunction, and it is a major factor in the increase in the costs of oral health care. It is a public health problem since it is highly prevalent and causes disability and social inequality [2].

M. Belluz (✉)
IRCCS Gavazzeni, Milan, Italy

E. V. Longhi
Department of Sexual Medical Center, San Raffaele Hospital, Milano, Italy

© Springer Nature Switzerland AG 2023
E. V. Longhi (ed.), *Managing Psychosexual Consequences in Chronic Diseases*,
https://doi.org/10.1007/978-3-031-31307-3_27

Prevention

In the context of prevention, gingivitis and periodontitis are best viewed as a continuum of a chronic inflammatory disease entity with periodontitis representing a perturbation of host-microbial homeostasis in susceptible individuals that leads to irreversible tissue destruction. Regular disruption and periodic removal of accumulating bacterial deposits at and below the gingival margin are a key component of the prevention of plaque-induced periodontal diseases. Individuals are often unable to accomplish this, so professional intervention is required. Prevention of gingivitis refers to the inhibition of the development of clinically detectable gingival inflammation or its recurrence. It is currently unknown whether low levels of gingival inflammation are compatible with the maintenance of oral health or should also be considered a risk for the development of periodontitis in susceptible individuals. Primary prevention of gingivitis aims to avoid the development of more severe and widespread forms of gingivitis that may ultimately convert to periodontitis.

Prevention of periodontitis may be primary or secondary. Primary prevention of periodontitis refers to preventing the inflammatory process from destroying the periodontal attachment; it consists of treating gingivitis through the disruption/removal of the bacterial biofilm and the consequent resolution of inflammation.

In addition, adjunctive interventions including pharmacological modification of the disease-associated biofilm and host modulation have been explored.

Secondary prevention of periodontitis refers to preventing the recurrence of gingival inflammation, which may lead to additional attachment loss in successfully treated periodontitis. Both at the population and at the individual subject level, prevention (and treatment) of gingivitis is a critical component for the prevention of periodontitis.

Furthermore, the control/management of risk factors for periodontitis such as smoking and diabetes forms an important part of the prevention of periodontitis.

Prevention of periodontal disease consists of patient-performed control of the dental biofilm and professional interventions. In developed countries, the above approaches have been used for several decades. Their application at the population level has been associated with an overall improvement in the levels of oral cleanliness and a decrease in gingival inflammation and in the prevalence of mild-to-moderate periodontitis [3]. In many of these countries, however, the prevalence of severe periodontitis has not decreased.

Traditionally, the diagnosis of the presence of periodontal diseases is based on the evaluation of clinical signs and symptoms and may be supported by evidence from radiographs. Gingival changes including color, contour, texture alterations, and the presence of bleeding on probing from the gingival tissues allow the diagnosis of plaque-induced gingival diseases. Non-plaque-induced gingival diseases may necessitate other investigations such as histopathology, microbiology, or serology to affect a diagnosis. Periodontitis is diagnosed by the presence of gingival changes as may be evidenced for gingivitis plus the presence of reduced resistance of the tissues to periodontal probing with a deeper gingival sulcus or "pocket," which reflects the loss of periodontal attachment [4].

It is important to recognize that "pockets" may have a horizontal and vertical dimension; thus, the clinician in carrying out their probing for attachment loss must be careful to evaluate furcation involvements. The detection of attachment loss in furcations demands a sound knowledge of tooth and furcation anatomy, particularly the sites of the furcation openings on multi-rooted teeth. Tooth mobility and migration must also be assessed. It is, however, important to realize that mobility is not by itself diagnostic of periodontitis and may be the result of occlusal trauma as may be migration of teeth, which may be segmental or single tooth migration. Mobility and migration solely related to periodontitis are usually late symptoms of the disease and are possibly of more importance in assessing prognosis and in treatment planning. Family history and factors, which modify risk, such as cigarette smoking, stress, drugs, or sex hormones, which affect the course of all types of periodontal diseases, need to be assessed and added to these primary descriptors to further describe the type of disease being diagnosed. Radiographs provide a secondary diagnostic tool and may demonstrate the presence of marginal bone loss, thus confirming the attachment loss. The role of radiographs in diagnosis will be addressed in another article in this supplement [5].

It is generally agreed that the healthy gingival crevice can range from 1 mm to 3 mm. In health, the distance from the cementoenamel junction to the alveolar bone crest is also variable and has a range of 1 mm to 3 mm. It must, however, be understood that attachment loss by itself does not constitute periodontitis, which is an inflammatory lesion in the periodontal tissues, and that health can exist in the presence of severe attachment loss and recession. Thus, a healthy periodontium can exist at different levels along the root as happens after successful treatment. The periodontal probe remains the primary diagnostic tool and is used to detect the presence of periodontal pockets as measured from the gingival margin to the base of the crevice and loss of attachment as measured from the cementoenamel junction to the base of the crevice. Measurements recorded by the probe, however, are not in fact the actual pocket depth or attachment level but the distance from a fixed reference point to where the probe tip penetrates the tissues. This measurement will depend upon the probing pressure used, the tiny size of the probe tip, angulation of the probe, the presence of subgingival deposits, and, most importantly, the presence or absence of inflammation in the tissues. Thus, clinical attachment level and probing depth changes recorded during treatment may not reflect a true change in fiber attachment levels but merely changes in the depth of penetration of the probe into the tissues caused by change in the above factors [6].

Once a diagnosis of disease has been made, the disease may be classified according to the criteria of the classification system. This process of diagnosis, while it may be valid for the diagnosis of periodontal disease for clinical management in dental practice, presents problems when trying to determine what constitutes periodontal disease in order to undertake clinical studies [7].

The problem is that our diagnosis is made upon an assessment of the destruction caused by the disease and not by an assessment of the presence of a destructive disease process within the periodontal tissues using the means usually used in assessing other diseases in medicine, such as the identification through biochemical markers, identification of responsible microbes, or identification by histopathology. As Caton [8] says "periodontitis by definition is inflammation of the supporting structures of the teeth – usually a progressive destructive change leading to loss of bone and periodontal ligament. Periodontal disease activity refers to the stage of the disease characterized by loss of supporting bone and tissue attachment. This implies the natural history of periodontal disease is marked by periods of active destruction and relative quiescence, even though the periodontal tissues remain relatively inflamed."

Sexuality and Quality of Life

Eke et al. [9] used this national survey sample of adults aged 30 years and older with recourse to full-mouth periodontal examination: clinical attachment level and probing depth for six sites, per tooth. Following adjustment for the effects of age, the prevalence of periodontitis was significantly higher in men than in women (56.4% versus 38.4%) [10].

We are speaking therefore of "sexual dimorphism of periodontitis prevalence."

What Do We Mean by Sexual Dimorphism?

In the clinical field, it means the systematic difference that exists between individuals belonging to the same species but of different sex. In the human species in terms of physical structure, males are on average heavier and stronger than females, whereas females have a larger structure and conformation of the pelvis, have a different distribution of fat mass, and emit a higher frequency voice.

Selecting older male patients, between 65 and 74 years of age, 18.3% (SE 2.5) were extensively proven to be diagnosed with severe periodontitis, compared with 5.6% (SE 1.3) of women.

There is more, however. During the 2017 World Workshop Classification of Periodontal Disease, two risk factors for a diagnosis of severe periodontitis were found: smoking and diabetes [11].

An important difference between the sexes and thus sexual dimorphism may lie in the different immune responses between men and women [12]. Compared with women, men produce a higher volume of inflammatory cytokines [13] in many infection and sepsis scenarios. Meanwhile, women generally form protective humoral and cell-mediated immune responses to antigenic challenge [14]. Gender differences in immunity are manifested in variations in the incidence of autoimmune disorders, susceptibility to infectious diseases, and vaccine response: This has been extensively reviewed by Klein et al. [15].

In addition, scientific studies have reported female anxiety toward oral hygiene to be higher than male anxiety, leading them to exercise more meticulous oral care [16–18].

In this regard, the study by Gurlek et al. [19] investigated the possible relationship between periodontal status and sexual dysfunction in perimenopausal women. The research was conducted on a sample of 106 participants. After the assessment of participants' sexual functioning with the Female Sexual Function Index (FSFI), periodontal status was assessed.

Participants were divided into two groups based on periodontal status. Patients with periodontitis were grouped according to stage and extent of disease in addition to the frequency of gingival bleeding.

A significant correlation emerged: Total FSFI scores and scores from the domains of arousal, lubrication, orgasm, satisfaction, and pain were significantly lower in patients with periodontitis ($p < 0.05$).

But What Role Does Anxiety Play in These Patients?

Genco et al. evaluated the association between stress, distress, and coping behaviors with periodontal disease [20].

The sample examined comprised 1426 subjects aged 25–74 years in Erie County, NY. Subjects were asked to complete a series of five psychosocial questionnaires measuring psychological traits and attitudes; daily-life events and their emotional impact; chronic stress or mood disorders; distress; and coping styles and strategies.

A clinical assessment of supragingival plaque, gingival bleeding, subgingival tartar, probing depth, clinical attachment level (CAL), and radiographic alveolar ridge height (ACH) was added to these assessments and eight putative bacterial pathogens were measured from the subgingival flora.

Result? Stress, coupled with economic stresses and mental distress (to the point of depression), is a significant risk indicator for periodontal disease, which is more severe in male adults with diabetes and heavy smokers.

Some studies have gone further. Saini et al. [21] questioned the correlation between oral sex, oral health, and orogenital infections. Especially since an injury in the mouth, bleeding gums, lip sores, or cracked skin increase the chances of infection. Given the possibility that oral sex can be practiced by people of all sexual orientations, the first to engage in it would seem to be adolescents who often use sexual practices unrelated to coitus, including oral sex [22]. Studies indicate that between 14% and 50% of adolescents have had oral sex before their first experience with intercourse [23], that more adolescents have had oral sex than vaginal sex, [24] and that few adolescents who engage in oral sex use barrier protection [25].

Adults and adolescents often underestimate the extent to which oral sex can be a mode of transmission for syphilis, [26] gonorrhea, [27] herpes, [28] HIV, [29] chlamydia, and HPV. The surgeon general's report on oral health highlights that the mouth serves as a window to many systemic diseases and infections that can affect an individual's immune status [30]. In particular, carious dentinal lesions can serve as a reservoir for Candida organisms in both HIV-positive and HIV-negative persons, but are more common in HIV-infected persons, and in immunocompromised patients [31].

Scholars therefore recommend the use of condoms or dental barriers when performing or receiving sexual intercourse with a partner whose STD status is unknown. (An improvised dental barrier can be made from a condom.) Thus, the study by Saini et al. emphasizes that oral sex involves giving or receiving oral stimulation to the male and female genitalia or anus. This practice was evaluated by the study as the most frequent in the transmission of sexual diseases as opposed to vaginal sex.

Conclusion

Although oral hygiene is often viewed as a weapon against diseases such as tooth decay and tartar buildup, the consequences affect a broader spectrum of disease relationships. Both in relation to sexual transmission and to influencing the immune system, especially with the practice of oral sex and relations with unfamiliar partners. The role of the psychosexologist even in this area is not to be underestimated and should help the patient to develop a greater understanding of their own health.

References

1. Kassebaum NJ, Bernable E, Dahiya M, Bhandari B, Murray CJ, Marcenes W. Global burden of severe periodontitis in 1990–2010: a systematic review and meta-regression. J Dent Res. 2014;93:1045–53.
2. Baehni P, Tonetti MS, on behalf of Group 1 of the European Workshop on Periodontology. Conclusions and consensus statements on periodontal health, policy and education in Europe: a call for Periodontology on Effective Prevention of Periodontal and Peri-Implant Diseases. action–consensus view 1. Consensus report of the 1st European Workshop on Periodontal Education. Eur J Dent Educ. 2010;14:1.
3. Eke PI, Dye BA, Wei L, Thornton-Evans GO, Genco RJ, CDC Periodontal Disease Surveillance workgroup: James Beck (University of North Carolina, Chapel Hill, USA), Gordon Douglass (Past President, American Academy of Periodontology), Roy Page (University of Washin). Prevalence of periodontitis in adults in the United States: 2009 and 2010. J Dent Res. 2012;91:914–20.
4. Listgarten MA. Pathogenesis of periodontitis. J Clin Periodontol. 1986;13:418–30.
5. Corbet EF. Radiographs in periodontal disease diagnosis and management. Aust Dent J. 2009;54(1 Suppl):S27–43.
6. Fowler C, Garrett S, Crigger M, Egelberg J. Histologic probe position in treated and untreated human periodontal tissues. J Clin Periodontol. 1982;9:373–85.

7. Preshaw PM. Definitions of periodontal disease in research. J Clin Periodontol. 2009;36:1–2.
8. Caton J. Periodontal diagnosis and diagnostic aids. In: Proceedings of the world workshop in clinical periodontics. Chicago: American Academy of Periodontology; 1989. p. 1/5–1/22.
9. Eke PI, Wei L, Borgnakke WS, Thornton-Evans G, Zhang X, Lu H, et al. Prevalence of periodontitis in adults ≥ 65 years of age, in the USA. Periodontology. 2000;72(1):76–95.
10. Eke PI, Dye BA, Wei L, Thornton-Evans GO, Genco RJ. Prevalence of periodontitis in adults in the United States: 2009 and 2010. J Dent Res. 2012;91(10):914–20. Represents one of the first national epidemiological investigations using the full mouth periodontal examination protocol.
11. Tonetti MS, Greenwell H, Kornman KS. Staging and grading of periodontitis: framework and proposal for a new classification and case definition. J Periodontol. 2018;89:S159–72.
12. Shiau HJ, Reynolds MA. Sex differences in destructive periodontal disease: exploring the biological basis. J Periodontol. 2010;81(11):1505–17.
13. Horst R, Jaeger M, Smeekens SP, Oosting M, Swertz MA, Li Y, et al. Host and environmental factors influencing the individual responses of human cytokines. Cell. 2016;167(4):1111–24.
14. Jaillon S, Berthenet K, Garlanda C. Sexual dimorphism in innate immunity. Allerg Immunol Clin Rev. 2017;30:1–4.
15. Klein SL, Flanagan KL. Sex differences in immune responses. Nat Rev Immunol. 2016;16(10):626. Gender is a biological variable and should be considered in future immunological studies.
16. Woelber JP, Bienas H, Fabry G, Silbernagel W, Giesler M, Tennert C, et al. Oral hygiene-related self-efficacy as a predictor of oral hygiene behavior: a prospective cohort study. J Clin Periodontol. 2015;42(2):142–9.
17. Saatchi M, Abtahi M, Mohammadi G, Mirdamadi M, Binandeh ES. The prevalence of dental anxiety and fear in patients referred to the dental school of Isfahan, Iran. Dent Res J. 2015;12(3):248–53.
18. Carlsson V, Hakeberg M, Boman UW. Associations between dental anxiety, sense of consistency, oral health-related quality of life, and healthcare behavior: a Swedish National Cross-sectional Survey. BMC Oral Health. 2015;15(1):100.
19. Gurlek B, et al. Is sexual dysfunction associated with periodontal status in perimenopausal women ? A pilot study. Oral Dis. 2021;4(3):33–41.
20. Genco RJ, et al. Relationship between stress, distress and inadequate coping behaviors with periodontal disease. J Periodontol. 1991;70:711. https://doi.org/10.1902/jop.1999.70.7.711.
21. Saini R, et al. Oral sex, oral health and orogenital infections. J Glob Infect Dis. 2010;2(1):57–62. https://doi.org/10.4103/0974-777X.59252.
22. Conard LA, Blythe MJ. Sexual function, sexual abuse and sexually transmitted diseases in adolescence. Best Pract Res Clin Obste Gynaecol. 2003;17:103–16.
23. Schuster MA, Bell RM, Kanouse DE. Sexual practices of teenage virgins: genital sexual activities of high school students who have never had vaginal intercourse. Am J Public Health. 1996;86:1570–6.
24. Prinstein MJ, Meade CS, Cohen GL. Teen oral sex, peer popularity, and best friends perception of sexual behavior. J Pediatr Psychol. 2003;28:243–9.
25. Halpern-Felsher BL, Cornell JL, Kropp RY, Tschann JM. Oral versus vaginal sex among adolescents: perceptions, attitudes and behavior. Pediatrics. 2005;115:845–51.
26. Centers for Disease Control and Prevention (CDC). Transmission of primary and secondary syphilis by Oral sex - Chicago, Illinois, 1998-2002. MMWR Morb Mortal Wkly Rep. 2004;53:966–8.
27. Edwards S, Carne C. Oral sex and transmission of viral sexually transmitted diseases. Infect Sex Transm. 1998;74:6–10.
28. Jin F, Prestage GP, Mao L, Kippax SC, Pell CM, Donovan B, et al. Transmission of herpes simplex virus types 1 and 2 in a prospective cohort of HIV-negative gay men: a health study in men. J Infects Dis. 2006;194:561–70.

29. Hawkins DA. Oral sex and HIV transmission. Infect Sex Transm. 2001;77:307–8.
30. Saini R. Dental expression and role in palliative care. Indian J Palliat Care. 2009;15:26–9.
31. Jacob LS, Flaitz CM, Nichols CM, Hicks MJ. Role of dentinal carious lesions in the pathogenesis of oral candidiasis in HIV infection. J Am Dent Assoc. 1998;129:187–94.

Part XV
Ophthalmology

Vascular and Degenerative Retinal Diseases

Alfredo Pece, Federica Fossataro, and Elena Vittoria Longhi

The retina, consisting of ten layers, is the innermost tissue of the eye and serves to capture light stimuli from the outside, transforming them into electrical impulses, which, by definition, form the visual system. If the central zone of the retina, the macula region, is damaged, there may be important visual impairment. There are several chronic retinal diseases, and this chapter will analyze the most frequent diabetic retinopathy, age-related macular degeneration, and central and branch vein occlusion.

Diabetic Retinopathy

Diabetic retinopathy, a microvascular complication of diabetes mellitus, is among the leading causes of visual loss worldwide. Its prevalence is growing rapidly, and it is expected to affect more than six million people in the USA by 2030 [1].

Risk Factors

The duration of diabetes mellitus plays a key role in the incidence of retinopathy: After 5 years, only 1% of patients present ocular manifestations, but after 10 years the proportion rises to 25%, reaching 70% after 20 years [2]. Adequate

A. Pece (✉) · F. Fossataro
Eye Clinic, Melegnano Hospital, Milan, Italy

Fondazione Retina 3000, Milan, Italy
e-mail: pece.retina@mclink.it; federica.fossataro@unina.it

E. V. Longhi
Department of Sexual Medical Center, San Raffaele Hospital, Milano, Italy

© Springer Nature Switzerland AG 2023
E. V. Longhi (ed.), *Managing Psychosexual Consequences in Chronic Diseases*,
https://doi.org/10.1007/978-3-031-31307-3_28

glyco-metabolic control delays micro- and macrovascular complications related to diabetes, including ocular disorders. Other risk factors are hypertension, hyperlipidemia, diabetic nephropathy, pregnancy, and smoking.

Pathogenesis

Diabetic retinopathy is a microangiopathy in which small capillary vessels are extremely vulnerable to high glucose levels. The first alterations occur in the retinal capillaries, which present abnormal thickening of the basal membrane, loss of pericytes associated with proliferation, and subsequent loss of endothelial cells. This causes alterations to the internal blood–retinal barrier. Consequently, capillary occlusion with non-perfused areas, vascular hyperpermeability, and retinal neovascularization are the effects of microangiopathic damage to retinal vessels.

Clinical Signs

- **Microaneurysms:** Located in the posterior pole and in the medium and extreme retinal periphery, these are the first vascular alterations of diabetic retinopathy. They are protrusions of the vascular capillary walls, characterized by the loss of pericytes. Microaneurysms are seen in the superficial vascular plexus but in particular in the deep plexus. They are clinically evident on fundus examination as sharp-edged small red dots and are also visible on multimodal imaging.
- **Retinal Hemorrhages:** They are Small, roundish, or flame-like shapes localized at the posterior pole and in the middle periphery. They are considered superficial when located in the inner layers or intraretinal when they originate from the venous side of the capillaries and are located in the retinal middle layers.
- **Hard Exudates:** Located in the outer plexiform layer, these yellowish lesions consist of macrophages full of lipoproteins, which, due to the loss of capillary wall integrity, extravasate and accumulate around an area of retinal edema.
- **Intra-Retinal Microvascular Abnormalities (IRMA):** They are segmental dilations that link retinal arterioles to venules, bypassing the capillaries. They are often adjacent to areas of capillary hypoperfusion.
- **Edema:** This is the most common cause of visual impairment in diabetic patients. On ophthalmoscopic examination, the retina appears thickened and grayish. Diffuse edema is a consequence of increased capillary permeability with fluid accumulation between the outer plexiform layers and the inner nuclear layer. When the macula is involved, it may have a cystic appearance and this condition

is therefore called cystoid macular edema. It is frankly evident on OCT examination and gives a flower petal pattern on fluorescein angiography (FAG) [3].

- **Neovascularization:** When there is considerable retinal ischemia, new vessels can develop, initially thin and then gradually extending parallel to the increase in vascular caliber [4]. These can affect the optic disk, retina, and iris. Neovascularization is a sign of advanced, ischemic, and proliferative diabetic retinopathy and therefore calls for urgent treatment.

Ophthalmic Examination

Ophthalmological examination in diabetic patients involves, in the first instance, measuring the best corrected visual acuity (BCVA) and investigating the anterior and posterior segments with close fundus examination. Ophthalmologists examine an eye with diabetic retinopathy using optical coherence tomography (OCT), OCT angiography (OCTA), and FAG.

Treatments

Regardless of the treatment of diabetes and its contributing causes, **laser photocoagulation** is mainly employed to destroy the ischemic areas, avoiding the occurrence of neovascularization. Laser treatment exploits the thermal effect of a beam of coherent monochromatic light to create burns on the retina at the point where it is focused. In the early form of nonproliferative diabetic retinopathy, the laser impacts are directed on the microaneurysms and altered capillaries that cause edema and exudates. In an eye with papillary or retinal new vessels, or both, the rationale for treatment involves the destruction of the ischemic areas from which the stimulus for their formation comes.

Nowadays, however, when there is widespread macular edema the first treatment option is **intravitreal injections** of antivascular endothelial growth factor (VEGF) or, secondly, of a steroid, whose purpose is to ensure the disappearance of intraretinal fluid.

The surgical approach, **pars plana vitrectomy**, may be indicated when macular edema is associated with vitreoretinal tangential traction with thickening and traction of the posterior hyaloid, or in case of hemovitreous and/or tractional retinal detachment.

The patient must be fully aware of the situation in order to ensure the best possible visual outcome, so adequate glycemic control, abolition of cigarette smoking and hypertension, and hyperlipidemia under control are mandatory (Fig. 1).

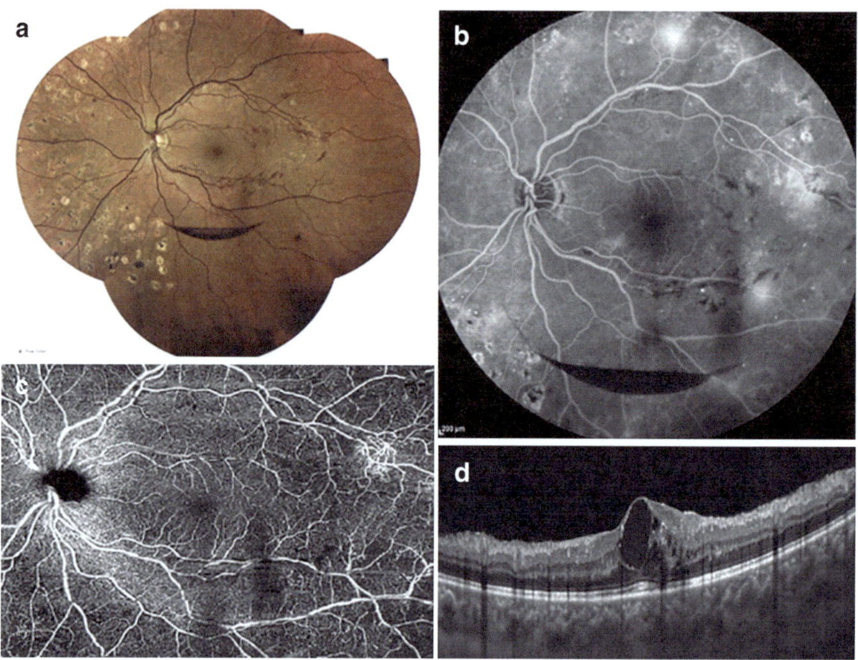

Fig. 1 A 53-year-old woman with diabetic retinopathy: Wide-field retinography shows hemorrhages and retinal neovascularization at the posterior pole. A sub-hyaloid hemorrhage is detected in the retinal inferior sector. Some laser spots are present in the retinal nasal and inferior sector (**a**). Fluorescein angiography shows points of hyperfluorescence due to retinal neovascularization and a half-moon-shaped hypofluorescence corresponding to the sub-hyaloid hemorrhage (**b**). No ischemic areas are observed, while florid neovascularization is detected along the superior–temporal vessels at optical coherence tomography (OCT) angiography (**c**). A wide intraretinal cyst is shown at OCT scan (**d**)

Age-Related Macular Degeneration

Age-related macular degeneration (AMD) is the leading cause of legal blindness among people over 60 years old in industrialized countries [5]. This degenerative disease affects the macular region, which contains the retinal area with the largest number of cones and rods, and is vital for the tasks of daily living such as reading, driving, and recognition of faces. Worldwide, by 2040, 288 million people will be affected by AMD.

Risk Factors

The disease most frequently affects people over 60 years old, age being the main risk factor. Additionally, AMD is more common among Caucasians than in people of other races. Heredity also plays an important role, with the risk of AMD three times higher when a relative has the disease. Cigarette smoking, hypertension or high cholesterol, obesity, poor quality of food, female sex, and light eye color are other predisposing factors.

Pathogenesis

AMD pathogenesis, which is multifactorial and involves metabolic, functional, genetic, and environmental factors, is still poorly understood [6]. The early stages of AMD involve the accumulation of extracellular deposits, called drusen, located between the retinal pigment epithelium (RPE) and Bruch's membrane. Drusen are made up of waste material that is not eliminated correctly and causes suffering and degeneration of the RPE and consequently of photoreceptors, increasing the risk of more advanced forms of AMD. Therefore, lipofuscin genesis, drusen, inflammation, and possible neovascularization specifically contribute to AMD.

Conventionally, this disease is divided into two forms: **dry AMD** (presenting drusen in the early stage and RPE atrophy in the late stage) and **wet AMD** (with exudation and macular neovascularization).

Symptoms

AMD is a progressive disease and can therefore get worse with time. The signs and symptoms of dry macular degeneration include progressive reduction in central vision, blurriness, difficulty in reading, and distorted vision.

Clinical Signs

- **Drusen**: They are localized deposits between the RPE and Bruch's membrane. Clinically, drusen are classified morphologically as hard or soft. Soft drusen are generally larger (>125 µm), have blurred edges, and tend to become confluent. Drusen typically cluster in the central macula, where the pathological abnormalities in AMD are most pronounced.
- **Pigment Epithelium Detachment (PED)**: This is caused by an alteration of the normal adhesion between the RPE and Bruch's membrane. The detachment may be **serous**, with a dome-shaped elevation with well-defined edges at fundus examination and an optically empty area underneath on OCT scan. **Fibrovascular** PED has a much more irregular elevation and contour than serous PED. It appears irregular at OCT examination, with fluid and visible fibrous proliferation. The latter presents diffuse and irregular reflectivity on OCT scan. **Drusenoid** PED, larger than 350 µm, results from the confluence of soft drusen and has jagged, irregular edges. OCT examination shows homogeneous hyper-reflectivity within drusenoid PED, with no fluid.

- **Geographic Atrophy**: There are confluent areas of RPE cell damage accompanied by overlying photoreceptor atrophy. Geographic atrophy can develop after drusen fade, in areas of RPE attenuation, following flattening of an RPE detachment, or after involution of choroidal neovascularization. The visible atrophy is usually accompanied by the atrophy of the underlying choriocapillaris.
- **Choroidal Neovascularization (CNV)**: It is a complex network of blood vessels that extends across Bruch's membrane from the choriocapillary layer to the sub-RPE and/or subretinal space. The current classification of CNV is based on the anatomical localization obtained with multimodal imaging and FAG, indocyanine green angiography (ICGA), and OCT. **Type 1 CNV**, the most common type of CNV in AMD, develops in the sub-RPE space. **Type 2 CNV** typically originates at the choroid and, crossing the RPE–Bruch's membrane complex, grows above the RPE, in the subretinal space. **Type 3 CNV**, also described as retinal angiomatous proliferation (RAP), originates from the retinal circulation or develops simultaneously, creating a retino-choroidal anastomosis, according to Freund et al. [7] Then, there is also **polypoidal vasculopathy**: This consists of polypoid lesions, which occur as focal dilations of blood vessels at the edge of a type 1 CNV and therefore grow in the sub-RPE space.

Ophthalmic Examination

Ophthalmological examination in AMD patients consists first in measuring their best corrected visual acuity (BCVA) and then doing the Amsler test. The next steps are a fundus examination and retinography, OCT and OCTA, and FAG and ICGA.

Treatment

Stopping cigarette smoking and protecting the eyes from the sun's rays by wearing sunglasses are helpful in slowing the progression of the condition. A healthy balanced diet rich in antioxidants can be beneficial, as may the addition of appropriate dietary supplements. However, there is no specific treatment yet for dry AMD. However, for the less common wet AMD, antivascular endothelial growth factor (**anti-VEGF**) intravitreal injections (IVTs) may halt or delay the progression of CNV and help preserve vision. The VEGF is involved in the formation of new blood vessels in the retina in people with wet AMD. Blocking the action of this vascular agent helps prevent the condition from progressing and may even partially reverse it. IVT anti-VEGF requires an injection every 4 weeks, considering the half-life of the drug, for the first three doses (the so-called loading phase), after which the timing may vary depending on the patient's response and on the therapeutic scheme followed by the ophthalmologist. In the past, there were different treatments, considered inappropriate nowadays, such as laser treatment and photodynamic therapy (Fig. 2).

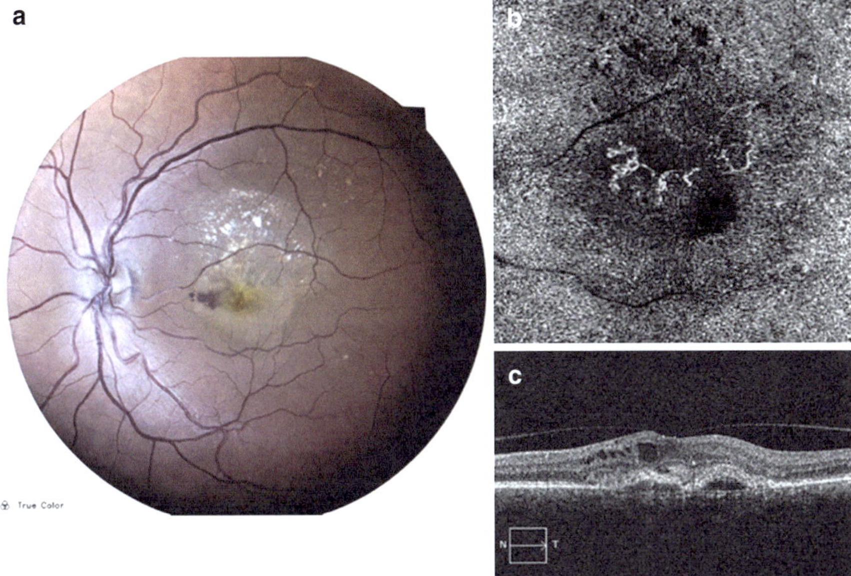

Fig. 2 A 68-year-old man with age-related macular disease complicated with choroidal neovascularization (CNV): Retinography of the posterior pole shows some hard drusen, exudates, intraretinal hemorrhage, and edema in the macular region, as a consequence of CNV (**a**). Optical coherence tomography (OCT) angiography highlights hyperreflective and thin vessels at the outer retina (**b**). Intraretinal cysts, pigment epithelium detachments, and outer retinal irregularities in the macular region associated with an increase in the normal macular thickness are observed at OCT scan (**c**)

Retinal Vein Occlusion

Retinal vein occlusion (RVO) is among the leading causes of visual impairment and one of the most common chronic retinal diseases. It is often due to an underlying systemic disease such as hypertension, chronic nephritis, or arteritis [8]. RVO can affect the main vein trunk consisting of the central retinal vein, thus causing the involvement of the whole retina; alternatively, it may only involve one of its branches—the temporal or nasal one, upper or lower one—causing localized damage to the specific sector normally supplied by the vessel occluded.

Risk Factors

Age is the most important risk factor, with RVO being frequent in patients over 40 years old or, more often, 60 [8]. Hypertension plays an essential role and is present in more than two-thirds of patients. Other risk factors are hyperlipidemia, diabetes mellitus, cigarette smoking, and glaucoma. Rarer causes such as thrombophilia, myeloproliferative disorders, inflammatory pathologies associated with occlusive periphlebitis, orbitopathy, and chronic renal failure should be included.

Pathogenesis

In the course of venous occlusion, there is an arteriosclerotic thickening of retinal arterioles, which causes venous loosening at an arteriovenous junction. This leads to vascular alterations such as loss of endothelial cells, turbulent blood flow, and thrombus formation. Once the venous occlusion occurs, venous pressure rises, and blood stagnates inside the vessels. This results in retinal hypoxia peripherally to the occlusion, which causes extravasation of the blood constituents and the release of mediators such as VEGF [9].

Clinical Signs and Ophthalmological Examination

RVO is typically associated with retinal vein dilation and tortuosity; variable degrees of hemorrhage from the optic nerve head to the extreme retinal periphery are found on fundus examination. Hemorrhages may be flame-shaped if they are located in the most inner layers, or present as deep blots. Often, they are associated with cotton wool spots and optic nerve head and macular edema, as a consequence of the release of mediators [9].

RVO is considered a branch retinal vein occlusion (**BRVO**) when these clinical signs are displayed on only half of the retina. The whole retina is typically involved in a central retinal vein occlusion (**CRVO**).

CRVO can be divided into two forms: non-ischemic CRVO, the most frequent, and ischemic CRVO. **Non-ischemic CRVO** is associated with sudden painless monocular vision loss and retinal hemorrhages, and fundus examination may reveal cotton wool spots with possible optic disk and macular edema. FAG shows delayed arteriovenous transit, with a masking effect due to retinal hemorrhages; capillary perfusion is within limits, and late leakage may be detected in the macular region and at the optic disk. OCT is also useful for assessing the presence and extent of macular edema. At the optic disk head, one may see collateral vessels, which constitute a compensatory mechanism generated by insufficient circulation at the nerve head. Most acute signs resolve within 6–12 months.

Ischemic CRVO is associated with sudden monocular vision loss and rarely with pain; it is attributable to neovascular glaucoma, especially if no previous reduction in visual acuity was reported. Extensive flame hemorrhages and cotton wool spots are visible throughout the retina, with possible optic disk edema. FAG shows delayed arteriovenous transit, with a masking effect due to retinal hemorrhages and extensive areas of capillary non-perfusion. These ischemic areas are responsible for retinal and iris neovascularization.

Considering the risk of neovascular glaucoma, which generally appears between 2 and 4 months from the acute event, gonioscopy may be advisable to rule out the presence of angular new vessels. OCT too is essential to assess the macular edema, which may be greater in ischemic CRVO than non-ischemic CRVO.

Acute signs usually resolve in 9–12 months, but macular alterations such as epiretinal membrane, persistent intraretinal cysts, and retinal pigment epithelium hyperplasia may persist even longer. Recently, ultra-wide-field OCTA has started to partly replace FAG, as it is a noninvasive and repeatable tool, without dye injection, for visualizing ischemic areas and retinal neovascularization.

Treatments

Laser photocoagulation is the standard of care for retinal neovascularization and ischemic areas and complications associated with RVO [10]. The aim of panretinal laser photocoagulation is to destroy the ischemic retina, leading to improvement of the blood supply to the remaining retina and delaying neovascular consequences. Before the advent of anti-VEGF therapy, laser photocoagulation was used to treat macular edema secondary to RVO [10]. Nowadays, the gold standard for treatment involves anti-VEGF intravitreal injections to lower the levels of VEGF released after RVO [11, 12]. However, some cases have responded less to anti-VEGF therapy and intravitreal steroid injections are proposed as the second treatment choice in order to reduce capillary permeability, which is the main cause of macular edema (Fig. 3).

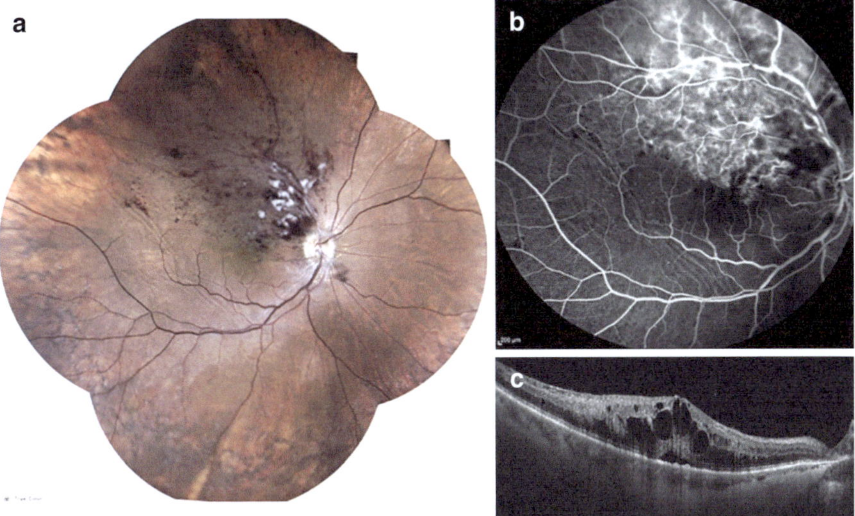

Fig. 3 A 78-year-old man with branch retinal vein occlusion: Wide-field retinography shows multiple flame-shaped retinal hemorrhages and hard exudates along the superior temporal vein and at the macular region (**a**). A widespread capillary dropout with extensive leakage and blockage by hemorrhages is observed at fluorescein angiography in the superior retinal sector and in the macular region (**b**). Cystoid macular edema with foveal neuroepithelium detachment is detected at OCT scan (**c**)

Conclusion (Quality of Life)

Cerebrovascular disease (CVD), including stroke, is one of the leading causes of death globally. The retina is an integral part of the brain, sharing embryological and vascular pathways, and researchers have evaluated the association between several retinal signs and CeVD [13].

Rim's clinical trial, Tyler Hyungtaek et al. [13], for example, tracked six databases (up to July 2019) assessing the link between retinal vascular signs and disease with CeVD. CeVD was classified into two groups: clinical CeVD (including clinical stroke, silent cerebral infarction, cerebral hemorrhage, and stroke mortality) and subclinical CeVD (including MRI-defined lacunar infarction and white matter lesions [WML]). Retinal vascular signs were classified into three groups: classical hypertensive retinopathy (including retinal microaneurysms, retinal micro hemorrhage, focal/generalized arteriolar narrowing, cotton wool spots, and arteriovenous notching), clinical retinal diseases (including diabetic retinopathy [DR], age-related macular degeneration [AMD], retinal vein occlusion, retinal artery occlusion [RAO], and retinal emboli), and retinal vascular imaging measurements (including retinal vessel diameter and geometry).

The results showed that hypertensive retinopathy was consistently associated with clinical CeVD and subtypes of subclinical CeVD including subclinical infarction of the great cerebral arteries, lacunar infarction, and WML. Certain clinical retinal diseases such as DR, retinal arterial and venous occlusion, and transient monocular vision loss were consistently associated with clinical CeVD. There is an increased risk of recurrent stroke immediately after RAO. Less consistent associations are observed with AMD. Retinal vascular imaging using semi-automated computer-aided software to measure retinal vascular caliber and other parameters (tortuosity, fractal size, and branching angle) showed strong associations with clinical and subclinical CeVD.

If we then examine degenerative maculopathy, we observe that it is not only related to the age of the patients, but also related to iatrogenic life habits such as cigarette smoking, being male, diabetes mellitus, alcohol abuse, sedentary life, prolonged and repeated exposure to very intense light, and diet low in omega-3 and vitamins

References

1. Rowley WR, Bezold C, Arikan Y, Byrne E, Krohe S. Diabetes 2030: I from yesterday, today, and future trends. Popul Health Manag. 2017;20(1):6–12.
2. Antonetti D, Klein R, Gardner TW. Diabetic retinopathy. N Engl J Med. 2012;366:1227–39.
3. Sakata K, Funatsu H, Harino S, Noma H, Hori S. Relationship between macular microcirculation and progression of diabetic macular edema. Ophthalmology. 2006;113:1385–91.
4. Durham JT, Herman IM. Microvascular modifications in diabetic retinopathy. Curr Diab Rep. 2011;11:253–64.

5. Friedman DS, O'Colmain BJ, Munoz B, et al. Prevalence of age-related macular degeneration in the United States. Arch Ophthalmol. 2004;122(4):564–72. Published correction appears in Arch Ophthalmol. 2011;129(9):1188.

6. Nowak JZ. Age-related macular degeneration (AMD): pathogenesis and therapy. Pharmacol Rep. 2006;58(3):353–63.

7. Freund KB, Zweifel SA, Engelbert M. Do we need a new classification for choroidal neovascularization in age-related macular degeneration? Retina. 2010;30(9):1333–49.

8. Schmidt-Erfurth U, Garcia-Arumi J, Gerendas B, et al. Guidelines for the Management of Retinal Vein Occlusion by the European Society of Retina Specialists (EURETINA). Ophthalmologica. 2019;242:123–62.

9. Ehlers JP, Fekrat S. Retinal vein occlusion: beyond the acute event. Surv Ophthalmol. 2011;56(4):281–99.

10. The Central Vein Occlusion Study Group. Natural history and clinical management of central retinal vein occlusion. Arch Ophthalmol. 1997;115(4):486–91.

11. Campochiaro PA, Heier JS, Feiner L, Gray S, Saroj N, et al. Ranibizumab for macular edema following branch retinal vein occlusion: six-month primary end point results of a phase III study. Ophthalmology. 2010;117:1102–12. e1101.

12. Clark WL, Boyer DS, Heier JS, et al. Intravitreal aflibercept for macular edema following branch retinal vein occlusion: 52-week results of the Vibrant study. Ophthalmology. 2016;123(2):330–6.

13. Rim TH, Teo AWJ, Yang HHS, Cheung CY, Wong TY. Retinal vascular signs and cerebrovascular disease. J Neuroophthalmol. 2020;40(1):44–59.

Part XVI
Orthopaedics and Traumatology

Osteoarthritis

Salvato Damiano, Placella Giacomo, Ometti Marco, Salini Vincenzo, and Elena Vittoria Longhi

Osteoarthritis (OA) is a degenerative joint disease characterized by deterioration of the articular cartilage. OA is a major cause of disability and chronic articular pain all over the world. With advances in modern medicine improving the prevention, diagnosis, and treatment of many diseases that were once life-threatening, the population is now living longer. This increased life expectancy has led to an increased prevalence of degenerative conditions including OA. Worldwide, arthritis is considered to be the fourth leading cause of disability [1]. In both the developed and developing worlds, osteoarthritis is one of the most important factors affecting disability-adjusted life years [2]. It is a progressive and debilitating condition that can affect both young and old people and is a highly prevalent condition, especially in the Western world. It has a radiological prevalence of up to 80% in subjects over the age of 65 years [3–5]. It is estimated that symptomatic osteoarthritis affects 10% of males and 18% of females over the age of 45 years [6]. Prevalence is likely to further increase given the increasing proportion of older people in society [3, 4]. Osteoarthritis affects one or several diarthrodial joints, including small joints (such as those in the hand) and large joints (especially the knee and hip joints). Diarthrodial joints join two adjacent bones that are covered by a layer of hyaline cartilage (specialized articular cartilage) and encased in a synovial capsule [7]. The bone, articular cartilage, and the thin region of calcified cartilage form a biocomposite, which is highly adapted to transfer loads during weight bearing and optimize joint motion. Alteration in the integrity of the individual joint tissues can occur either acutely associated with traumatic injury or can evolve over time through cell-derived or

S. Damiano · P. Giacomo (✉) · O. Marco · S. Vincenzo
Orthopedics and Traumatology Unit, IRCCS San Raffaele Hospital, Vita - Salute San Raffalele University, Milan, Italy
e-mail: salvato.damiano@hsr.it; placella.giacomo@hsr.it; ometti.marco@hsr.it; salini.vincenzo@hsr.it

E. V. Longhi
Department of Sexual Medical Center, San Raffaele Hospital, Milano, Italy

© Springer Nature Switzerland AG 2023
E. V. Longhi (ed.), *Managing Psychosexual Consequences in Chronic Diseases*,
https://doi.org/10.1007/978-3-031-31307-3_29

matrix-derived factors that alter the composition, structure, and material properties of this specialized part of the skeletal system. Although pathological processes are usually referred to the hyaline cartilage, all of the joint tissues are affected because of their intimate physical and functional association. OA is thus considered a whole joint disease. OA can be classified as primary (or idiopathic) and secondary (based on the attribution to recognized causative factors (e.g., trauma, surgery on the joint structures, and abnormal joints at birth) [8]. The etiology of primary OA is not fully understood yet. It is clear that it is linked to a combination of risk factors, with increasing age and obesity being the most prominent. Elevated body mass index (BMI) is related mainly to knee OA. Other risk factors for primary OA include articular malalignment, increased biomechanical loading of joints, genetics, and low-grade systemic inflammation. Numerous biochemical mediators such as growth factors, cytokines, metalloproteinases, and enzymes are involved in cartilage homeostasis. Disruption of this homeostasis has been the subject of research in recent years, and further findings in this field are expected to better understand OA disease [9].

Physical Examination and Diagnosis

Osteoarthritis is the most common degenerative joint disorder that affects one or several diarthrodial joints, including small joints (such as those in the hand) and large joints (such as the knee and hip joints). To date, OA remains challenging to diagnose [10]. Cardinal signs include pain, transient morning stiffness, and crepitus on joint motion (a grating sound or sensation produced in the joint) that leads to reduced range of motion and physical disability, thus impairing quality of life (QOL). Physical examination may reveal joint rigidity and palpable deformities (e.g., Heberden's nodes and Bouchard's nodes affecting distal and proximal inter-phalangeal joints, respectively) [11].

The clinical diagnosis of osteoarthritis can be made only if the patient has symptoms, and the prevention or alleviation of these is the goal of any intervention [8]. Indeed, symptoms are usually the reason that leads patients to seek medical attention outside screening or research programs. The issue of using symptoms to define the presence of osteoarthritis is that they can develop only once the disease is advanced and usually irreversible. This stage might follow a period of subclinical structural change. For disease modification, symptoms therefore have limited value in the diagnosis of early osteoarthritis, when intervention is more likely to be successful. Structural osteoarthritis can be defined as evident cartilage loss without inflammatory or crystal arthropathy, irrespective of whether the patient has symptoms. This definition aims to describe osteoarthritis at an early stage. Although cartilage changes might be preceded by changes within synovium and bone, articular cartilage degeneration seems to be the common endpoint [8].

Osteoarthritis is traditionally diagnosed with plain film radiography; features include narrowing of the joint space width, osteophyte formation, and the development of subchondral sclerosis and cysts. Scoring systems include those proposed by Kellgren and Lawrence [12] and the Osteoarthritis Research Society International [13]; however, joint space width alone is more sensitive and reliable than these systems [13, 14].

Conservative Treatment

Current medical treatment strategies for OA are aimed at pain reduction and symptom control rather than disease modification. Clinicians treating patients with joint OA face major challenges in recommending the most effective conservative therapies to postpone joint surgery as long as possible. A multidisciplinary, patient-centered combination of education, selfmanagement, exercise, weight loss with realistic goals, encouragement, and regular reassessment is recommended for individuals with OA [15]. Optimizing nutrition and maintaining a near-normal body mass index are critical for preventing OA. Weight loss has been shown to reduce the incidence of knee OA. Individuals who are overweight or obese should be provided with dietary advice because weight loss (usually ~10% of body weight) is associated with improved pain and function and might be associated with reduced progression of structural damage [16–20].

Multiple oral drugs have been recommended to improve symptoms of OA. Glucosamine and chondroitin sulfate and nonsteroidal anti-inflammatory drugs (NSAIDs), including cyclooxygenase-2 inhibitors, are the drugs most commonly prescribed for initial treatment. It must be considered that NSAIDs have a high incidence of side effects and gastrointestinal complications, so their use should be carefully balanced [21, 22].

Intra-articular injections are used extensively as a conservative treatment for OA for their efficacy. Different types of injections exist, and the main types are listed below.

Steroid Injections Steroid injections work by inhibiting the release of prostaglandins, which are the precursors to histamine—the primary inflammatory enzyme released by mast cells and basophils. It is believed that steroid longevity ranges from 2 to 4 weeks inside the joint, but the antalgic effect can last some months [23]. Repeating this type of injection too frequently is not recommended because of the degenerative effect of steroids on the cartilage and tendons [24].

Hyaluronic Acid Endogenous hyaluronan is the major hydrodynamic component of joint synovial fluid. Viscosupplementation enhances chondrocyte metabolism, decreases chondrocyte apoptosis, and stimulates the synthesis of endogenous hyaluronic acid, which decreases shear secondary to increased viscosity [25].

Stem Cells Mesenchymal stem cells are multipotent stromal cells that can differentiate into a variety of cell types, including osteoblasts ad chondrocytes. Stem cells have been isolated from bone marrow, adipose tissue, synovium, blood, and amniotic fluid. Bone marrow mesenchymal stem cells are the most extensively studied, but in recent years has been reported that adipose tissue stem cells have the most stability, are significantly pluripotential, and have increased chondrogenicity [10].

The rationale of using stem cells is to regenerate the articular cartilage. Mesenchymal stem cells appear to be the most helpful in younger patients with mild-to-moderate OA and, if used in the knee, with chronic patellar tendinosis [26]. Studies indicated that one of the main biological mechanisms of action is a strong anti-inflammatory effect, including on neurogenic inflammation [8].

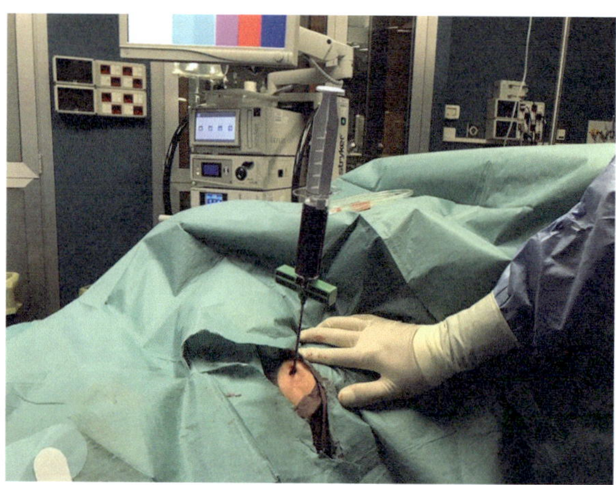

Surgical Treatment

Surgical indication and choice of treatment are based on symptoms (e.g., pain and knee function), OA stage, and patient-related factors such as age, level of physical activity, and patient's comorbidities. Radiological evidence of OA alone (joint space narrowing, osteophytes, etc.) does not justify surgical intervention, which is indicated only in combination with relevant symptoms when conservative treatment failed. Finally, it is the patient's degree of suffering, in correlation to radiological evidence of OA, which determines the time point of surgery [27].

Different surgical treatments are possible for OA.

Cartilage Repair Techniques Damaged articular cartilage has only limited or no healing capacity. Repair of the cartilage surface has therefore been proposed. However, cartilage repair is indicated only for focal cartilage defects, which can be seen as a precursor of OA. The different techniques can be divided into bone marrow stimulating techniques like abrasion, drilling, or microfracture and replacement techniques like mosaicplasty or osteochondral allograft transplantation [28].

Osteotomies They are used mainly for knee OA. Osteotomies are an accepted method for the treatment of unicompartmental OA with associated varus or valgus deformity. Osteotomies around the knee modify the weight-bearing axis of the lower extremity [29]. The aim is to unload the damaged compartment and to transfer the weight load from the affected areas by slightly overcorrecting it into a valgus or varus axis to reduce pain, slow the degenerative process, and delay joint replacement [30–32]. This was the most widely used technique for a long time. In the 1980s and 1990s, osteotomy around the knee lost importance due to the improvement and diffusion of knee arthroplasty. Compared with arthroplasty, osteotomy was considered a demanding procedure with a less predictable outcome and associated with more complications [27].

Joint Arthroplasty Joint arthroplasty is a well-accepted, effective method for the treatment of advanced OA, especially for the hip and the knee. Owing to its irreversible nature, joint arthroplasty is recommended only in patients for whom other treatment modalities have failed or are contraindicated. Regarding the knee joint, arthroplasty could be unicompartmental—involving just half of the joint, usually the medial one—or total. One advantage of unicompartmental knee arthroplasty includes a less invasive surgical technique [33].

One of the principal concerns about surgical interventions such as arthroplasty relates to the cost implications surrounding it. It may be argued that avoiding or delaying these surgical procedures may have a positive impact on health budgets through savings. However, it should be noted that delaying such a procedure may have a detrimental effect on the quality of life of patients and may lead to additional costs [34].

The durability of prosthetic components can be estimated at about 15–20 years nowadays [27].

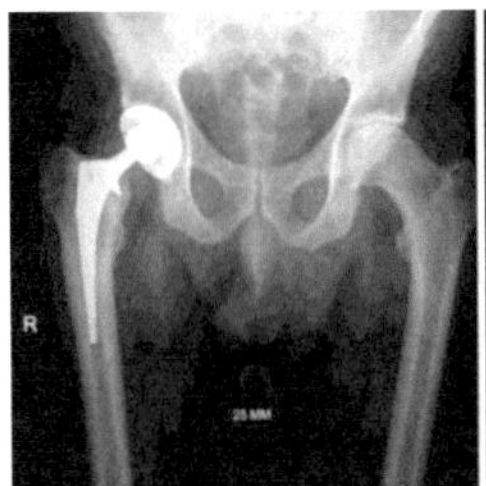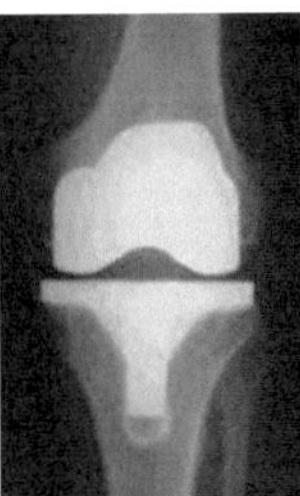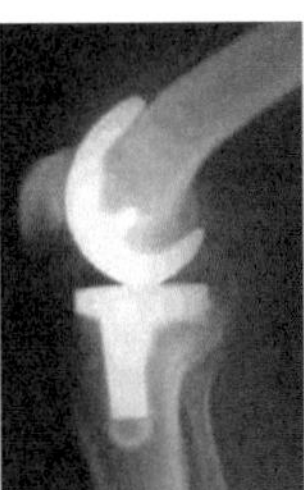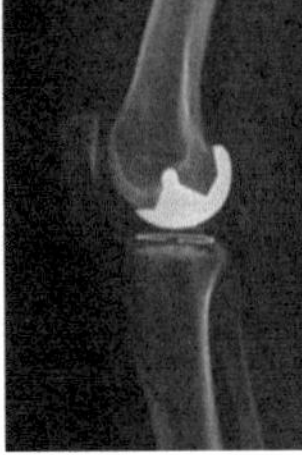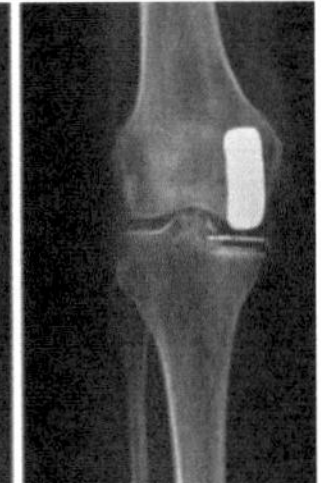

Sexuality and Quality of Life

The study by Salvato KF et al. [35] involved 91 elderly people of both sexes (age: 70.36 ± 5.57 years) from the EELO project, each with self-reported osteoarthritis of the knee or hip, confirmed by radiographic analysis. Pharmacotherapy data were assessed by a structured questionnaire, and quality of life was analyzed by the SF-36 questionnaire at the time of initial diagnosis and 2 years after the start of pharmacological treatment. All domains of quality of life were grouped into physical and mental components for further data analysis.

A statistically significant decrease in health-related quality of life was observed (Wilcoxon's test, $p < 0.05$). However, a slight decrease in physical components was observed in the chondroitin/glucosamine-treated group compared to other groups, according to the Kruskal–Wallis test ($p = 0.007$). On the other hand, no influence of drug treatment on the mental components of health-related quality of life was observed. Anxiety and mood swings, dependent on the perception of pain, whether more persistent or more bearable, were present in all respondents.

The research of Bernad-Pineda et al. [36] is even more detailed: A multicenter observational and cross-sectional study was conducted in which 628 traumatologists or rheumatologists evaluated 1849 patients with knee and/or hip osteoarthritis, aged $\geq$50 years, and representative of 49 Spanish provinces. Each researcher evaluated three patients and also completed the SF-12v2 health questionnaire. Patients completed the WOMAC and SF-12v2 questionnaires.

The patients were 68.5 ± 9.5 years of age, and 61.5% had osteoarthritis of the knee, 19% had osteoarthritis of the hip, and 19.5% had osteoarthritis of both sites. According to both patients and researchers, older patients and those who had both knee and hip osteoarthritis had a worse quality of life. The physical health perceived by the researchers was better than that reported by the patients (36.74 ± 8.6 and 35.21 ± 8.53, respectively, $p < 0.001$), and the mental health scores given by both doctors and patients were similar. The whole sample reported difficulty in movement, poor physical endurance, impatience, irritability, anhedonia, and generalized anxiety disorder.

Similarly, a study by Escobar et al. [37] sought to validate a translated version of the Western Ontario and McMaster Universities Osteoarthritis Index (WOMAC) questionnaire in Spanish patients with hip or knee osteoarthritis (OA). The WOMAC questionnaire and the SF-36 were administered to a sample of 269 patients on the waiting list for hip or knee replacement.

For this reliability study, another sample of 58 patients who had received the WOMAC twice within 15 days was recruited. The reactivity study was carried out by sending the two questionnaires to all patients once again, 6 months after surgery; reactivity was measured by means of the paired t-test, effect size I, and standardized response mean. The coefficients obtained for the item-scale correlation of pain area were 0.74 or higher, 0.91 or higher for stiffness, and 0.61 or higher for function. When measuring test–retest reliability, the coefficients ranged from 0.66 to 0.81. Internal consistency produced Cronbach's alpha ranging from 0.81 to 0.93. The responsiveness showed an effect size I ranging from 1.5 to 2.2 in patients undergoing hip replacement; for those undergoing knee replacements, the range was 1 to 1.8. The mean standardized response ranged from 1.3 to 1.9 for patients with hip OA; those with knee OA ranged from 0.8 to 1.5.

While validating the effectiveness of the questionnaires used in this study, a German study by Rosemann et al. [38] examined the validity of a translated and culturally adapted version of the Arthritis Impact Measurement Scales 2, Short Form (AIMS2-SF), in patients with osteoarthritis (OA) in primary care.

A structured procedure was used for the translation and cultural adaptation of the AIMS2-SF into German. The questionnaire was administered to 220 primary care patients with OA of the knee or hip. Test–retest reliability was tested in 35 randomly selected patients, who received the questionnaire a second time after 1 week. The physical scale of the original AIMS2-SF was divided into an "upper body limitations" scale and a "lower body limitations" scale.

With values between 0.52 and 0.97 for Pearson's r, the item-scale correlations were reasonably good. Significant effects occurred in the upper limb scale (33.8%). Principal factor analysis confirmed the postulated three-factor structure with physical, physiological, and social dimensions explaining 49.8, 14.1, and 6.4% of the variance, respectively. The external validity assessment revealed satisfactory correlations with the corresponding WOMAC scales (Western Ontario and McMaster Universities Arthrosis Index). The correlation with the physician's rating was high in the scales dominated by physical factors, but rather low in the health areas dominated by psychological or social factors. The external validity assessment revealed satisfactory correlations with the corresponding WOMAC (Western Ontario and McMaster Universities Arthrosis Index) scales.

None of these scales examined sexual desire, the type of intimacy experienced (affectionate, passionate, and coital), the precariousness of a sex life conditioned by pain, and anticipatory anxiety about experiencing physical discomfort or frustration.

In addition to the Arthritis Impact Measurement Scales 2 (AIMS2), many other measures allow arthritis researchers to collect data on physical disability, its determinants, and outcomes, which are useful for comparing disease and health conditions. The Organization for Economic Co-operation and Development (OECD) Long-Term Disability (LTD) questionnaire is one of the first broad-based measures developed to assess physical disability. It is a precursor to more recent measures such as the EQ-5D developed by the European Group on Quality of Life and the WHO Disability Assessment Programme II (WHODASII) and finally the Late-Life Function and Disability Instrument (LLFDI), in full and abbreviated versions.

Conclusion

Each of these questionnaires helps researchers to understand the outcome of therapies and surgery in the treatment of osteoarthritis. The fact remains that few clinicians support their expertise with a multidisciplinary approach and targeted interviews to understand the psychological, emotional, and life motivation difficulties related to this pathology. In this case, the sexologist could be a facilitator in the process of understanding the physical, intrapsychic, and relational pain with the external world of these patients. Sexuality does not only include sexual intercourse per se, and in these cases, there is limited interest in this area. Caregivers often complain about the nursing and affective burden in assisting their relatives and describe their altered behavior, impatience, poor adherence to therapy, dissatisfaction, and the resignation of some patients in the face of pain. The multidisciplinary consideration of each individual patient could perhaps limit dropout and intra-familial and social–relational tensions. Isolation from the friendship nucleus and that from recreational activities because of the limitations imposed by the pathology exacerbate the perception of the pathology and its chronic inevitability.

Chronic pain and stiffness of the body are the main factors of this condition, from both the physical and psycho-sexological points of view. For these reasons, some patients experience guilt and anger and discontinue treatment due to a lack of trust in the Specialists and themselves. Changes in lifestyle seem insurmountable: interruption or limitation of work activity, inability to manage the family, lack of sexual desire, abandonment of hobbies, and sports activities. The literature shows that sexual difficulties most frequently reported by sexually active women are related to sexual arousal (32%) and orgasm achievement (27%), while for men it is mostly erectile dysfunction (39%). In both genders, hypotonia of desire (11%) and infrequency of sexual intercourse (8%) are described.

References

1. Fransen M, Bridgett L, March L, et al. The epidemiology of osteoarthritis in Asia. Int J Rheum Dis. 2011;14(2):113–21.
2. Brooks PM. Impact of osteoarthritis on individuals and society: how much disability? Social consequences and health economic implications. Curr Opin Rheumatol. 2002;14(5):573–7.
3. Peat G, McCarney R, et al. Knee pain and osteoarthritis in older adults: a review of community burden and current use of primary health care. Ann Rheum Dis. 2001;60(2):91–7.
4. Gupta S, Hawker GA, et al. The economic burden of disabling hip and knee osteoarthritis (OA) from the perspective of individuals living with this condition. Rheumatology. 2005;44(12):1531–7.
5. Issa S, Sharma L. Epidemiology of osteoarthritis: an update. Curr Rheum Rep. 2006;8(1):7–15.
6. Zhou Q, Yang W, Chen J, et al. Metabolic syndrome meets osteoarthritis. Nat Rev Rheumatol. 2012;8:729–37.
7. Goldring SR, Goldring MB. Kelly's textbook of rheumatology. In: Firestein GS, Budd RC, Gabriel SE, McInnes IB, O'Dell JR, editors. Saunders; 2013. p. 1–19.
8. Glyn-Jones S, Palmer AJR, Agricola R, Price AJ, Vincent TL, Weinans H, Carr AJ. Osteoarthritis. Lancet. 2015;386:376–87.
9. Sellam J, Berenbaum F. Is osteoarthritis a metabolic disease? Joint Bone Spine. 2013;80:568–73.
10. Freitag J, et al. Mesenchymal stem cell therapy in the treatment of osteoarthritis: reparative pathways, safety and efficacy - a review. BMC Musculoskelet Disord. 2016;17:230. https://doi.org/10.1186/s12891-016-1085-9.
11. Arden N, Cooper C. Osteoarthritis handbook. In: Arden N, Cooper C, editors. Taylor and Francis; 2006. p. 1–22.
12. Kellgren JH, Lawrence JS. Radiological assessment of osteo-arthrosis. Ann Rheum Dis. 1957;16:494–502.
13. Altman RD, Gold GE. Atlas of individual radiographic features in osteoarthritis, revised. Osteoarthr Cartil. 2007;15(Suppl A):A1–56.
14. Gossec L, Jordan JM, Lam MA, et al. Comparative evaluation of three semi-quantitative radiographic grading techniques for hip osteoarthritis in terms of validity and reproducibility in 1404 radiographs: report of the OARSI-OMERACT Task Force. Osteoarthr Cartil. 2009;17:182–7.

15. Gossec L, Jordan JM, Mazzuca SA, et al. Comparative evaluation of three semi-quantitative radiographic grading techniques for knee osteoarthritis in terms of validity and reproducibility in 1759 X-rays: report of the OARSI-OMERACT task force. Osteoarthr Cartil. 2008;16:742–8.
16. Fernandes L, et al. EULAR recommendations for the non pharmacological core management of hip and knee osteoarthritis. Ann Rheum Dis. 2013;72:1125–35.
17. Felson DT, Zhang Y, Anthony JM, Naimark A, Anderson JJ. Weight loss reduces the risk for symptomatic knee osteoarthritis in women. The Framingham Study. Ann Intern Med. 1992;116:535–9.
18. Teichtahl AJ, et al. Weight change and change in tibial cartilage volume and symptoms in obese adults. Ann Rheum Dis. 2015;74:1024–9.
19. Hunter DJ, et al. The intensive diet and exercise for arthritis (IDEA) trial: 18 month radiographic and MRI outcomes. Osteoarthr Cartil. 2015;23:1090–8.
20. Messier SP, et al. Effects of intensive diet and exercise on knee joint loads, inflammation, and clinical outcomes among overweight and obese adults with knee osteoarthritis: the IDEA randomized clinical trial. JAMA. 2013;310:1263–73.
21. De Vos BC, Landsmeer MLA, van Middelkoop M, et al. Long-term effects of a lifestyle intervention and oral glucosamine sulphate in primary care on incident knee OA in over- weight women. Rheumatology (Oxford). 2017;56(8):1326–34.
22. Runhaar J, Deroisy R, van Middelkoop M, et al. The role of diet and exercise and of glucosamine sulfate in the prevention of knee osteoarthritis: further results from the Prevention of Knee Osteoarthritis in Over- weight Females (PROOF) study. Semin Arthritis Rheum. 2016;45(4 Suppl):S42–8.
23. Bodick N, Lufkin J, Willwerth C, et al. An intraarticular, extended-release formulation of triamcinolone acetonide prolongs and amplifies analgesic effect in patients with osteoarthritis of the knee: a randomized clinical trial. J Bone Joint Surg Am. 2015;97(11):877–88.
24. Tillander B, et al. Effect of steroid injections on the rotator cuff: an experimental study in rats. J Should Elbow Surg. 1999;8:271–4.
25. Bagga H, Burkhardt D, Sambrook P, March L. Long-term effects of intraarticular hyaluronan on synovial fluid in osteoarthritis of the knee. J Rheumatol. 2006;33(5):946–50.
26. Bradley J. Biologics for the knee: what re- ally works and what I do in my practice. Paper presented at: American Academy of Orthopaedic Surgeons Specialty Day; New Orleans, LA; 2018.
27. Rönn K, Reischl N, Gautier E, Jacobi M. Current surgical treatment of knee osteoarthritis. Arthritis. 2011;2011:454873, 9 pages. https://doi.org/10.1155/2011/454873.
28. Widuchowski W, Lukasik P, Kwiatkowski G, et al. Isolated full thickness chondral injuries. Prevalence and outcome of treatment. A retrospective study of 5233 knee arthroscopies. Acta Chir Orthop Traumatol Cechoslov. 2008;75(5):382–6.
29. Maquet PG. Biomechanics of the knee: with applications of the pathogenesis and the surgical treatment of osteoarthritis. 2nd ed. New York, NY: Springer; 1984.
30. Coventry MB. Osteotomy of the upper portion of the tibia for degenerative arthritis of the knee. A preliminary report. J Bone Joint Surg. 1965;47:984–90.
31. Maquet P. Valgus osteotomy for osteoarthritis of the knee. Clin Orthop Relat Res. 1976;120:143–8.
32. Fujisawa Y, Masuhara K, Shiomi S. The effect of high tibial osteotomy on osteoarthritis of the knee. An arthroscopic study of 54 knee joints. Orthop Clin N Am. 1979;10(3):585–608.
33. Borus T, Thornhill T. Unicompartmental knee arthroplasty. J Am Acad Orthop Surg. 2008;16(1):9–18.
34. Kamaruzaman H, et al. Cost-effectiveness of surgical interventions for the management of osteoarthritis: a systematic review of the literature. BMC Musculoskelet Disord. 2017;18:183. https://doi.org/10.1186/s12891-017-1540-2.
35. Salvato KF, Santos JP, Pires-Oliveira DA, Costa VS, Molari M, Fernandes MT, Poli-Frederico RC, Fernandes KB. Análise da influência da farmacoterapia sobre a qualidade de vida em idosos com osteoartrite. [Analysis of the influence of pharmacotherapy on the quality of life of seniors with osteoarthritis]. Rev Bras Reumatol. 2015;55(1):83–8. Portuguese.

36. Bernad-Pineda M, de Las Heras-Sotos J, Garcés-Puentes MV. Calidad de vida en pacientes con artrosis de rodilla y/o cadera. [Quality of life in patients with knee and hip osteoarthritis]. Rev Esp Cir Ortop Traumatol. 2014;58(5):283–9. Spanish.
37. Escobar A, Quintana JM, Bilbao A, Azkárate J, Güenaga JI. Validation of the Spanish version of the WOMAC questionnaire for patients with hip or knee osteoarthritis. Western Ontario and McMaster Universities Osteoarthritis Index. Clin Rheumatol. 2002;21(6):466–71.
38. Rosemann T, Körner T, Wensing M, Schneider A, Szecsenyi J. Evaluation and cultural adaptation of a German version of the AIMS2-SF questionnaire (German AIMS2-SF). Rheumatology (Oxford). 2005;44(9):1190–5.

Osteoporosis

Marcella Montini, Alessandra Ana Maria Pagani, Silvio Sporeni, and Elena Vittoria Longhi

Osteoporosis is a systemic skeletal disease associated with an increased risk of fracture and characterized by reduced bone mass and qualitative alterations in bone structure (in both macro- and micro-architecture). Cases of osteoporosis appearing after menopause (postmenopausal) or with advancing age (senile) are defined as primary. Juvenile osteoporosis is commonly used to indicate the forms of osteoporosis that are found in childhood and adolescence: These pathologies are mostly due to genetic mutations that can involve quantitative or qualitative alterations of the connective component of the bone (as in osteogenesis imperfecta) or an altered osteoblastic activity majorly affecting the trabecular bone. On the other hand, secondary osteoporosis can be caused by a large number of pathologies and drugs (Tables 1 and 2). Osteoporosis is not a disease affecting only women, indeed, about 20% of all hip fractures occur in males and the incidence of vertebral fractures is about half that of females. However, contrary to the prevalence, in affected males mortality and morbidity from vertebral and femoral fractures are higher than in affected females [1].

M. Montini (✉)
Humanitas Gavazzeni, Bergamo, Italy

A. A. M. Pagani
ASST Papa Giovanni XXIII, Bergamo, Italy
e-mail: apagani@asst-pg23.it

S. Sporeni
San Matteo Hospital, Pavia, Italy
e-mail: silvio.sporeni@humanitas.it

E. V. Longhi
Department of Sexual Medical Center, San Raffaele Hospital, Milano, Italy

© Springer Nature Switzerland AG 2023
E. V. Longhi (ed.), *Managing Psychosexual Consequences in Chronic Diseases*,
https://doi.org/10.1007/978-3-031-31307-3_30

"""

Table 1 Osteoporosis-associated pathologies

Endocrine pathologies	Hematological pathologies	Gastroenterological pathologies	Rheumatic pathologies
Renal pathologies	Neurologic pathologies	Genetic pathologies	Others (COPD, amyloidosis, AIDS, sarcoidosis, depression)

Table 2 Osteopenazing drugs

Pharmacological class	Active substance
Glucocorticoids	• Hydrocortisone • Prednisone • Dexamethasone
Aromatase inhibitors	• Letrozole • Anastrozole • Exemestane
SSRI (selective serotonin reuptake inhibitors)	• Citalopram • Fluoxetine • Paroxetine
Proton-pump inhibitors (PPI)	• Esomeprazole • Omeprazole • Lansoprazole
H2 inhibitors	• Ranitidine • Cimetidine
Thiazolidinediones	• Rosiglitazone • Pioglitazone
Thyroid supplementation therapy	• Levothyroxine
Anticoagulants	• Heparin • Warfarin
GnRH	• Leuprolide • Goserelin
Loop diuretics	• Furosemide
Antiretrovirals	• Efavirenz • Nevirapine • Tenofovir • Protease inhibitors
Calcineurin inhibitors	• Cyclosporine A (high doses) • Tacrolimus

Osteoporosis Evaluation

Nowadays bone mass and, in particular, bone mineral density (BMD) can be accurately measured in g/cm2 of projected bone surface through densitometric studies. It must be noted that 60–80% of bone mechanical strength is consequential to BMD, and this is the reason why it has become a pivotal measurement in the evaluation of osteoporosis.

The densitometric diagnosis of osteoporosis, according to the WHO (World Health Organization) guidelines, is based on the evaluation of mineral density with the dual-energy X-ray absorptiometry (DXA) technique, compared to the average of healthy adults [2]. The unit of measurement is represented by the standard deviation from the average peak of bone mass (T-score). To interpret the results of the BMD, the WHO advises to adopt the following definitions:

1. Normal BMD is defined by a T-score between +2.5 and − 1.0 SD.
2. Osteopenia (low BMD) is defined at a T-score between −1.0 and − 2.5 SD.
3. Osteoporosis is defined by a T-score lower than −2.5 SD.
4. Overt osteoporosis is defined by a T-score lower than −2.5 SD and by the simultaneous presence of one or more fragility fractures.

It should be noted that this is only a densitometric diagnosis that can be translated into a clinical diagnosis only after an overall differential clinical evaluation. The individual fracture risk and the decision to initiate or not a drug treatment are influenced by other factors, both skeletal and extra-skeletal.

Overall Fracture Risk Assessment

In the last decade, the scientific community developed algorithms, such as FRAX and DeFRA, which can calculate the risk over the next 10 years of the main fragility fractures (vertebral, femoral, humeral, and carpal) by integrating the information deriving from the measurement of BMD with that deriving from the presence of other clinical risk factors. Risk assessment, with or without the aid of these algorithms, must be based on information that is easily available and accessible.

Based on these considerations and to overcome some of FRAX limitations, DeFRA was developed in Italy: an algorithm derived from FRAX based on data reporting the risk of fracture specifically in the Italian population and improving the stratification of some variables already present in FRAX (e.g., location and number of previous fractures, comorbidities), in order to improve the prediction of fracture risk [3].

It is mandatory to continuously and frequently update the tools for the definition of fracture risk with data deriving from clinical studies, which, over time, can identify new clinical risk factors, as in the case of diabetes and aromatase inhibitors, or allow a better interpretation of risks deriving from already known factors [4].

TBS (Trabecular Bone Score)

The TBS is software that, applied to the DXA, exposes the degree of inhomogeneity of the vertebral bone, providing indirect information on the trabecular micro-architecture. Studies published so far show that TBS improves the ability to predict fracture risk compared to BMD alone. This application has been approved by the FDA (Food and Drug Administration).

The TBS represents only the trabecular bone distribution; for this reason, it is not affected by quantitative changes in the bone matrix. During the BMD analysis, the TBS can be printed in the following 10 seconds and can be retrospectively analyzed in any examination performed with the densitometer. A reduced TBS is indicative of a weak micro-architecture, indicating an increased risk of fracture. In order to define reference values, an international working group has provided the following ranges (dimensionless unit of measurement) valid for female subjects in the post-menopausal phase: $\geq$1350 normal; 1349–1201 partially degraded micro-architecture; and $\leq$ 1200 degraded micro-architecture [5].

QCT (Quantitative Computed Tomography)

Due to its ability to separate trabecular from cortical BMD, QCT allows to measure both the total and compartmental volumetric BMD (g/cm3) at the vertebral and femoral levels [6, 7].

Epidemiology

Osteoporosis is a socially impacting disease. Its incidence increases with age until it affects the majority of the population beyond the eighth decade of life. In Italy, it has been estimated that there are about 3.5 million women and one million men suffering from osteoporosis. Since the percentage of the Italian population over the age of 65 will increase by 25% in the next 20 years, we are expecting a proportional increase in the incidence of osteoporosis [8].

Therapy

The main therapy regarding secondary osteoporosis is based on the resolution of the causing disease.

As follows there are the main therapeutical approaches in the treatment of osteoporosis:

1. Dietary calcium intake implementation.
2. Vitamin D supplementation.
3. Physical activity.
4. Medical therapy.
5. Surgical interventions: vertebroplasty and kyphoplasty.

Calcium Intake and Diet

The recommended dietary allowance of calcium varies depending on age between 800 and 1500 mg/day [9]. If necessary, it is preferable to increase calcium intake through diet and then through supplementation, since the risk of non-oxalic kidney stones may increase with supplements, while it decreases with diet. Moreover, the calcium supplement safety profile has been questioned for a possible increase in calcium vascular calcifications and cardiovascular risk: Recent data have not confirmed the relationship between calcium intake and cardiovascular diseases, and for this reason, it is recommended to resort to supplements only when dietary correction is not sufficient [10].

An increase in protein intake in subjects with inadequate consumption reduces the risk of fractures of the femur in both sexes. An adequate protein intake (1.0–1.2 g/kg/day with at least 20–25 g of noble proteins per meal) associated with resistance physical exercises (muscle strengthening exercises) is able to increase muscle mass and strength, improving bone health as well.

Other micronutrients such as zinc, silicon, vitamin K, vitamin E, vitamin B6, vitamin B12, and magnesium, which are at the base of a balanced diet, also seem to have a protective role on bone and muscle.

Vitamin D Supplementation

To maintain adequate vitamin D status is preferable the use of fractionated doses (daily, weekly, or monthly) of cholecalciferol. It is well demonstrated that sufficient plasma levels (> 30 ng/mL) of 25OHD (25 OH vitamin D) are able to improve the response to osteoporosis drug therapy.

The most physiological supplementation approach is the daily one; however, in order to improve adherence to treatment, the use of equivalent weekly or monthly doses is justified from a pharmacological point of view.

Calcifediol [25 (OH) D3] induces a more rapid increase in the levels of 25OHD compared to cholecalciferol, due to the different pharmacokinetics and lower distribution volume; consequently, 25OHD3 can be indicated in the case of 25-hydroxylation deficiency.

Calcitriol [1–25 (OH) 2D3] is indicated in conditions of 1-alpha-hydroxylase enzyme deficiency (e.g., moderate-to-severe renal insufficiency, hypoparathyroidism, and mutations of the 1-alpha-hydroxylase enzyme encoding gene) or of intestinal malabsorption [3, 11].

With the updated knowledge, it cannot be assumed that calcium and vitamin D supplementation alone is an effective treatment for osteoporosis, even if all patients must be guaranteed an adequate intake of both. While a sufficient intake of calcium can be obtained with the diet, this is not feasible for vitamin D, which must be supplemented exogenously.

Medical Therapy

Anti-Catabolic Drugs

Bisphosphonates

1. Aminobisphosphonates have a potency of 10 to 1000 times higher than those not containing an amino group. The mainly used drugs belonging to this category are as follows:

   (a) Alendronate (70 mg/week) and risedronate (35 mg/week or 75 mg × 2 days/month) efficacy for the prevention of vertebral and non-vertebral fractures (including those of the femur) has been extensively documented.
   (b) Ibandronate (150 mg/month p.o).
   (c) Zoledronate (5 mg/iv/year) was approved for the treatment of osteoporosis based on a study clearly documenting a reduction in the risk of vertebral, non-vertebral, and hip fractures after 3 years of treatment.

   Alendronate, risedronate, and zoledronate have also been approved for the treatment of male and glucocorticoid-induced osteoporosis (GIO).

   In order to minimize the risk of subtrochanteric fracture in patients undergoing therapy with bisphosphonates, it may be useful:

   (a) To consider periods of "drug holiday," after careful evaluation of the risk-to-benefit ratio.
   (b) To correct and monitor other risk factors for atypical fracture (e.g., chronic use of glucocorticoids, hypovitaminosis D, chronic use of proton-pump inhibitors, and presence of skeletal diseases other than osteoporosis) [12].

   A very rare adverse event in patients undergoing bisphosphonates therapy is the ONJ (osteonecrosis of the jaw or osteomyelitis of the jaw). The risk to develop ONJ during treatment increases if the patient undergoes oral interventions with exposure to the bone tissue. Other individual risk factors for this adverse event are diabetes, immunosuppression, steroid use, smoking, and alcohol consumption.

   Based on the available data, a risk reassessment should be made after 5 years of treatment with alendronate, ibandronate, or risedronate and after 3 years with zoledronate.

   A 12- to 24-month suspension of treatment (drug holiday) appears beneficial in patients on oral bisphosphonate therapy for more than 5 years at low risk of fractures. Instead, it is recommended to continue treatment uninterruptedly for up to 10 years in patient at a higher risk.
2. Non-Aminobisphosphonates.

   Clodronate (200 mg/i.m./2–4 weeks) is predominantly eliminated by the kidney; therefore, adequate fluid intake must be ensured during the whole treatment. For the aminobisphosphonates, this drug has been associated with rare cases of ONJ [13].

Denosumab

Denosumab is a human monoclonal antibody capable of neutralizing RANKL (receptor activator of the nuclear factor B ligand), a cytokine, which, by interacting with the RANK receptor on the membrane of mature pre-osteoclasts and osteoclasts, affects their recruitment, maturation, and survival. The pivotal trials were conducted using 60 mg subcutaneous injection of denosumab every 6 months.

Denosumab has been proven effective in reducing the risk of fracture in breast cancer patients treated with aromatase inhibitors and in prostate cancer patients treated with antiandrogens. Unlike bisphosphonates, discontinuation of denosumab treatment is followed by a sharp increase in bone turnover and a rapid loss of BMD. Therefore, if discontinuation of denosumab is considered, it is generally recommended to immediately start another therapy with antiresorptive agents. Treatment with denosumab can sometimes cause hypocalcemia, which must be addressed and prevented with adequate calcium and vitamin D supplementation. Rare cases of ONJ and atypical femoral fractures have been observed in post-registration studies.

Hormone Replacement Therapy (HRT)

In postmenopausal women, treatments with estrogen, alone or in combination with progestins, and with tibolone are able to reduce bone turnover and increase bone mass.

Selective Estrogen Receptor Modulators (SERMs)

SERMSs are synthetic compounds able to bind the estrogen receptor and produce agonist effects on bone and liver and antagonist effects on breast and genitourinary tissues. Raloxifene and bazedoxifene are the SERMs currently approved in Italy for the prevention and treatment of osteoporosis. In the pivotal MORE study [14], raloxifene (60 mg/day) reduced the incidence of new vertebral fractures; however, no improvement was observed in non-vertebral and femoral ones. Bazedoxifene (20 mg/ day) significantly reduced the risk of vertebral and non-vertebral (excluding femoral) fractures in women at high risk treated for 3–5 years. SERMs, like HRT, are associated with an increased risk of thromboembolic events and are therefore not recommended in patients who have already had or are at an increased risk of venous thrombosis [15].

Anabolic Drugs

Teriparatide

The administration of the 1–34 parathormone (PTH) active fragment (also known as teriparatide) stimulates both bone formation and resorption, with particularly evident prevalence of bone neoformation (anabolic window) in the first 12 months of treatment. The major beneficial effects of treatment on BMD values were observed in trabecular bone, with a slight improvement of fracture resistance in the cortical bone due to structural remodeling. Teriparatide (20 µg/s.c./day) has been shown to reduce vertebral and non-vertebral fractures in postmenopausal women, but its administration cannot exceed a total of 24 months.

Teriparatide is contraindicated in patients with hyperparathyroidism, Paget's disease of the bone, severe renal insufficiency, primary or metastatic cancer of the skeleton or in patient who underwent previous skeletal radiotherapy [7].

Double-Acting Drugs

Strontium Ranelate

Treatment with strontium ranelate has been associated with an increased risk of myocardial infarction and thromboembolic events; therefore, it is contraindicated in patients with known or current ischemic heart diseases, peripheral arterial diseases, cerebrovascular diseases, or uncontrolled arterial hypertension. The densitometric increases observed during therapy are about 50% related to the greater molecular weight of strontium compared to calcium [16].

Romosozumab

Romosozumab (105 mg/s.c./2 × day simultaneously in two different sites per month × 12 months) is a humanized monoclonal antibody directed against sclerostin, a glycoprotein secreted by osteocytes, which plays a fundamental role as an inhibitor of osteoblastic activity. Its main effect is to increase the activity of osteoblasts and new bone formation; however, studies have also shown an inhibitory effect on osteoclasts and, consequently, an antiresorptive activity. In the pivotal study, romosozumab was shown to be able to reduce the incidence of vertebral fractures and significantly increase BMD, already after just one year of therapy. The major contraindication criteria are cardiovascular events. The clinical application of this drug has been approved in Italy in 2020 by the AIFA (Agenzia Italiana del Farmaco), effectively becoming a treatment choice [17–19].

Vertebroplasty and Kyphoplasty

Vertebroplasty and kyphoplasty are both surgical procedures based on the injection of cement in fractured vertebrae to restore their supporting capacities. The major difference between the two is that in vertebroplasty the cement is injected at high pressure with a greater risk of leakage and pulmonary embolism, while in kyphoplasty the cement is introduced at low pressure, after the introduction of a balloon, which is subsequently swollen within the vertebral body, resulting in a lower risk of leakage.

Given the possible risks associated and the uncertain long-term benefits, these procedures are recommended only for patients with intractable pain lasting weeks [20].

Fracture Liaison Service (FLS)

FLS is a diagnostic–therapeutic pathway, implemented within healthcare facilities, with the aim of reducing the treatment gap in patients with osteoporotic fractures and improving communication between the various healthcare professionals involved. They represent the most common, economically and clinically effective coordinated model for secondary fracture prevention.

Developed for the first time in the UK at the end of the 90 s, they are also spreading in Italy, with some experiences already active and others being defined and implemented nowadays [21, 22].

Sexuality and Quality of Life

Osteoporosis is a widespread disease: It is estimated that over 200 million people are affected worldwide. In Italy, it affects about 5,000,000 people, over 80% of whom are postmenopausal women. Osteoporosis causes almost 100,000 admissions for femoral neck fractures in Italy every year, with serious consequences in terms of social costs: Mortality within 1 year of fracture is 20%, while 30% of patients suffer permanent disability with 40% losing the ability to walk independently [23].

To this end, in 2021 the North American Menopause Society (NAMS) set out its clear position on the management of osteoporosis in postmenopausal women [24].

NAMS enlisted a panel of clinical experts in the field of metabolic bone disease and/or women's health to review and update the 2010 NAMS position statement and recommendations based on new evidence and clinical judgments. The panel's recommendations were reviewed and approved by the NAMS Board of Trustees.

Postmenopausal bone loss, related to estrogen deficiency, is the leading cause of osteoporosis other than advanced age, genetics, smoking, thinness, and many diseases and medications that compromise bone health. An assessment of these risk factors to identify candidates for osteoporosis screening and recommending non-pharmacological measures such as good nutrition (especially adequate intake of protein, calcium, and vitamin D), regular physical activity, and avoidance of smoking and excessive alcohol consumption is appropriate for all postmenopausal women.

For women at high risk of osteoporosis, particularly perimenopausal women with low bone density and other risk factors, estrogen or other therapies are available to prevent bone loss. For women with osteoporosis and/or other fracture risk factors (including advanced age and previous fractures), the main goal of therapy is to prevent new fractures. This is achieved by combining non-pharmacological measures, drugs to increase bone density and improve bone strength, and strategies to reduce the risk of falling.

The recent study by Angın et al. [25] investigated the effects of clinical Pilates exercises on bone mineral density (BMD), physical performance, and quality of life (QOL) in postmenopausal osteoporosis.

A total of 41 patients were recruited and divided into two groups: the Pilates group and the control group. The subjects were assessed for BMD in the lumbar region. The level of physical performance was measured. The level of pain intensity was assessed with the visual analog scale. *QUALEFFO-41* was used to assess QOL.

Results BMD values increased in the Pilates group ($p < 0.05$), while they decreased in the control group ($p < 0.05$). The results of the physical performance test showed significant increases in the Pilates group ($p < 0.05$), while there was no change in the control group ($p > 0.05$). The level of pain intensity in the Pilates group was significantly decreased after exercise ($p < 0.05$), while it was unchanged in the control group. There were significant increases in all QOL parameters in the Pilates group. In contrast, some QOL parameters showed decreases in the control group ($p < 0.05$).

The study by Küçükçakır et al. [26] also evaluated the effects of the Pilates exercise program on pain, functional status, and quality of life in women with postmenopausal osteoporosis. The study was conducted as a randomized, prospective, controlled, single-blind study. *Seventy women (age range, 45–65 years) diagnosed with postmenopausal osteoporosis were included.*

Patients were randomly assigned to two groups (home exercise group and Pilates). Patients in the Pilates exercise group underwent a supervised Pilates exercise program twice a week for 1 year. Patients in the home exercise group were asked to perform a home exercise program consisting of chest extension exercises. The patients were evaluated at baseline and after 1 year of participation in the exercise programs.

The visual analog scale for pain, six-minute walk, and sit-to-stand tests for functional status and the *QUALEFFO-41 and Short Form-36 (SF-36)* questionnaire for quality of life were used. Patients were also asked to report the number of falls during the investigation.

At the end of the study, the results of 60 patients were analyzed. A significant improvement was noted in all assessment parameters at the end of the exercise program in the Pilates exercise group. With the exception of *QUALEFFO* (pertaining to leisure activities, physical role limitation subscales SF-36, and emotional role limitation), at the end of the program a significant improvement was noted in all other evaluation parameters in the control group. The Pilates group showed a slight improvement in mood and physical movement disorder, while the group following the home exercise regime showed lower QOL levels.

The socialization and playful aspect of the Pilates group exercises could have influenced the stimulation of a psychic feeling of gratification despite movement limitations and pain.

There is more. Scientific literature has also investigated the issue of osteoporosis prevention after breast cancer diagnosis.

Recently, a group of experts in the UK developed guidelines for the prevention of bone loss. The main recommendations concern bone loss in women who enter premature menopause before the age of 45 due to cancer surgery or who are receiving hormone suppression therapy [27].

As they are at high risk of significant bone loss, these women should have a baseline dual-energy X-ray absorptiometry (DXA) assessment of BMD. Since randomized clinical trials in postmenopausal women indicate that bisphosphonates prevent bone loss and accelerate bone turnover associated with aromatase inhibitor therapy, their use is recommended as the main preventive therapy, together with a healthy lifestyle and adequate calcium and vitamin D intake.

Conclusion

Osteoporosis is a common disorder in postmenopausal women. The management of skeletal health in postmenopausal women involves assessment of risk factors for fracture, changes in diet and lifestyle, and the use of drug therapy for patients at significant risk of osteoporosis or fracture. For women with osteoporosis, ongoing management is required. Treatment decisions are made continuously throughout a postmenopausal woman's life. Decisions must be individualized and should include the patient in the shared decision-making process. This is not to give up on sexuality: restriction of movement, hypoactive libido, and vaginal dryness often appear to be limiting factors; however, one should never forget one's sexual role and identity.

References

1. Abrahamsen B, Van Staa T, Ariely R, Olson M, Cooper C. Excess mortality following hip fracture: a systematic epidemiological review [Internet]. Osteoporos Int. 2009 [cited 2021 May 24];20:1633–1650. Available from: https://pubmed.ncbi.nlm.nih.gov/19421703/.
2. WHO. WHO Study Group. Assessment of fracture risk and its application to screening for postmenopausal osteoporosis. World Health Organ Tech Rep Ser. 1994;1994(843):1–129.
3. Rossini M, Adami S, Bertoldo F, Diacinti D, Gatti D, Giannini S, et al. Linee guida per la diagnosi, la prevenzione ed il trattamento dell'osteoporosi. Reumatismo. 2016;68(1):1–42.
4. Pothuaud L, Carceller P, Hans D. Correlations between grey-level variations in 2D projection images (TBS) and 3D microarchitecture: applications in the study of human trabecular bone microarchitecture. Bone [Internet]. 2008 [cited 2021 May 26];42(4):775–87. Available from: https://pubmed.ncbi.nlm.nih.gov/18234577/.
5. Hernlund E, Svedbom A, Ivergård M, Compston J, Cooper C, Stenmark J, et al. Osteoporosis in the European Union: medical management, epidemiology and economic burden: a report prepared in collaboration with the International Osteoporosis Foundation (IOF) and the European Federation of Pharmaceutical Industry Associations (EFPIA). Arch Osteoporos [Internet] 2013 [cited 2021 May 24];8(1–2). Available from: https://pubmed.ncbi.nlm.nih.gov/24113837/.

6. Brunader R, Shelton DK. Radiologic bone assessment in the evaluation of osteoporosis [Internet], vol. 65, American Family Physician; 2002 [cited 2021 Apr 4]. Available from: www.aafp.org/afp.

7. Rossini M, Adami S, Bertoldo F, Diacinti D, Gatti D, Giannini S, et al. Guidelines for the diagnosis, prevention and management of osteoporosis. Reumatismo. 2016;68(1):1–39.

8. Hernlund E, Svedbom A, Ivergård M, Compston J, Cooper C, Stenmark J, et al. Osteoporosis in the European Union: medical management, epidemiology and economic burden: a report prepared in collaboration with the International Osteoporosis Foundation (IOF) and the European Federation of Pharmaceutical Industry Associations (EFPIA). Arch Osteoporos [Internet]. 2013 [cited 2021 Apr 1];8(1–2). Available from: https://pubmed.ncbi.nlm.nih.gov/24113837/.

9. Cosman F, de Beur SJ, LeBoff MS, Lewiecki EM, Tanner B, Randall S, et al. Clinician's Guide to Prevention and Treatment of Osteoporosis. Osteoporos Int [Internet]. 2014 [cited 2021 Apr 8];25(10):2359–81. Available from: https://pubmed.ncbi.nlm.nih.gov/25182228/.

10. Tsourdi E, Zillikens MC, Meier C, Body JJ, Gonzalez Rodriguez E, Anastasilakis AD, et al. Fracture risk and management of discontinuation of denosumab therapy: a systematic review and position statement by ECTS. J Clin Endocrinol Metab [Internet] 2021 [cited 2021 May 24];106(1):264–281. Available from: https://pubmed.ncbi.nlm.nih.gov/33103722/.

11. Khundmiri SJ, Murray RD, Lederer E. PTH and vitamin D. Compr Physiol. 2016;6(2):561–601.

12. Gralow JR, Biermann JS, Farooki A, Fornier MN, Gagel RF, Kumar RN, et al. NCCN task force report: bone health in cancer care [Internet]. J Natl Compr Cancer Netw. 2009 [cited 2021 Apr 22];7. Available from: https://pubmed.ncbi.nlm.nih.gov/19555589/.

13. McCloskey E, Paterson AH, Powles T, Kanis JA. Clodronate. Bone [Internet]. 2020 [cited 2021 Apr 8];143. Available from: https://pubmed.ncbi.nlm.nih.gov/33127577/.

14. Agnusdei D, Iori N. Raloxifene: results from the MORE study. J Musculoskelet Neuronal Interact [Internet]. 2000;1(2):127–32. Available from: http://www.ncbi.nlm.nih.gov/pubmed/15758505.

15. Yavropoulou MP, Makras P, Anastasilakis AD. Bazedoxifene for the treatment of osteoporosis. Expert Opin Pharmacother [Internet]. 2019 [cited 2021 Apr 8];20(10):1201–10. Available from: https://www.tandfonline.com/doi/full/10.1080/14656566.2019.1615882.

16. Rossini M, Adami G, Adami S, Viapiana O, Gatti D. Safety issues and adverse reactions with osteoporosis management [Internet], vol. 15. Expert Opinion on Drug Safety. Taylor and Francis Ltd; 2016 [cited 2021 Apr 8]. p. 321–2. Available from: https://pubmed.ncbi.nlm.nih.gov/26699669/.

17. Cosman F, Crittenden DB, Adachi JD, Binkley N, Czerwinski E, Ferrari S, et al. Romosozumab treatment in postmenopausal women with osteoporosis. N Engl J Med [Internet]. 2016 [cited 2021 May 24];375(16):1532–43. Available from: https://pubmed.ncbi.nlm.nih.gov/27641143/.

18. Cosman F, Crittenden DB, Ferrari S, Khan A, Lane NE, Lippuner K, et al. FRAME study: the foundation effect of building bone with 1 year of romosozumab leads to continued lower fracture risk after transition to denosumab. J Bone Miner Res [Internet] 2018 [cited 2021 May 24];33(7):1219–1226. Available from: https://pubmed.ncbi.nlm.nih.gov/29573473/.

19. Saag KG, Petersen J, Brandi ML, Karaplis AC, Lorentzon M, Thomas T, et al. Romosozumab or Alendronate for Fracture Prevention in Women with Osteoporosis. N Engl J Med [Internet]. 2017 [cited 2021 May 24];377(15):1417–27. Available from: https://pubmed.ncbi.nlm.nih.gov/28892457/.

20. Chandra R V., Maingard J, Asadi H, Slater LA, Mazwi TL, Marcia S, et al. Vertebroplasty and kyphoplasty for osteoporotic vertebral fractures: what are the latest data? [Internet], vol. 39.American Journal of Neuroradiology; 2018 [cited 2021 Apr 10]. p. 798–806. Available from: https://pubmed.ncbi.nlm.nih.gov/29170272/.

21. Fuggle NR, Kassim Javaid M, Fujita M, Halbout P, Dawson-Hughes B, Rizzoli R, et al. Fracture risk assessment and how to implement a fracture liaison service. In: 2021 [cited 2021 May 26]. p. 241–56. Available from: https://pubmed.ncbi.nlm.nih.gov/33347219/.

22. Chadha M, Shingare A, Prasanth A, Chauhan P, Shah NF. Fracture liaison service: prevention by coordination [Internet], vol. 22. Ind J Endocrinol Metab. Wolters Kluwer Medknow

Publications; 2018 [cited 2021 May 26]. p. 719–21. Available from: https://pubmed.ncbi.nlm.nih.gov/30766806/.

23. Greco EA, Migliaccio S, Marcocci C, et al. Therapeutic appropriateness in osteoporosis. Endocrinologist. 2017;18:153–8.

24. Management of osteoporosis in postmenopausal women: the 2021 position statement of the North American Menopause Society. Menopause. 2021;28(9):973–97.

25. Angın E, Erden Z, Can F. The effects of clinical pilates exercises on bone mineral density, physical performance and quality of life of women with postmenopausal osteoporosis. J Back Musculoskelet Rehabil. 2015;28(4):849–58.

26. Küçükçakır N, Altan L, Korkmaz N. Effects of Pilates exercises on pain, functional status and quality of life in women with postmenopausal osteoporosis. J Bodyw Mov Ther. 2013;17(2):204–11.

27. Reid DM. Prevention of osteoporosis after breast cancer. Maturitas. 2009;64(1):4–8. https://doi.org/10.1016/j.maturitas.2009.07.008. Epub 2009 Aug 25. PMID: 19709826.

Part XVII
Psychiatry

Persistent Depressive Disorder (Dysthymia) and Recurrent Unipolar Major Depressive Disorder

Irene Pinucci, Massimo Pasquini, and Elena Vittoria Longhi

Historical Background/Introduction

The term depression comes from the Latin *"depressio"* and indicates a state of dejection perceived by the subject accompanied by extreme suffering and discomfort. *"Melancholia"* (*melas* means black and *cholé* means bile), the term historically used to describe this condition, was first introduced by Hippocrates in the treatise *On the Nature of Man* [1] based on the humoral theories of Alcmaeon of Croton and then resumed by Galen, who described a melancholic temperament characterized by a black bile excess. This belief was still solid in the sixteenth century, when the French physician Andreas Laurentius related the cause of this pathology to the "coldness and darkness of this humor." In the nineteenth century, Pinel eventually proposed a new theory discontinuing the connection between humor and black bile and describing four new mental disorders, which included Melancholia and Mania [2]. Kraepelin unified all types of affective disorders in the unitary concept of manic-depressive illness, which included "periodic circular insanities," "mania," and "melancholy" [3]. In opposition to this view, Wernicke distinguished five different types of melancholia, going back to taking into consideration the possibility of single episodes of melancholia [4]. Nowadays, the term melancholic represents a subtype of major depressive disorder.

I. Pinucci · M. Pasquini (✉)
Department of Human Neurosciences, SAPIENZA University of Rome, Rome, Italy
e-mail: irene.pinucci@uniroma1.it; massimo.pasquini@uniroma1.it

E. V. Longhi
Department of Sexual Medical Center, San Raffaele Hospital, Milano, Italy

© Springer Nature Switzerland AG 2023
E. V. Longhi (ed.), *Managing Psychosexual Consequences in Chronic Diseases*,
https://doi.org/10.1007/978-3-031-31307-3_31

Clinical Manifestation

Core symptoms that constitute the current definition of depression include depressed mood and anhedonia (reduced ability to experience pleasure from natural rewards) accompanied by neurovegetative symptoms (abnormalities in appetite and sleeps), sexual dysfunction, feelings of worthlessness, alterations in psychomotor skills and in cognitive area, and recurrent thoughts of death.

Epidemiological investigations show how depressive disorder has the highest lifetime prevalence of any psychiatric disorder. Lifetime prevalence for major depressive disorder varies between 5% and 17%. This type of episode can be resolved completely or partially in about two-thirds of cases and is not resolved in about a third. Dysthymia has 3–6% lifetime prevalence and an age of onset at about 20 years. Recurrent brief depressive disorder has an estimated lifetime prevalence of 16% [5].

Patients suffering from depressive disorders frequently describe a feeling of depression, hopelessness, guilt, worthlessness, and inadequacy, sometimes accompanied by a pervasive state of concern, irritability, loss of appetite, weight loss, and insomnia. Typical manifestation of this syndrome is asthenia, agitation or psychomotor slowing (mutism and stupor), and, on the cognitive level, memory gaps, and, with difficulty concentrating, decreased libido. Recurrent ideas of death and suicide are found in the most severe depressions [6]. It is not uncommon for patients to report having lost the ability to feel emotions and hopes for healing; in some cases, these beliefs can assume a delusional nature, especially of a nihilistic type (delusion of guilt, ruin, bodily denial, Cotard delusion) or hypochondriac type. Hallucinations may also be present in the form of accusatory voices or visions of deceased people, accompanied by a strong sense of guilt. If present, both delusions and hallucinations are usually mood-congruent.

Definition and Classification of DSM-5

The DSM-5, introduced in 2013, classifies depressive disorders and bipolar disorders separately, removing the broad category of mood disorders [6].

Among the five symptoms necessary for the diagnosis of a major depressive episode, the DSM-5 signals the depressed mood and the loss of pleasure or interest and then lists a series of other symptoms of the abovementioned areas associated with nuclear symptoms, which must be present for at least 2 weeks.

The DSM-5 includes a new classification of chronic depression introducing persistent depressive disorder (dysthymia), which represents a consolidation of DSM-IV-defined chronic major depressive disorder and dysthymic disorder. This change was caused by the evidence showing the difficulty of differentiating the two diagnoses and their frequent co-occurrence [7]. Persistent depressive disorder is diagnosed when a depressed mood and two or more between a list of six symptoms (poor appetite/overeating, insomnia/hypersomnia, low energy/fatigue, low self-esteem, poor concentration or difficulty making decisions, and feelings of hopelessness) are present for at least 2 years (Table 1). During this period, any symptom-free interval must last no longer than 2 months (Table 2).

Table 1 Persistent depressive disorder (dysthymia) diagnostic criteria according to DSM-5

A. Depressed mood for most of the day, for more days than not, as indicated by either subjective account or observation by others, for at least 2 years **Note**: In children and adolescents, mood can be irritable and duration must be at least 1 year
B. Presence, while depressed, of two (or more) of the following: 1. Poor appetite or overeating 2. Insomnia or hypersomnia 3. Low energy or fatigue 4. Low self-esteem 5. Poor concentration or difficulty making decisions 6. Feelings of hopelessness
C. During the 2-year period (1 year for children or adolescents) of the disturbance, the individual has never been without the symptoms in criteria A and B for more than 2 months at a time
D. Criteria for a major depressive disorder may be continuously present for 2 years
E. There has never been a manic episode or a hypomanic episode, and criteria have never been met for cyclothymic disorder
F. The disturbance is not better explained by a persistent schizoaffective disorder, schizophrenia, delusional disorder, or other specified or unspecified schizophrenia spectrum and other psychotic disorder
G. The symptoms are not attributable to the physiological effects of a substance (e.g., a drug of abuse and medication) or another medical condition (e.g., hypothyroidism)
H. The symptoms cause clinically significant distress or impairment in social, occupational, or other important areas of functioning

Table 2 Major depressive disorder diagnostic criteria according to DSM-5

A. Five (or more) of the following symptoms have been present during the same 2-week period and represent a change from previous functioning; at least one of the symptoms is either (1) depressed mood or (2) loss of interest or pleasure **Note:** Do not include symptoms that are clearly attributable to another medical condition 1. Depressed mood most of the day, nearly every day, as indicated by either subjective report (e.g., feels sad, empty, and hopeless) or observation made by others (e.g., appears tearful). (**note**: In children and adolescents, can be an irritable mood) 2. Markedly diminished interest or pleasure in all, or almost all, activities most of the day, nearly every day (as indicated by either subjective account or observation) 3. Significant weight loss when not dieting or weight gain (e.g., a change of more than 5% of body weight in a month), or decrease or increase in appetite nearly every day. (**note:** In children, consider failure to make expected weight gain) 4. Insomnia or hypersomnia nearly every day 5. Psychomotor agitation or retardation nearly every day (observable by others, not merely subjective feelings of restlessness or being slowed down) 6. Fatigue or loss of energy nearly every day 7. Feelings of worthlessness or excessive or inappropriate guilt (which may be delusional) nearly every day (not merely self-reproach or guilt about being sick) 8. Diminished ability to think or concentrate, or indecisiveness, nearly every day (either by subjective account or as observed by others) 9. Recurrent thoughts of death (not just fear of dying), recurrent suicidal ideation without a specific plan, or a suicide attempt or a specific plan for committing suicide
B. The symptoms cause clinically significant distress or impairment in social, occupational, or other important areas of functioning
C. The episode is not attributable to the psychological effects of a substance or to another medical condition

Pathophysiology

Several factors are involved in the pathophysiology of depressive disorder such as life events, genetics, neurotransmitters, and neuroendocrine alterations. No single mechanism seems to be able to explain every aspect of this disease. Premorbid personality traits and psychosocial and biological stressors could contribute to the development of a depressive disorder and eventually of a persistent/recurrent form. The depressogenic role of scarce coping resources when facing stressful life events was recently introduced by Tellenbach, who described a personality vulnerable to the development of depression (melancholia) called Typus Melancholicus [8]. The constitutive traits of this personality are orderliness, conscientiousness, hyper/heteronomy, and intolerance to ambiguity, and they represent the nucleus through which the vulnerability to depressive syndrome is expressed. Typus Melancholicus is considered a fundamental construct for understanding the premorbid and intermorbid personality structure liable to the previously defined "endogenous depression." In this regard, it is important to notice that within the current nosographic classification, the "endogenous" and "reactive" opposition was abandoned. In the most recent edition of the Classification of Mental and Behavioural Disorders of the World Health Organization (ICD-10), the adjective "endogenous" was replaced by the term "somatic" and was used to characterize the depressive episode under the symptomatological point of view. Major depressive disorder with Melancholia is a subtype that is interpreted as a clinico-descriptive value, beyond any etiopathogenetic implication.

On the other hand, according to the cognitive model of personality, a depressive personality style is well documented and results to be often undiagnosed or misdiagnosed as a dysthymic disorder. Bowlby named "avoidant" certain attachment behaviors that would lead to a pattern of dysfunctional organization together with early trauma experiences [9]. Children without a secure-base attachment figure are prone to a constant self-referral with a lack of social interactions that emphasize their sense of loneliness. Thus, personal identity will be based on emotional reactions to the experience of loss that return in feelings of desperation, anger, and hopelessness. The depressive personality organization entails a "self-meaning" of loneliness and a particular sensitivity to every loss situation that could happen during life.

In a more complex conception, it is believed that between a stressful event, a personality trait, and a mood disorder there is an interactive—rather than casual—connection, in which a series of genetic, biological, psychological, and environmental factors are involved. Constitutional predisposition and stressing factors are considered complementary based on a psycho-socio-biological model, which allows a unified interpretation of the adaptive process in their dynamic becoming.

Among the identified involved factors, several studies have highlighted how coping styles and the defense mechanisms used by individuals play a fundamental role in the development of depressive symptomatology. More in detail, research has shown that coping styles mainly based on avoidance mechanisms and immature or primitive defense mechanisms are more correlated with anxiety and depressive disorders. The complex interaction between coping styles and defense mechanisms could provide further elements to better understand how individuals relate to the disease.

Coping skills are the turning point to understand how similar stimuli can elicit different responses even from a neurobiological point of view. Following a stressful life event, many neurotransmitters, hormones, and cytokines work in order to produce a stress response aimed at maintaining homeostasis. The hypothalamic–pituitary–adrenal axis (HPA), in response to stress and modulated by amygdala and prefrontal cortex, cooperate with the nervous and immune system for the fight or flight reaction. Major depression is strongly associated with hyperactivity of the HPA [10–12] and an increased amount of plasma cortisol. Cortisol imbalance is due to the increased CRH production of the hypothalamus, which communicates with the sympathetic system as an acute response determining a release of adrenalin and noradrenalin in response to a perceived dangerous event. An anxiolytic response balancing the fight or flight CRH response is activated by peptides called urocortins. Both CRH and urocortins are regulated by glucocorticoids. Cortisol hyperproduction and CRH overdrive determine an alteration in the balance of monoamines and neuronal atrophy in the amygdala and in several areas of the prefrontal cortex. While an acute stress response activates the monoamines, the chronic stress response determines a reduced activity of serotoninergic, dopaminergic, and noradrenergic neurons.

The "monoamine hypothesis," positing that depression is caused by decreased monoamine function in the brain, derives from the observation made in the mid-twentieth century that the anti-hypertension drugs that would reduce the amount of monoamine could cause depression in a subset of patients. Such theory was supported by the evidence of a "mood elevation" caused by monoamine oxidase inhibitors (MAOIs) and by tricyclic drugs, which increased the availability and excitatory effect of neurotransmitters. Today's antidepressant drugs offer lower rates of side effects, but their efficacy is still linked to the increase in monoamine transmission. Although these drugs produce immediate increases in monoamine transmission, weeks of treatment are required in order to establish mood-enhancing properties. These characteristics led to hypothesis that their efficacy could be linked to secondary neuroplastic changes involving transcriptional and translational changes mediating cellular and molecular plasticity [13].

Studies investigating the genetic contribution to the development of a depressive disorder showed a higher-than-chance incidence of depression among first-degree relatives. Twin studies suggest that genes account for 40–50% of the susceptibility to major depressive disorder in the population [14]. The most accepted hypothesis suggests that different genes interact with the environment increasing the individual's susceptibility [15].

The role of functional polymorphisms in a small set of genes, which could be involved in monoaminergic neurotransmission and in the development and resistance to treatment of depressive disorder, was studied. Most of them are implicated in the synthesis, degradation, or neurotransmission of serotonin (5-HT). Current research comprises the loci encoding the serotonin transporter SLC6A4 and its methylation [16, 17], the limiting enzyme for dopamine synthesis called tyrosine hydroxylase (TH) [18], the serotonin 2A receptor (5HTR2A), and the tryptophan hydroxylase 1 (TPH1) [19]. Other genes that have been studied are involved in dopamine catabolism (COMT) [20] and the dopamine receptor (DRD4). Regarding dysthymia and recurrent depressive disorder, some studies recently focused on the role of TCF4 gene [21] and circadian clock genes [22] on their etiopathogenesis.

It is noticed that a recent study on large samples focused on 18 genes empirically identified as commonly studied in the last 25 years and do not support previous depression candidate genes findings. It was posited that early hypotheses about depression candidate genes were incorrect and that the large number of associations reported are likely to be false positive [23].

Following works studying the adaptive functions of anxiety, an expanding body of literature has focused on functional explanation of depressive disorder, proposing mood states as the target for an evolutionary analysis. According to these views, depression serves as a method for, de-escalation, energy conservation and for bonding to caregiver. The social risk hypothesis, integrating the over mentioned theories, suggests that depressive phenomena can be considered a defensive psychobiological response to increased risk of exclusion from social contexts vital to dealing with adaptive, socio-reproductive challenges [24].

Assessment

Besides the abovementioned DSM-5 classification, also the International Classification of Diseases (ICD) relies on the presence of a number of key symptoms. Recurrent depressive disorder can be diagnosed when repeated episodes of depression are present without any episode of mania; dysthymia can be diagnosed when a depression of mood is not sufficiently severe or prolonged to diagnose a depressive disorder that lasts at least several years [25]. It is important to notice that a fundamental approach to diagnose a depressive syndrome is the clinical evaluation. Besides the formerly mentioned symptoms, clinical manifestations can be found in signs such as deceleration and reduction in the speech rate, scarce facial expression, frequent crying, and poor care of one's appearance. Activation and anxiety could be present, and affective involvement could be exaggerated or poor. In some cases, somatization is the principal mean of expression of depressive syndrome, especially in elderly patients [26] or some ethnocultural groups [27, 28]. Once depressive syndrome is diagnosed, several tools can be used to assess its severity and to measure the outcomes of the interventions. The Beck Depression Inventory (BDI) [29], the Montgomery–Åsberg Depression Rating Scale (MADRS) [30], and the Hamilton Depression Scale HAM-D [31] are administered by a mental health professional, while the Zung Self-Rating Depression Scale [32] is a self-administered tool. It is also important to provide an in-depth investigation into the suicidal ideation and behavior of patients presenting a depressive syndrome. The

Columbia Suicide Severity Rating Scale (C-SSRS) [33] represents a fundamental tool for its exploration.

Treatments

In 2009, the National Institute for Health and Care Excellence published guidelines for the recognition and management of depression in adults, updated in 2018. The proposed stepped-care model provides a sequence of interventions starting from the most effective and less intrusive one (assessment, support, psychoeducation, active monitoring, and referral for further assessment and interventions) to evolve, when necessary, into more targeted interventions. Step 3 and step 4 are dedicated to mild-to-severe forms of depression resistant to treatment for which proposed therapies start from medication, high-intensity psychological interventions, combined treatment, and collaborative care for step 3 with the addition of ECT, crisis service, and multiprofessional and inpatient care in addition for step 4.

In 2016, the Canadian Network for Mood and Anxiety Treatment published an update of the evidence-based clinical guidelines for the treatment of depressive disorder published in 2009 [34]. The first of the six sections is dedicated to psychological treatments, which are especially indicated in moderately severe and low-risk cases, depending on patient preferences, and availability of treatment, with the exclusion of psychotic depression. CANMAT guidelines report studies that showed the comparison in the efficacy of specific models of psychological treatments and propose a list of recommendations. The efficacy in comparison with control groups—and not to other psychological treatments—is expressed by the first- to third-line treatments.

Cognitive-behavioral therapy (CBT), interpersonal therapy (IPT), and behavioral activation (BA) are first-line acute treatments, while CBT together with mindfulness-based cognitive therapy (MBCT) are first-line maintenance treatments. Either CBT or IPT combined with SSRIs or TCAs shows more effectiveness compared to psychological treatment alone and psychological treatment with a placebo or with antidepressants alone [35, 36] (Table 3).

Starting from the mid-twentieth century, pharmacotherapy for depressive symptoms has been founded on the enhancement of monoaminergic neurotransmission, but newer antidepressant agents target different brain systems such as melatonin, NMDA receptors, or GABA. Available antidepressants act on postsynaptic and pre-synaptic receptors and neurotransmitter transporters, and they may be classified according to many aspects, notably based on their principal pharmacological action as in the proposed Table 4. Pharmacodynamics and pharmacokinetics of different classes go beyond the scope of this paper.

The effectiveness of continuation and maintenance treatments for persistent depressive disorder was recently investigated. Ten studies were described comparing pharmacological (SSRIs, MOIs, SNDRIs, TCAs), placebo, and psychological therapies in seven different combinations. Five studies showed to favor continuation

Table 3 Recommendation for psychological treatment for acute and maintenance treatments of major depressive disorder. Partly adapted from CANMAT guidelines

	Acute treatment	Maintenance treatment (relapse prevention)
Cognitive-behavioral therapy (CBT)	First line	First line
Interpersonal therapy (IPT)	First line	Second line
Behavioral activation (BA)	First line	Second line
Mindfulness-based cognitive therapy	Second line	First line

Table 4 Principal pharmacological actions

Class	Drugs
TCAs	Amitriptyline, clomipramine, doxepin, imipramine, nortriptyline, trimipramine
MAOIs	Tranylcypromine, moclobemide, phenelzine
SSRIs	Citalopram, escitalopram, fluoxetine, fluvoxamine, paroxetine, sertraline
SNRIs	Desvenlafaxine, duloxetine, levomilnacipran, milnacipran, venlafaxine
NDRIs	Bupropion
SMSs	Vortioxetine
Others	Mirtazapine, trazodone, agomelatine, tianeptine, sulpiride/amisulpride, mianserin

and maintenance pharmacotherapy as an effective treatment to prevent relapse and recurrence in persistent depressive disorder compared to placebo. Nevertheless, this primary outcome did not reach significance when only studies with a low risk of bias were included. An appropriate duration of assumption was not drawn emphasizing the need for further studies. Concerning psychotherapy, it was assumed that maintained active psychotherapy has a positive effect on depression outcomes and on relapse or recurrence rate of depression. No statistically significant differences were found when comparing combined psychological and pharmacological continuation and maintenance therapy with therapies alone [37]. It is important to notice that most antidepressants cause sexual dysfunctions [38].

Conclusions

Although recurrent unipolar major depressive disorder and persistent depressive disorder represent two manifestations of chronic forms of depression, these disorders stand out in intrinsic fundamental differences regarding their clinical presentation and etiopathogenesis. While the former shares some aspects with unipolar but also with bipolar disorder in which etiopathogenesis is more easily reported to neurobiological causes than to life events, the latter represents a personality trait characterizing a life path. As described in 1963, a depressive personality determines a feeling of a "little of the normal joy of living" in people "inclined to be lonely and solemn, to be gloomy, submissive, pessimistic, and self-deprecatory (…) prone to express regrets and feelings of inadequacy and hopelessness" [39]. Such a description of depressive personality is consistent with more recent studies showing how being anxious, pessimistic, and shy could be related to future depressive symptoms, while being responsible, purposeful, and resourceful could be a marker of executive functions that protect a person from depression [40].

Sexuality and Quality of Life

While there is statistical evidence that sexuality is practiced from adolescence [41], it seems likely that sexually active adolescents often use birth control inconsistently, have multiple sexual partners, and use alcohol or drugs at the time of sex.

These behaviors are often associated with mood disorders and depression. Approximately 14% of adolescents have experienced at least one episode of major depression, resulting in a serious impairment of emotional stability: at home, at school, or at work, in intimate relationships or in social life [42]. All the more so since the percentage has risen considerably due to the COVID 19 pandemic and the resulting emotional fragility.

The scientific literature associates the phenomena of adolescent depression with family events experienced at an early age [43].

For example, early parental separation (before age 5) can prompt multi-partner sexual behavior in adolescence, while early father absence anticipates higher rates of sexual activity among 16-year-old female adolescents [44].

The timing of parental relationship instability may also predict increased psychological distress among children and adolescents [45].

When an individual's parents separate in early childhood, they tend to have poorer well-being as pre-adolescents than those whose parents separated later in childhood [46].

Depressive symptoms associated with the experience of parental separation during childhood may also worsen over time as individuals reach adolescence and early adulthood.

Accordingly, studies have shown *early emotional instability, sexual behavior, and depression in adolescents.*

A study conducted by Kelly L. Donahue BA et al., [47] assessed 585 children (52% male; 81% Caucasian) and their families. Assessments were conducted annually, and those who moved after the initial assessment were followed up by mail or telephone. At age 24, 83% of the original sample ($N = 484$) continued to participate in the assessments.

The study started from the hypothesis that parental relationship instability before the age of 5 years would be associated with a higher probability of reporting early sexuality (SP) at the age of 16 years and a higher probability of experiencing a major depressive episode (MDE) between the ages of 13 and 18 years.

The following were assessed: (a) less parental awareness of activities, (b) parents with little interaction with children, (c) exposure to numerous transitions in the parental relationship (change of city, job, new marriage, etc.) during development, or (d) fewer available caregivers (grandparents and friends).

Methods of the Survey

At the age of 12, using a 3-point scale, adolescents rated how much their parents knew about their friends, shopping, after-school activities, and leisure time [48]. At age 13, interviewers asked primary caregivers (94% mothers, 3% fathers, and 3% others) a series of 35 questions about their adolescents' homework, school experiences, entertainment choices, and peer relationships. The interviewers rated how knowledgeable the parent was in each of the four domains, using a five-point scale.

At the age of 12, adolescents reported on their pubertal development in terms of height growth, body hair growth, and skin changes; facial hair growth and deepening of the voice (boys); and breast growth and menstruation (girls).

Results: At the age of 16 years, more than one-third of participants reported SP during the previous year. The prevalence of sexual activity at this age is in line with rates found in larger population-based samples [49, 50]. Between the ages of 13 and 18, 16% of participants had at least one MDE, consistent with estimates from recent epidemiological studies.

The identification of individuals most at risk of pathological outcomes, such as those experiencing parental separation or divorce prematurely, could help sexologists and psychiatrists to build a personalized treatment model for each adolescent experiencing depression and deviant sexual behavior [51].

And the Adults?

Depression in adults can lead to hypersexuality, compulsive sexual behavior (often also indicative of bipolar disorder), psychosocial distress, relationship, and work problems [52].

Some articles in the literature have investigated the relationship between hypersexuality and trauma in veterans, highlighting various forms of sexual compulsivity or problematic sexuality associated with traumatic life experiences [53].

In this regard, it has been hypothesized that hypersexuality may arise more generally from PTSD symptom (abuse, traumatic death of a parent, abandonment, violence, etc.).

This would explain how in the case of depression, adult hypersexual behavior is acted out in order to cope with internal suffering caused by trauma in the past and related to psychopathological symptoms.

There Is More

Drawing on the pandemic period, some studies have assessed the interaction between depression, sexuality, and alcohol abuse.

Specifically, Ellesse-Roselee Akré et al. collected, from May 21 to July 15, 2020, 3245 adults living in the five major metropolitan areas of the United States (Atlanta, Georgia; Chicago, Illinois; New Orleans, Louisiana; New York, New York; and Los Angeles, California) [54].

Participants were categorized as straight cisgender or LGBTQ+ (i.e., lesbian, gay, bisexual and transgender people, and men who have sex with men and women who have sex with women who do not identify as lesbian, gay, bisexual, or transgender).

The age groups examined were 18–26, 27–49, 50–64, and ≥65 years. They were subdivided by gender (male and female), race/ethnicity (African American/Black, Asian, Hispanic/Latino, White), educational level (below high school, high school diploma, some college or associate or technical degree, and bachelor's degree or higher), household income in relation to the federal poverty level (FPL; according to the US Department of Health and Human Services) relationship status (married or partnered; in a romantic relationship; widowed; and single, divorced, or separated); health insurance (uninsured, private, public, and other); and city of residence (Atlanta, Chicago, Los Angeles, New Orleans, and New York City).

The results showed more frequent psychological distress and alcohol abuse in times of pandemic among LGBTQ+ and heterosexual cisgender people. Heterosexuals reported hypoactive craving and increased eating compulsivity, frustration, anhedonia, memory and sleep disturbances, and mild depression.

Megan E Patrik et al. [55] confirmed in a study from spring 2019 to autumn 2020 that the young adults studied (1244) reported stress, economic difficulties, mood disorders, autoerotic compulsivity, and drug use to cope with the COVID-19 pandemic.

In particular, 15.7% of the sample reported marijuana use, 8.9% reported increased use of some type of substance, and 8.2% reported increased use of alcohol. About 1% reported smoking more cigarettes, using prescribed and/or non-prescribed medication for mood disorders. [56, 57].

Staying with the pandemic theme, studies [58] have also shown a lowering of mood and sexual frequency with a significant drop in female sexual function index (FSFI) scores in adult pregnant women.

We refer to hypoactive desire, disturbance of arousal, lubrication, orgasm, satisfaction, and pain, with negative effects on the quality of life of affected women.

Data show a reduction of up to 64% in interest in sexual activity after childbirth. The return to sexual activity occurs on average 4 months after childbirth, varying from 1 month to 2 years.

Therefore, the importance of assessing women's sexual health in one of the countries most affected by COVID-19 has become apparent, especially during a vulnerable period with regard to sexual dysfunction, such as puerperium [59].

It appears that sexual dysfunction in the third trimester of pregnancy is linked to the fear of hurting the fetus, triggering mechanisms of low self-esteem, mood disorders, and relationship problems [60, 61].

Conclusion

Depression, sexuality, and quality of life remain a triad that must be investigated with the utmost care and by means of a multi-specialist criterion: psychiatric and psychosexological. The complementary anamnesis would allow the patient to learn the causes of his or her behavior and to associate the pharmacological therapy with a process of re-evaluation of himself or herself and of his or her weaknesses. Any hyposexual or hypersexual behavior would take on more relevance in the individual's life, limiting the use of alcohol and substances.

References

1. Adams F. The genuine works of Hippocrates. South Med J. 1922;15:519.
2. Pinel P. A treatise on insanity. Cadell and Sheffiels; 1806.
3. Kreaepelin E. Kompendium der Psychiatrie: Zum Gebrauch für Studierende und Ärzte (Compendium of psychiatry: for the use of students and physicians); 1883.
4. Wernicke C. Grundriss der Psychiatrie in klinischen Vorlesungen (Foundation of psychiatry in clinical lectures); 1894.
5. Sadock BJ. Kaplan & Sadock's synopsis of psychiatry: behavioral sciences/clinical psychiatry. 11th ed. Wolters Kluwer Health; 2015.
6. American Psychiatric Association (APA). DSM 5; 2013.
7. Lam RW, McIntosh D, Wang J, Enns MW, Kolivakis T, Michalak EE, Sareen J, Song WY, Kennedy SH, MacQueen GM, Milev RV, Parikh SV, Ravindran AV. Canadian Network for Mood and Anxiety Treatments (CANMAT) 2016 clinical guidelines for the management of adults with major depressive disorder: section 1. Disease burden and principles of care. Can J Psychiatr. 2016;61:510–23.
8. Tellenbach H. Melancholy. Duquesne U. Pittsburgh; 1961.
9. Bowlby J. Attachment and loss: attachment, vol. 1. New York: Basic Books; 1969.
10. Nemeroff C. The corticotropin-releasing factor (CRF) hypothesis of depression: new findings and new directions. Mol Psychiatry. 1996;1:336–42.
11. Holsboer F. The corticosteroid receptor hypothesis of depression. Neuropsychopharmacology. 2000;23:477–501.
12. Pariante CM. Depression, stress and the adrenal axis. J Neuroendocrinol. 2003;15:811–2.
13. Krishnan V, Nestler EJ. The molecular neurobiology of depression. Nature. 2008;455:894–902.
14. Anguelova M, Benkelfat C, Turecki G. A systematic review of association studies investigating genes coding for serotonin receptors and the serotonin transporter: II. Suicidal behavior. Mol Psychiatry. 2003;8:646–53.
15. Kendler KS. The structure of the genetic and environmental risk factors for six major psychiatric disorders in women. Arch Gen Psychiatry. 2011;52:374.
16. Lam D, Ancelin ML, Ritchie K, Freak-Poli R, Saffery R, Ryan J. Genotype-dependent associations between serotonin transporter gene (SLC6A4) DNA methylation and late-life depression. BMC Psychiatry. 2018;18:282.

17. Lotrich FE, Pollock BG. Meta-analysis of serotonin transporter polymorphisms and affective disorders. Psychiatr Genet. 2004;14:121–9.
18. Serretti A, Macciardi F, Verga M, Cusin C, Pedrini S, Smeraldi E. Tyrosine hydroxylase gene associated with depressive symptomatology in mood disorder. Am J Med Genet. 1998;81:127–30.
19. Zill P, Baghai TC, Zwanzger P, Schüle C, Eser D, Rupprecht R, Möller H-J, Bondy B, Ackenheil M. SNP and haplotype analysis of a novel tryptophan hydroxylase isoform (TPH2) gene provide evidence for association with major depression. Mol Psychiatry. 2004;9:1030–6.
20. Antypa N, Drago A, Serretti A. The role of COMT gene variants in depression: bridging neuropsychological, behavioral and clinical phenotypes. Neurosci Biobehav Rev. 2013;37:1597–610.
21. Mossakowska-Wójcik J, Orzechowska A, Talarowska M, Szemraj J, Gałecki P. The importance of TCF4 gene in the etiology of recurrent depressive disorders. Prog Neuropsychopharmacol Biol Psychiatry. 2018;80:304–8.
22. Kovanen L, Kaunisto M, Donner K, Saarikoski ST, Partonen T. CRY2 genetic variants associate with dysthymia. PLoS One. 2013;8:e71450.
23. Border R, Johnson EC, Evans LM, Smolen A, Berley N, Sullivan PF, Keller MC. No support for historical candidate gene or candidate gene-by-interaction hypotheses for major depression across multiple large samples. Am J Psychiatry. 2019;176:376–87.
24. Allen NB, Badcock PBT. Darwinian models of depression: a review of evolutionary accounts of mood and mood disorders. Prog Neuropsychopharmacol Biol Psychiatry. 2006;30:815–26.
25. ICD-10. Tenth revision of the international classification of diseases, Chapter V (F): mental and behavioural disorders. Clinical descriptions and diagnostic guidelines; 1992.
26. Drayer RA, Mulsant BH, Lenze EJ, Rollman BL, Dew MA, Kelleher K, Karp JF, Begley A, Schulberg HC, Reynolds CF. Somatic symptoms of depression in elderly patients with medical comorbidities. Int J Geriatr Psychiatry. 2005;20:973–82.
27. Raguram R, Weiss MG, Channabasavanna SM, Devins GM. Stigma, depression, and somatization in South India. Am J Psychiatry. 1996;153:1043–9.
28. Becker SM. Detection of somatization and depression in primary care in Saudi Arabia. Soc Psychiatry Psychiatr Epidemiol. 2004;39:962–6.
29. Beck AT, Ward CH, Mendelson M, Mock J, Erbaugh J. An inventory for measuring depression. Arch Gen Psychiatry. 1961;4:561–71.
30. Montgomery SA, Asberg M. A new depression scale designed to be sensitive to change. Br J Psychiatry. 1979;134:382–9. https://doi.org/10.1192/bjp.134.4.382.
31. Hamilton M. A rating scale for depression. J Neurol Neurosurg Psychiatry. 1960;23:56–62.
32. Zung WKW. A self-rating depression scale. Arch Gen Psychiatry. 1965;12:63–70.
33. Posner K, Brown GK, Stanley B, Brent DA, Yershova KV, Oquendo MA, Currier GW, Melvin GA, Greenhill L, Shen S, Mann JJ. The Columbia-suicide severity rating scale: initial validity and internal consistency findings from three multisite studies with adolescents and adults. Am J Psychiatry. 2011;168:1266–77.
34. Parikh SV, Quilty LC, Ravitz P, Rosenbluth M, Pavlova B, Grigoriadis S, Velyvis V, Kennedy SH, Lam RW, MacQueen GM, Milev RV, Ravindran AV, Uher R. Canadian Network for Mood and Anxiety Treatments (CANMAT) 2016 clinical guidelines for the management of adults with major depressive disorder: section 2. Psychological treatments. Can J Psychiatry. 2016;61:524–39.
35. de Maat SM, Dekker J, Schoevers RA, de Jonghe F. Relative efficacy of psychotherapy and combined therapy in the treatment of depression: a meta-analysis. Eur Psychiatry. 2007;22:1–8.
36. Cuijpers P, De Wit L, Weitz E, Andersson G, Huibers MJH. The combination of psychotherapy and pharmacotherapy in the treatment of adult depression: a comprehensive meta-analysis. J Evidence-Based Psychother. 2015;15:147–68.
37. Machmutow K, Meister R, Jansen A, Kriston L, Watzke B, Härter MC, Liebherz S. Comparative effectiveness of continuation and maintenance treatments for persistent depressive disorder in adults. Cochrane Database Syst Rev. 2019;2019:CD012855.
38. Gregorian R, Golden K, Bahce A, Goodman C, Kwong WJ, Kahn Z. Antidepressant-induced sexual dysfunction. Ann Pharmacother. 2002;36:1577–89.

39. Noyes AP, Kolb LC. Modern clinical psychiatry; 1963.
40. Cloninger CR, Svrakic DM, Przybeck TR. Can personality assessment predict future depression? A twelve-month follow-up of 631 subjects. J Affect Disord. 2006;92(1):35–44.
41. Centers for Disease Control and Prevention juvenile risk behavior surveillance: United States 2007 coordination Center for Health Information and Services, Atlanta, GA; 2007.
42. Administration of Substance Abuse and Mental Health Services Results from the 2004 national survey on drug use and health. Rockville, MD: National Results Substance Abuse and Mental Health Services Administration; 2005.
43. Bates JE, Alexander DB, Oberlander S, et al. History of sexual activity at the age of 16 and 17 in a community sample followed by the age of 5. In: Bancroft J, editor. Childhood sexual development. Bloomington, IN: Indiana University Press; 2003. p. 206–38.
44. Ellis BJ, Bates JE, Dodge KA, et al. Does the absence of the father expose the daughters to a particular risk for early sexual activity and adolescent pregnancy? Child Dev. 2003;74:801–21.
45. Amato PR, Malone PS, Castellino DR, et al. The consequences of divorce for adults and children. J Marriage Fam. 2000;62:1269–87.
46. Allison PD, Furstenberg FF, McRae C. How marriage breakdown affects children: age and gender variations. Dev Psychol. 1989;25:540–9.
47. Donahue KL, et al. Early exposure to parental relationship instability: implications for sexual behavior and depression in adolescence. J Adolesc Health. 2010;47(6):547–54.
48. Kerr M, Statin H, et al. What parents know, how they know and different forms of adolescent adaptation: further support for a reinterpretation of monitoring. Dev Psychol. 2000;36:366–80.
49. McGue M, Iacono WG. The association of early adolescent problem behavior with adult psychopathology. Am J Salute Behav. 2005;162:1118–9.
50. Santelli JS, Lindberg LD, Finer LB, Singh S. Explain the recent decline in teen pregnancies in the United States: the contribution of abstinence and the improvement of contraceptive use. Am J Public Health. 2007;97:150–6.
51. Zietsch BP, Verweij KJ, Bailey JM, et al. Genetic and environmental influences on risky sexual behavior and its relationship with personality. Behav Genet. 2010;40:12–21.
52. Ciocca G, et al. Hypersexuality: the controversial mismatch of psychiatric diagnosis. J Psychopath. 2018;24:187–91.
53. Turban JL, Shirk SD, Potenza MN, Hoff RA, Kraus SW. Posting sexually explicit images or videos of oneself online is associated with impulsivity and hypersexuality, but not psychopathology measures in a sample of U.S. veterans. J Sex Med. 2020;17:163–7.
54. Akré E-R, et al. Depression, anxiety and alcohol use among LGBTQ + people during the COVID-19 pandemic. Am J Public Health. 2021;111(9):1610–9.
55. Patrik ME, et al. Substance use to cope with the COVID 19 pandemic: US national data at age 19. J Adolesc Health. 2021;68(2):277–83.
56. Carlo NE, et al. Increased symptoms of mood disorder, perceived stress and alcohol use among college students during the COVID 19 pandemic. Psychiatry Res. 2021;296:113706.
57. Rhew IC, et al. The frequency of marijuana use, but not alcohol, is associated with greater loneliness, psychological distress and less prosperity among young adults. Alcohol Addiction. 2021;218:108404.
58. Zanardo V, et al. Psychological impact of quarantine measures for COVID-19 in northeastern Italy on mothers immediately after giving birth. Int J Gynaecol Obstet. 2020;150(2):184–8. https://doi.org/10.1002/ijgo.13249.
59. Schiavi MC, et al. Love in the time of COVID-19: analysis of sexual function and quality of life during social distancing measures in a group of Italian women of reproductive age. J Sex Med. 2020;17(8):1407–13. https://doi.org/10.1016/j.jsxm.2020.06.006.
60. Jawed-Wessel S, Sevick E. The impact of pregnancy and childbirth on sexual behaviors: a systematic review. J Sex Res. 2017;54(4–5):411–23. https://doi.org/10.1080/00224499.201 6.1274715.
61. Yuksel B, Ozgor F. Effect of the COVID-19 pandemic on female sexual behavior. Int J Gynecol Obstet. 2020;150:98–102. https://doi.org/10.1002/ijgo.13193.

Autism and Sexuality

Flavia Caretto, Carlo Hanau, and Elena Vittoria Longhi

Introduction

The word autism, derived from the Greek "autòs," which means "self," was first used in psychiatry by Eugen Bleuler in 1911, in order to describe one of the symptoms of schizophrenia in one of its phases, consisting of turning in on oneself and isolation.

In 1943, the pediatric psychiatrist Leo Kanner [1] took up this definition to define the pathological condition of 11 children described by him, whose appearance had been precocious, within 3 years of age.

Despite having noted and meticulously described an enormous range of behavioral anomalies, Kanner was particularly struck by the loneliness these children seemed to actively seek at an age when such an attitude is totally unusual. Kanner correctly hypothesized in his first work that the cause of this behavior, which being innate cannot be psychogenic, is "an innate inability to communicate." "We must, then, assume that these children have come into the world with innate inability to form the usual, biologically provided affective contact with people…omissis… For here we seem to have pure-culture examples of *inborn autistic disturbances of affective contact.*"

This hypothesis was corroborated by Anne Freud and S. Dann [2].

F. Caretto
CulturAutismo Onlus, Rome, Italy

C. Hanau (✉)
Association Cimadori for Italian Research on Down Syndrome, Autism and Brain Damage (A.P.R.I.), OdV, ETS, Bologna, Italy

Programming of Social and Health Services, The University of Modena and Reggio Emilia, Modena, Italy

E. V. Longhi
Department of Sexual Medical Center, San Raffaele Hospital, Milano, Italy

© Springer Nature Switzerland AG 2023

E. V. Longhi (ed.), *Managing Psychosexual Consequences in Chronic Diseases*,
https://doi.org/10.1007/978-3-031-31307-3_32

Kanner moved away from this first correct hypothesis in the following years, after noting that the families bringing autistic children were generally well-to-do and with a high cultural level, even in the mother, often engaged in work outside their home. Kanner [3], influenced by psychoanalysis at that time dominant [4], made the rash deduction that their parents (especially the mother defined as a refrigerator mother) were the psychogenic cause of their children's autism. In 1949, he wrote "They were left neatly in refrigerators which did not defrost. Their withdrawal seems to be an act of turning away from such a situation to seek comfort in solitude." In 1969, Kanner retracted his hypothesis of the refrigerator mother, which was definitively falsified in 1987 by Sanua [5] with an epidemiological investigation. Biological research on what previously seemed to be a psychogenic problem took off only at the beginning of the century, accounting for why there are no drugs for autism today.

Main Medical Characteristics of Autism

The chronicity of autism in the cases studied by Kanner is demonstrated by his study on the distant evolution of the 11 children described in 1943 [6]. Those adults were no longer people withdrawn into themselves, but with presumed good hidden potential, they were persons with severe mental disabilities. They showed impairment in all areas of development and moreover with very serious psychotic elements. He repeated the observation on about a hundred cases he subsequently diagnosed and found them institutionalized and totally dependent, with the exception of some of them, self-sufficient and able to carry out a job diligently, but with elective deficiencies in the ability to socialize; no one was married or lived in a couple, so the problem of genetic transmission did not arise.

Let us consider people with autism that allows married life, and subsequent epidemiological research studies have shown the possibility of family transmission and the highly significant higher frequency of an ever-increasing number of transmissible or "de novo" genetic anomalies. Since the end of the last century, genetic research has increasingly found various rare or very rare forms of genes or combinations of genes, or CNV (copy number variation), which can cause autism.

Anatomopathological investigations on the brains of deceased people with autism have found an excess of synaptic connections. This is due to the lack of pruning, which should begin between the 18th and 20th weeks of intrauterine life [7].

The choice of the term autism has generated confusion and led to the creation of successive names, first of all: Kanner's syndrome; even today, when the causes cannot be referred to, which in most cases remain unknown, autism is defined on the basis of the behaviors observed by Kanner. They are included in the International Statistical Classification of Diseases and Related Health Problems, officially adopted and translated in the countries of the world and also used for administrative and accounting purposes.

The ICD-10 CM (https://www.icd10data.com/ICD10CM/Codes/F01-F99/F80-F89/F84-/F84.0) will give way to ICD-11 in 2022 (ICD-11 (who.int)), where the code 299.00 of the ICD-9 and the code F84 of the ICD-10 CM will be replaced by 6A02, which separately classifies the types of autism of the spectrum (https://www.findacode.com/icd-11/code-437815624.html). F84.5 Asperger's syndrome is classified as 6A02.0.

Autism spectrum disorder is characterized by persistent deficits in the ability to initiate and to sustain reciprocal social interaction and social communication and by a range of restricted, repetitive, and inflexible patterns of behavior, interests, or activities that are clearly atypical or excessive for the individual's age and sociocultural context. The onset of the disorder occurs during the developmental period, typically in early childhood, but symptoms may not become fully manifest until later, when social demands exceed limited capacities. Deficits are sufficiently severe to cause impairment in personal, family, social, educational, occupational, or other important areas of functioning and are usually a pervasive feature of the individual's functioning observable in all settings, although they may vary according to social, educational, or other contexts. Individuals along the spectrum exhibit a full range of intellectual functioning and language abilities.

Inclusion Autistic Disorder; Exclusion Rett Syndrome (LD90.4)
Sections/Codes in this Section (6A02-6A02)

- Autism spectrum disorder without disorder of intellectual development and with mild or no impairment of functional language (6A02.0).
- Autism spectrum disorder with disorder of intellectual development and with mild or no impairment of functional language (6A02.1).
- Autism spectrum disorder without disorder of intellectual development and with impaired functional language (6A02.2).
- Autism spectrum disorder with disorder of intellectual development and with impaired functional language (6A02.3).
- Autism spectrum disorder with disorder of intellectual development and with absence of functional language (6A02.5).
- Other specified autism spectrum disorder (6A02.Y).
- Autism spectrum disorder, unspecified (6A02.Z).

In scientific publications, the classification of DSM-5 [8] is widely used, which brings together all autisms in the "autism spectrum disorder" (ASD) class. Inside this class, various specifications are prescribed together with a global index to be 1–3 in order to take into account the severity and complexity of needs. Inside DSM-5, the following terms are removed:

- Asperger's syndrome, which in DSM-IV represented the borderline of autism, where language is often presented in an early and refined way, where IQ is normal or even above normal, and where early diagnosis within 3 years is very difficult.
- Rett syndrome, the genes that cause it have been found. They are MECP2, CDKL5, or FOXG1.

In current diagnostics, if the laboratory finds one of the dozens of rare genetic syndromes known because there is an incidence of autistic behavior significantly higher than that of the general population, the diagnosis of autism takes second place. Conversely, it happens when the concomitant diagnosis is ADHD or epilepsy, which are considered minor pathologies or otherwise treatable with health care, as well as psychoeducational interventions.

The characteristics of autism manifest themselves very differently from person to person, also in relation to the level of general skills, the presence and degree of intellectual impairment, and the educational path taken [9]. Since within this condition the differences between people are truly remarkable, we prefer to speak of "autisms" in the plural or, according to the English-speaking scientific literature, of ASD to identify a great variety of characteristics (as for the "spectrum" of the light).

ESCAP (European Society for Child and Adolescent Psychiatry) advises psychiatrists and neuropsychiatrists belonging to European scientific societies to direct their diagnostic and therapeutic interventions to cases in which autistic behavior is a problem [10].

For people who have only some behaviors included in the autism spectrum, but do not register reductions in quality of life, the diagnosis of autism spectrum can be considered a stigmatizing and unacceptable false positive, since usually for some it can be a pride. These conditions cannot be defined as "global developmental disorders of psychological development," but rather atypical neurodevelopment, outside the norm in the statistical sense. They are part of the great variability of human species. They do not constitute a problem for the person himself, and indeed, they can constitute a quality appreciated also by people, which nevertheless requires to be educated in order to recognize and respect differences.

Autism can be taken as one of the examples of a situation in which medicine, not knowing the causes, made the mistake of believing that it was a psychogenic pathology, caused by the inadequacy of motherly love. Even today, there is little scientific knowledge on the etiopathogenesis of the majority of autism cases. This is the first cause, for which there are no effective health intervention tools, and other than those of special education, which can ignore the knowledge of the causes.

From the first description of autism made by Kanner to today, 78 years have passed. Diagnoses of Global Developmental Disorders of Psychological Development (ICD-10), Pervasive Disorder of Psychological Development (DSM-IV), and the Autism Spectrum (DSM-5) undergo an enormous and continuous increase everywhere. Such an increase is due to both the real increase in the phenomenon and the improvement of social attention and the expansion of diagnostics for autism. In the USA, (https://www.cdc.gov/ncbddd/autism/addm.html), in 2016, there was in the average one case for every 54 8-year-olds, albeit with great variations from one state to another. Those with intellectual disabilities, which were almost all at the time of Kanner, have dropped to a third of the total (https://www.cdc.gov/ncbddd/autism/addm-community-report/index.html). The age at the first diagnosis has decreased, favoring the appearance of cases also of the disappearance of ASD (https://pubmed.ncbi.nlm.nih.gov/30187843/).

In Italy, nowadays, *quotidianosanità.it* [11], which reports the National Autism Observatory of the Higher Institute of Health ISS), as well as the US CDC, estimates that the prevalence in Italy of the diagnosis of primary school pupils included in the spectrum is almost one for every 77 children between 7 and 9 years of age.

According to the Italian Statistics Institute [12], which lists all certified disabilities for which school support is required, the prevalence of "Global developmental disorders of psychological development" (F 84 in ICD-10) continues to grow more than all other forms of disability, approaching 1% of students in 2019–2020 [13].

The growth is due both to the increase in the phenomenon and to the greater attention that is paid to this condition.

Main Tools for the Diagnosis of Autism

Autistic behaviors can be found in about one-third of cases of "Neurodevelopmental disorders," where all the major mental abnormalities of childhood are found, regardless of the biological and genetic diagnosis, which would be useful for distinguishing cases that require qualitative and quantitative resource details. Effective psycho-pedagogical interventions, such as those recommended by Guideline No. 21 on autism, issued by ISS, can ignore the etiology of the disorder. They must begin as early as possible, even before a definitive diagnosis.

The differences in the development of people with autism are particularly evident in two large areas: The first area concerns interaction and social communication and the second area concerns interests, sensory aspects, and other behavioral peculiarities.

These characteristics find different expressions at different ages, in males and females. They rely upon many personal characteristics, hence requiring the ASD concept class. In any case, all people in the spectrum exhibit different behaviors, at least in the years of very early childhood; among these characteristics, there are, for example, odd relations with people.

With the growth, what actually characterizes this group of people is the way of perceiving and processing information. The way of processing social information appears qualitatively different from what is expected of a typical person.

The assessment and diagnosis in the autism spectrum are conducted in relation to two broad categories: the characteristics of autism, or symptoms, on the one hand, and abilities on the other. The symptom part of the assessment must be based on international criteria for diagnosis. Traditionally, practitioners have employed tests to support clinical observations. These tests must evaluate the symptoms present "at the time" and those present "historically," in the frame of contexts other than the clinical one. The most used test is the ADOS, which consists of a direct and standardized observation of the person. It is accompanied by ADI, a meticulous interview with the people who know the person the best, usually his parents. The ADOS is not the only test that can be used. It does not include the population of adolescents and adults with cognitive and verbal difficulties; CARS is generally used in such a case, an observational assessment that does not require a standardized context. To evaluate the aspects related to skills, on the other hand, two types of measures are used. Tests that indicate the age of development or the IQ (the classic intelligence scales), which may include verbal language, are enrolled. They may include verbal language or not include it. Functional tests (such as the Denver Scale, the PEP scale, and the TTAP) and adaptive tests (such as the Vineland or ABAS scales) may be exploited. A retest after some time must be planned. The functional and adaptive tests allow for a definition of the objectives useful for the educational intervention, which are identified on the basis of the emerging or potential skills detected.

The cognitive profile of people with neurodiversity characteristics is always different from that of people with neurotypical characteristics. Both in the first and in the second group of people, there are cases with cognitive deficit: The type of basic neurological organization determines its manifestation. People with cognitive difficulties, if they are autistic, have some specific characteristics, and if they are not, they have others.

In about 30% of people with autism, a qualitative difference in the "way" of thinking, which generally manifests itself in the IQ tests of a single individual with a distribution of scores wider than one would expect, is detected. Moreover, an IQ lower than 70 is detected, a score that marks the presence of cognitive difficulties.

Adults with the characteristics of autism spectrum are often under-employed or do not work. They do not live independently, even when this would be possible. They do not have a social support network and are afflicted with anxiety and mental health problems.

Autism and Sexuality

Regarding **autism, affectivity, and sexuality**, people with autism show a whole range of sexual behaviors [14].

To understand the peculiarities of the affective development of children in the spectrum, it is useful first to take into consideration the particularities of attention and joint emotion [15], perception [16], and the tendency to focus on details generally considered of little or no relevance by people with typical development [17].

The earliest particularities related to the affective sphere are observed in joint attention and in the first expressions of attachment. In persons with ASD mechanisms of attachment, or the creation and development of emotional bonds, atypical paths are followed. Different forms are compared to what happens in people with typical development. It is the expression of attachment that is different from what was expected, and not the attachment itself [18].

In developing bonds, both with their family members and with unfamiliar people, people with autism can experience greater difficulties than non-autistic ones. Since joint attention is the basis of sharing and sharing is the basis of intimacy, this greater difficulty can also be experienced in romantic and/or sexual relationships.

Unlike what happens in neurotypical children, sensations and emotions of autistic children are not confirmed in the interaction with neurotypical adults. ASD persons feel many difficulties in joint attention. Neurotypical interlocutors generally "intuitively grasp" emotions. ASD children do not, hence, provide explicit explanations on these. Children with autism, including those with normal intellectual and speech abilities, may have difficulty naming, describing, and mimicking emotions. These children undergo more complex stresses than non-autistic ones from the social and non-social world. The difficulty in cognitively manipulating emotional concepts often manifests itself, at a behavioral level, in a poor capacity for self-regulation.

Growing up, people with autism may find it difficult to grasp the thoughts and emotions of neurotypical interlocutors. Autistic people have a kind of "innate" and general difficulty in forming a theory of mind and also display a deficit of "empathy."

We know today that this is not completely true, or rather that it is an incomplete definition. It is true that people with autism do not have a typical theory of mind as much as non-autistic people. This also applies to empathy: People with autism do not have empathy toward people, as non-autistic people do not have empathy toward those with autism.

Due to the mutual misunderstanding between autistic and neurotypical, adolescents and adults with autism have a greater risk of engaging in inappropriate sexual behavior and sexual victimization than their typically developing peers [19].

As for adolescents and adults with autism without intellectual and language impairment, these people appear to have more hypersexual and paraphilic fantasies and behaviors than the general population [20]. This observation is mainly driven, in literature studies, by observations from male participants.

Women with autism are usually more socially adapted and show fewer symptoms. They are more able to "mask" the characteristics of the spectrum and personal suffering, mimicking what they observe in neurotypical contexts [21, 22].

In recent years, the finding that women with autism are capable of this "masking" has led to a reassessment of the percentages of males and females within the spectrum in DSM-5 [8]. It states that autism "in females without concomitant intellectual impairment or without language delays may not be recognized" (p. 66). This suggests that, in relation to autism and sexuality, studies should focus on the male and female gender separately.

Pecora [23] carried out a meta-analysis to consider the impact that sexual experiences can have, over time, on the sexual/romantic functioning of autistic people "without intellectual and verbal impairment." Females show higher levels of sexual understanding, and they are prone to more adverse sexual experiences than males with the same characteristics and neurotypical counterparts. Males reported greater desire and commitment to both solitary and dyadic sexual contact.

It should be considered that within the spectrum there are people who define themselves as "asexual," who are not interested in aspects related to sexuality.

Additionally, some studies have identified among transgender people a higher rate of autism diagnosis, with estimates ranging from 6% to 13%.

Other studies have found that people with autism also have a higher rate of gender dysphoria or gender variance, often in co-occurrence with mental health problems, which include suicide attempt. It is important that evaluations for autism routinely take into account gender variance and that clinical evaluations of young people referring to gender variance are also important [24, 25].

There is growing recognition that autistic women exhibit more sexual and gender identities than their non-autistic counterparts. Likewise, autistic women are also at greater risk for adverse sexual experiences. As higher rates of sexual victimization are observed in individuals with different sexual identities in the broader population, the rates of negative sexual experiences among autistic women remain unclear [19].

People with the Characteristics of the Autism Spectrum Who Also Have an Intellectual Impairment

In the last century, almost all of the cases diagnosed in F 84 of the ICD-10 presented both behavioral problems and cognitive deficits from an early age. The presence of severe disability was clear to everyone. Some sexual misbehaviors may appear at prepuberal age, such as self-stimulation of the genitals or compulsive masturbation in public. When they occur in children, these behaviors are not considered highly problematic, and they create great discomfort when the person enters adolescence. Attempts are made to decrease the frequency by intervening psychologically or pharmacologically. The best option would be to prevent these behaviors through a good education in sexuality and affectivity. It should be remembered that some antipsychotics widely used for problem behaviors, such as risperidone, act on prolactin in males, hence reducing sexual manifestations.

People within the spectrum who also have an intellectual disability are about 30% of the total diagnosed in the United States [26]. They face much difficulty in implementing an age-appropriate intervention, or that changes, for example, in the use of educational materials, according to the age of the person with autism: A permanent "infantilization" is generally observed, as if the person were "younger than" and only "younger" instead of different. The infantilization of adults included in the spectrum is often observed in clothing and self-care, in the failure to teach skills of personal autonomy, and in the welcoming social response to age-inappropriate behaviors, such as hugging strangers or kissing them.

An extreme form of tolerance is sometimes reserved for problematic behaviors with sexual components. They are "ignored" until it is no longer possible to do so, or when they are well-established and very problematic. It is very difficult to deal, emotionally and operationally, both as parents and as professionals, with these behaviors. They include compulsive masturbation or particular forms of sexual interest. Little space is given to prevention through adequate education.

Autistic People as Victims or Perpetrators of Sex Offenders

People in the spectrum, whatever their type of functioning, are frequently subjected to different forms of abuse, including sexual abuse.

Reynolds [27, 28] states that the figures for sexual assault attempted violence and harassment in the general population of boys and girls under the age of 18 double if the person has a developmental disability. Counting how many people with autism are sexually harassed is not easy. Note that violence is not disclosed or reported by autistic people.

In the event that harassment or violence is suspected, the protected hearing should follow a series of principles, currently only hypothesized, to adapt to the characteristics of the autistic person, ensuring authentic listening [27, 28].

Some characteristics of people with autism favor abusers, such as the difficulty in asking for help, in revealing what happened immediately. They are unable to explicitly reject an unwelcome interaction. They cannot understand when it is violence. They cannot realize that can be refused sexual interaction.

Early education in knowledge and respect for oneself, adequate self-esteem, and good communication skills, together with a correct affective and sexual education, help to reduce abuse.

This is also true when men with autism are viewed as potential abusers. Creaby Attwood and Allely [29] considered some legal cases in which offenders were in the autism spectrum. This study suggests that the difficulty in developing appropriate and consenting sexual relationships, as a result of impaired social cognition, may increase the risk of sexual offenses.

A recent study [30] suggests that people in the spectrum who commit crimes engage more frequently in crimes against the person and sexual offenses, than other types of crimes such as property, traffic, and drug-related crimes. To date, there is little empirical knowledge on the reasons why men with autism commit sex offenses more frequently. Understanding their reasons is the key to developing and implementing effective interventions to reduce both initial crime and recidivism. In the aforementioned study [30], semi-structured interviews were conducted with nine autistic sex offenders in prisons and probation services in England and Wales. Thematic analyses revealed five main themes (social difficulties, misunderstandings, sexual and relationship deficits, and inadequate control and imbalance). The main reasons for the crime were difficulties in social skills, lack of perspective or a weak "central coherence," misunderstanding of the seriousness of their behaviors, and lack of appropriate relationships.

Need for Emotional and Sexual Education

The latest studies highlight the need to develop sex and relationship education interventions that are tailored to the needs of autistic individuals. This may address both the reasons reported by the abusers themselves for the offense and their lack of sexual knowledge and awareness.

Adequate emotional and sexual education could prevent at least some of the sexual abuses.

We must implement effective sex education programs to foster the development of a healthy sexual identity and relationships that meet the needs of each individual. The need for an appropriate and specific education for people in the spectrum is shared. Many references are now available to implement a psychoeducational intervention on affectivity and sexuality from childhood. Dealing with these issues in the scholastic and habilitation field remains a difficult task [31].

Psychoeducational intervention in this area is not actually simple or intuitive, but it is possible and should be determined by guidelines that establish its "policy."

In any case, it facilitates the recognition of one's rights and the integration of one's sexual preferences in the development of one's identity and personality. It improves the knowledge of the "mechanics" linked to sexual activities, personal safety from abuse and sexually transmitted diseases, and conscious pregnancy.

In some countries of the world, part of the educational function in this area is carried out at the institutional level. In addition, some countries have an educational figure, the "sex assistant," who deals with issues related to both education and operational aspects related to the healthy expression of sexuality.

Nowadays, practicing educational activities on this front is possible: Educators and health personnel have extensive reference literature. If made operational, such literature allows to prevent serious suffering for individuals, their families, and collectivity. While respecting cultural differences, awareness of this information should be widespread (http://www.culturautismo.it) [32–36].

References

1. Kanner L. Autistic disturbances of affective contact. Nerv Child. 1943;2:217–50. http://mail.neurodiversity.com/library_kanner_1943.pdf
2. Freud A, Dann S. An experiment in group upbringing. Psychoanal Study Child. 1951;6:127–68.
3. Kanner L. Problems of nosology and psychodynamics of early infantile autism. Am J Orthopsychiatry. 1949;19:416–26.
4. Maestrini E, Mariani Cerati D. L'autismo: una condizione genetica. Autismo oggi, n.25, novembre 2013; 2013.
5. Sanua VD. Infantile autism and parental socioeconomic status. Child Psychiatry Hum Dev. 1987;17(3):189–98.
6. Kanner L. How far can autistic children go in matters of social adaptation? J Autism Child Schizo. 1972;2(1):9–33.
7. De la Torre-Ubieta L, Won H, Stein J, et al. Advancing the understanding of autism disease mechanisms through genetics. Nat Med. 2016;22:345–61. https://doi.org/10.1038/nm.4071.
8. APA American Psychiatric Association. DSM Manuale diagnostico e statistico dei disturbi mentali—Quinta Edizione. Milano: Raffaello Cortina; 2013 (it 2014).
9. Hanau C.. Autismo, criteri diagnostici e prevalenza: una riflessione critica—QI—Questioni e idee in psicologia—Il magazine online di Hogrefe Editore; 2020.
10. Fuentes J, Hervás A, Howlin P, et al. ESCAP practice guidance for autism: a summary of evidence-based recommendations for diagnosis and treatment. Eur Child Adolesc Psychiatry. 2020;30:961. https://doi.org/10.1007/s00787-020-01587-4.
11. Pecora LA, Hooley M, Sperry L, Mesibov GB, Stokes MA. Sexuality and gender issues in individuals with autism spectrum disorder. Child Adolesc Psychiatr Clin N Am.

2020;29(3):543–56. Quotidianosanità.it 01/04/2021. https://www.quotidianosanita.it/scienza-e-farmaci/articolo.php?articolo_id=94245.

12. ISTAT. L'inclusione scolastica degli alunni con disabilità. 2020. https://www.istat.it/it/archivio/251409.

13. Hanau C. Il numero degli allievi certificati per disabilità continua a salire, "Scienza dell'Amministrazione Scolastica". Anno. 2021;15(1):38–40.

14. Turner D, Briken P, Schöttle D. Autism-spectrum disorders in adolescence and adulthood: focus on sexuality. Curr Opin Psychiatry. 2017;30(6):409–16.

15. Mundy P. Autismo e attenzione congiunta: fondamenti evolutivi, neuro scientifici e clinici. Roma: Giovanni Fioriti; 2016 (it. 2019).

16. Bogdashina O. Le percezioni sensoriali nell'Autismo e nella sindrome di Asperger. Crema: Uovonero; 2003 (it. 2011).

17. De Clercq H. Il labirinto dei dettagli: iperselettività cognitiva nell'Autismo. Trento: Erickson; 2003 (it 2006).

18. Caretto F, Lonigro A. Autismo e attaccamento: modelli di analisi e considerazioni operative. Autismo e Disturbi dello Sviluppo. 2006;4(3):370–92.

19. Pecora LA, Hancock GI, Hooley M, Demmer DH, Attwood T, Mesibov BG, Stokes MA. Gender identity, sexual orientation and adverse sexual experiences in autistic females. Mol Autism. 2020;11(1):57.

20. Schöttle D, Briken P, Tüscher O, Turner D. Sexuality in autism: hypersexual and paraphilic behavior in women and men with high-functioning autism spectrum disorder. Dialogues Clin Neurosci. 2017;19(4):381–93.

21. Attwood S, Powell J. Making sense of sex: a forthright guide to puberty, sex and relationships for people with Asperger's syndrome. London: Jessica Kingsley; 2008. It. Attwood T. Guida completa alla Sindrome di Asperger. Milano: Edra; 2019.

22. Di Biagio L. Donne in blu: l'Autismo femminile. Viareggio: Dissensi; 2018.

23. Pecora LA, Mesibov GB, Stokes MA. Sexuality in high-functioning autism: a systematic review and meta-analysis. J Autism Dev Disord. 2016;46(11):3519–56.

24. Butter E. Identità di genere e Autismo. 2019. https://www.autismspeaks.org/expert-opinion/gender-identity-and-autism.

25. Van DerMiesen AIR, Hurley H, De Vries ALC. Gender dysphoria and autism spectrum disorder: a narrative review. Int Rev Psychiatry. 2016;28(1):70–80.

26. ADDM Network Autism and Developmental Disabilities Monitoring Network. Community report ADDM community report on autism 2018 (cdc.gov); 2018.

27. Reynolds KE. Sexuality and severe autism: a practical guide for parents, caregivers and health educators. London: Jessica Kingsley; 2013.

28. It. Reynolds KE. Sessualità e Autismo: Guida per genitori, caregiver e educatori. Trento: Erickson; 2013 (it. 2014).

29. Creaby-Attwood A, Allely CS. A psycho-legal perspective on sexual offending in individuals with autism spectrum disorder. Int J Law Psychiatry. 2017;55:72–80.

30. Payne KL, Maras K, Russel AJ, Brosnam MJ. Self-reported motivations for offending by autistic sexual offenders. Autism. 2020;24(2):307–20.

31. Caretto F. Affettività e sessualità nelle persone con Autismo. Autismo e Disturbi; 2005.

32. Brenner J, Pan Z, Mazefsky C, Smith KA, Gabriels R. Behavioral symptoms of reported abuse in children and adolescents with autism spectrum disorder in inpatient settings. J Autism Dev Disord. 2018;48(11):3727–35.

33. Di Biagio L. Neurodivers Amanti: la sessualità vissuta dagli autistici. Viareggio: Dissensi; 2019.

34. Mandell DS, Walrath CM, Manteuffel B, Sgro G, Pinto Martin JA. The prevalence and correlated of abuse among children with autism served in comprehensive community-based mental health setting. Child Abuse Negl. 2005;29(12):1359–72.

35. Matthews E. Il significato di età, stato e genere per gli adulti con Autismo. In: Morgan H. (a cura di) Adulti con Autismo: bisogni, interventi e servizi. Trento: Erickson; 1996 (it. 2003).

36. Mundi P. A review of joint attention and social-cognitive brain systems in typical development and autism spectrum disorder. Eur J Neurosci. 2018;47(6):497–514.

Suggested Reading

Posar A, Visconti P. The thousand faces of autism spectrum disorder. Turk Pediatri Ars. 2018;53(4):273–4. https://doi.org/10.5152/TurkPediatriArs.2018.18066. PMID: 30872936; PMCID: PMC6408186.

Posar A, Visconti P. Long-term outcome of autism spectrum disorder. Turk Pediatri Ars 2019;54(4):207–212. https://doi.org/10.14744/TurkPediatriArs.2019.16768. PMID: 31949411; PMCID: PMC6952468.

Posar A, Visconti P. Autism in 2016: the need for answers. J Pediatr (Rio J). 2017;93(2):111–119. https://doi.org/10.1016/j.jped.2016.09.002. Epub 2016 Nov 9. PMID: 27837654.

Maenner MJ, Warren Z, Williams AR, Amoakohene E, Bakian AV, Bilder DA, Durkin MS, Fitzgerald RT, Furnier SM, Hughes MM, Ladd-Acosta CM, McArthur D, Pas ET, Salinas A, Vehorn A, Williams S, Esler A, Grzybowski A, Hall-Lande J, Nguyen RHN, Pierce K, Zahorodny W, Hudson A, Hallas L, Mancilla KC, Patrick M, Shenouda J, Sidwell K, DiRienzo M, Gutierrez J, Spivey MH, Lopez M, Pettygrove S, Schwenk YD, Washington A, Shaw KA. Prevalence and characteristics of autism Spectrum disorder among children aged 8 years - autism and developmental disabilities monitoring network, 11 sites, United States, 2020. MMWR Surveill Summ. 2023;72(2):1–14. https://doi.org/10.15585/mmwr.ss7202a1. PMID: 36952288; PMCID: PMC10042614.

Caretto F. Autismo, affettività e sessualità. Giornale Italiano dei disturbi del neurosviluppo. 2023;8(1):36–44.

Murtas Caretto, Zanini. Caratteristiche della sessualità e disturbi della risposta sessuale. In: Caretto F, Murtas I, Autismo e Psicoterapia: l'intervento cognitivo e comportamentale per adolescenti e adulti. Carocci: Roma; 2022.

Murtas I. Intervento sulla sessualità. In: Caretto F, Murtas I, editors. Autismo e Psicoterapia: l'intervento cognitivo e comportamentale per adolescenti e adulti. Carocci: Roma; 2022.

Part XVIII
Rare Disease

Ehlers–Danlos Syndrome

Alessandra Bassotti and Elena Vittoria Longhi

Definition

With Ehlers–Danlos syndrome (EDS), we indicate a heterogeneous group of relatively rare inherited connective tissue disorders that share common joint hypermobility, skin hyperextensibility, and generalized tissue fragility. The overall prevalence ratio of EDS has been estimated at 1:500–10,000, with no sex or ethnic differences. However, it is likely that some individuals with milder manifestations of the disease do not come to medical attention and thus go undetected. The most common types of EDS are the hypermobile type (prevalence: 1:500–1:20,000), the classic type (prevalence: 1:20,000–40,000), the kyphoscoliotic type (prevalence: 1:100,000), and the vascular type (prevalence: 1–9:100,000). The other types are very rare and currently described only in a few familiar clusters.

Interested Population (Enrollment Criteria)

Clinical, imaging, and laboratory criteria must be applied in order to confirm or rule out the diagnosis. The diagnostic procedures should be applied in the following cases:

1. Subjects with suspected clinical manifestations and family EDS occurrence.
2. Sporadic cases with at least one of the following clinical manifestations:

A. Bassotti (✉)
IRCCS Policlinico, Ehlers-Danlos Center, Milan, Italy
e-mail: alessandra.bassotti@policlinico.mi.it

E. V. Longhi
Department of Sexual Medical Center, San Raffaele Hospital, Milano, Italy

© Springer Nature Switzerland AG 2023

E. V. Longhi (ed.), *Managing Psychosexual Consequences in Chronic Diseases*,
https://doi.org/10.1007/978-3-031-31307-3_33

- Frequent joint subluxation/luxation and positive Beighton score.
- Skin hyperextensibility associated with atrophic scars, poor wound healing, and easy bruising following relatively minor trauma, especially over pressure points (knees, elbows) and areas prone to trauma (shins, forehead, and chin).
- Arterial dissection/aneurysm, organ rupture, and uterus rupture.
- Early progressive scoliosis associated with hypotonia or other skeletal malformations such as pectus excavatum, knee valgus, congenital clubfoot, and pes planus/valgus.
- Other suspected symptoms, especially in the adult, may include disabling joint pain, visceroptosis, and vascular abnormalities such as aneurysm or stroke history.

Since the expression of EDS phenotypes can be time-dependent, where there is no reasonable clinical suspicion, 1- or 2-year follow-up period is indicated. Even those with minor criteria must be reviewed over time, to confirm or rule out the diagnosis with certainty.

Clinical Manifestations

The main clinical features of EDS are present in the skin, joints, and neuromuscular level.

The mucocutaneous involvement is certainly one of the cardinal features of the syndrome. The skin is usually soft, velvety, doughy, and hyperelastic. Blood vessel fragility increases the risk of bleeding, hematomas, and bruising, even spontaneously. Typically, we have delayed scar formation with enlarged and atrophic scars, defined as "cigarette paper," occasionally with accumulations of hemosiderin. In classic EDS, molluscoid pseudotumors and solid subcutaneous spherules are characteristic. Other skin manifestations include atrophic striae, abdominal and post-surgical hernias, and varicosities of the lower extremity at young age. On the mucous side, abnormal bluish sclera, frequent nose bleeding, and increased tendency toward gum disease (gingivitis and periodontitis) in the absence of oral cavity pathology are frequent. The oral mucosa may be thin, easily tear, and give rise to mouth ulcers (classical and hypermobile EDS).

Joint hypermobility is certainly another distinctive feature of these syndromes. Investigating joint hypermobility essentially consists in measuring the range of motion of the joints. In EDS, joint hypermobility is frequently congenital (nontraumatic) and generalized, although in some types, such as in the vascular type, may be present only in the extremities. The **_Beighton score_** is a popular and simple screening system to quantify joint laxity and hypermobility.

The neuromuscular aspects of EDS have recently been acquired [1] increasing importance. Mild muscle hypotonia is a frequent feature of probable congenital (or prenatal) origin that is responsible, at least in part, for of the characteristic orthopedic abnormalities such as flexible flat feet, big toes, valgus knees and elbows, mild scoliosis, and high arched palate. It is possible to find a lack of strength in various muscle areas or muscular hypotrophy, the latter usually in the thenar and hypothenar eminences and in the interosseous muscles. Joint contractures of myogenic origin, such as camptodactyly and clubfoot, are possible, although rare, and usually associated with some specific variants of the syndrome, such as the vascular form. It is possible to find a lack of strength in various muscle areas or muscular hypotrophy, the latter usually in the thenar and hypothenar eminences and in the interosseous muscles. The most relevant neurological element on physical examination is proprioceptive impairment, in the absence of other signs of vestibular dysfunction, which determines space dispersion. The sensory function is usually intact, although some patients report areas of hypoesthesia or dysesthesia. The combination of congenital (mild) hypotonia and proprioception defects sometimes results in a slight psychomotor developmental delay with the absence of crawling, walking on toes, first steps alone >14 months, and motor awkwardness.

Main Symptoms Divided by Organs

Musculoskeletal System: recurrent sprains and dislocations, slow healing of joint trauma, tendinitis, recurrent synovitis and tenosynovitis, chronic-recurrent arthralgia, chronic-recurrent myalgia, including cramp-like pain, ruptures of muscles, and tendons.

Nervous System: neuropathic pain, hyperalgesia, allodynia, paraesthesia, dysesthesia, local anesthetic resistance, chronic-recurrent mixed headache, oropharyngeal dysphagia, recurrent dysphonia, mood disorders, anxiety, personality, depression, and selective cognitive impairment.

Sense Organs: hyperacusis, dizziness, tinnitus/tinnitus, myopia, corneal and sclera fragility (rupture of the cornea and eyeball), and hypo/hyperosmia.

Skin and Mucous Membranes: easy to bruise, skin and gingival fragility, rhinorrhea, slow and poor healing, xerophthalmia, xerostomia, hypohidrosis/diaphoresis, palmoplantar hyperhidrosis, and vaginal dryness.

Cardiovascular System: orthostatic intolerance, cold and/or sudden changes in temperature, recurrent tachycardia and palpitations, Raynaud's phenomenon, acrocyanosis, ruptures of vessels, aneurysms, and dissections.

Gastrointestinal System: symptoms of gastroesophageal reflux, heartburn, abdominal swelling and/or fullness, recurrent abdominal pain, alterations of the hives, and ruptures of the colon and spleen.

Genitourinary System: stress urinary incontinence symptoms, neurological bladder symptoms, menstrual cycle changes, less/metrorrhagia, dysmenorrhea, dyspareunia, vulvodynia, and pelvic prolapse.

2017 International EDS Classification

The Ehlers–Danlos syndrome (EDS) is currently classified in a system of 13 subtypes, as outlined in Table 1, each of them has a set of clinical criteria that help guide diagnosis; a patient's physical signs and symptoms will be matched up to the major and minor criteria to identify the subtype that is the most complete fit.

Table 1 EDS type chart from https://www.ehlers-danlos.com/eds-types/

Name of EDS subtype	IP[a]	Genetic basis	Protein involved
Classical EDS (cEDS)	AD	Major: *COL5A1, COL5A2*	Type V collagen
		Rare: *COL1A1* c.934C > T, p.(Arg312Cys)	Type I collagen
Classical-like EDS (clEDS)	AR	*TNXB*	Tenascin XB
Cardiac valvular EDS (cvEDS)	AR	*COL1A2* (biallelic mutations that lead to *COL1A2* NMD and absence of pro α2(I) collagen chains)	Type I collagen
Vascular EDS (vEDS)	AD	Major: *COL3A1*	Type III collagen
		Rare: *COL1A1* c.934C > T, p.(Arg312Cys) c.1720C > T, p.(Arg574Cys) c.3277C > T, p.(Arg1093Cys)	Type I collagen
Hypermobile EDS (hEDS)	AD	Unknown	Unknown
Arthrochalasia EDS (aEDS)	AD	*COL1A1, COL1A2*	Type I collagen
Dermatosparaxis EDS (dEDS)	AR	*ADAMTS2*	ADAMTS-2
Kyphoscoliotic EDS (kEDS)	AR	*PLOD1*	LH1
		FKBP14	FKBP22
Brittle cornea syndrome (BCS)	AR	*ZNF469*	ZNF469
		PRDM5	PRDM5
Spondylodysplastic EDS (spEDS)	AR	*B4GALT7*	β4GalT7
		B3GALT6	β3GalT6
		SLC39A13	ZIP13
Musculocontractural EDS (mcEDS)	AR	*CHST14*	D4ST1
		DSE	DSE
Myopathic EDS (mEDS)	AD or AR	*COL12A1*	Type XII collagen
Periodontal EDS (pEDS)	AD	*C1R*	C1r

[a] Inheritance pattern: *AD* autosomal dominant, *AR* autosomal recessive

Laboratory Finding

Once the diagnosis is suspected, genetic confirmation should be performed. This procedure is not available for variants for which the causative gene is not known. Ultrastructural examination and electrophoresis of dermal collagens require a skin biopsy and may be technically inaccessible. The most used method to confirm is molecular investigation, although a negative result generally does not exclude the diagnosis made clinically. In specific circumstances, laboratory tests on skin biopsy can be considered preliminary to the molecular study if there are significant clinical doubts in selecting the gene (or genes) to be analyzed. The identification of the causative mutation, unlike other laboratory confirmation methods, offers the possibility of prenatal diagnosis and presymptomatic testing in family members at risk.

In the presence of bruising, a PT, PTT, INR dosage, and blood count with formula are useful for differential diagnosis from coagulopathies.

Due to the higher incidence and precocity of osteoporosis in some patients with Ehlers–Danlos syndrome, it is recommended to periodically monitor the blood parameters involved in bone remodeling (BONE PROTOCOL). The bone protocol includes a blood dosage of total calcium, phosphorus, albumin, parathyroid hormone, alkaline phosphatase with isoenzymes, 25 (OH) vitamin D, osteocalcin, Ctx telopeptide, and creatinine. The protocol also provides for 24-h urine collection with a dosage of deoxypyridinoline, urinary calcium, urinary phosphorus, and urinary creatinine.

Evaluations Following Initial Diagnosis

The following diagnostic investigations are recommended in Ehlers–Danlos syndrome:

- **Abdomen ultrasound** in both standing and supine position for all EDS subtypes in order to evaluate visceroptosis and great vessel dilatations.
- **Supra-aortic trunk echo-**Doppler (TSA) for all EDS subtypes in order to evaluate the dimensions and course of the blood vessels.
- **Baseline transthoracic echocardiogram** to evaluate the structure of heart valves and measures of the aortic diameter for dilatations.
- **Magnetic resonance angiograph** (MRA)/computed tomography angiography (CTA) total body for the detection of small aneurysms and dissections in young adults in the presence of clinical criteria or family history for vascular EDS.
- **Bone densitometry** (column and femur) for all EDS patients, due to a higher prevalence rate of osteoporosis compared with healthy individuals.
- **Spine or district radiography** in the presence of column scoliosis or other skeletal deformities.
- **Complete eye examination** in all forms of EDS for early detection of eye abnormalities.
- **Use of the Beighton score** for a joint mobility evaluation.

- **Chronic pain assessments** for all patients with certain pain severity, accordingly to the numeric rating scale (NRS).
- **Physiotherapy assessment and rehabilitation** in all patients with neuromuscular and muscular pain involvement.

Molecular Diagnostics

It should be noted that molecular genetic testing has considerable weight and value in the diagnosis, in consideration of the patient's family history and the type of EDS suspected. In fact, it is emphasized that some EDS types have a high percentage of detection of genetic mutations and an exact genotype–phenotype assessment; in these cases, the genetic analysis has an effective diagnostic value to confirm the clinical suspicion. However, there are other pathogenic variants where the causative genes are not yet known or only hypothesized. Diagnosis in these cases is obtained clinically, and genetic analysis can only help to confirm and direct the diagnosis. The identification of the causal mutation in the gene involved allows, if required, a prenatal molecular diagnosis of the disease.

Additional Diagnostic Tools

A skin biopsy can be useful for EDS diagnosis. By analyzing collagen synthesis by fibroblasts in vitro, we can evaluate the effect of the causative gene. It should be noted that the test involves a skin biopsy and is therefore more invasive than a blood sample or a urine sample: Its usefulness must be assessed case by case. The screening of collagens produced in vitro by fibroblasts can be useful for the diagnosis in EDS of the arthrochalasia, dermatosparaxis, and vascular and classic forms (collagen V but also, in rare cases, type collagen I, especially where the genetic investigation is negative). The biochemical data can be helpful, for example, in the differential diagnosis between classic and vascular forms of Ehlers–Danlos or in cases of Ehlers–Danlos characterized by extreme rarity (such as arthrochalasia and dermatosparaxis or Cyphoscoliotic with negative urine test). It should be emphasized that for dermatosparaxis form it would be more appropriate to perform an electron microscopy of the biopsy for the presence of hieroglyphic collagen fibers, a hallmark of the syndrome. The biochemical investigation is also useful, once the molecular defect has been identified, to verify the phenotypic effect of the genetic mutation.

Treatment of Manifestations

There are no specific guidelines for the treatment of EDS, but it is possible to manage many of the symptoms with support and advice. Treatment and management of patients with EDS should use a multidisciplinary approach that focuses on the prevention of disease progression and subsequent complications as there is no cure for the disease. Specialists generally manage specific care within the field of which the patient has concerning pathology, e.g., the monitoring of cardiovascular concerns by a cardiologist; likewise, musculoskeletal pathology is monitored and treated by an orthopedist; geneticist or family medicine provider acts as the primary provider referring the patient to these specialists.

Treatment of EDS typically consists of the management of specific signs and symptoms and lifestyle adjustments to prevent injury/complications. The therapy of patients suffering from Ehlers–Danlos syndrome must first of all be divided into pharmacological and non-pharmacological and must address all the different clinical aspects by which EDS is characterized.

Pharmacological Therapy

- Pain management (NSAIDs/opioids, pregabalin, and gabapentin and triptans).
- Cardiovascular management (b-blockers).
- Management of asthenia and dysautonomia (corticosteroids and vasopressors, in particular midodrine, and some dietary supplements, with regard to fermented papaya extracts and coenzyme Q10).

Non-pharmacological Therapy

- Rehabilitation program.
- Physical therapy (TECAR therapy, cryotherapy, idrotherapy, TENS).
- Physiokinesis therapy.
- Acupuncture.
- Cognitive and behavioral therapy.
- Articulation tutors.
- Occupational therapy.

Surgery

Particular attention should be reserved to even small interventions that require local anesthesia, as for the EDS patients a greater dose of anesthetic drug may be needed. People with EDS may experience local anesthetic resistance, defined as the failure to provide pain prevention, more often than the general population.

Due to the risk of bleeding and tissue fragility, it is absolutely necessary that the sutures are made with nonresorbable material and with isolated stitches.

Do not use skin glue or metal staples for the external stitches, keep the stitches longer, and remove them after 2 weeks.

In the case of lacerated wounds, especially in children, the use of skin glue or Steri-Strip is preferred.

Emergency Situations

It is good to keep in mind when managing therapy that emergency situations are possible in EDS and may require specialist emergency intervention. In particular, some examples are given as follows:

- In vascular EDS and classic variant EDS with vascular ruptures, in the kyphoscoliotic type and in the tortuous artery syndrome, acute pain in any anatomical region (especially if in the thoracic and abdominal area) and/or loss of consciousness and/or ischemia of a limb, which they can lay down for the dissection of a vase.
- Intolerable exacerbation of musculoskeletal pain and/or headaches, even after administration of painkillers, for all variants of EDS.
- Acute ocular pain with or without loss of vision in patients with kyphoscoliotic type and brittle cornea syndrome.
- Need for non-deferrable surgical intervention for any reason even not related to the underlying disease for all variants of EDS.
- Childbirth for all variants of EDS, especially those at the highest risk of vascular ruptures.

Prognosis

The prognosis depends on the type of Ehlers–Danlos syndrome and the individual. Life expectancy can be shortened for those with vascular Ehlers–Danlos syndrome due to the possibility of organ and vessel rupture. Life expectancy is usually not affected by the other types. There can be a wide or narrow range of severity within a family, but each person's case of Ehlers–Danlos syndrome will be unique. While there is no cure for the Ehlers–Danlos syndrome, there is treatment for symptoms, and there are preventive measures that are helpful for most.

Sexuality and Quality of Life

EDS affects more women (70%) than men (30%). Patients complain of pelvic floor disorders dyspareunia (painful intercourse), pelvic organ prolapse (where internal organs protrude from the vagina), and urinary incontinence (loss of bladder control), dysfunction of arousal and orgasm. In some cases, dysmenorrhea (painful menstrual cycle) and menorrhagia (severe bleeding during menstruation) are complained of, which may affect the desire for and frequency of sexual intercourse [2].

Some studies have reported vulvodynia (chronic pain or burning sensation outside the vagina) or labial edema (swelling of the vaginal lips), which can make intercourse painful and anxiety-inducing [3].

Pelvic floor weakness also occurs in men mostly involving erectile dysfunction and cryptorchidism (problems with testicles not descending), hypogonadism (not producing enough testosterone and/or sperm), tight foreskin, and testicular torsion (twisting of the testicles) [4].

There Is More

Patients with EDS are also at a relatively high risk of mental disorders, such as anxiety and mood disorders, accompanied by headaches, muscle aches, neuralgia, abdominal pain, and general malaise [5]. Depressive symptoms in patients with EDS were first reported in 2003 [6].

As patients with EDS and depression frequently experience pain [7], one could hypothesize both physical pain (as in dislocation) and psychological pain, caused by the mood disorder [8]. In addition, chronic pain in such patients may lead to negative emotions because of the psychological burden. A large-scale population-based study in Sweden found that patients with EDS report a higher risk of mood and developmental disorders than the general population [9].

A study by Samantha Aliza Hershenfeld et al. [10] highlighted psychiatric disorders and their relationship with systemic manifestations in a group of 106 patients with classic-type EDS and hypermobility.

Psychiatric disorders were found in 42.5% of the EDS cohort, with 22.7% of patients having two or more psychiatric diagnoses. Anxiety and depression were most commonly reported, with frequencies of 23.6% and 25.5%, respectively. A number of other psychiatric diagnoses were also identified. Abdominal pain [odds ratio (OR): 7.38], neuropathic pain (OR: 4.07), migraine (OR: 5.21), joint pain (OR: 2.85), and fatigue (OR: 5.55) were significantly associated with the presence of a psychiatric disorder. The presence of any painful symptom was significantly associated with having a psychiatric disorder (OR: 9.68). Muscle pain (OR: 2.79), abdominal pain (OR: 5.78), neuropathic pain (OR: 3.91), migraine (OR: 2.63), and fatigue (OR: 3.78) were strongly associated with having an anxiety or mood disorder.

Again, the literature indicates [11] that vascular Ehlers–Danlos syndrome (vEDS) is characterized by arterial, bowel, and/or uterine fragility; thin, translucent skin; easy bruising; characteristic facial appearance (thin vermilion lips, micrognathia, narrow nose, prominent eyes), and an aged appearance in the extremities, particularly the hands.

Vascular dissection or rupture, gastrointestinal perforation, and organ rupture are the presenting signs in most adults with vEDS. Arterial rupture may be preceded by an aneurysm, arteriovenous fistulae, or dissection, but may also occur spontaneously. The majority (60%) of people with vEDS who are diagnosed before the age of 18 years are identified because of positive family history. Infants may present with clubfoot, hip dislocation, limb deficits, and/or amniotic bands. Approximately half of the children tested for vEDS in the absence of positive family history have a major complication at a mean age of 11 years. Four minor diagnostic features—distal joint hypermobility, easy bruising, thin skin, and clubfeet—are more often present in those children diagnosed without major complications.

With regard to podiatric abnormalities, a study by Inmaculada C Palomo-Toucedo [12] studied 38 individuals with hypermobile or classic EDS. The type of foot was classified according to the footprint and the Foot Posture Index. In all patients, a high degree of pain, disability, intensity of fatigue, and low quality of life were observed. According to the footprint, 20% presented flat feet, 47% normal feet, and 33% hollow feet. It seems clear that in these patients the quality of life was very reduced and a cause of psychophysical discomfort.

Conclusion

The complexity of Ehlers–Danlos syndrome (EDS) modifies in no small way the quality of life of patients and their caregivers. The latter must be followed by specialists in general to obtain the most information to understand, over and above the pain, the physical, psychological, and relational factors of the patient, excluding affective aspects.

The psychosexologist in these cases can be a facilitator of communication doctor–patient–family, but also a support to the patient and relatives about the sexual development of the individual and the sexual role.

Despite scarce studies, psychological factors associated with EDS hypermobility type that potentially influence chronic pain and disability have been identified. These are cognitive problems and attention to body sensations, negative emotions, and unhealthy activity patterns (hypo/hyperactivity).

As in other chronic pain conditions, these aspects should be more explored in the EDS hypermobility type and integrated into chronic pain prevention and management programs. Implications for rehabilitation physicians should be aware that joint hypermobility may be associated with other health problems and, in its presence, suspect an inherited connective tissue disease such as Ehlers–Danlos syndrome (EDS) type hypermobility, in which chronic pain is one of the most frequent and disabling symptoms. It is necessary to explore patients' psychosocial functioning as part of the overall management of chronic pain in EDS hypermobility type, especially when they do not respond to biomedical approaches as psychological factors may work against rehabilitation and so in self-image.

References

1. Voermans et al. Neuromuscular involvement in various types of Ehlers-Danlos syndrome. Ann Neurol. 2009;65(6):687–97.
2. Malfait F, Francomano C, Byers P, Belmont J, Berglund B, Black J, et al. The 2017 international classification of Ehlers-Danlos syndromes. Am J Med Genet C Med Genet Semin. 2017;175(1):8–26.
3. Mayer K, Kennerknecht I, Steinmann B. Genetic card of clinical utility for: types of Ehlers-Danlos I-VII syndrome and variants—update 2012. Eur J Hum Genet. 2013;21(1):118. https://doi.org/10.1038/ejhg.2012.162.
4. Baeza-Velasco C, Bulbena A, Polanco-Carrasco R, Jaussaud R. Cognitive, emotional, and behavioral considerations for chronic pain management in the hypermobility type of Ehlers-Danlos syndrome: a narrative review. Disabil Rehabil. 2016;22:1–9.
5. Hershenfeld SA, Wasim S, McNiven V, et al. Psychiatric disorders in Ehlers-Danlos syndrome are frequent, diverse and strongly associated with pain. Rheumatol Int. 2016;36(3):341–8. https://doi.org/10.1007/s00296-015-3375-1.
6. Sienaert P, De Hert M, Houben M, et al. Safe ECT in a patient with Ehlers-Danlos syndrome. J ECT. 2003;19(4):230–3. https://doi.org/10.1097/00124509-200312000-00010.
7. Doan L, Manders T, Wang J. Neuroplasticity underlying the comorbidity between pain and depression. Neural Plast. 2015;2015:16. https://doi.org/10.1155/2015/504691.504691.
8. Li J. Comorbidity with pain and depression: a preclinical perspective. Behav Brain Res. 2015;276:92–8.
9. Cederlöf M, Larsson H, Lichtenstein P, Almqvist C, Serlachius E, Ludvigsson JF. National population-based cohort study of psychiatric disorders in individuals with Ehlers-Danlos syndrome or hypermobility syndrome and their siblings. BMC Psychiatry. 2016;16(207):207. https://doi.org/10.1186/s12888-016-0922-6.
10. Hershenfeld SA, et al. Psychiatric disorders in Ehlers-Danlos syndrome are frequent, diverse and strongly associated with pain. Reumatol Int. 2016;36(3):341–8. https://doi.org/10.1007/s00296-015-3375-1. Epub 2015 ottobre 3.
11. Adam MP, Ardinger HH, Pagon RA, et al., editors. GeneReviews® [Internet] Seattle (WA): University of Washington; 1993–2022.
12. Palomo-Toucedo IC, et al. Podiatry alterations in Ehlers-Danlos syndrome. Med Clin. 2020;154(3):94–7. https://doi.org/10.1016/j.medcli.2019.05.06. Epub 2019 giu 27.

Suggested Reading

Malfait F, Francomano C, Byers P, Belmont J, et al. The 2017 classification of the Ehlers-Danlos syndromes. Am J Med Genet C Semin Med Genet. 2017;175c:8–26.
Mantle D, Wilkins RM, Preedy V. A novel therapeutic strategy of Ehlers-Danlos syndrome based on nutritional supplements. Med Hypotheses. 2005;64:279–83. Received 6 Aug 2003; Accepted 18 Jul 2004.
Frankm M, Adham S, Seigle S, et al. Vascular Ehlers-Danlos syndrome. J Am Coll Cardiol. 2019;73(15):1948.

Malek S, Koster DV. The role of cell adhesion and cytoskeleton dynamics in the pathogenesis of the Ehlers-Danlos syndromes and hypermobility spectrum disorders. Coventry: Division of Biochemical Sciences, Centre for Mechanochemical Cell Biology, Warwick Medical School, University of Warwick; 2021. https://doi.org/10.3389/fcell.2021.649082.

Talarico R, Aguilera S, Alexander T, et al. The impact of COVID-19 on rare and complex connective tissue diseases: the experience of ERN ReCONNET. Nat Rev Rheumatol. 2021;17:177.

Kang J, Hanif M, Mirza E, Jaleel S. Ehlers-Danlos syndrome in pregnancy: a review. Eur J Obstet Gynecol Reprod Biol. 2020;255:118–23. 0301-2115|2020 Elsevier B.V A.

Kohn A, Chang C. The relationship between hypermobile Ehlers-Danlos syndrome (hEDS), postural orthostatic tachycardia syndrome (POTS), and mast cell activation syndrome (MCAS). Springer; 2019.

Malfait F, Wenstrup R, De Paepe A. Classic Ehlers-Danlos syndrome. NHI. U.S National Library of Medicine. Created 29 May 2007; Updated 26 Jul 2018. GeneReviews. Seattle: University of Washington.

Tinkle BT, Levy HP. Symptomatic joint hypermobility. The hypermobile type of Ehlers-Danlos syndrome and the hypermobility spectrum disorders. Med Clin N Am. 2019;103:1021–33. 0025-7125/19/Published by Elsevier Inc. https://doi.org/10.1016/j.mcna.2019.08.002.

Levy HP. Hypermobile Ehlers-Danlos syndrome. Created 22 Oct 2004; Revised 21 June 2018. NIS U.S. National Library of Medicine. Bookshelf. https://ncbi.nlm.nih.gov/books/.

Baumann M, Giunta C, Krabichler B, Rüschendorf F, Zoppi N, Colombi M, Bittner RE, Quijano-Roy S, Muntoni F, Cirak S, Schreiber G, Zou Y, Hu Y, Romero NB, Carlier RY, Amberger A, Deutschmann A, Straub V, Rohrbach M, Steinmann B, Rostásy K, Karall D, Bönnemann CG, Zschocke J, Fauth C. Mutations in FKBP14 cause a variant of Ehlers-Danlos syndrome with progressive kyphoscoliosis, myopathy, and hearing loss. Am J Hum Genet. 2012;90:1–16.

De Paepe A, Malfait F. The Ehlers–Danlos syndrome, a disorder with many faces. Clin Genet. 2012;82:1–11.

Symoens S, Delfien S, Malfait F, Callewaert B, De Backer J, Vanakker O, Coucke P, De Paepe A. Comprehensive molecular analysis demonstrates type V collagen mutations in over 90% of patients with classic EDS and allows to refine diagnostic criteria. Hum Mutat. 2012;33(10):1485–93.

Castori M, Sperduti I, Celletti C, Camerota F, Grammatico P. Symptom and joint mobility progression in the joint hypermobility syndrome (Ehlers-Danlos syndrome, hypermobility type). Clin Exp Rheumatol. 2011;29:998–1005.

Burkitt-Wright EMM, Spencer HL, Daly SB, Manson FDC, Zeef LAH, Urquhart J, Zoppi N, Bonshek R, Tosounidis I, Mohan M, Madden C, Dodds A, Chandler KE, Banka S, Au L, Clayton-Smith J, Khan N, Biesecker LG, Wilson M, Rohrbach M, Colombi M, Giunta C, Black GCM. Mutations in PRDM5 in brittle cornea syndrome identify a novel pathway regulating extracellular matrix development and maintenance. Am J Hum Genet. 2011;88:767–77.

Dworkin RH, Durk DC, et al. Evidence-based clinical trial design for chronic pain pharmacotherapy: a blueprint for action. Pian. 2011;152:S107 15.

Mayer K, Kennerknecht I, Steinmann B. Clinical utility gene card for: Ehlers–Danlos syndrome types I–VII. Eur J Hum Genet. 2010;18.

Attal A, Cruccu G, Baron R, Haanpa M, Hansson P, Jensen TS, Nurmikko T. EFNS guidelines on the pharmacological treatment of neuropathic pain: 2009 revision. Eur J Neurol. 2009;2010

Plancke A, Holder-Espinasse M, Rigau V, Manouvrier S, Claustres M, Van Kien PK. Homozygosity for a null allele of COL3A1 results in recessive Ehlers-Danlos syndrome. Eur J Hum Genet. 2009;17:1411–6.

Malfait F, Symoens S, Coucke P, Nunes L, De Almeida S, De Paepe A. Total absence of the alpha2(I) chain of collagen type I causes a rare form of Ehlers-Danlos syndrome with hypermobility and propensity to cardiac valvular problems. J Med Genet. 2006;43:e36.

Part XIX
Rheumatology

Rheumatoid Arthritis

Elena Bartoloni, Roberto Gerli, and Elena Vittoria Longhi

Introduction to Chronic Joint Diseases

Rheumatoid arthritis (RA) and osteoarthritis (OA) represent the most frequent chronic articular diseases characterized by a diametrically opposite etiopathogenesis and clinical picture. Indeed, the first one is the prototype of chronic inflammatory articular diseases, mainly involving women in middle age, being the second the typical example of chronic degenerative joint conditions, thus affecting almost exclusively elderly subjects. Osteoarthritis represents the most common chronic articular disorder affecting about 3.3–3.6% of the population aged above 60 years, and prevalence raises with age. It has been estimated that the lifetime risk of having symptomatic knee OA is about 45% in both sexes and about 60% in obese subjects. On the other hand, incidence rates of RA are higher in northern Europe and North America compared with southern Europe. In North America and northern Europe, RA affects 0.4–1% of the population; in southern Europe, it affects 0.3–0.7% of the population. The female-to-male ratio is 2–3:1, and the prevalence of RA increases with age.

As chronic diseases, both are characterized by a considerably high social and economic impact mainly due to long-term joint damage, poorer quality of life, articular disability, activity and working limitations, healthcare use, and, consequently, relevant costs for society. In this setting, both diseases are characterized by high economic burden. Several studies highlighted that, although the major advances in the management of RA due to the introduction of biologic therapies led to a significant decrease in direct costs over time, as costs related to hospitalization, indirect

E. Bartoloni · R. Gerli (✉)
Rheumatology Unit, Department of Medicine and Surgery, University of Perugia, Perugia, Italy
e-mail: elena.bartolonibocci@unipg.it; roberto.gerli@unipg.it

E. V. Longhi
Department of Sexual Medical Center, San Raffaele Hospital, Milano, Italy

© Springer Nature Switzerland AG 2023

E. V. Longhi (ed.), *Managing Psychosexual Consequences in Chronic Diseases*,
https://doi.org/10.1007/978-3-031-31307-3_34

costs referred to productivity losses, caregivers, lost production due to sick leave, reduced work performance, and early retirement still account for up to 80% of total costs, with work disability accounting for the majority [1]. On the other hand, cost estimates for OA are highly variable and differ according to body location, being higher for hip and knee and lower for hand OA. Hip and knee OA alone are major contributors to the rise in socioeconomic burdens having a notable impact on patient mobility and articular function. Moreover, because of the chronic nature of the disease and the need for total replacement joint surgery during the disease course for the majority of subjects, direct costs for OA are still considerably high and represent the major contributors to the rise in socioeconomic burden related to this chronic disease. Nevertheless, nonsurgical interventions, although characterized by lower direct costs, may exert relevant economic impacts including sick leave from work and the need for joint devices or splints, which may be highly expensive [2].

Of consequence, deeper knowledge of disease pathogenesis represents an essential need in order to reach an early diagnosis, introduce specific treatment, and, as consequence, prevent or delay articular damage. Despite recent research advances, RA etiopathogenesis has not been completely elucidated yet. Surely, the interaction between a specific genetic background and environmental factors represents the main trigger for disease development. Genome-wide analyses of single nucleotide polymorphisms have identified the human leukocyte antigen D-related B1 gene (HLA-DRB1) as the most relevant disease-susceptible gene in association with other genes, including the protein tyrosine phosphatase non-receptor type 22 (PTPN22), the cytotoxic T-lymphocyte antigen-4 (CTLA4), the signal transducer and activator of transcription 4 (STAT4), and the peptidylarginine deiminase 4 (PADI4). Among environmental and occupational factors, smoking represents the strongest airway exposure conferring a higher risk of developing the disease in susceptible individuals, in particular in subjects carrying certain alleles of HLADRB, named "shared epitope" alleles, and with anti-cyclic citrullinated peptide protein (anti-CCP) antibody positivity. Moreover, changes in composition and function of the gut microbiome with altered gut mucosal permeability and chronic gingivitis by *Porphyromonas gingivalis* have been related to epigenetic modifications, breakdown of immune tolerance to antigens and autoimmunity induction, and finally leading to disease development. Autoreactive T and B lymphocytes accumulate in the synovial membrane, the main target of RA, where it induces a strong inflammatory environment characterized by angiogenesis, synoviocyte proliferation, and production of pro-inflammatory cytokines, such as tumor necrosis factor-α, interleukin-1, and interleukin-6, which contribute to in situ inflammatory synovial infiltrate. Furthermore, cytokine-stimulated synoviocytes produce matrix metalloproteinases (MMP) and fibroblast and inflammatory cells lead to osteoclast generation resulting in bone juxta-articular erosions, the hallmark feature of RA [3].

The pathogenic mechanisms underlying OA are an interplay of risk factors, mechanical stress, and abnormal joint mechanics [4]. A genetic background has been also identified in OA, a disease mainly affecting the cartilage and subchondral bone, especially in the primary form. Variant alleles of some specific genes expressed in cartilage, as gene variant of growth differentiation factor (GDF) 5, have been linked to an increased risk to develop hip or knee OA. Subsequently, a dysregulated balance between anabolic and pathologic catabolic forces, including traumatic meniscal tears, ligament damage, osteochondral defects, and direct cartilage trauma, contributes to the initiation of osteochondral unit damage. Different factors, including obesity, cigarette smoking, local trauma, muscle weakness or imbalance, work-related habits, physical activity, and hormonal menopausal changes, contribute to accelerate articular OA damage. The early stage of OA is characterized by a variable degree of synovial inflammation, with resident macrophages and lymphocyte, which trigger inflammatory and catabolic damage, and by inflammatory cytokines and complement components detectable in the synovial fluid. These processes are also regulated by a complex network of chemokines, neuropeptides, and proteolytic enzymes. In the subsequent phases, pathologic damage extends to the subchondral bone with angiogenesis and remodeling of the subchondral bone plate by osteoclasts and osteoblasts, which contribute to the initial formation of osteophytes. In later stages, osteoclasts perpetuate damage within the calcified cartilage and osteoblast infiltration contributes to novel deposition of bone tissue, finally contributing to osteophyte growth, fissures and cartilage erosions, reduced chondrocyte density, and end-stage subchondral sclerosis. In the final stages of OA damage, different proteases and the collagenases MMP-1, MMP-3, MMP-9, and MMP-13 contribute to cartilage extracellular matrix degradation. Fragments and cleavage products derived by extracellular matrix degradation induce local recruitment of inflammatory cells, enhance phagocytic functions, and elicit cytokine, in particular IL-1, TNF, IL-6, and, to a minor extent, IL-15, IL-17, and IL-18, and chemokine release by inflammatory cells, thus perpetuating chondral and subchondral bone damage. Finally, osteoclast activity and osteoblast infiltrate in the calcified cartilage contribute to subchondral damage and novel bone deposit resulting in end-stage OA [4].

Main Medical Characteristics of Rheumatoid Arthritis and Osteoarthritis

The most common clinical presentation of RA is an insidious onset of a symmetric, additive, polyarthritis of small hand joints, including proximal interphalangeal (PIP) and metacarpophalangeal (MCP) and metatarsophalangeal joints and wrists. Some patients may present with monoarticular joint involvement, mainly involving the knees. Articular involvement is often associated with characteristic morning stiffness, often lasting more than an hour, and flexor tenosynovitis. In addition, patients often complain of systemic symptoms, such as low-grade fever, malaise, fatigue, and weight loss. Up to 35% of patients develop, generally in the later stages of the disease, rheumatoid nodules on the extensor surface of elbows and on hands. Late in the disease course, characteristic articular deformities, including "boutonniere" (PIP flexion and DIP extension) and "swan neck" (DIP flexion and PIP extension) deformities, MCP subluxation, and ulnar deviation, may occur, usually in patients with long-standing and not properly treated disease [3, 5].

As a systemic inflammatory disease, RA may be characterized, in up to 40% of patients, by a wide range of extra-articular manifestations, usually observed during the disease course and identifying a subset of patients with more severe disease associated with poorer prognosis. In this setting, almost each organ or anatomic system may be involved and more frequent manifestations include rheumatoid skin vasculitis, neutrophilic dermatoses, rheumatoid nodulosis, peripheral nerve involvement as multiplex neuritis or sensory symmetric neuropathy, interstitial lung disease, ocular involvement including keratoconjunctivitis sicca, scleritis, episcleritis, and peripheral ulcerative keratitis, pericarditis, and renal amyloidosis. Moreover, in recent years, cardiovascular disease emerged as a leading cause of higher mortality risk in these patients [3, 5].

On the other hand, the clinical picture and rate progression of OA may vary according to the involved joint and for each individual [6]. The most characteristic symptoms include a gradual, progressive, and localized articular pain typically worsening with prolonged activity and reducing at rest, often associated with joint stiffness and reduced articular mobility. Patients may also experience bony swelling, joint deformity, and articular instability. Although OA is most commonly reported in the knee, it can occur in any articular site and multiple joints are affected in up to 25% of individuals. In addition to the knee, the spine is frequently involved, in particular at cervical and lumbar levels. Symptoms may vary according to the location of the pathological process and include occipital pain often with headache or buttock pain with or without nerve root compression. However, although knee and spine OA are the most frequent forms, symptomatic hand OA is estimated more prevalent. Patients with hand OA complain of decreased function, reduced grip strength, stiffness, and pain, often activity-related. Hallmarks of hand OA include bony enlargements at the distal IP (Heberden nodules), at PIP (Bouchard nodules), and involvement of the first carpometacarpal (CMC) joint, frequently all occurring in the same patient. Non-modifiable risk factors, such as age, sex, genetics, menopause status, and ethnicity, and modifiable risk factors, including occupation, mechanical use, diet, and smoking, have been demonstrated to contribute to hand OA pathogenesis [6, 7].

Main Tools for the Diagnosis of Rheumatoid Arthritis and Osteoarthritis

Specific laboratory tests are essential in confirming the diagnosis of RA. Rheumatoid factor (RF), an immunoglobulin (Ig) M binding the Fc part of IgG, can be detected, in general at medium to high titer, in about 80% of patients with established disease. However, RF is not specific to the disease as it can be detected in patients with systemic autoimmune diseases, in subjects with an infective condition, in about 15% of elderly individuals, and up to 5% of healthy subjects. High titer of RF does not correlate with disease activity, but RA patients with serum positivity for RF are characterized by a more severe disease, with a higher risk of joint erosions and extra-articular involvement. The specificity of RF for disease diagnosis increases in subjects with concomitant positivity for anti-CCP antibodies. Anti-CCP antibodies are nearly as sensitive as RF, but their specificity is remarkably higher, also in patients with early disease. Moreover, positivity for anti-CCP has been correlated with more aggressive disease characterized by a higher risk of radiographic damage and extra-articular systemic involvement, as interstitial lung disease. Both antibodies have no diagnostic value for assessing disease activity. In this setting, laboratory evaluation of systemic inflammation requires the determination of erythrocyte sedimentation rate and C-reactive protein, which are both elevated in patients with active disease. The RA classification criteria published by the American College of Rheumatology and the European League Against Rheumatism in 2010 have been validated, in subjects with at least one joint with clinical synovitis no better explained by other diseases, to classify patients as RA and to allow prompt introduction of specific therapy. These criteria attribute a different score according to RF, anti-CCP and inflammatory index titer, disease duration, and type and number of involved joints. Six or more points are necessary to establish the diagnosis [8].

In addition to a thorough history and physical examination, radiographic imaging is an important diagnostic tool, in particular in patients with OA. Typical radiographic findings in OA include joint space narrowing, osteophytes, subchondral sclerosis, and subchondral cysts. In RA, radiographic imaging allows to detect the characteristic juxta-articular erosions. In these patients, articular damage may be quantified by the evaluation of the findings of the total Sharp score, a scoring system that is calculated at different joints (wrists, fingers, and toes) and attributes a numerical score according to joint space narrowing, indicating cartilage absorption and bone erosions. Recently, advanced imaging techniques, including magnetic resonance imaging and musculoskeletal ultrasound, emerged as the important toll in the diagnostic workup of RA patients. These techniques, improving the detection of subtle areas of synovial inflammation, bone marrow edema, and joint damage, allow earlier disease diagnosis, thus influencing decision-making in the management of RA.

Main Nonsurgical and Surgical Treatments

Treatment for RA has made many advances in the last 30 years since the introduction of conventional synthetic disease-modifying anti-rheumatic drugs (DMARDs). Therapeutic strategies should be evaluated according to a comprehensive assessment of disease activity, imaging findings, extra-articular involvement, and presence of comorbidities. The therapeutic goal for RA patients is disease remission or achievement of a low-disease activity status according to internationally validated composite activity indices in order to prevent future joint erosive damage [9–11].

The standard initial management after disease diagnosis requires the introduction of conventional synthetic DMARDs, such as hydroxychloroquine or methotrexate, in association with glucocorticoid therapy. According to international recommendations, methotrexate should be considered as the first therapeutic choice, unless contraindicated. It exerts its anti-inflammatory and disease-modifying effects by controlling lymphocyte and synoviocyte proliferation. Adverse drug effects include liver toxicity, gastrointestinal intolerance, and myelosuppression, especially in elderly patients. Sulfasalazine and leflunomide may be recommended when methotrexate use is contraindicated. When no improvement is observed within 3 months or when no remission is achieved within 6 months, the introduction of biological DMARDs or Janus kinase (JAK) inhibitors, as monotherapy or in association with methotrexate, is recommended. Biologic drugs with different mechanisms, including anti-TNFα (infliximab, etanercept, adalimumab, golimumab, and certolizumab), IL-6-targeting drugs (tocilizumab and sarilumab), T cell-selective co-stimulation modulator abatacept, and JAK inhibitors (baricitinib, tofacitinib), allow disease remission in more than half of the patients and have been demonstrated to delay or, in some cases, to prevent the progression of joint damage [9–11].

Initial treatment of OA rests on nonsurgical interventions, which have the final goal to reduce pain and improve articular mobility [6]. International OA guidelines recommend patient education, lifestyle interventions of physical activity, exercise, and weight loss, and physical therapies as the first-line treatment options in patients with symptomatic OA. Pharmacological therapies, such as nonsteroidal anti-inflammatory drugs (oral or topical), paracetamol, and intra-articular glucocorticoid injections, are often prescribed in association with physical therapy to reduce joint pain and stiffness and to optimize the clinical effects of exercise. Intra-articular corticosteroid injection may be useful for symptomatic knee OA to reduce local inflammation. In some patients, intra-articular hyaluronic acid (HA) injections represent another option for knee osteoarthritis. Local administration of HA into the joint acts as a lubricant and is particularly recommended for long-term treatment as has been demonstrated to achieve more durable effects in comparison with corticosteroid and a more favorable safety profile than repeated corticosteroid injections. Surgical treatments, including osteotomy, unicompartmental knee arthroplasty, or total knee arthroplasty, are typically indicated only in patients with end-stage OA not responding to medical or non-medical conservative therapies [6].

Sexuality and Quality of Life

Even though chronic diseases such as rheumatoid arthritis (RA) are known to affect the quality of sexual life, sexual dysfunction is still underdiagnosed. There are two reasons for this: Patients of both sexes do not report the disorder at all due to shame or frustration and clinicians rarely address this issue. They prefer to discuss the pharmacological treatment of joint disease, quality of life, fatigue, and pain [12].

Sexual dysfunction is still underdiagnosed, for two reasons: (1) Patients do not report the disorder because of shame or frustration and (2) this topic is rarely called out by physicians. Rheumatologists are increasingly willing to discuss areas that are not directly related to drug treatment of joint disease, such as quality of life, fatigue, and patient education; however, sexuality is rarely addressed.

Clinical experience mostly shows premature ejaculation in men and dyspareunia in women. In both mood hypotonia and sexual desire, disorder seems to be the underlying conditions.

A study conducted by Almeida PH et al. [13] assessed the prevalence of sexual dysfunction in women followed at the outpatient rheumatology clinic of the Hospital Universitário de Brasília and the Hospital das Clínicas da Universidade de São Paulo who had diagnoses of systemic lupus erythematosus; rheumatoid arthritis; systemic sclerosis; antiphospholipid antibody syndrome; and fibromyalgia.

The Female Sexual Function Index (FSFI), obtained by applying a 19-item questionnaire assessing six domains (sexual desire, arousal, vaginal lubrication, orgasm, sexual satisfaction, and pain), was used for the survey.

Previous studies [14, 15] have shown that 36–70% of men living with rheumatoid arthritis report impaired sexual health attributed to the disease. In addition, a tendency for reduced ability to conceive was present in patients living with ARD, and this was attributed to sexual problems [16].

That is not all. Decreased libido, erectile dysfunction (inability to have or maintain an erection sufficient to have sexual intercourse over a period of at least 6 months), and premature ejaculation [17] are the discomforts most frequently reported by patients with rheumatoid arthritis. Consequent emotional disorders are anxiety, frustration, anhedonia, insomnia, and depression.

Considering the male pathophysiology, erectile dysfunction in ARDs has been linked to endothelial dysfunction. Strong evidence accumulated in recent years supports the idea that erectile function is an exceptional surrogate indicator of systemic health in general and vascular performance in particular [18].

The study by Yasser El Miedany et al. [19] traced another factor that plays an important role in erectile dysfunction among men with ARD: the link between cardiovascular health risk and erectile dysfunction [20].

Unfortunately, this finding is not always considered in cardiovascular diseases such as hypertension, ischemic heart disease, dyslipidemia, diabetes mellitus, and insulin resistance/metabolic syndrome complex. However, there are guidelines for the treatment of men with erectile dysfunction who are known to have cardiovascular disease [21].

Another issue is fertility: A systemic research conducted by Tiseo et al. [22] evaluated the potential alteration of male fertility in a variety of rheumatic diseases. The results showed that frequency and severity varied among different rheumatic diseases: Systemic lupus erythematosus would affect gonadal function by impairing spermatogenesis mainly due to anti-sperm antibodies and cyclophosphamide therapy.

Patients with Behçet's disease, gout, and ankylosing spondylitis, including those on anti-TNF therapy in the latter disease, do not appear to have impaired fertility, whereas in dermatomyositis the potential for fertility is hampered by disease activity and alkylating agents. Data from rheumatoid arthritis revealed that gonadal dysfunction was observed as a consequence of disease activity and anti-spermatozoa antibodies.

The presence of multiple anti spermatozoa antibodies can induce sperm immobilization and agglutination, blocking sperm–egg interaction. This may also prevent implantation or cause arrested embryo development [23]. In patients with rheumatoid arthritis who experience difficulty conceiving, impaired gonadal function with elevated LH/FSH levels has been linked to a higher incidence of ASA [24].

Another major factor for gonadal dysfunction is drug treatment. Some drugs, such as nonsteroidal anti-inflammatory drugs in women and sulfasalazine/methotrexate in men, can cause reversible infertility, whereas after treatment with alkylating agents such as cyclophosphamide-CYC and chlorambucil, irreversible infertility has been observed on some occasions in both sexes [25].

It seems that sexual dysfunction is closely related to disease activity, its medical treatment, and associated comorbidities.

But How Can the Rheumatologist and Sexologist Accompany the Patient with Rheumatoid Arthritis to a Program of Sexual Rehabilitation?

With regard to the clinician: Panus et al. [26] described a strategy to approach and offer guidance on sexual function, called PLIS-SIT (permission, limited information, specific strategies, and intensive therapy). Permission is to ask the patient-specific questions about sexual dysfunction; the second step is to provide information about sexual dysfunction. The third step is to develop specific strategies for each problem. In cases of arthritic men who develop impotence, usually of psychogenic origin, phosphodiesterase inhibitors can be used on level "A" evidence in cases of organic, psychogenic, and pharmacologic erectile dysfunction [27].

Regardless of the outcome of drug therapies, the sexologist should accompany the patient's medication intake with an individualized sexological course. More often than not, the sexologist is only consulted after a negative pharmacological outcome.

Conclusion

Although the scientific literature has traced a relevant frequency of male and female sexual dysfunctions in patients with rheumatoid arthritis, it still remains difficult to introduce into the therapeutic process of clinical care an adequate sexual history of the patient and the partner.

There is not only one type of erectile dysfunction, premature ejaculation, hypoactive desire, etc., there is a different type of dysfunction for each type of patient and couple. An erectile dysfunction, for example, in a couple's parenting project is not the same as an erectile deficit in a hypertensive man with rheumatoid arthritis.

Each individual and couple history reveals a different approach to sexuality that must also be respected during sexological rehabilitation for sexual dysfunction.

Doctors and nurses should educate the patient in a team-based process where the sexologist can act as the facilitator of a therapeutic process, built "on the patient and the couple" and not only on standardized research protocols.

References

1. Hsieh PH, Wu O, Geue C, McIntosh E, McInnes IB, Siebert S. Economic burden of rheumatoid arthritis: a systematic review of literature in biologic era. Ann Rheum Dis. 2020;79:771–7.
2. Bowden JL, Hunter DJ, Deveza LA, Duong V, Dziedzic KS, Allen KD, Chan PK, Eyles JP. Core and adjunctive interventions for osteoarthritis: efficacy and models for implementation. Nat Rev Rheumatol. 2020;16:434–47.
3. Figus FA, Piga M, Azzolin I, McConnell R, Iagnocco A. Rheumatoid arthritis: extra-articular manifestations and comorbidities. Autoimmun Rev. 2021;20:102776.
4. Grässel S, Zaucke F, Madry H. Osteoarthritis: novel molecular mechanisms increase our understanding of the disease pathology. J Clin Med. 2021;10:1938.
5. Conforti A, Di Cola I, Pavlych V, Ruscitti P, Berardicurti O, Ursini F, Giacomelli R, Cipriani P. Beyond the joints, the extra-articular manifestations in rheumatoid arthritis. Autoimmun Rev. 2021;20:102735.
6. Jang S, Lee K, Ju JH. Recent updates of diagnosis, pathophysiology, and treatment on osteoarthritis of the knee. Int J Mol Sci. 2021;22:2619.
7. Plotz B, Bomfim F, Sohail MA, Samuels J. Current epidemiology and risk factors for the development of hand osteoarthritis. Curr Rheumatol Rep. 2021;23:61.
8. Wu CY, Yang HY, Luo SF, Lai JH. From rheumatoid factor to anti-citrullinated protein antibodies and anti-carbamylated protein antibodies for diagnosis and prognosis prediction in patients with rheumatoid arthritis. Int J Mol Sci. 2021;22:686.
9. Koga T, Kawakami A, Tsokos GC. Current insights and future prospects for the pathogenesis and treatment for rheumatoid arthritis. Clin Immunol. 2021;225:108680.
10. Blaess J, Walther J, Petitdemange A, Gottenberg JE, Sibilia J, Arnaud L, Felten R. Immunosuppressive agents for rheumatoid arthritis: a systematic review of clinical trials and their current development stage. Ther Adv Musculoskelet Dis. 2020;12:1759720X20959971.
11. Shams S, Martinez JM, Dawson JRD, Flores J, Gabriel M, Garcia G, Guevara A, Murray K, Pacifici N, Vargas MV, Voelker T, Hell JW, Ashouri JF. The therapeutic landscape of rheumatoid arthritis: current state and future directions. Front Pharmacol. 2021;12:680043.
12. Tavares PH. How the rheumatologist can guide the patient with rheumatoid arthritis on sexual function. Rev Bras Reumatol. 2015;55(5):458–63. https://doi.org/10.1016/j.rbr.2014.08.009. Epub 24 Oct 2014.
13. Zautra AJ, Hoffman JM, Matt KS, Yocum D, Potter PT, Castro WL, et al. An examination of individual differences in the relationship between interpersonal stress and disease activity among women with rheumatoid arthritis. Arthritis Care Ris. 1998;11:271–9. https://doi.org/10.1002/art.1790110408.
14. World Health Organization. International classification of functioning, disability and health. Geneva: OMS Library Cataloging-in-Publication Data; 2001. https://psychiatr.ru/download/1313?view=name=CF_18.pdf.
15. Sariyildiz MA, Batmaz I, Dilek B, Bozkurt M, Karakoc M, Çevik R, et al. The impact of ankylosing spondylitis on female sexual functions. Int J Res. 2013;25:104–8. https://doi.org/10.1038/ijir.2012.42.

16. Bourg M, Ruyssen-Witrand A, Bettiol C, Parinaud J. Fertility and sexuality of women with inflammatory arthritis. Eur J Obstet Gynecol Reprod Biol. 2020;251:199–205. https://doi.org/10.1016/j.ejogrb.2020.05.068.
17. Bal S, Bal K, Turan Y. Sexual functions in ankylosing spondylitis. Rheumatol Int. 2011;31:889–94. https://doi.org/10.1007/s00296-010-1406-5.
18. Jannini EA. MS = MS: the interface between systems medicine and sexual medicine to address NCDs in a gender-dependent manner. Sex Med Rev. 2017;5(3):349–64. https://doi.org/10.1016/j.sxmr.2017.04.002.
19. El Miedany Y, Palmer D. Rheumatology-driven pregnancy clinic: male perspective. Clin Reumatol. 2021;40(8):3067–77.
20. Sansone A, Mollaioli D, Ciocca G. Tackling male sexual and reproductive health in the wake of the COVID-19 epidemic. J Endocrinol Investig. 2020; https://doi.org/10.1007/s40618-020-01350-1.
21. Billups K. Sexual dysfunction and cardiovascular disease: integrative concepts and strategies. Am J Cardiol. 2005;96(12):57–61. https://doi.org/10.1016/j.amjcard.2005.10.007.
22. Tiseo BC, Cocuzza M, Bonfá E, Srougi M, Clovis A. Alteration of male fertility potential in rheumatic diseases: a systematic review. Int Braz J Urol. 2016;42(1):11–21. https://doi.org/10.1590/S1677-5538.IBJU.2014.0595.
23. Arap MA, Vicentini FC, Cocuzza M, Hallak J, Athayde K, Lucon AM, et al. Late hormone levels, sperm parameters and presence of antisperm antibodies in patients treated for testicular torsion. J Androl. 2007;28:528–32. https://doi.org/10.2164/jandrol.106.002097.
24. Haas GG Jr. The inhibitory effect of sperm-associated immunoglobulins on cervical mucus penetration. Fertil Steril. 1986;46:334–7. https://doi.org/10.1016/S0015-0282(16)49538-5.
25. Fu L, Xiong DK, Ding XP, Li C, Zhang LY, Ding M, et al. Genetic screening for chromosomal abnormalities and Y-chromosome microdeletions in infertile Chinese men. J Assist Reprod Genet. 2012;29:521–7. https://doi.org/10.1007/s10815-012-9741-y.
26. Panush SR, Mihailescu GD, Gornisiewicz MT, Sutaria HS. Sex and arthritis. Bull Rheum Dis. 2000;49:1–4.
27. Heidelbaugh JJ. Management of erectile dysfunction. Am Fam Physician. 2010;81:305–12.

Part XX
Sexuality

Genital Lichen

Simone Ribero, Alice Ramondetta, Elena Stroppiana, Maria Teresa Fierro, and Elena Vittoria Longhi

Genital Lichen Planus

Lichen planus is a relatively uncommon inflammatory dermatologic condition that can affect the skin, mucosa, nails, and scalp. Approximately 50% of women and 25% of men with cutaneous disease have genital involvement. Mucous membrane disease is usually more persistent.

Four distinct forms of the disease are described: papulosquamous lichen planus, erosive lichen planus, hypertrophic lichen planus, and lichen planopilaris.

Lichen is more common in women, generally arising in the sixth decade, but the incidence and prevalence of vulvar disease have not been clearly established. It seems to affect 0.5–2% of the population; estimates have varied based on geographic location and diagnostic criteria [1].

Lichen planus probably represents T-cell-mediated damage to epidermal cells that express altered self or foreign antigens on their surface, but the exact etiology is unknown. The disorder is often associated with other autoimmune diseases [2]. Infectious triggers, particularly hepatitis C viral infections, may be associated with mucosal lichen planus.

S. Ribero (✉) · A. Ramondetta · E. Stroppiana · M. T. Fierro
Dermatology Clinic, University of Turin, Turin, Italy
e-mail: simone.ribero@unito.it; estroppiana@cittadellasalute.to.it; mariateresa.fierro@unito.it

E. V. Longhi
Department of Sexual Medical Center, San Raffaele Hospital, Milano, Italy

© Springer Nature Switzerland AG 2023

E. V. Longhi (ed.), *Managing Psychosexual Consequences in Chronic Diseases*,
https://doi.org/10.1007/978-3-031-31307-3_35

Main Medical Features

Women with vulvar lichen planus frequently complain about vulvar pain, burning, pruritus, soreness, or dyspareunia (sometimes with post-coital bleeding) [3]. Signs and symptoms of vulvar lichen planus can be constant or intermittent, while a minority of women are asymptomatic or have only minimal symptoms.

Four types of lichen planus can be observed: papulosquamous lichen planus, erosive lichen planus, hypertrophic lichen planus, and lichen planopilaris [4, 5].

Papulosquamous lichen planus—this variant of lichen planus consists of small, intensely pruritic papules with a violaceous color that appears usually on the mons pubis and the labia majora and minora in women or the glans penis and shafts in men. Penile plaques are frequently annular. It could be associated with milky striae on the inner side of the labia [6]. The resolution of papulosquamous lesions is often characterized by post-inflammatory hyperpigmentation [7].

Erosive lichen planus—erosive lichen planus is the most common type of vulvar lichen planus, and it involves much more frequently women than men. Desquamative, erosive, and chronic dermatitis often also affects the vagina. Recurrent exacerbations, slow healing, and scarring are common. The latter can cause significant anatomic disruption, including severe stenosis of the vagina and urethral obstruction. Dyspareunia, apareunia, difficulty in urination, and dysuria are the major symptoms. Lesions are characterized by well-demarcated, brightly erythematous patches or erosions with white striae or a serpentine, white border along the margin (Wickham striae). The lesions may occur on the labia minora and vestibule as isolated lesions on an otherwise normal vulva, or they may be associated with marked architectural destruction, including loss of the labia minora and narrowing of the introitus (Fig. 1a).

The vulvovaginal–gingival syndrome is a variant of erosive lichen planus that involves the epithelium of the vulva, vestibule, vagina, and mouth; additional sites (e.g., skin and esophagus) may also be involved [8]. Although all three areas can be affected, the lesions may not be concurrent. The gingival mucosa usually shows erosions, white plaques, or a whitish and lace-like reticular pattern. Scarring and stricture formation are a major cause of long-term morbidity [9].

Hypertrophic lichen planus—hypertrophic lichen planus characteristically exhibits whitish hyperkeratotic, rough lesions on the perineum and perianal region, on the vulva or shaft of the penis [10].

Lichen planopilaris—follicular keratotic papules are limited to the labia majora and the mons pubis, but may also be seen on the scalp and the trunk and in the axillae.

Main Tools for the Diagnosis

The diagnosis of genital lichen planus is primarily based on the recognition of characteristic clinical manifestations.

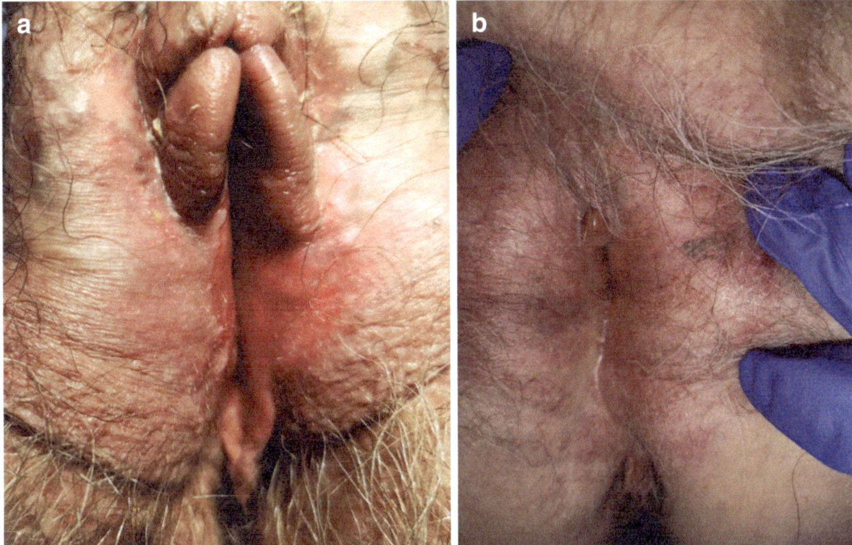

Fig. 1 (**a**) Vulval erosive lichen planus: brightly erythematous erosions with white border along the margin. (**b**) Vulval lichen sclerosus: depigmentation, hyperpigmentation, and sclerosis leading to almost complete loss of labia minora

However, if there is any uncertainty regarding the clinical diagnosis, a biopsy of lesions suspicious of erosive or papulosquamous lichen planus should be performed to rule out other disorders. It is usually indicated in patients with suspected hypertrophic lichen planus because this variant can closely resemble squamous cell carcinoma.

In addition to the examination of the genital area, the physical examination of patients with suspected lichen planus should include the observation of other mucosal and cutaneous surfaces, including the oral cavity, scalp, nails, anus, and entire skin surface.

The identification of classic histologic features of lichen planus in biopsy specimens from patients with clinical manifestations suggestive of lichen planus confirms the diagnosis. Classic histologic features include the following:

- Irregular acanthosis of the epidermis (in sites of keratinized skin)
- Vacuolar change in the epidermal basal cell layer
- A band-like dermal lymphocytic infiltrate in the upper dermis
- Apoptotic keratinocytes scattered within the epidermis

Immunofluorescence studies are typically reserved for erosive presentations to rule out autoimmune blistering disease. If performed, direct immunofluorescence of genital lichen planus may show ragged staining of the basement membrane zone, suggesting deposition of fibrinogen, IgM, cytoid bodies, and, occasionally, granular IgG or IgA [11].

Main Treatment

Data on the treatment of genital lichen planus are limited. The approach to treatment is predominantly managed by uncontrolled studies and reports of clinical experience.

Hypertrophic and papulosquamous genital lichen planus are more responsive to therapy than the erosive variant. A 2-week course of a moderate or superpotent (clobetasol 0.05% ointment) topical corticosteroid is usually adequate to obtain complete remission or significant improvement of the disease.

Hyperkeratotic lesions may fail to treat with topical corticosteroids due to the limited ability of the drugs to penetrate a thickened stratum corneum. Intralesional corticosteroid injections may be useful for these cases.

The treatment of erosive lichen planus of the vulva is challenging. Most commonly, at first line, treatment starts with a daily application of superpotent topical corticosteroid ointment until remission. The goal of the maintenance phase is to ensure improvement while reducing the frequency and potency of topical corticosteroid treatment to minimize the risk for local corticosteroid side effects (like skin atrophy, although the vulvar area is relatively resistant to corticosteroid side effects).

As a second-line therapy, topical tacrolimus (a topical calcineurin inhibitor) is a valid alternative local therapy. However, high-quality data on the efficacy of topical tacrolimus for this indication are lacking like for the oral lichen planus.

Patients who present with severe erosive lichen planus, which limits the application of topical therapy due to pain, may benefit from an alternative initial approach to treatment. Initiating treatment with a systemic glucocorticoid can be beneficial for these patients (a 4–6-week course of oral prednisone, 40–60 mg/day, tapered over 4–6 weeks or intramuscular triamcinolone 1 mg/kg, may be given as a single dose or as a series of injections separated by 1 month).

For refractory disease, a variety of systemic immunomodulatory and immunosuppressive agents (e.g., methotrexate, mycophenolate mofetil, hydroxychloroquine, acitretin, minocycline, and cyclosporine) have been tested in individual patients, but data are not sufficient to confirm the efficacy of the mentioned molecules.

Genital involvement by lichen planus can lead to anatomic distortion and functional limitations secondary to the formation of adhesions and scarring. Dilators and surgery can be useful for improving these complications after mucosal inflammation is resolved with medical therapy. Postectomy can be a treatment option for prepuce lichen in order to resolve the chronic inflammatory phimotic state. Follow-up care is necessary to maintain benefit after these procedures.

Emerging therapy—photodynamic therapy (PDT) may be an emerging treatment option for genital lichen planus.

Adjunctive measures—although medical therapy is the mainstay of treatment of genital lichen planus, other interventions play important roles in patient management, like patient education and psychological support or counseling should be provided if needed.

Genital Lichen Sclerosus

Introduction

Lichen sclerosus is a chronic inflammatory disease that preferentially affects the anogenital region, although any cutaneous site may be affected; 15–20% of patients with genital lichen sclerosus will have an extragenital disease. Its incidence ranges from 1/300 (0.3%) to 1/1000 individuals (0.1%). Several elements have been hypothesized responsible for the pathogenesis, such as hormonal, traumatic (local friction or rubbing and scratching may induce lesions of lichen sclerosus through the Koebner phenomenon), infectious (Borreliosis), and genetic factors. However, the most accepted hypothesis to date is that of autoimmune pathogenesis, in consideration of frequently associated autoimmune diseases (e.g., autoimmune thyroiditis: 12–30%, alopecia areata: 9%, and vitiligo: 6%).

Main Medical Features

Pruritus or soreness is the most typical symptom, shared by both male and female patients, and dyspareunia or dysuria is frequently reported. Rarely, this disorder may be entirely asymptomatic. The characteristic clinical findings are hypopigmented and atrophic skin, erythema, fissures, disepithelization, bleeding suffusions, and telangiectasias (Fig. 1b). The scrotum, if involved, may present atrophy or lichenification. For both, there may be perianal involvement, but this appears more frequent in women due to anatomical contiguity. Architectural changes are common and differ between men and women based on the different anatomy. In men, we observe narrowing of the urethral meatus, reabsorption of the frenulum, synechiae of the balanopreputial sulcus, and narrowing of the foreskin with phimosis that can be reduced or not (Fig. 2). In women, there is incarceration of the clitoris, reabsorption of the labia minora, fusion of the labia minora with the labia majora, and narrowing of the vaginal ostium due to the scarring tendency of lichen sclerosus.

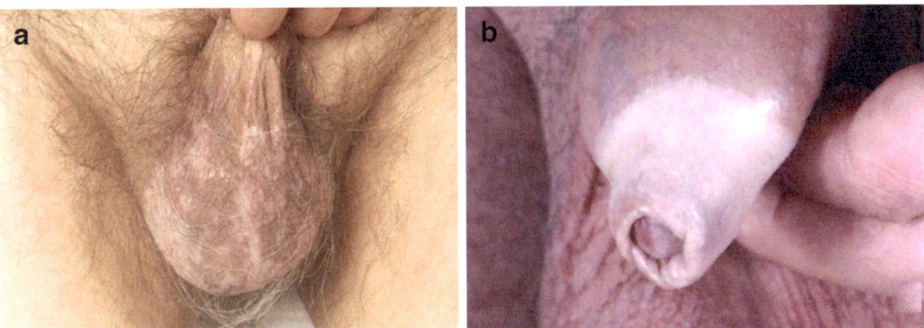

Fig. 2 (**a**) Lichen sclerosus of the scrotum: depigmentation and sclerosis of the skin of the scrotum. (**b**) Lichen sclerosus prepuce: depigmentation and severe sclerosis leading to phimosis

Main Tools for the Diagnosis

For lichen sclerosus, the diagnosis is evenly established by a combination of clinical and histologic findings. From a histological point of view, alterations of the epidermis are nonspecific (atrophy and acanthosis can be observed), but the diagnostic clue concerns the dermis, which shows horizontalization of the dermoepidermal junction with underlying lympho-monocyte infiltrate and specially the presence of a hyaline band at the level of the superficial layer. Occasionally, despite marked clinical changes, the disease cannot be confirmed histologically and repeat biopsies over time may be needed to establish the diagnosis [12].

Main Treatment

The main aim of therapy for lichen sclerosus is to bring the disease under control as quickly as possible with the fewest side effects. With early treatment, long-term sequelae such as destruction of anatomic structures and progression to squamous cell carcinoma may be prevented.

For initial treatment, a daily application of potent topical corticosteroids such as clobetasol propionate 0.05% ointment for 3 months is prescribed. Subsequently, the corticosteroid is tapered over 2 weeks and clinical remission is maintained by limited (typically twice weekly) application of a corticosteroid. Soap substitutes and emollients based on vitamin E must be constantly used, from the beginning, both in association with the topical steroids, and as a maintenance therapy for a long time after stopping the steroid. Several case series have demonstrated success with topical calcineurin inhibitors; however, the risk of long-term treatment of lichen sclerosus with topical calcineurin inhibitors is unknown.

Longitudinal evaluation is essential for patients with lichen sclerosus because both men and women are at increased risk of developing genital SCCs; prospective studies have in fact, respectively, highlighted a risk of developing a squamous cell carcinoma of 3–7% in women and 4–8% in men. Non-healing fissures, ulcers, hyperkeratotic lesions, or nodules must be examined histologically.

Platelet-rich plasma for lichen sclerosus has shown promising results in both males and females.

For longstanding lichen sclerosus in which narrowing of the introitus has resulted in dyspareunia, surgical refashioning with the division of adhesions may be helpful. Vaginal dilators may also be needed, as well as psychosexual counseling. Men may need surgery such as circumcision, meatoplasty (often after using urethral dilators), or reconstructive surgery of the urethra and glans penis.

Sexuality and Quality of Life

Lichen sclerosus (LS) and lichen planus (LP) are immunologically mediated diseases with a preference for the genitalia in patients of both sexes.

For example, vulvovaginal–gingival syndrome has been described as a distinctive pattern of erosive multi-mucosal lichen planus (LP) and is a clinical triad of vulvar, vaginal, and gingival LP. It can lead to sequelae such as vaginal and urethral stenosis that can have serious implications for quality of life. The oral mucosa is the most implicated in LP and up to 1–2% of the general population can be affected [13]. Approximately 25% of women with oral LP also have vulvovaginal involvement [14]. Mucosal LP (MLP) of the genital skin is usually located on the glans in males and on the vulva and vagina in females [15].

In a retrospective study, the frequency of vulvar LP was found to be 3.7% in the population attending a vulvar clinic [16].

Vulvovaginal–gingival syndrome (VVGS) has been described as a distinctive pattern of erosive multi-mucosal LP characterized by a triad of vulvar, vaginal, and gingival LP [17]. In a recent study of a large series of VVGS patients, 90% of cases were found to develop genital fibrosis and stenosis, but there are only a few reports of isolated vulvar LP leading to stenosis [18]. Vaginal and urethral stenosis can have a significant negative impact on the patient's quality of life.

The basic principles of the management of vulvar LS and vulvovaginal LP are the same and involve explaining the disease, emphasizing the chronic nature of the condition, and outlining treatment options. The main difference between the two conditions is that LP has a propensity to involve the mucous membranes, including the mouth and vagina, which are rarely affected in LS [19].

This disease affects the oral mucosa with an estimated prevalence of 0.5–3% and a female-to-male ratio of 1.5–3. The age of onset is generally between 30 and 60 years, and the disease also has a much-debated premalignant potential [20].

The possible malignant transformation of LP is a highly controversial topic [21]. Although the risk is low, the monitoring of patients with the disease has provided evidence of its potential malignancy [22]. Modifying some of the criteria outlined above, Warnakulasuriya et al. [23] included PLO as a potentially malignant disorder and most researchers recommend indefinite monitoring of patients with PLO, aiming at early detection of potential malignancy.

In general, the average duration of discomfort reported by patients with PLO was 1–3 months. Other studies report times between 3 and 12 months or even longer (up to 21 months) [24].

Some clinical studies indicate that the prevalence of smoking and alcohol consumption among patients with PLO makes no significant clinical and diagnostic difference compared to the general population [25]. However, smoking and alcohol consumption appear in 27% of the patient groups analyzed (although no significant correlation between smoking and PLO has been identified) in the literature.

Furthermore, of 131 patients [26] presenting with skin lesions, the most commonly affected areas were the flexural surfaces of the body, accounting for 60.1% of cases. White patches associated with striae were observed in 45% of these cases. Purple papules (hyperpigmented spots) were present in 37.40% of the subjects. The itching was the most commonly reported symptom (85.4%), followed by pain (25.9%). The mean time of evolution of the skin lesions was 18 months, ranging from a minimum of 1 month to a maximum of 13 years. These data showed a small difference between patients presenting with both cutaneous and oral LP and patients presenting with cutaneous LP alone.

Of these 131 patients with cutaneous lichen planus, 19% (n = 25) also had oral lesions. Of the patients presenting with both cutaneous and oral lichen planus (n = 25), 12% (n = 3) had skin lesions before the appearance of the oral lesions.

Although stress and depression are commonly regarded as factors in the onset and evolution of LP, this cannot be categorically confirmed. The literature regarding this issue remains controversial, as it is difficult to establish whether mental disorders precede the onset of these chronic painful lesions or are a consequence of the distress suffered. Among the sample in the study by Cassol-Spanemberg J et al. [26], 48% of patients (45% of whom were taking anxiolytics) reported psychological problems such as stress, anxiety, and depression, with no significant differences between subgroups. However, a study including psychometric assessment found a higher level of anxiety among patients with PLO than among control patients [27]. In another study [28], 25% of the patients clearly identified a stressful situation prior to the appearance of skin lesions and 8% suffered from some form of depressive disorder.

Several studies point to the presence of emotional problems, stress, anxiety, and/or depression as being responsible for triggering the disease and also for triggering relapses [29]. Current figures show that 41% of patients with oral lesions associated the outbreak with some stressful event.

It has long been suggested that patients with PLO have a higher incidence of diabetes than the general population, and it is estimated that the incidence of PLO in the diabetic population is 1.6% [30]. Lopez-Jornet et al. [31] found type 2 diabetes in 11.5% of a sample of patients with PLO. A study by Tovaru et al. [32] evaluated 633 patients with OLP, of whom 10% had type 2 diabetes. Another study [28] noted that 10% of patients evaluated with PLO were diagnosed with diabetes mellitus and 30% reported a family history of diabetes.

Lastly, Kaplan et al. [33], in a study of 171 patients, showed that the prevalence of carcinoma was 5.8% and that malignant transformation can occur in any clinical form of OLP, although the process of malignant transformation is still unclear [34].

A study by Khoo LS [35] mainly investigated the implications of male genital lichen. This was a prospective study of 467 male patients attending a public clinic for sexually transmitted diseases. The results showed various dermatoses that were anatomical variants: pearly penile papules in 67 patients [14.3%], sebaceous hyperplasia in 16 [3.4%], Tyson's glands in 32 [7%] and penile melanosis in 13 [2.8%]) or pathological conditions (balanitis in 45 [9, 6%], eczema in 10 [2.1%], traumatic ulcers in 10 [2.1%], folliculitis and furunculosis in 8 [1.7%], scabies nodules in 7 [1.5%], genital candidiasis in 7 [1.5%], and lichen (6.7%). Fifty percent of patients with Tyson's glands also had pearly papules of the penis. Most of the anatomical variants were incidental findings, whereas the majority of patients with pathological dermatoses had these lesions. A lack of familiarity with these dermatoses may cause unnecessary anxiety to the patient and physician, resulting in inappropriate treatment.

A further study by Cassol-Spanemberg J et al. [26] analyzed the clinical histories of 274 patients all of whom had histological confirmation of lichen planus verified by a pathologist. The sample of patients was selected from those attending the Dental Hospital of the University of Barcelona, Faculty of Dentistry (Bellvitge University Campus), or the Sagrat Cor Hospital, Barcelona. Among patients with cutaneous LP (47.8%), the most commonly affected areas were the flexural surfaces of the body, representing 60.1% of cases. Twenty-four percent of patients ($n = 55$) correlated the onset of injury with previous stress events. Of the 131 subjects with skin lesions, 19% ($n = 25$) also had oral lichen planus (OLP). Of the total sample, 53.6% ($n = 147$) of patients had oral lesions. The systemic diseases most commonly associated with this patient sample were psychological problems such as stress, anxiety, and depression (48%), hypertension (27%), gastric problems (12%), and diabetes (9.7%). A family history of lichen planus was found in only two cases (0.72%) of a total of 274.

The total sample included 208 women (75.91%) and 66 men (24.08%), showing statistically significant differences ($p \leq 0.005$). Age ranged from 28 to 94 years, with a mean age of 56.40 years (SD ± 14.34). Age and gender showed no significant differences between the two subgroups.

A family history of PLO was found in only two patients (0.72%) of a total of 274. However, it is important to note that medical records show the presence of a family member with the same disease, as genetic predisposition is thought to be an element involved in the etiopathogenesis of PLO [36].

Although a family history of this disease is rare, Huang C et al. [37] analyzed nine consecutive family histories of FBLP with 36 affected individuals presenting to the Department of Dermatology at Wuhan Union Hospital, a tertiary referral hospital in central China. Parameters analyzed included age of onset, gender predilection, lesion distribution, nail and mucosal involvement, clinical course, and inheritance pattern.

Thirty-six of 85 individuals in the nine families were diagnosed with genital bullous lichen (42.4%): Female patients were more likely to be affected than males (58.3% vs 35.7%, G(chi 2) = 3.99, $p < 0.05$). Bimodal disease onset was found, with a peak at 1–3 years and another at 13–17 years. The shin is the most affected area (97%) followed by the upper limbs, thighs, and genitals. Involvement of the torso is relatively rare. Only a minority of cases involve the oral mucosa. The disease tends to follow a chronic and progressive course. Hereditary transmission is autosomal dominant with variable penetrance.

The scientific province has sought to investigate further. Although this pathology is rare, Luis-Montoya P et al. [38] conducted a retrospective investigation of a sample of children attending the Department of Dermatology, "Dr Manuel Gea González" General Hospital, Tlalpan, Mexico.

A total of 235 patients with a clinical and histological diagnosis of lichen planus observed over a period of 22 years and 7 months were studied. Twenty-four (10.2%) of these patients were children (aged 15 years or less). The ratio of males to females was 1:1.2. The main clinical picture was classic lichen planus (43.5%). Mucosal and nail involvement was rare. No family history of lichen planus or systemic disease was detected. In the international literature, the frequency of lichen planus ranged from 2.1% to 11.2% of the pediatric population. In most studies, no significant gender predominance was identified. Most patients presented with the classic variety of lichen planus. Reported mucosal involvement was rare, except in India and Kuwait. The frequency of nail involvement ranged from 0% to 16.6%. Little evidence of systemic disease or family history was found.

Conclusion

This clinical picture reveals significant implications of the disease on the sexual life of patients of both sexes and their quality of life in general. To what extent has the efficacy of the therapies and the stress implicit in the lack of results or their achievement been investigated?

In a systematic study, Cooper SM [39] recorded the clinical features, symptomatic response to treatment, and resolution of clinical signs in a large sample of women with erosive lichen planus of the vulva. A mean follow-up of 72 months was conducted in a university and district hospital in Oxfordshire, England.

One hundred and fourteen adult women with a definite clinical diagnosis of erosive lichen planus of the vulva had received topical corticosteroids with or without other topical preparations and systemic treatments as part of their normal care.

The quality of symptomatic response to individual treatments (good, partial, or poor), overall symptomatic response to treatment and with time (good, partial, no change, or worse), vulvar sign response (total, partial, moderate, less, equal, or worse), and the presence or absence of moderate or severe scarring were investigated.

Results

The mean age at onset of vulvar symptoms was 56.9 years. First-line therapy was an ultra-potent topical corticosteroid in 89 women (78%), of whom 63 (71%) were symptom-free during treatment. Overall and with time, 86 women (75%) improved with treatment, and of these, 62 (54%) were symptom-free (good response), and 24 (21%) had a partial response. Eighteen (16%) had no change, and 10 (9%) had worsened. The global response of vulvar signs was recorded in 113 patients. Only 10 (9%) of these had complete resolution of clinical signs except for scarring, with 57 (50%) showing resolution of erosions. Squamous cell carcinoma developed in three women (3%). It can therefore be seen that these patients, both men and women, although they may achieve improvement, will continue to suffer from inadequacy and the inability to enjoy a rewarding and continuous intimate life [40–47].

Sexological counseling could help these patients to rediscover a new body image and to find new variables of enjoyment and intimacy, even where the physical scars of the pathology and the atrophy of the tissues bring to mind a sense of inadequacy, low esteem, pain, anxiety, and body dysmorphism.

References

1. Schlosser BJ. Lichen planus and lichenoid reactions of the oral mucosa. Dermatol Ther. 2010;23:251.
2. Cooper SM, Ali I, Baldo M, Wojnarowska F. The association of lichen sclerosus and erosive lichen planus of the vulva with autoimmune disease: a case-control study. Arch Dermatol. 2008;144:1432.
3. Simpson RC, Thomas KS, Leighton P, Murphy R. Diagnostic criteria for erosive lichen planus affecting the vulva: an international electronic-Delphi consensus exercise. Br J Dermatol. 2013;169:337.
4. Neill SM. Erosive lichen planus: diagnosis and management. Syllabus of the post-graduate course. International Society for the Study of Vulvovaginal Disease; 1999.
5. Grunwald MH, Zvulunov A, Halevy S. Lichen planopilaris of the vulva. Br J Dermatol. 1997;136:477.
6. Ridley CM, Neill SM. Non-infective cutaneous conditions of the vulva. In: Ridley CM, Neill SM, editors. The vulva. Oxford: Blackwell Science; 1999. p. 121.
7. Ball SB, Wojnarowska F. Vulvar dermatoses: lichen sclerosus, lichen planus, and vulval dermatitis/lichen simplex chronicus. Semin Cutan Med Surg. 1998;17:182.
8. Rogers RS III, Eisen D. Erosive oral lichen planus with genital lesions: the vulvovaginal-gingival syndrome and the peno-gingival syndrome. Dermatol Clin. 2003;21:91.
9. Setterfield JF, Neill S, Shirlaw PJ, Theron J, Vaughan R, Escudier M, et al. The vulvovaginal gingival syndrome: a severe subgroup of lichen planus with characteristic clinical features and a novel association with the class II HLA DQB1*0201 allele. J Am Acad Dermatol. 2006;55:98.
10. Lewis FM. Vulval lichen planus. Br J Dermatol. 1998;138:569.
11. Helander SD, Rogers RS III. The sensitivity and specificity of direct immunofluorescence testing in disorders of mucous membranes. J Am Acad Dermatol. 1994;30:65.
12. Funaro D. Lichen sclerosus: a review and practical approach. Dermatol Ther. 2004;17(1):28.
13. Scully C, Hegarty A. The oral cavity and lips. In: Burns T, Breathnach SM, Cox N, Griffiths C, editors. Rook's handbook of dermatology. 8th ed. Singapore: Wiley Blackwell; 2010. p. 69.1–69.129.
14. Goldstein AT, Metz A. Vulvar lichen planus. Clin Obstet Gynecol. 2005;48:818–23.
15. Wagner G, Rose C, Sachse MM. Clinical variants of lichen planus. J Dtsch Dermatol Ges. 2013;11:309–19.
16. Micheletti L, Preti M, Bogliatto F, Zanotto-Valentino MC, Ghiringhello B, Massobrio M. Vulval lichen planus in the practice of a vulvar clinic. Br J Dermatol. 2000;143:1349–50.
17. Pelisse M, Leibowitch M, Sedel D, Hewitt J. A new vulvovaginogingival syndrome. Erosive plurimucosal lichen planus. Ann Dermatol Venereol. 1982;109:797–8.

18. Setterfield JF, Neill S, Shirlaw PJ, Theron J, Vaughan R, Escudier M, et al. Vulvovaginal gingival syndrome: a severe subgroup of lichen planus with characteristic clinical features and a novel association with the HLA DQB1 * 0201 class II allele. J Am Acad Dermatol. 2006;55:98–113.

19. McPherson T, Cooper S. Vulval lichen sclerosus and lichen planus. Dermatol Ther. 2010;23(5):523–32. https://doi.org/10.1111/j.1529-8019.2010.01355.x. PMID: 20868406.

20. Robledo-Sierra J, van der Waal I. How general dentists might manage a patient with oral lichen planus. Med Oral Patol Oral Cir Bucal. 2018;23:e198–202.

21. Krupaa RJ, Sankari SL, Masthan KM, Rajesh E. Oral lichen planus: an overview. J Pharm Bioallied Sci. 2015;7:S158–61.

22. Shailaja G, Kumar JV, Baghirath PV, Kumar U, Ashalata G, Krishna AB. Estimation of the rate of malignant transformation in cases of oral epithelial dysplasia and lichen planus using the immunohistochemical expression of the markers Ki-67, p53, BCL-2 and BAX. Dent Res J (Isfahan). 2015;12:235–42.

23. Patil S, Rao R, Raj T. Role of miRNA in the malignant transformation of oral lichen planus. J Contemp Dent Pract. 2015;16–21

24. Gorouhi F, Davari P, Fazel N. Cutaneous and mucosal lichen planus: a comprehensive review of clinical subtypes, risk factors, diagnosis, and prognosis. World Sci J. 2014;2014:742826.

25. Sandhu SV, Sandhu JS, Bansal H, Dua V. Oral lichen planus and stress: an evaluation. Contemp Clin Dent. 2014;5:352–6.

26. Cassol-Spanemberg J, Blanco-Carrión A, Rodríguez-de Rivera-Campillo ME, Estrugo-Devesa A, Jané-Salas E, López-López J. Cutaneous, genital and oral lichen planus: a descriptive study of 274 patients. Med Oral Patol Oral Cir Bucal. 2019;24(1):e1–7. Published 1 Jan 2019. https://doi.org/10.4317/medoral.22656.

27. Nadendla LK, Meduri V, Paramkusam G, Pachava KR. Association of salivary cortisol and anxiety levels in patients with lichen planus. J Clin Diagn Res. 2014;8:ZC01–3.

28. Giménez-Garcia R, Pérez-Castrillón JL. Lichen planus and associated diseases: a clinical-epidemiological study. Actas Dermosifiliogr. 2004;95:154–60.

29. Munde AD, Karle RR, Wankhede PK, Shaikh SS, Kulkurni M. Demographic and clinical profile of oral lichen planus: a retrospective study. Contemp Clin Dent. 2013;4:181–5.

30. Jelinek JE. Skin manifestations of diabetes mellitus. Int J Dermatol. 1994;34:605–17.

31. López-Jornet P, Parra-Perez F, Pons-Fuster A. Association of autoimmune diseases with oral lichen planus: a cross-sectional clinical study. J Eur Acad Dermatol Venereol. 2014;28:895–9.

32. Tovaru S, Parlatescu I, Gheorghe C, Tovaru M, Costache M, Sardella A. Oral lichen planus: a retrospective study on 633 patients from Bucharest, Romania. Med Oral Patol Oral and Cir Bucal. 2013;18:e201–6.

33. Kaplan I, Ventura-Sharabi Y, Gal G, Calderon S, Anavi Y. The dynamics of oral lichen planus: a retrospective clinicopathological study. Pathol Neck Head. 2012;6:178–83.

34. Warnakulasuriya S, Johnson NW, van der Wall I. Nomenclature and classification of potentially malignant disorders of the oral mucosa. Oral J Pathol Med. 2007;36:575–80.

35. Khoo LS, Cheong WK. Common genital dermatoses in male patients attending a public sexually transmitted disease clinic in Singapore. Ann Acad Med Singap. 1995;24(4):505–9. PMID: 8849177.

36. Sandhu K, Handa S, Kanwar AJ. Familial lichen planus. Pediatric dermatol. 2003;20:186.

37. Huang C, Chen S, Liu Z, Tao J, Wang C, Zhou Y. Familial bullous lichen planus (FBLP): Pedigree analysis and clinical characteristics. J Cutan Med Surg. 2005;9(5):217–22.

38. Luis-Montoya P, Domínguez-Soto L, Vega-Memije E. Lichen planus in 24 children with review of the literature. Pediatr Dermatol. 2005;22(4):295–8.

39. Cooper SM, Wojnarowska F. Influence of treatment of erosive lichen planus of the vulva on its prognosis. Arch Dermatol. 2006;142(3):289–94.

40. Ribero S, Stieger M, Quaglino P, Hongang T, Bornstein MM, Naldi L, et al. Efficacy of topical tacrolimus for oral lichen planus: real-life experience in a retrospective cohort of patients with a review of the literature. J Eur Acad Dermatol Venereol. 2015;29(6):1107–13.

41. Simpson RC, Littlewood SM, Cooper SM, Cruickshank ME, Green CM, Derrick E, et al. Real-life experience of managing vulval erosive lichen planus: a case-based review and U.K. multi-centre case note audit. Br J Dermatol. 2012;167:85.
42. Nelson DM, Peterson AC. Lichen sclerosus: epidemiological distribution in an equal access health care system. J Urol. 2011;185(2):522–5.
43. Meyrick Thomas RH, Ridley CM, McGibbon DH, Black MM. Lichen sclerosus et atrophicus and autoimmunity—a study of 350 women. Br J Dermatol. 1988;118(1):41–6.
44. Kirtschig G, Becker K, Günthert A, Jasaitiene D, Cooper S, Chi CC, Kreuter A, et al. Evidence-based (S3) Guideline on (anogenital) Lichen sclerosus. J Eur Acad Dermatol Venereol. 2015;29(10):e1–43.
45. Virgili A, Minghetti S, Borghi A, Corazza M. Long-term maintenance therapy for vulvar lichen sclerosus: the results of a randomized study comparing topical vitamin E with an emollient. Eur J Dermatol. 2013;23(2):189–94.
46. Neill SM, Lewis FM, Tatnall FM, Cox NH. British Association of Dermatologists' guidelines for the management of lichen sclerosus 2010. Br J Dermatol. 2010;163(4):672.
47. Casabona F, Gambelli I, Casabona F, Santi P, Santori G, Baldelli I. Autologous platelet-rich plasma (PRP) in chronic penile lichen sclerosus: the impact on tissue repair and patient quality of life. Int Urol Nephrol. 2017;49(4):573–80.

HIV

Stefano Buttò and Elena Vittoria Longhi

Acquired immunodeficiency syndrome (AIDS) is a life-threatening chronic condition caused by the human immunodeficiency virus (HIV). HIV infection continues to be a major public health issue with an estimated 38 million people living with HIV at the end of 2019, worldwide [1].

HIV is a retrovirus, which holds its genetic information in a single-stranded RNA molecule. When HIV enters a human cell, it releases its RNA and an enzyme called reverse transcriptase (RT) makes a DNA copy of the virus' RNA. The resulting HIV DNA (the provirus) integrates into the DNA of the infected cell. This is a reverse process to the one used by human cells, which make an RNA copy of the DNA. For this, HIV is referred to as a retrovirus, indicating this reverse transcription process from RNA into DNA.

HIV Variability

HIV is characterized by extensive genetic diversity that is due to its high replication rate, the error-prone RT, and the recombination events that may occur during virus replication. Based on genetic characteristics and differences among the viral antigens, HIV is classified into types 1 and 2 (HIV-1, HIV-2), which are estimated to be more than 55% genetically distinct. Worldwide, the predominant virus is HIV-1 that accounts for around 95% of all infections, whereas HIV-2 virus is concentrated in West Africa and in other countries with links to West Africa. HIV-2 is less infectious

S. Buttò (✉)
"Surveillance and Pathogenesis of HIV Variants and Associated Co-infections"-National Center for HIV/AIDS Research-Istituto Superiore di Sanità, Roma, Italy
e-mail: stefano.butto@iss.it

E. V. Longhi
Department of Sexual Medical Center, San Raffaele Hospital, Milano, Italy

© Springer Nature Switzerland AG 2023
E. V. Longhi (ed.), *Managing Psychosexual Consequences in Chronic Diseases*,
https://doi.org/10.1007/978-3-031-31307-3_36

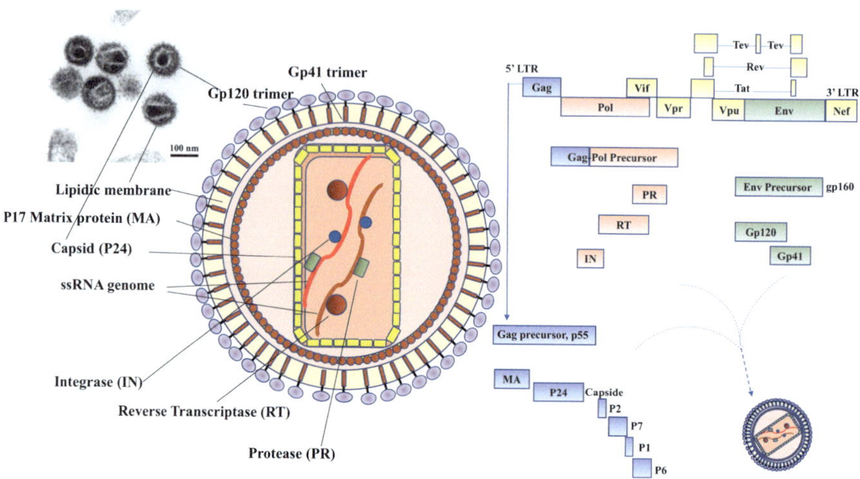

Fig. 1 Structure of the HIV virion and genome organization

and progresses more slowly than HIV-1, although, without treatment, similarly to HIV-1, the HIV-2 infection progresses to AIDS and death [2, 3]. Both HIV-1 and HIV-2 are further divided into groups and subtypes. Focusing only on HIV-1, it includes four groups: M (main), O (outlier), N (non-M, non-O), and P [4], which have different geographic distributions. The M group further splits into 10 subtypes (A through L) [5], as well as more than 100 circulating recombinant forms (CRF), including complex forms (cpx) [6].

HIV predominantly attacks cells that express the CD4 receptor on their surface, such as CD4+ T helper lymphocytes and monocytes/macrophages. These cells are important, as they play a central role in the immune response, in particular, the CD4+ T helper lymphocytes are key in coordinating the immune response by stimulating other immune cells, such as macrophages, B lymphocytes (B cells), and CD8+ T lymphocytes (CD8+ cells), to fight infections from different pathogens and the generation of tumors. Thus, by destroying CD4 cells, HIV weakens the immune system, leaves the infected individual exposed to the attacks of many other infectious pathogens, and favors the onset of tumors. Many of the complications caused by HIV infection, including death, are usually due to these other infections and tumors, and not directly to HIV infection.

HIV Structure

In the electron microscopy (EM), the viral particle has a rounded shape with a diameter between 100 and 120 nm (Fig. 1a, b).

Externally, we can distinguish a pericapsid envelope (the "envelope"), which covers a capsid or core. The envelope consists of a phospholipid bilayer to which the viral glycoproteins gp120 and gp41 are anchored. The bilayer is not viral in its nature, but derives from the cytoplasmic membrane of the host cell, which the virion acquires during budding, in the final stages of replication. Therefore, on the envelope there are both viral proteins (gp120 and gp41) and surface antigens of the host cell, such as antigens of the class I and II major histocompatibility complex and adhesion molecules (adhesins). As regards the proteins of viral origin, at the level of the external surface there are structures formed by homotrimers, whose individual components are in turn made up of two associated protein subunits, both produced by the *env* gene, the gp120 and the gp41. Thus, each spike visible in the electron microscope is a heterodimer trimer, composed of an external homotrimer glycoprotein gp120 and a homotrimer transmembrane glycoprotein gp41 (Fig. 1a, b). The matrix protein (p17) lies at the inner face of the lipid bilayer. More internally, at the EM the capsid is evident as a bar-shaped electron-dense structure, composed of p24 (Fig. 1a, b). The structure encloses and protects two strands of single-stranded RNA, each one 9.2 kb long, with positive polarity with which some molecules of RT, integrase, and protease viral enzymes are associated (Fig. 1b).

Like all retroviruses, the HIV genome contains three structural genes organized, from 5' end to the 3' end, as *gag* (group-specific antigen), *pol* (polymerase), and *env* (envelope) (Fig. 1c). During replication (see below), the *gag* and *pol* genes are initially transcribed into a single mRNA, which is translated into a 180 kDa polyprotein (p180), and subsequently cleaved by a viral protease. A 55-kDa protein (p55) and the three associated enzymatic function proteins (protease, RT, and integrase) are thus formed from the cut of the precursor. Cleavage of the p55 precursor gives origin to the matrix protein (p17), the capsid protein (p24), and the p15 that is further cleaved during virion assembly into p9 and p7 that are needed for correct insertion of virion RNA into the capsid (Fig. 1c). The *env* gene is translated into a precursor protein that is rapidly glycosylated to reach the weight of 160 kDa (gp160). From this protein, the two envelope proteins gp120 and gp41 originate due to cleavage by a cellular protease (Fig. 1c).

In addition to the genes encoding for the structural proteins, the HIV genome also contains six regulatory and accessory genes: The former ones are represented by *tat* and *rev*, while the latter ones are by *nef*, *vpr*, *vif*, and *vpu*. The products of these genes play an essential role in the viral replication cycle and in the synthesis of related macromolecules. Briefly, the Tat protein is expressed very early after infection and promotes the expression of HIV genes. The Rev protein ensures the export from nucleus to cytoplasm of the correctly processed messenger and genomic RNA. The Vpr protein is involved in the arrest of the cell cycle. This protein also enables the reverse-transcribed DNA to gain access to the nucleus in non-dividing cells such as macrophages. Vpu is a protein necessary for the correct release of virus particle, whereas the Vif protein enhances the infectiveness of progeny virus particles. Finally, the Nef protein has multiple functions including cellular signal transduction and the downregulation of the CD4 receptor on the cell surface to allow virus budding in the late stages of the virus replication cycle.

The replication cycle of HIV consists of several phases that are schematically described in Fig. 2.

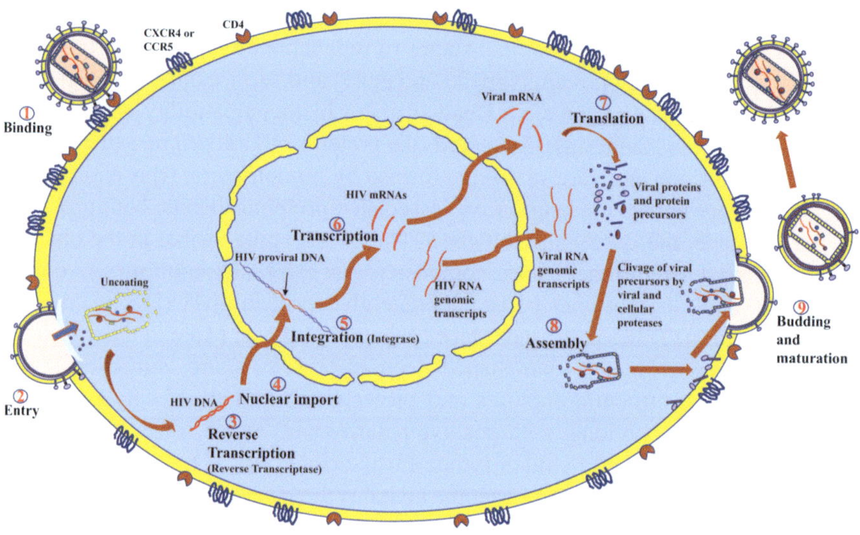

Fig. 2 Replication cycle of HIV

After binding and entry into the host cell (Fig. 2, steps 1 and 2), the single-strand viral RNA is transcribed into DNA by reverse transcriptase (step 3). Once the DNA molecule is formed, it is transported into the nucleus and integrated into the cellular genome (steps 4 and 5). The integrated HIV DNA is then transcribed to mRNA by the cell's transcriptional apparatus. The translation of the viral proteins (step 7) causes new viral particles to form (step 8), containing the RNA genome of the virus, which will be released by budding from the infected cell (step 9).

More in detail, the first step (Fig. 2, step 1) of the replication cycle consists of the interaction between the proteins of the viral envelope and the surface receptors of the host cell. In particular, the viral gp120 binds with high affinity to the CD4 receptor present on T helper lymphocytes (considered the target cell of election) and on monocytes/macrophages. However, the presence of the CD4 receptor alone is not sufficient for HIV to infect the cell. The mechanism needs the presence of co-receptors. These co-receptors have been identified among the chemokine receptors; in particular, the interaction between gp120 and the CXCR4 chemokine receptor is necessary for the infection of T lymphocytes, while that with CCR5 chemokine receptor for the infection of monocytes/macrophages. The described events are the main mechanism of entry of HIV, although the virus can use alternative mechanisms and can infect different types of cells.

Once the virus is bound to the cell surface, a fusion occurs between the viral and the cell membranes. This is possible due to conformational changes in the gp120 that occur as a consequence of the binding with cellular receptors, which lead to the exposure and activation of gp41, whose direct interaction with the cell membrane through its terminal NH2 portion (a fusogenic peptide) determines the fusion of the viral envelope with the lipid bilayer of the target cell (Fig 2, step 2). Once the fusion has taken place, the virus capsid penetrates the target cell, while the glycoprotein coating of the envelope remains outside the cell. Once inside the cell, the capsid undergoes an uncoating process through which the protein coating of the core is degraded and the RNA genome and viral enzymes are released in the cell's cytoplasm. The retro-transcription process takes place in the nucleoprotein complex (the RNA genome and the enzymes) and requires the action of the RT that "retrotranscribes" the viral single-strand RNA into DNA (Fig. 2, step 3). The viral DNA (called provirus) and the associated p17 and integrase proteins form the so-called pre-integration complex. This complex is transported to the nucleus (Fig. 2, step 4), where the viral DNA integrates into the cellular genome, thanks to the intervention of the associated integrase protein (Fig. 2, step 5). Integration is random and can occur at any point in the cellular DNA, although some preferential sites have been described. At this point, the viral DNA can duplicate itself with each division with the genetic material of the cell, making the infection permanent and the integrated provirus a stable element. In this case, viral DNA remains associated with the cell's genome without necessarily undergoing transcription and this state of latency can persist for months or even years. It is when the cell is activated by other immune cells, or antigens, or mitogens, or cytokines that HIV genes become to be expressed. The viral Tat protein controls the HIV transcription [7]. The process starts with a short and abortive transcription of the provirus by the RNA polymerase II of the cell, with the short transcripts that are translocated to the cytoplasm where they are translated into the Tat and Rev proteins [8]. Tat enters again the nucleus and activates the RNA polymerase II-driven transcription elongation by several mechanisms [9–12] that lead to the transactivation of HIV gene expression (Fig. 2, step 6). When there is no activation of the above complex, the infected cell becomes latent, and therefore, these cells are called viral reservoirs [13–17]. The HIV genome is transcribed by the host RNA polymerase II into viral mRNAs, which can be un-spliced, singly spliced, or multiply spliced. The multiply spliced mRNAs are translated into the accessory and regulatory proteins, the singly spliced into the envelope precursor (*env*), and the un-spliced mRNAs into Gag or they serve as the genomic RNA [18] (Fig. 2, step 7). Thus, the first class of mRNA is produced during the early stages of viral replication, while the mRNAs for structural proteins are produced later thanks to the action of the regulatory proteins.

The assembly of the HIV viral particle (Fig. 2 step 8) takes place in the cytoplasm, where the increased levels of proteins and viral genomes start the process. The initial stage involves the association of the Gag and Gag-Pol protein precursors with the inner portion of the cell plasma membrane after a myristylation. The Env glycoproteins are synthesized as a polyprotein precursor from a singly spliced mRNA on the rough endoplasmic reticulum. Concomitant with translation, the Env precursor is glycosylated to generate a gp160 protein and each gp160 monomer associates with other two gp160 monomers to form a trimer. This facilitates the trafficking of gp160 to the Golgi complex, where each gp160 monomer is cleaved by cellular furin or furin-like proteases to yield mature gp120 and gp41. These proteins then traffic through the secretory pathway to the cellular plasma membrane, where are incorporated as trimeric spikes into virus particles during the budding process.

The final step of the life cycle of HIV is the maturation of the virion, which occurs within the budding virion and continues after budding. Maturation consists of cleavage of the Gag precursor by the viral protease in an ordered manner to produce the p24, the p17, and the other structural proteins (Fig. 2 step 9).

Pathogenesis of HIV Infection

Transmission of HIV infection requires contact with a body fluid that contains the virus or cells infected with the virus. HIV can be present in almost all body fluids, but transmission occurs primarily through blood, sperm, vaginal secretions, and breast milk. Therefore, HIV is usually transmitted through (1) sexual contact with an infected person, when the mucous membranes that line the mouth, vagina, penis, or rectum are exposed to body fluids that contain HIV, such as sperm or vaginal secretions, as it can happen during unprotected sexual intercourse; (2) injection of contaminated blood, i.e., when needles are shared during drug injection or a health-care professional is accidentally stung with a needle contaminated by HIV; (3) transfer from infected mother to fetus before or during birth, or after birth to the newborn through breast milk; and (4) medical procedures, such as transfusion of blood containing HIV, surgery performed with inadequately sterilized instruments, or transplant of infected tissues or organs.

HIV belongs to the Lentivirus genus of the Retroviridae family. Infections with lentiviruses typically show a chronic course of the disease, with a long period of clinical latency (years), persistent viral replication, and involvement of the central nervous system. Left untreated, HIV infection causes progressive and critical damage to the immune system, rendering the host susceptible to potentially fatal opportunistic infections and cancers.

Following infection with HIV, after approximately 2–4 weeks, more than 50% of individuals develop a transient, symptomatic illness, also known as primary or acute HIV syndrome, with symptoms generally resembling those of influenza or mononucleosis [19] (Fig. 3).

The most common signs and symptoms include fever, fatigue, rash, headache, lymphadenopathy, pharyngitis, myalgia, arthralgia, aseptic meningitis, retro-orbital pain, weight loss, depression, gastrointestinal distress, night sweats, and oral or genital ulcers. Generally, symptoms last between 7 and 10 days and rarely longer than 14 days.

After 10–12 days from infection, the virus starts multiplying at high rates and the HIV-RNA can be detectable in the blood by RT-PCR amplification methods, with the peak of viremia occurring approximately two weeks after the initial detection of viral RNA [20]. The phase from the infection and the appearance of HIV-RNA in the blood is referred to as eclipse period, where no markers of HIV infection are evident. Considering the sexual transmission at the genital mucosa as the most common mode of HIV-1 infection, in the acute phase, soon after virus entry in the body, the Langerhans' cells, i.e., tissue dendritic cells found in the lamina propria

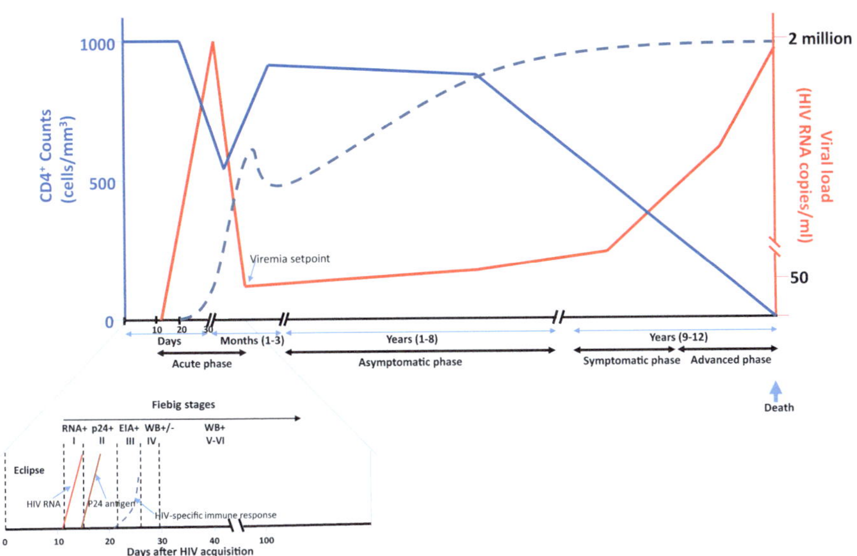

Fig. 3 Natural course of the untreated HIV infection

subjacent to the cervicovaginal epithelium, are the first targets of the virus. For their role in the immune response, these cells meet the CD4+ T lymphocytes and infect them. Within two days after infection, virus is detected in the draining internal iliac lymph nodes, where, in about 10 days, the virus and the infected cells can enter into the bloodstream and be disseminated to other organs including lymph nodes, the gut-associated lymphoid tissue, the spleen, and the brain [21]. In the gut, the mucosal tissue is seriously damaged by the cytopathic effects of HIV replication, resulting in the loss of the gut barrier integrity and, therefore, allowing passage of pathogens and immunostimulatory molecules from the gut lumen into the lamina propria and into the systemic circulation, thus continuously promoting a local and systemic inflammatory response.

The onset of viremia is a critical time point in the natural history of HIV infection, because it indicates that the infected individual has the potential of transmitting the infection [22–24] and provides the first chance to diagnose the infection in the blood sample by detecting the presence of either the virus RNA, using reverse transcriptase polymerase chain reaction amplification techniques, or the p 24 antigen, by fourth-generation enzyme-linked immunosorbent assays (ELISAs) [25–28]. Thus, the period from infection to the appearance of the first marker of infection is referred to as "window period," where no HIV diagnostic test gives positive results.

The high levels of HIV-1 viremia are normally short-lived, since starting from the third week after infection the host generates strong humoral and cellular immune responses that partly control viral replication. These responses are characterized by high levels of inflammatory cytokines and chemokines (the "cytokine storm") [29]. Consequently, viremia starts declining by several orders of magnitude until it reaches a lower steady level (viral set point) or drops under the detection level

(Fig. 3) [30]. The presence of HIV-specific antibodies is detected by both third-generation ELISA and Western blotting (WB) assay. The time of the appearance of the first HIV-specific antibodies has been estimated by detecting their presence in sequential samples from patients with accurate information on the time of HIV infection. Seroconversion has been observed to occur in a period ranging from 3 to 5 weeks, with an average of 22 days [31]. Several factors associated with innate and acquired antiviral immunity can influence viral replication and the establishment of a viral set point during this phase of infection. However, the role of the virus-specific cell-mediated immune response, in particular of the specific CD8+ T-cell cytotoxic activity, seems to be central in the initial control of virus replication at this stage of the infection, before the appearance of anti-HIV binding and/or neutralizing antibodies [32–35]. Thus, the primary HIV infection phase can be defined as the interval from the detection of the virus HIV-RNA in the plasma (the end of the eclipse period) until the establishment of a stable plasma HIV-RNA level (viral set point) in the presence of evolving anti-HIV antibody reactivity [36]. During acute HIV-1 infection, the number of CD4+ T cells dramatically declines, in association with high viremia levels, before the onset of the antiviral immune response [37]. When the HIV-specific immune response starts raising, HIV viremia drops and CD4+ T cells raise again (Fig. 3), although to levels lower than those present before infection, suggesting the persistence of virus-associated pathogenic effects. In addition, qualitative functional impairment of immune responses to HIV and other antigens can be detected [38–41], indicating that the virus induces, very early after infection, a dysfunction of CD4+ T cells and of other cells of the immune system. In particular, the retention of the virus in lymphoid tissues induces a sustained and chronic immune activation that causes damages to the lymphoid tissue architecture and limits the access to homeostatic factors, thus contributing to the immune cell loss. Finally, early after infection, the HIV genome is established as a latent virion in CD4+ T cells in different tissues, thus generating viral reservoirs [42].

In order to better characterize the stages occurring in the acute phase, Fiebig et al identified six stages based on viral replication and evolving antibody responses [20]. After the eclipse period, Fiebig stage 1 is described as the period where, during ramp-up viremia, only HIV-1 RNA in the blood can be detected (Fig. 3). About 7 days later, fourth-generation EIA tests start detecting the p24 antigen and this phase is identified as Fiebig stage II. Within about 5–10 days after the p24 antigen appearance, HIV-1-specific antibodies start being detected by third-generation EIA tests and this event marks the beginning of the Fiebig stage III that typically occurs 1–2 weeks after the onset of the acute retroviral symptoms. Fiebig stage IV represents the development of an indeterminate WB test, and this occurs a few days after the sensitive EIA tests show positive results. Conversion to a clearly positive WB test characterizes Fiebig stages V (positive WB) and VI (WB with the expression of all HIV proteins) (Fig. 3).

A few weeks after the onset of acute infection, a long clinically asymptomatic period begins, generally associated with low HIV viremia levels and absence of symptoms (Fig. 3). This event reflects primarily the antiviral action exerted by both innate and adaptive immune responses [43]. Neutralizing antibodies are generated, which are able to prevent cell infection [44], whereas other HIV-specific antibodies favor the elimination of infected cells by a mechanism known as antibody-dependent cellular cytotoxicity (ADCC), mediated by T lymphocytes and natural killer cells [45]. HIV-specific T lymphocytes promote the elimination of infected cells by antigen-specific cytotoxic mechanisms [32]. Although the presence of a strong immune response, HIV continuously replicates in the body compartments, counteracting antiviral immunity and inducing a state of chronic systemic inflammation, which, in turn, is responsible for the weakening of the immune system. There are several reasons why antiviral immunity is not able to eradicate the infection; however, the persistence of the integrated virus in lymphoid compartments (reservoir), with low expression of virus antigens and the high frequency of mutations within virus genome, which leads to the virus to escape from the immune response, are the most effective mechanisms. Thus, virus replication keeps occurring in the lymphoid compartment, and transitory peaks of HIV viremia can be detected in plasma in the absence of symptoms related to the infection [43]. In some individuals, HIV viremia is not detectable for many years, indicating the occurrence of efficient control of the infection. These individuals are termed as elite "controllers" [46, 47] and are intensely studied with the aim of understanding the mechanisms involved in the control of HIV infection.

In the course of the asymptomatic period, HIV-associated pathogenic effects persist and induce a slow but progressive loss of CD4+ lymphocytes and impairment of the immune system [43] (Fig. 3). The progression of the disease is characterized by the destruction of the lymphoid tissue architecture, which is a consequence of the virus replication and of the chronic activation of the cells of the immune system. This leads to an increase in virus diffusion to surrounding CD4+ T cells and favors HIV-1 spread within local, regional, and the entire lymphoid environment. Particularly, at this stage HIV infection is associated with an extensive replication in the gut lamina propria and the submucosa and in draining lymph nodes, with local depletion of CD4+ T cells [48, 49]. The further progression of the disease depends on the capacity of the host to contain virus replication and to reconstitute the pool of memory T cells within the mucosa-associated lymphoid tissue or lymph nodes. In the absence of virus containment, the destruction of the lymphoid system proceeds and the CD4+ T-cell number continues to drop to levels <200 cells/μl, which are associated with the risk of onset of opportunistic infections by bacteria, viruses, fungi, and parasites and tumors, as a consequence of a serious impairment of the immune system. The most common opportunistic infections, which define the AIDS stage, are caused by Pneumocystis pneumonia, Candida albicans, Cytomegalovirus, Herpes zoster, or enteropathic parasites (Cryptosporidium and Giardia species, Cystoisospora belli), which can determine life-threatening diseases [50]. This phase is usually characterized by diffuse lymph node swelling, severe reduction in body weight, fever, and respiratory and gastrointestinal symptoms. Neoplastic diseases, such as Kaposi's sarcoma and lymphomas, most likely emerging as a consequence of the immunodeficiency status, also severely weaken the organism, worsening the clinical course of the disease [51]. A progressive encephalopathy, induced by HIV or other opportunistic infections, can be present, also associated with a severe invalidation and increased risk of mortality. About 30–40% of patients can show symptoms or signs of dementia (AIDS dementia complex) caused by neuronal damage by HIV. These include slowed thinking and expression, difficulty concentrating, apathy, slow movements, ataxia, and weakness, together with abnormal neurologic signs that include paraparesis, lower-extremity spasticity, ataxia, extensor plantar responses, mania, or psychosis.

During the advanced phase, the number of CD4+ T cells continues to decrease (Fig. 3), and anemia and marked lymphopenia are frequently detected. In the absence of treatment, the mean time from the infection onset to AIDS-related death is approximately 11 years (Fig. 3). Of course, the progression of the disease is extremely variable, depending on the infecting virus isolate and the antiviral response of the host. In fact, besides the above described "Elite Controllers," who can adequately control HIV infection, infected individuals are classified, based on the infection course, with non-standardized definitions as "Progressors," "Rapid Progressors," "Non Progressors," and "Long Term Non-Progressors." It is evident that this distinction is based mainly on clinical evaluation and mirrors the individual response to HIV infection.

HIV Infection Treatment and Prevention

To date, there is no therapy capable of completely eradicating HIV infection, due to the presence of a reservoir of latently infected CD4$^+$ T cells that are able to produce infectious viruses once activated, on which the antiretroviral therapy has no effect [52–54]. Thus, the virus reservoir is the major barrier to virus eradication. However, there are effective antiretroviral drugs capable of controlling viral replication, suppressing it to undetectable levels, and preventing or severely limiting the progression of the disease and the emergence of AIDS. Current drugs are effective in both adults and children. In particular, in HIV-infected children an early commencement of an antiretroviral therapy made of a combination of different drugs (combination antiretroviral therapy, cART) has resulted in a dramatic control of neurocognitive disorders that are a common event in children, although they remain vulnerable to cognitive impairment and psychological disorders [55].

Drugs have been developed for each critical step of HIV replication. Virus entry into the cell can be inhibited by drugs able to block the mechanism of membrane fusion, such as enfuvirtide, which binds the gp41 protein, or to prevent the binding of HIV to CD4, such as ibalizumab, a monoclonal anti-CD4-antibody, and maraviroc that binds to the cell's CCR5-receptor, thus preventing entry of HIVs that use this co-receptor. Many drugs, which have the RT enzyme as a target, have been developed since 1987, year of the approval of the first antiretroviral against HIV, the azidothymidine (AZT), for human administration, by the US FDA. These drugs belong to either the class of nucleoside reverse transcriptase inhibitors (NRTIs) or the non-nucleoside reverse transcriptase inhibitors (NNRTIs). Associated with the drugs of the class of protease inhibitors (PI), these are the main components of the highly active anti-retroviral therapy (HAART), a cART that drastically limits the generation of drug-resistance virus variants, compared to monotherapy. A more recently developed class of drugs is that of integrase inhibitors (INSTI) that block the virus-specific enzyme integrase, thereby preventing viral DNA from being integrated into the cellular genome. The very broad HIV variability is responsible for changes in the genetic structure of HIV that affect the ability of drugs to block the replication of the virus. Therefore, all current antiretroviral drugs, including newer classes, are at risk of becoming partly or fully inactive because of the emergence of drug-resistant virus strains, even when administered as a cART. Thus, a major public health issue, worldwide, is to limit the generation and spreading of antiretroviral drug-resistant HIV variants, which can be responsible for the increased numbers of HIV infections and HIV-associated morbidity and mortality.

Despite significant advances in HIV treatment, HIV transmission remains common and public health strategies to prevent HIV infection are necessary. These include the promotion of safer sexual practices, expanded HIV testing, and administration of HIV therapy to HIV-infected people, in order to decrease viral load in blood, thus decreasing the risk of transmission. However, these strategies do not eliminate the risk of HIV transmission. Therefore, other strategies foresee the implementation of combined biomedical, behavioral, and structural interventions [56]. The term "combined prevention" includes different prevention methods that can interfere with the sexual transmission of the virus. Among these, there is the use of antiretrovirals in HIV-negative people, and this identifies pre-exposure prophylaxis (PrEP) and post-exposure prophylaxis (PEP), as biomedical interventions. In particular, PEP is used after behaviors at risk of acquiring HIV infection, i.e., a sexual intercourse without using condoms, or in case of condom failure, whereas Prep is used before exposure to the virus, in all cases where the likelihood of committing HIV risk behaviors is high.

Right now, preventive vaccines against HIV have been ineffective. The reasons are the great HIV variability that provides the virus the ability of outwitting the immune system and the still not clear understanding of the mechanisms of the HIV immune pathogenesis. Thus, therapeutic vaccines against HIV are being developed, which could help control infection and delay the progression of the disease. They work by eliciting the immune system against HIV-infected cells and therefore should prevent or limit HIV replication. These vaccines are thought to be administered to people who are already HIV-positive but who have healthy immune systems. In addition, combining ART with a therapeutic vaccine could elicit or boost cellular and humoral immune responses that could control viral replication and purge the HIV reservoir that the current antiretroviral drugs fail to adequately reach. Combinatorial interventions for developing novel HIV-1 therapeutic vaccines are on the way and open new perspectives for a functional cure for HIV infection [57].

Sexuality and Quality of Life

The literature often refers to "sexual marathons" (i.e., prolonged sexual activity over hours and even days) in the practice of homosexual intercourse. Semple et al. [58] conducted an exploratory study of a sample of 341 HIV-positive men who consumed methamphetamines during these relationships. Eighty-four percent of respondents reported having marathon sex while conditioned by the mind-altering effects of methamphetamines. MSM who had engaged in sexual marathons and those who had not were compared in terms of baseline characteristics, methamphetamine use variables, alcohol and illicit drug use, sexual risk behavior, and psychosocial factors.

From an HIV prevention perspective, a sexual marathon, particularly if it involves prolonged anal intercourse, is considered high risk because of the increased likelihood of condom breakage and of tearing of the delicate rectal tissue, events that may facilitate the transmission of HIV and sexually transmitted infections (STIs). Oral sex, while having a lower potential for HIV transmission, can cause HIV infection through lesions in the mouth, which are more likely to occur during prolonged sexual activity [59].

The rates of unprotected receptive and insertive anal intercourse during the marathon were reported to be 93% and 72%, respectively. Of MSM who had engaged in marathon sex, receptive oral sex without a condom and unprotected insertive (giving) oral sex were reported as 90% and 97%, respectively. These results point to sex marathons as a possible contributor to increased HIV/STI rates in the gay and bisexual community [60].

In Semple's study [58], the majority of participants were Caucasian (57%), had never married (82%), had a two-year college degree or less (77%), were unemployed (74%), and lived alone or with other adults in a sexual relationship (63%). The mean age was 37.1 years. The most frequent methods of methamphetamine use were smoking (80%) and snorting (78%). The mean amount of methamphetamine used in the previous 30 days was 5.8 grams (SD = 11.9).

Participants were asked: "When you are high on methamphetamine, how often do you practice marathon sex?" The answers were coded on a 5-point scale ranging from 1 (never) to 5 (always). The response categories were narrowed to create two groups: (1) those who engaged in marathon sex and (2) those who did not engage in marathon sex.

The amount of methamphetamine used was measured as the number of grams consumed in the previous 30 days. Frequency of methamphetamine use was measured by two items: "In the past 30 days, on how many days did you consume methamphetamine?" and "On a typical day, how many times did you consume methamphetamine?" Uncontrolled use was assessed using the following question: "Are you an uncontrolled user of amphetamines?"

The total number of sexual partners was measured by counting all persons with whom the participant had had anal or oral intercourse during the previous 2 months. Within this total, five categories of partner type were distinguished: stable (e.g., spouse and steady); other regular partners (e.g., boyfriend); casual (e.g., one-night stand); anonymous (e.g., someone in the park); and paid partners. The total number of each partner type was calculated. In addition, for each type of partner, participants were asked how many times in the previous two months they had engaged in receptive anal sex, insertive anal sex, receptive oral sex, insertive (given) oral sex, and insertive vaginal sex.

Sixty-seven percent of the respondents reported engaging in receptive anal sex without a condom some of the time, most of the time, or all of the time. Using the same response categories, 58% reported having insertive anal sex without a condom, 88% reported receptive oral sex without a condom, and 87% reported insertive oral sex without a condom. Other high-frequency activities associated with marathon sex included masturbation (23.0%), watching pornographic films (16.7%), using toys or dildos (13.3%), and fisting (10.0%).

In addition, those who had participated in sex marathons were significantly more likely to report using methamphetamine to "get pumped up" for sex, to meet sexual partners, and to enhance sexual pleasure than those who did not. The sex marathon group had also used significantly more illicit drugs in the previous 2 months and were more likely to have used amyl nitrate and sildenafil [61].

A more recent study by Sullivan et al. [62] investigated the emotional, relational, and health difficulties of HIV-positive patients (PLWH) in disclosing their HIV status to new (non-HIV) sexual partners. It found that substance use at the time of sex was associated with a lower likelihood of disclosing HIV status to first-time partners and that viral suppression moderated the relationship between substance use and condom use in PLWH [63].

In all of this, it is useful to consider that over one million people are living with HIV in the United States, with an estimated 38,739 new infections in the United States and its six dependent territories in 2017 (Centers for Disease Control and Prevention). Men who have sex with men (MSM) are disproportionately affected by HIV in the United States, particularly young black MSM (Centers for Disease Control and Prevention). HIV diagnosis rates among black and Hispanic men increased by 87% between 2005 and 2014 (Centers for Disease Control and Prevention). The continuing HIV crisis among MSM requires an understanding of their current prevention needs and new interventions to address the risk of HIV transmission.

A recent study by Horvath [64] also emphasized the need for biomedical HIV prevention strategies: In particular, TasP treatment and pre-exposure prophylaxis (PrEP) [65] were found to be the primary tools to control the HIV epidemic in the United States.

The study determined four separate definitions for a high-risk sexual encounter among participants who had reported anal intercourse in the previous 3 months [66]:

1. First, they identified HIV-positive men who had reported CAS with HIV-negative or unknown HIV-positive partners among those ($n = 281$) who had reported anal intercourse in the previous 3 months (Definition 1).

2. Second, they identified HIV-positive men with a non-suppressed viral load ($\geq$200 copies/mL) who had had one or more episodes of CAS with HIV-negative or unknown HIV-positive partners (Definition 2).
3. Third, they identified HIV-positive men who had had CAS with HIV-negative or unknown partners, at least one of whom was not using PrEP (Definition 3).
4. Fourth, in the most restrictive definition of risk, they identified HIV-positive men who were not virally suppressed and who had had CAS with HIV-negative or unknown HIV-positive partners, at least one of whom was not using PrEP (Definition 4). Definitions 2, 3, and 4 were restricted to include only men who had reported CAS in the previous 3 months ($n = 118$).

There is More [67]

A sample of 609 men were interviewed while attending a gay pride festival in Atlanta, Georgia. Participants completed a questionnaire assessing demographic information, Internet use, gay acculturation, AIDS awareness, attitudes toward condoms, overall substance use, and sexual behavior. A substantial majority of men (75%) reported using the Internet to access gay-oriented websites. One-third of the sample (34%) reported having met a sexual partner through the Internet. Men who met sexual partners online reported higher rates of methamphetamine use ($M = 8.38$, SD $= 19.39$) than men who did not meet partners in this way ($M = 3.13$, SD $= 4.99$, $p < 0.001$). Men who met partners via the Internet also reported higher rates of unsafe sexual behavior, including unprotected receptive anal intercourse ($p < 0.05$) and unprotected insertive anal intercourse ($p < 0.01$). The high prevalence of Internet use as a method of meeting sexual partners suggests that sexual networks may be forming on the Internet. Thus, the Internet offers opportunities for new HIV primary prevention interventions.

HIV and COVID-19

The study by Zapata et al. [68] sought to highlight the voices of young sexual minority men (YSMM) aged 17–24 years on the perceived impact of the pandemic on HIV prevention (among a diverse national sample of YSMM who participated in synchronous online focus group discussions between April and September 2020). Forty-one YSMM described the negative effects of the COVID-19 pandemic on HIV testing and prevention services, including limited and interrupted access to HIV testing, HIV pre-exposure prophylaxis (PrEP), and HIV post-exposure prophylaxis. The challenges associated with COVID-19 have been compounded by the ongoing pre-COVID-19 barriers encountered by YSMM in the United States.

For example,

1. Many YSMM moved home with their families, forcing men to avoid HIV prevention services for fear of putting relatives at risk.
2. YSMM also took care not to put their family at greater risk of COVID-19 by avoiding clinical appointments.

3. YSMM who sought HIV prevention services, including access to PrEP, faced significant barriers, including limited availability of appointments and services that were not tailored to YSMM.

Further efforts are needed to support YSMM's re-engagement in HIV prevention during and after the COVID-19 era.

Future Perspectives

Despite enormous progress in the treatment of HIV/AIDS, its spread and prevalence are persistent public health problems in the United States and around the world; marginalized populations (such as the poor and/or members of racial/ethnic and/or sexual minorities) bear a disproportionate mental and physical burden due to the virus. Global HIV targets focus on the "90–90–90" target, which calls on health systems to increase awareness among people living with HIV (PLWH) so that 90% can:

1. Learn about HIV and its symptoms
2. Receive sustained antiretroviral therapy (ART)
3. Achieve HIV viral suppression

Andersson et al. [69] and Lazarus et al. [70] fittingly called for a "4th 90," however, to go beyond viral suppression to ensure that PLWH enjoys a high quality of life. This step is crucial now that PLWH are seeking treatment and living longer. PLWH must experience less stigma to achieve a high quality of life [70].

Young black men (in the USA) who have sex with men (MSM) face numerous barriers, including medical and social stigma, including in accessing pre-exposure prophylaxis (PrEP) to HIV, as well as in finding a supportive community [71]. Similar individuals who are already living with HIV experience trauma due to stigma and a subsequent cascade of medical and social consequences from an HIV diagnosis [72]. Therefore, individuals who are already disadvantaged by their intersectional identity may be even more severely affected by an HIV diagnosis, such as a poor black woman who uses drugs while living with HIV compared to a black woman who is healthy and resourceful while living with HIV [73].

When individuals are subjected to HIV stigma in both institutional and social contexts, the unique combination of exposure to such discrimination can lead individuals to withdraw from society [74]. In this regard, the individuals in the studies cited here described their feelings toward society as a whole with words such as "forgotten," "separated," and "excluded" and how HIV stigma made them feel alone and isolated.

Lesbian, bisexual, queer, and transgender (LBQT) women living with HIV have been described as invisible and under-researched. However, social and structural contexts of violence and discrimination exacerbate the risk of HIV infection among LBQT women.

Logie [75] conducted two focus groups; one focus group was conducted with HIV-positive lesbian, bisexual, and queer women ($n = 7$) and the second with HIV-positive transgender women ($n = 16$). Participants were recruited using purposive sampling. Focus groups were digitally recorded and transcribed verbatim. Thematic analysis was used to analyze the data to improve understanding of the factors influencing the well-being of LBQT HIV-positive women.

Accounts given by female respondents with HIV recalled social exclusion and verbal violence from society: multiple barriers to HIV care and support, including discriminatory and incompetent treatment by health workers. The under-representation of LBQT women in HIV research further contributed to marginalization and exclusion. Participants expressed a willingness to participate in HIV research that would develop over time.

In addition: A meta-analysis of US-based studies synthesized weighted averages across 29 studies to estimate HIV prevalence rates and reported that rates among transgender women ranged from 11.8% (self-assessment) to 27.7% (HIV test results) [76].

Conclusion

Transactional sex (i.e., selling sex for money, drugs, a place to stay, or other survival needs) is a behavior associated with some negative health outcomes, including HIV acquisition and transmission [77]. Most of the research on transactional sex has focused on women [78], while much less has been published on sex work among gay, bisexual, and other men who have sex with men (MSM), who are disproportionately affected by HIV. In 2017, MSM accounted for 70% of new HIV infections, while in 2016, 72% of those living with HIV were attributed to male-to-male sexual contact. It is important to note that MSM who engage in transactional sex run additional risks of acquiring and/or transmitting HIV and are more likely to be newly diagnosed with sexually transmitted infections (STIs), report poly-drug use, and also have had six or more male anal sex partners in the previous 60 days [79].

A recent cross-sectional surveillance study sampling MSM in 20 metropolitan areas of the United States reported that 7% of MSM had engaged in transactional sex, while an online study of MSM found that 12.5% had reported sexual transactions in the previous 60 days [80]. Another respondent-driven cross-sectional sampling study sampling men who injected drugs found that 15% of heterosexually identified men and 60% of gay and bisexual men reported transactional sex, suggesting that MSM who inject drugs may be more likely to engage in transactional sex than those who do not inject drugs [78]. In addition, bisexual men were found to have a higher prevalence of such encounters than both heterosexual and gay MSM [81].

If we then look at drug use, 22% of respondents (a total of 35,532 through an online questionnaire) reported having used drugs in their lifetime [81]. In the previous 90 days, 40% reported not having used drugs, 25% reported using one drug,

12% reported using two drugs, and 23% reported using three or more drugs. When evaluating different types of drugs that HIV-positive MSM reported using in the previous 90 days, it was found that 32% reported using stimulants, 21% reported using downers, 11% reported using opioids, 11% reported using hallucinogens, 43% reported using poppers, and 1% reported using synthetic drugs.

What can be said? World studies, despite progress in preventive and curative therapies, show a social, psychological, and life motivation distress that is still underestimated. Many studies highlight the phenomenon of HIV, but there is still a lack of global development of care and treatment centers able to take care of the individual and not just the pathology.

References

1. https://www.unaids.org/en/resources/fact-sheet. Accessed 11 May 2021.
2. Azevedo-Pereira JM, Santos-Costa Q. HIV interaction with human host: HIV-2 as a model of a less virulent infection. AIDS Rev. 2016;18(1):44–53.
3. Campbell-Yesufu OT, Gandhi-Perrin RT. Update on human immunodeficiency virus (HIV)-2 infection. Clin Infect Dis. 2011;52(6):780–7. https://doi.org/10.1093/cid/ciq248.
4. Santoro MM, Perno CF. HIV-1 genetic variability and clinical implications. ISRN Microbiol. 2013;2013:481314. https://doi.org/10.1155/2013/481314.
5. Yamaguchi J, Vallari A, McArthur C, Sthreshley L, Cloherty GA, Berg MG, Rodgers MA. Brief report: complete genome sequence of CG-0018a-01 establishes HIV-1 subtype L. J Acquir Immune Defic Syndr. 2020;83(3):319–22. https://doi.org/10.1097/QAI.0000000000002246.
6. CRFs. https://www.hiv.lanl.gov/content/sequence/HIV/CRFs/CRFs.html. Accessed 11 May 2021.
7. Dayton AI, Sodroski JG, Rosen CA, Goh WC, Haseltine WA. The trans-activator gene of the human T cell lymphotropic virus type III is required for replication. Cell. 1986;44(6):941–7. https://doi.org/10.1016/0092-8674(86)90017-6.
8. Kao SY, Calman AF, Luciw PA, Peterlin BM. Anti-termination of transcription within the long terminal repeat of HIV-1 by tat gene product. Nature. 1987;330(6147):489–93. https://doi.org/10.1038/330489a0.
9. Karn J, Stoltzfus CM. Transcriptional and posttranscriptional regulation of HIV-1 gene expression. Cold Spring Harb Perspect Med. 2012;2(2):a006916. https://doi.org/10.1101/cshperspect.a006916.
10. Asamitsu K, Okamoto T. The Tat/P-TEFb protein-protein interaction determining transcriptional activation of HIV. Curr Pharm Des. 2017;23(28):4091–7. https://doi.org/10.2174/1381612823666170710164148.
11. Asamitsu K, Fujinaga K, Okamoto T. HIV Tat/P-TEFb interaction: a potential target for novel anti-HIV therapies. Molecules. 2018;23(4):933. https://doi.org/10.3390/molecules23040933.
12. Nekhai S, Jeang K-T. Transcriptional and post-transcriptional regulation of HIV-1 gene expression: role of cellular factors for Tat and Rev. Future Microbiol. 2006;1(4):417–26. https://doi.org/10.2217/17460913.1.4.417.
13. Donahue DA, Kuhl BD, Sloan RD, Wainberg MA. The viral protein Tat can inhibit the establishment of HIV-1 latency. J Virol. 2012;86(6):3253–63. https://doi.org/10.1128/JVI.06648-11.
14. Kumar A, Herbein G. The macrophage: a therapeutic target in HIV-1 infection. Mol Cell Ther. 2014;2:10. https://doi.org/10.1186/2052-8426-2-10.
15. Kamori D, Ueno T. HIV-1 Tat and viral latency: what we can learn from naturally occurring sequence variations. Front Microbiol. 2017;8:80. https://doi.org/10.3389/fmicb.2017.00080.

16. Khoury G, Darcis G, Lee MY, Bouchat S, Van Driessche B, Purcell DFJ, Van Lint C. Adv Exp Med Biol. 2018;1075:187–212. https://doi.org/10.1007/978-981-13-0484-2_8.
17. Hendricks CM, Cordeiro T, Gomes AP, Stevenson M. The interplay of HIV-1 and macrophages in viral persistence. Front Microbiol. 2021;12:646447. https://doi.org/10.3389/fmicb.2021.646447. eCollection 2021.
18. Emery A, Swanstrom R. HIV-1: to splice or not to splice, that is the question. Viruses. 2021;13(2):181. https://doi.org/10.3390/v13020181.
19. Cohen MS, Shaw GM, McMichael AJ, Haynes BF. Acute HIV-1 infection. N Engl J Med. 2011;364(20):1943–54. https://doi.org/10.1056/NEJMra1011874.
20. Fiebig EW, Wright DJ, Rawal BD, Garrett PE, Schumacher RT, Peddada L, Heldebrant C, Smith R, Conrad A, Kleinman SH, Busch MP. Dynamics of HIV viremia and antibody seroconversion in plasma donors: implications for diagnosis and staging of primary HIV infection. AIDS. 2003;17(13):1871–9. https://doi.org/10.1097/00002030-200309050-00005.
21. Kahn JO, Walker BD. Acute human immunodeficiency virus type 1 infection. N Engl J Med. 1998;339(1):33–9. https://doi.org/10.1056/NEJM199807023390107.
22. Busch MP, Satten GA. Time course of viremia and antibody seroconversion following human immunodeficiency virus exposure. Am J Med. 1997;102(5B):117–24. https://doi.org/10.1016/s0002-9343(97)00077-6.
23. Ling AE, Robbins KE, Brown TM, Dunmire V, Thoe SY, Wong SY, Leo YS, Teo D, Gallarda J, Phelps B, Chamberland ME, Busch MP, Folks TM, Kalish ML. Failure of routine HIV-1 tests in a case involving transmission with preseroconversion blood components during the infectious window period. JAMA. 2000;284(2):210–4. https://doi.org/10.1001/jama.284.2.210.
24. Kopko PM, Fernando LP, Bonney EN, Freeman JL, Holland PV. HIV transmissions from a window-period platelet donation. Am J Clin Pathol. 2001;116(4):562–6. https://doi.org/10.1309/GBLA-NL8D-3277-XUP1.
25. Lindbäck S., Thorstensson R., Karlsson AC, von Sydow M., Flamholc L., Blaxhult A., Sönnerborg A., Biberfeld G., Gaines H. Diagnosis of primary HIV-1 infection and duration of follow-up after HIV exposure. Karolinska Institute Primary HIV Infection Study Group. AIDS 2000; 14(15): 2333-2339. doi: https://doi.org/10.1097/00002030-200010200-00014.
26. Hecht FM, Busch MP, Rawal B, Webb M, Rosenberg E, Swanson M, Chesney M, Anderson J, Levy J, Kahn JO. Use of laboratory tests and clinical symptoms for identification of primary HIV infection. AIDS. 2002;16(8):1119–29. https://doi.org/10.1097/00002030-200205240-00005.
27. Holodniy M, Busch M. Establishing the diagnosis of HIV infection. In: Dolin R, Masur H, Saag M, editors. AIDS therapy. 2nd ed. New York: Churchill Livingstone; 2002. p. 3–20.
28. Nguyen KA, Busch MP. Evolving strategies for diagnosing human immunodeficiency virus infection. Am J Med. 2000;109(7):595–7. https://doi.org/10.1016/s0002-9343(00)00611-2.
29. Stacey AR, Norris PJ, Qin L, Haygreen EA, Taylor E, Heitman J, Lebedeva M, DeCamp A, Li D, Grove D, Self SG, Borrow P. Induction of a striking systemic cytokine cascade prior to peak viremia in acute human immunodeficiency virus type 1 infection, in contrast to more modest and delayed responses in acute hepatitis B and C virus infections. J Virol. 2009;83(8):3719–33. https://doi.org/10.1128/JVI.01844-08.
30. Little SJ, McLean AR, Spina CA, Richman DD, Havlir DV. Viral dynamics of acute HIV-1 infection. J Exp Med. 1999;190(6):841–50. https://doi.org/10.1084/jem.190.6.841.
31. Buttò S, Raimondo M, Fanales-Belasio E, Suligoi B. Suggested strategies for the laboratory diagnosis of HIV infection in Italy. Ann Ist Super Sanita. 2010;46(1):34–41. https://doi.org/10.4415/ANN_10_01_05.
32. Bangham CRM. CTL quality and the control of human retroviral infections. Eur J Immunol. 2009;39(7):1700–12. https://doi.org/10.1002/eji.200939451.
33. Koup RA. Virus escape from CTL recognition. J Exp Med. 1994;180(3):779–82. https://doi.org/10.1084/jem.180.3.779.
34. Borrow P, Lewicki H, Hahn BH, Shaw GM, Oldstone MB. Virus-specific CD8+ cytotoxic T-lymphocyte activity associated with control of viremia in primary human

immunodeficiency virus type 1 infection. J Virol. 1994;68(9):6103–10. https://doi.org/10.1128/JVI.68.9.6103-6110.1994.

35. Price DA, Goulder PJ, Klenerman P, Sewell AK, Easterbrook PJ, Troop M, Bangham CR, Phillips RE. Positive selection of HIV-1 cytotoxic T lymphocyte escape variants during primary infection. Proc Natl Acad Sci U S A. 1997;94(5):1890–5. https://doi.org/10.1073/pnas.94.5.1890.

36. Prins HAB, Verbon A, Boucher CAB, Rokx C. Ending the epidemic: critical role of primary HIV infection. Neth J Med. 2017;75(8):321–7.

37. Vanhems P, Lambert J, Cooper DA, Perrin L, Carr A, Hirschel B, Vizzard J, Kinloch-de LS, Allard R. Severity and prognosis of acute human immunodeficiency virus type 1 illness: a dose-response relationship. Clin Infect Dis. 1998;26(2):323–9. https://doi.org/10.1086/516289.

38. Rosenberg YJ, Anderson AO, Pabst R. HIV-induced decline in blood CD4/CD8 ratios: viral killing or altered lymphocyte trafficking? Immunol Today. 1998;19(1):10–7. https://doi.org/10.1016/s0167-5699(97)01183-3.

39. Lichterfeld M, Kaufmann DE, Yu XG, Mui SK, Addo MM, Johnston MN, Cohen D, Robbins GK, Pae E, Alter G, Wurcel A, Stone D, Rosenberg ES, Walker BD, Altfeld M. Loss of HIV-1-specific CD8+ T cell proliferation after acute HIV-1 infection and restoration by vaccine-induced HIV-1-specific CD4+ T cells. J Exp Med. 2004;200(6):701–12. https://doi.org/10.1084/jem.20041270.

40. Douek DC. Disrupting T-cell homeostasis: how HIV-1 infection causes disease. AIDS Rev. 2003;5(3):172–7.

41. Lange CG, Lederman MM, Medvik K, Asaad R, Wild M, Kalayjian R, Valdez H. Nadir CD4+ T-cell count and numbers of CD28+ CD4+ T-cells predict functional responses to immunizations in chronic HIV-1 infection. AIDS. 2003;17(14):2015–23. https://doi.org/10.1097/00002030-200309260-00002.

42. Henrich TJ, Hanhauser E, Marty FM, Sirignano MN, Keating S, Lee T-H, Robles YP, Davis BT, Li JZ, Heisey A, Hill AL, Busch MP, Armand P, Soiffer RJ, Altfeld M, Kuritzkes DR. Ann Intern Med. 2014;161(5):319–27. https://doi.org/10.7326/M14-1027.

43. Ford ES, Puronen CE, Sereti I. Immunopathogenesis of asymptomatic chronic HIV infection: the calm before the storm. Curr Opin HIV AIDS. 2009;4(3):206–14. https://doi.org/10.1097/COH.0b013e328329c68c.

44. Stamatatos L, Morris L, Burton DR, Mascola JR. Neutralizing antibodies generated during natural HIV-1 infection: good news for an HIV-1 vaccine? Nat Med. 2009;15(8):866–70. https://doi.org/10.1038/nm.1949.

45. Chung A, Rollman E, Johansson S, Kent SJ, Stratov I. The utility of ADCC responses in HIV infection. Curr HIV Res. 2008;6(6):515–9. https://doi.org/10.2174/157016208786501472.

46. Baker BM, Block BL, Rothchild AC, Walker BD. Elite control of HIV infection: implications for vaccine design. Expert Opin Biol Ther. 2009;9(1):55–69. https://doi.org/10.1517/14712590802571928.

47. Saksena NK, Rodes B, Wang B, Soriano V. Elite HIV controllers: myth or reality? AIDS Rev. 2007;9:195–207.

48. Brenchley JM, Schacker TW, Ruff LE, Price DA, Taylor JH, Beilman GJ, Nguyen PL, Khoruts A, Larson M, Haase AT, Douek DC. CD4+ T cell depletion during all stages of HIV disease occurs predominantly in the gastrointestinal tract. J Exp Med. 2004;200(6):749–59. https://doi.org/10.1084/jem.20040874.

49. Mehandru S, Poles MA, Tenner-Racz K, Horowitz A, Hurley A, Hogan C, Boden D, Racz P, Markowitz M. Primary HIV-1 infection is associated with preferential depletion of CD4+ T lymphocytes from effector sites in the gastrointestinal tract. J Exp Med. 2004;200(6):761–70. https://doi.org/10.1084/jem.20041196.

50. Brooks JT, Kaplan JE, Holmes KK, Benson C, Pau A, Masur H. HIV-associated opportunistic infections–going, going, but not gone: the continued need for prevention and treatment guidelines. Clin Infect Dis. 2009;48(5):609–11. https://doi.org/10.1086/596756.

51. Clifford GM, Franceschi S. Cancer risk in HIV-infected persons: influence of CD4(+) count. Future Oncol. 2009;5(5):669–78. https://doi.org/10.2217/fon.09.28.
52. Chun TW, Stuyver L, Mizell SB, Ehler LA, Mican JA, Baseler M, Lloyd AL, Nowak MA, Fauci AS. Presence of an inducible HIV-1 latent reservoir during highly active antiretroviral therapy. Proc Natl Acad Sci U S A. 1997;94(24):13193–7. https://doi.org/10.1073/pnas.94.24.13193.
53. Finzi D, Hermankova M, Pierson T, Carruth LM, Buck C, Chaisson RE, Quinn TC, Chadwick K, Margolick J, Brookmeyer R, Gallant J, Markowitz M, Ho DD, Richman DD, Siliciano RF. Identification of a reservoir for HIV-1 in patients on highly active antiretroviral therapy. Science. 1997;278(5341):1295–300. https://doi.org/10.1126/science.278.5341.1295.
54. Wong JK, Hezareh M, Günthard HF, Havlir DV, Ignacio CC, Spina CA, Richman DD. Recovery of replication-competent HIV despite prolonged suppression of plasma viremia. Science. 1997;278(5341):1291–5. https://doi.org/10.1126/science.278.5341.1291.
55. Bartlett AW, Williams PCM, Jantarabenjakul W, Kerr SJ. State of the mind: growing up with HIV. Paediatr Drugs. 2020;22(5):511–24. https://doi.org/10.1007/s40272-020-00415-1.
56. UNAIDS: Combination HIV prevention: tailoring and coordinating biomedical, behavioural and structural strategies to reduce new HIV infections A UNAIDS discussion paper. 2010. https://www.unaids.org/sites/default/files/media_asset/JC2007_Combination_Prevention_paper_en_0.pdf. Accessed 11 May 2021.
57. Moretti S, Cafaro A, Tripiciano A, Picconi O, Buttò S, Ensoli F, Sgadari C, Monini P, Ensoli B. HIV therapeutic vaccines aimed at intensifying combination antiretroviral therapy. Expert Rev Vaccines. 2020;19(1):71–84. https://doi.org/10.1080/14760584.2020.1712199.
58. Semple SJ, Zians J, Strathdee SA, et al. Sex marathons and methamphetamine use among HIV-positive men who have sex with men. Arch Sex Behav. 2009;38:583.
59. AMMAR. Creating a research and development agenda for rectal microbicides that protect against HIV infection: seminar report. 2003. http://www.microbicide.org/microbicideinfo/reference/amfar.report.on.rectal.microbicides.pdf. Accessed 24 January 2007.
60. Worth H, Zablotska I. Associations between crystal methamphetamine use and potentially dangerous sexual activity among gay men in Australia. Arch Sex Behav. 2007;36:646–54.
61. Shoptaw S, Reback CJ, Freese TE. Patient characteristics, HIV serostat and risk behaviors among gay and bisexual males seeking treatment for methamphetamine abuse and addiction in Los Angeles. J Addict Dis. 2002;21:91–105.
62. Sullivan MC, Cruess DG, Huedo-Medina TB, et al. Substance use, HIV serostat disclosure, and sexual risk behavior in people living with HIV: an event-level analysis. Arch Sex Behav. 2020;49:2005–18.
63. Bird JD, Eversman M, Voisin DR. "You can't trust everyone": the impact of sexual risk, partner type, and perceived partner reliability on HIV disclosure decisions among HIV-positive black gay and bisexual men. Cult Health Sex. 2017;19(8):829–43.
64. Horvath KJ, Lammert S, Martinka A, et al. Definizione del rischio sessuale nell'era della prevenzione biomedica dell'HIV: implicazioni per la ricerca e la pratica sull'HIV. Arch Sex Behav. 2020;49:91–102.
65. Ning C, Huang J, Liang H. Pre-exposure prophylaxis for the prevention of HIV infection in high-risk populations: a meta-analysis of randomized controlled trials. PLoS ONE. 2014;9(2):e87674. https://doi.org/10.1371/journal.pone.0087674.
66. Rodger AJ, Cambiano V, Bruun T, Vernazza P, Collins S, Degen O, et al. Risk of transmission of HIV through condomless sex in serodifferent gay couples with HIV-positive partner receiving suppressive antiretroviral therapy (PARTNER): final results of a prospective, multicentre observational study. Lancet. 2019;393:2428–38.
67. Benotsch EG, Kalichman S, Cage M. Men who met sexual partners via the Internet: prevalence, predictors, and implications for HIV prevention. Arch Sex Behav. 2002;31:177–83.
68. Zapata JP, Dang M, Quinn KG, et al. COVID-19 related disruptions in HIV testing and prevention among young sexual minority men aged 17-24: a qualitative study using synchronous online focus groups, April-September 2020. Arch Sex Behav. 2022;51:303–14.

69. Andersson GZ, Reinius M, Eriksson LE, Svedhem V, Esfahani FM, Deuba K, Rao D, Lyatuu GW, Giovenco D, Ekstrom AM. Stigma-reducing interventions in people living with HIV to improve health-related quality of life. HIV Lancet. 2020;7(2):e129–40. https://doi.org/10.1016/s2352-3018(19)30343-1.

70. Lazarus JV, Safreed-Harmon K, Barton SE, Costagliola D, Dedes N, Del Amo Valero J, Gatell JM, Baptista-Leite R, Mendao L, Porter K, Vella S, Rockstroh JK. Beyond HIV viral suppression: the new frontier of quality of life. BMC Med. 2016;14(1):94. https://doi.org/10.1186/s12916-016-0640-4.

71. Quinn K, Bowleg L, Dickson-Gomez J. Fear of being black plus fear of being gay: the effects of intersectional stigma on PrEP use among young black gay, bisexual and other men who have sex with men. Soc Sci Med. 2019;232:86–93.

72. Mgbako O, Benoit E, Iyengar NS, Kuhner C, Brinker D, Duncan DT. "Like a time bomb": the persistence of trauma in the HIV diagnosis experience among black men having sex with men in New York City. BMC Public Health. 2020;20(1):1–14. https://doi.org/10.1186/s12889-020-09342-9.

73. Logie CH, James L, Tharao W, Loutfy MR. "We don't exist": a qualitative study of the marginalization experienced by HIV-positive, lesbian, bisexual, queer and transgender women in Toronto, Canada. J Int AIDS Soc. 2012;15(2):17392. https://doi.org/10.7448/ias.15.2.17392.

74. Johnson Shen M, Freeman R, Karpiak S, Brennan-Ing M, Seidel L, Siegler EL. The intersectionality of stigmas among key HIV-infected older populations: a thematic analysis. Clin Gerontol. 2019;42(2):37–149.

75. Logie CH, James L, Tharao W, Loutfy MR. We do not exist: a qualitative study on the marginalization experienced by HIV-positive lesbian, bisexual, queer and transgender women in Toronto, Canada. 2012. https://doi.org/10.7448/IAS.15.2.17392.

76. Herbst JH, Jacobs ED, Finlayson TJ, McKleroy VS, Neumann MS, Crepaz N. Estimating HIV prevalence and risk behaviors of transgender people in the United States: a systematic review. Behav Against AIDS. 2008;12(1):1–17.

77. Javanbakht M, Ragsdale A, Shoptaw S, Gorbach PM. Transactional sex among men who have sex with men: differences in substance use and HIV status. Urban Health J. 2019;96:429–41.

78. Walters SM, Rivera AV, Reilly KH, Anderson BJ, Bolden B, Wogayehu A, Braunstein S. Sex swapping between people injecting drugs in the New York metropolitan area: the importance of local context, gender, and sexual identity. AIDS Behav. 2018;22(9):2773–87.

79. Bond KT, Yoon IS, Houang ST, Downing MJ, Grov C, Hirshfield S. Transactional sex, substance use, and sexual risk: earnings direction comparison for a us sample of men who have sex with men based on the internet. Res Sex Soc Policy. 2019;16:255–67.

80. Nerlander LM, Hess KL, Sionean C, Rose C, Thorson A, Broz D, Paz-Bailey G. Sex swapping and HIV infection among men who have sex with men: 20 US cities, 2011. AIDS Behav. 2017;8:2283–94.

81. Friedman MR, Dodge BM. The role of syndemics in explaining health disparities among bisexual men: a blueprint for a theoretically informed perspective. In: Understanding the HIV/AIDS epidemic in the United States. Cham: Springer; 2016. p. 71–98.

Sexually Transmitted Diseases and COVID-19

Matteo Bassetti, Laura Magnasco, Federica Portunato, and Elena Vittoria Longhi

Sexually transmitted disease (STD) refers to a disease that has developed after an infection acquired by sexual contact. Human immunodeficiency virus (HIV), hepatitis B virus (HBV), hepatitis C virus (HCV), atypical bacteria, and syphilis can follow a chronic course, causing long-term complications. Prevention and early diagnosis are key factors to prevent the physical and psychological impact of these diseases [1] and have been strongly empowered during the last decades with promising results, but the COVID-19 pandemic could reverse these achievements.

SARS-CoV-2 is transmitted mainly by droplets and is highly transmissible from an infected person [2]. Despite the restrictive measures (physical distancing, hand hygiene, travel restrictions, and quarantine) adopted by many countries to prevent transmission and to reduce the burden on healthcare facilities [3], healthcare systems were overwhelmed by patients often requiring intensive care, and most services collapsed, compromising the access to care for patients with chronic conditions [4]. Moreover, this pandemic caused a dramatic reduction in public health surveillance programs and screening services, including those for STDs [5].

In this chapter, we will briefly describe the main STDs, their symptoms, and treatment and how COVID-19 impacted their management.

M. Bassetti (✉) · L. Magnasco · F. Portunato
Clinica Malattie Infettive, Università degli Studi di Genova e IRCCS Policlinico San Martino, Genova, Italy
e-mail: matteo.bassetti@hsanmartino.it; Laura.Magnasco@hsanmartino.it

E. V. Longhi
Department of Sexual Medical Center, San Raffaele Hospital, Milano, Italy

© Springer Nature Switzerland AG 2023
E. V. Longhi (ed.), *Managing Psychosexual Consequences in Chronic Diseases*,
https://doi.org/10.1007/978-3-031-31307-3_37

Atypical Bacteria

Intracellular bacteria, such as *Chlamydia trachomatis*, *Mycoplasma genitalium*, and *Ureaplasma urealyticum* and *parvum,* are the main causative pathogens of non-gonococcal urethritis (NGU) in men and of cervicitis or salpingitis in women. They can determine recurrent or persistent NGU, as well as chronic complications, such as prostatitis, orchitis, and epididymitis in men and pelvic inflammatory disease (PID) in women. Acute infection is asymptomatic or paucisymptomatic in females, while it manifests with dysuria, pruritus, and purulent discharge in men [6]. Perineal pain and low-grade fever can present in the case of prostatitis, while PID causes chronic abdominal pain and can lead to infertility [7]. *C. trachomatis* is the etiological agent of *lymphogranuloma venereum* (LGV), which initially causes a genital indolent and ulcerated vesicle that develops in painful lymphadenopathy with frequent drainage of exudate. If not treated, it can lead to elephantiasis or chronic fistulas.

If microscopic testing of a smear of urethral secretion shows >5 polymorphonucleated cells per high-power field, nucleic acid amplification tests should be performed to reach a definitive diagnosis.

For NGU, a single administration of 1000 mg of azithromycin, alternatives are a 7-day course of fluoroquinolones (although emerging resistance is an issue) or doxycycline [6] that should be preferred in non-urethral localizations of disease, such as proctitis in men [8]. In LGV, therapy should last 21 days, and surgery might be needed when chronic complications such as fistulas ensue [9]. Given the polymicrobial nature of PID in the majority of cases, the treatment is based on combination therapy with ceftriaxone, metronidazole, and doxycycline [10].

During the COVID-19 pandemic, the US CDC compared the mean weekly count of *Chlamydia* cases during weeks 1–11 and 12–40 of 2020, reporting a decrease of 20.2%. This effect was less pronounced for gonorrhea (−3.0%), whereas an opposite trend was observed for primary and secondary syphilis (+5.5%) [11]. In a survey performed between 2019 and 2020 in California [12], the weekly number of bacterial STDs reported declined sharply in conjunction with the stay-at-home order and did not return to prior baseline levels by the summer of 2020 (−31% for *C. trachomatis*, −19% for late syphilis, −15% for primary and secondary syphilis, −14% for early non-primary non-secondary syphilis, and −13% for gonorrhea).

In Italy, a decrease in the diagnosis of non-acute STIs was reported, even if the number of acute bacterial infections associated with men who have sex with men (MSM) increased. In fact, the comparison of diagnosis of STIs made between 15 March and 14 April 2020, with 2019 reported a slight increase in secondary syphilis and gonorrhea, suggesting that lockdown and social distancing did not inhibit risky behaviors [13].

Chronic Bacterial Prostatitis

Chronic bacterial prostatitis is a chronic or recurrent infection of the prostate, with or without accompanying symptoms of prostatitis [14]. Little is known about the precise epidemiology, mainly because a clear definition of chronic infection is missing, because symptoms frequently overlap with other noninfectious conditions and are nonspecific (perineal pain, irritable bowel syndrome, dysuria, urgency, increased frequency, decreased libido, erectile dysfunction, ejaculation disorders, and anxiety) [15].

The presence of recurrent urinary tract infection and isolation of an etiologically recognized organism (*Escherichia coli*, *Klebsiella* spp., *Proteus mirabilis*, *Enterococcus faecalis* and *Pseudomonas aeruginosa*, *Chlamydia*, and *Mycoplasma*) from prostatic fluid or urine allows the putative diagnosis, once differential diagnosis are excluded. Urine analysis and culture, four-glass urine test, screening for STDs, and prostate-specific antigen dosing in blood are helpful tools for diagnosis. Moreover, imaging studies such as trans-rectal ultrasound, cystoscopy, or prostate MRI can be employed [15].

Treatment of chronic prostatitis aims at treating the causative agent with specific antibiotic treatment and at the relief of pain. Antibiotic therapy with good penetration in prostate tissue, such as quinolones, trimethoprim, macrolides, or doxycycline, should be protracted for 4–6 weeks [16].

Because of its chronic course and the nonspecific symptoms, during the SARS-CoV-2 pandemic many infections went unnoticed, despite the effort of some centers that proposed in-house appointments and telemedicine to avoid losing patients to follow-up [17].

HIV

HIV is the causative agent of acquired immunodeficiency syndrome (AIDS) and causes a gradual development of severe immunodeficiency, being $CD4^+$ T-lymphocytes as its main target.

Clinical manifestations can be divided into those deriving from the damage to the different organs (brain, kidney, gut, and bone marrow) and those from the destruction of immune cells, leading to opportunistic infections caused by a wide array of bacteria and fungi [18].

HIV infection progresses unnoticed before leading to overt AIDS, making screening in asymptomatic patients fundamental. The point-of-care test for HIV is based on serology and detection of HIV antigens, whereas to confirm viral replication and to evaluate the degree of immunodeficiency HIV-RNA and CD4+ cell count are used [19].

The treatment of HIV infection is based on antiretroviral therapy (ART), consisting of a combination of drugs from different classes with activity against replicating enzymes of the virus [20]. Since HIV infection is chronic and cannot be eradicated, ART is a lifelong therapy.

The COVID-19 pandemic posed several challenges to HIV testing, threatening the reach of UNAIDS' 90-90-90 target globally [21]. Moreover, maintaining the continuum of care during the pandemic was challenging, social distancing and isolation hindered ART continuation, and the restriction of hospital visits led to psychological pressure among people living with HIV [22].

In a retrospective cohort study, secondary data from the AIDS Healthcare Foundation Global Quality Program compared records of a number of screening tests from 1 January 2020 to 31 August 2020, with 2019 [23]. The authors observed an overall reduction in all four continents involved of 35.4%. Some countries like Indonesia, Nepal, and Cambodia report an astonishing decrease of 368%, 85%, and 65%, respectively. An overall increase of 9.52% in the percentage of positive tests in all continents was reported, suggesting a potential prioritization of testing among individuals at higher risk or those presenting with overt AIDS-related symptoms. In the near future, facilities should be prepared to face an increase in the number of HIV late presenters due to this delayed access to care.

Viral Hepatitis

HBV and HCV are responsible for chronic infection of the liver. HBV is a DNA virus, whose genome integrates into hepatic cells and causes persistent latent infection: Only 10% of people infected in adulthood develop chronic infection [24], whereas 80–90% of HCV patients (RNA virus) progress to a chronic course [25]. Both viruses are transmitted through contact with infected blood, vertically, or after sexual intercourse (sexual transmission is less efficient for HCV).

Hepatitis can range from an asymptomatic elevation of liver enzymes to a severe form of cirrhosis with liver failure, portal hypertension, and hepatic encephalopathy and could finally cause hepatocellular carcinoma. Moreover, both viruses can be responsible for extrahepatic manifestations such as vasculitis or lymphoma [26, 27].

The diagnosis of chronic HBV infection is based on the persistence of detection of HBV surface antigen (HBsAg) for more than 6 months from acute infection. The presence of HBV-DNA in the blood is a marker of active replication and infectiousness [28]. For HCV, the point-of-care test is the detection of anti-HCV antibodies, whereas the diagnosis is based on the detection of HCV-RNA in blood after 6 months from infection. [29].

The treatment of HBV chronic infection is indicated only in selected patients and can be based either on a 48-week course of subcutaneous interferon or on lifelong administration of oral nucleoside analogs (mainly tenofovir or entecavir), even if the best tool available against HBV is vaccination [28]. For HCV, different and well-tolerated direct antiviral agents are available for oral treatment that lead to a complete cure [29].

The COVID-19 pandemic jeopardized the results of HCV elimination and the WHO goal of HCV eradication by 2030 [30]. A recent study performed in British Columbia assessed the weekly changes in HCV antibodies, HCV-RNA, and genotype testing episodes from January 2008 to December 2020 [31]. The authors demonstrated that, following the imposition of public measures, the average weekly HCV testing and first-time HCV diagnosis rates fell by 62.3 per 100,000 population and by 2.9 episodes per 1,000,000 population, respectively. Although these rates rebounded to near pre-restriction level by December 2020, further assessment will be required to understand the impact of this disruption on the HCV cascade of care. With regard to HBV, the Institute for Health Metrics and Evaluation in Washington showcased a drop in global vaccination coverage in 2020 to levels as low as those seen in the 1990s: Reduced availability and provision of HBV vaccines will have detrimental effects on the incidence of HBV during infancy and childhood, increasing the chances of chronicity in the generation to come [32]. It is therefore fundamental to reactivate the Hepatitis Prevention and Treatment Programs to screen and diagnose viral hepatitis in a timely fashion to provide prompt treatment.

The massive impact that the COVID-19 global pandemic has had on public health infrastructure undermined the prevention and control of communicable diseases such as HIV, viral hepatitis, and STDs. In fact, most of the STD staff have been redeployed to guarantee the COVID-19 public health response [33] and the reduction in diagnostic capability of laboratories leads to a decline in early diagnosis of STDs [34].

A recent survey developed by the WHO European Region reported a decrease of over 50% in testing volume for HIV, HBV, HCV, and STDs during the period March to May 2020 compared to 2019 (Fig. 1) [35].

Unfortunately, women, children, adolescents, and other vulnerable and neglected populations are at higher risk for the detrimental impacts of the COVID-19 "second

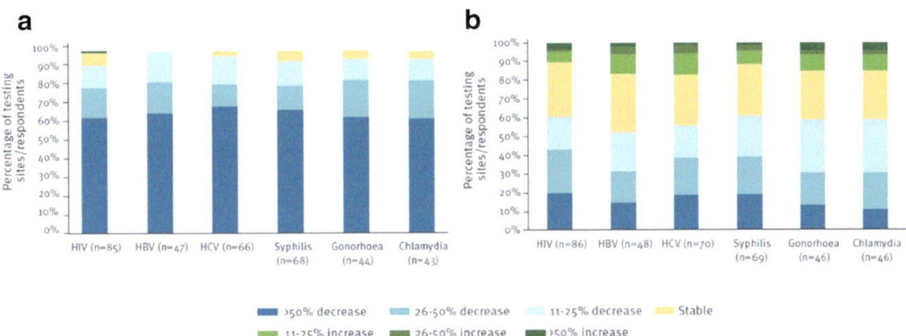

Fig. 1 (**a**) Changes in testing volume, March–May 2020 compared to March to May 2019. (**b**) Changes in testing volume, June–August 2020 compared to March to May 2019. Reproduced from Simoes D, Stengaard AR, Combs L, et al. Impact of the COVID-19 pandemic on testing services for HIV, viral hepatitis and sexually transmitted infections in the WHO European Region, March to August 2020. Eurosurveillance 2020. Reproduced under the terms of the Creative Commons Attribution (CC BY 4.0) Licence

hit" [36]. Therefore, in the coming years, we should expect a rise in HIV late presenters, as well as new HCV and HBV infections and an upsurge in STDs.

The CDC recently published new guidance for STD programs and included recommendations such as the expansion of the use of telehealth and home-based STD testing and stressed the importance of prevention and vaccination to obtain proper control of STDs [37].

The COVID-19 pandemic highlighted the weaknesses of our healthcare system and demonstrated that despite the incredible potential of modern medicine, infectious diseases still represent a serious threat that could be effectively faced only with adequate prevention strategies. In fact, until large-scale SARS-CoV-2 vaccination coverage is not achieved, most of the efforts put in place to halt STDs would be vanished by the persistence of SARS-CoV-2 circulation, especially in resource-limited settings.

References

1. Workowski KA, Bachmann LH, Chan PA, Johnston CM, Muzny CA, Park I, et al. Sexually transmitted infections treatment guidelines, 2021. MMWR Recomm Rep. 2021;70(4):1–187.
2. Guo Y-R, Cao Q-D, Hong Z-S, Tan Y-Y, Chen S-D, Jin H-J, et al. The origin, transmission and clinical therapies on coronavirus disease 2019 (COVID-19) outbreak - an update on the status. Mil Med Res. 2020;7(1):11.
3. World Health Organization. Considerations in adjusting public health and social measures in the context of COVID-19: interim guidance, 16 April 2020. Geneva: World Health Organization; 2020. Report No.: WHO/2019-nCoV/Adjusting_PH_measures/2020.1. Available from https://apps.who.int/iris/handle/10665/331773.
4. Fekadu G, Bekele F, Tolossa T, Fetensa G, Turi E, Getachew M, et al. Impact of COVID-19 pandemic on chronic diseases care follow-up and current perspectives in low resource settings: a narrative review. Int J Physiol Pathophysiol Pharmacol. 2021;13(3):86–93.
5. Li G, Tang D, Song B, Wang C, Qunshan S, Xu C, et al. Impact of the COVID-19 pandemic on partner relationships and sexual and reproductive health: cross-sectional, online survey study. J Med Internet Res. 2020;22(8):e20961.
6. Moi H, Blee K, Horner PJ. Management of non-gonococcal urethritis. BMC Infect Dis. 2015;15(1):294.
7. Scholes D, Satterwhite CL, Yu O, Fine D, Weinstock H, Berman S. Long-term trends in chlamydia trachomatis infections and related outcomes in a US managed care population. Sex Transm Dis. 2012;39(2):81–8.
8. Dombrowski JC, Wierzbicki MR, Newman LM, Powell JA, Miller A, Dithmer D, et al. Doxycycline versus azithromycin for the treatment of rectal chlamydia in men who have sex with men: a randomized controlled trial. Clin Infect Dis. 2021;73(5):824–31. https://doi.org/10.1093/cid/ciab153.
9. de Vries HJ, de Barbeyrac B, de Vrieze NH, Viset JD, White JA, Vall-Mayans M, et al. 2019 European guideline on the management of lymphogranuloma venereum. J Eur Acad Dermatol Venereol. 2019;33(10):1821–8.
10. Curry A, Williams T, Penny ML. Pelvic inflammatory disease: diagnosis, management, and prevention. AFP. 2019;100(6):357–64.
11. Crane MA, Popovic A, Stolbach AI, Ghanem KG. Reporting of sexually transmitted infections during the COVID-19 pandemic. Sex Transm Infect. 2021;97(2):101–2.

12. Johnson KA, Burghardt NO, Tang EC, Long P, Plotzker R, Gilson D, et al. Measuring the impact of the COVID-19 pandemic on sexually transmitted diseases public health surveillance and program operations in the State of California. Sex Transm Dis. 2021;48(8):606–13.

13. Cusini M, Benardon S, Vidoni G, Brignolo L, Veraldi S, Mandolini PL. Trend of main STIs during COVID-19 pandemic in Milan, Italy. Sex Transm Infect. 2021;97(2):99.

14. Krieger JN, Nyberg L, Nickel JC. NIH consensus definition and classification of prostatitis. JAMA. 1999;282(3):236–7.

15. Rees J, Abrahams M, Doble A, Cooper A. Diagnosis and treatment of chronic bacterial prostatitis and chronic prostatitis/chronic pelvic pain syndrome: a consensus guideline. BJU Int. 2015;116(4):509–25.

16. Pirola GM, Verdacchi T, Rosadi S, Annino F, Angelis MD. Chronic prostatitis: current treatment options. RRU. 2019;11:165–74.

17. Boehm K, Ziewers S, Brandt MP, Sparwasser P, Haack M, Willems F, et al. Telemedicine online visits in urology during the COVID-19 pandemic-potential, risk factors, and patients' perspective. Eur Urol. 2020;78(1):16–20.

18. Moylett EH, Shearer WT. HIV: clinical manifestations. J Allergy Clin Immunol. 2002;110(1):3–16.

19. Cornett JK, Kirn TJ. Laboratory diagnosis of HIV in adults: a review of current methods. Clin Infect Dis. 2013;57(5):712–8.

20. NIH. What's new in the guidelines? 2021. Available from https://clinicalinfo.hiv.gov/en/guidelines/adult-and-adolescent-arv/whats-new-guidelines.

21. Joint United Nations Programme on HIV/AIDS (UNAIDS). 90-90-90 an ambitious treatment target to help end the AIDS epidemic [Internet]. 2014. Available from https://www.unaids.org/sites/default/files/media_asset/90-90-90_en.pdf.

22. Jiang H, Zhou Y, Tang W. Maintaining HIV care during the COVID-19 pandemic. Lancet HIV. 2020;7(5):308–9.

23. Rick F, Odoke W, van den Hombergh J, Benzaken AS, Avelino-Silva VI. Impact of coronavirus disease (COVID-19) on HIV testing and care provision across four continents. HIV Med. 2021;23(2):169–77.

24. Tang LSY, Covert E, Wilson E, Kottilil S. Chronic hepatitis B infection: a review. JAMA. 2018;319(17):1802–13.

25. Spearman CW, Dusheiko GM, Hellard M, Sonderup M. Hepatitis C. Lancet. 2019;394(10207):1451–66.

26. Cacoub P, Saadoun D. Extrahepatic manifestations of chronic HCV infection. N Engl J Med. 2021;384(11):1038–52.

27. Virlogeux V, Trépo C. Extrahepatic manifestations of chronic hepatitis B infection. Curr Hepatol Rep. 2018;17(3):156–65.

28. Lampertico P, Agarwal K, Berg T, Buti M, Janssen HLA, Papatheodoridis G, et al. EASL 2017 clinical practice guidelines on the management of hepatitis B virus infection. J Hepatol. 2017;67(2):370–98.

29. Pawlotsky J-M, Negro F, Aghemo A, Berenguer M, Dalgard O, Dusheiko G, et al. EASL recommendations on treatment of hepatitis C 2018. J Hepatol. 2018;69(2):461–511.

30. World Health Organization. Global health sector strategy on viral hepatitis 2016-2021. Towards ending viral hepatitis. Geneva: World Health Organization; 2016. Report No.: WHO/HIV/2016.06. Available from https://apps.who.int/iris/handle/10665/246177.

31. Binka M, Bartlett S, Velásquez García HA, Darvishian M, Jeong D, Adu P, et al. Impact of COVID-19-related public health measures on HCV testing in British Columbia, Canada: an interrupted time series analysis. Liver Int. 2021;41(12):2849–56.

32. Rehman ST, Rehman H, Abid S. Impact of coronavirus disease 2019 on prevention and elimination strategies for hepatitis B and hepatitis C. World J Hepatol. 2021;13(7):781–9.

33. COVID-19 and the state of the STD field |NCSD [Internet]. 2021. Available from https://www.ncsddc.org/resource/covid-19-and-the-state-of-the-std-field/.

34. Guidance and resources during disruption of STD clinical services [Internet]. 2021. Available from https://www.cdc.gov/std/prevention/disruptionGuidance.htm.
35. Simões D, Stengaard AR, Combs L, Raben D. EuroTEST COVID-19 impact assessment consortium of partners. Impact of the COVID-19 pandemic on testing services for HIV, viral hepatitis and sexually transmitted infections in the WHO European Region, March to August 2020. Euro Surveill. 2020;25(47):2001943.
36. Nundy S, Kaur M, Singh P. Preparing for and responding to Covid-19's 'second hit'. Healthc Forum. 2020;8(4):100461.
37. CDC. STI treatment guidelines [Internet]. Centers for Disease Control and Prevention. 2021. Available from https://www.cdc.gov/std/treatment-guidelines/default.htm.

Part XXI
Urology

Male Sexual Pain and Chronic Prostatitis: A New Point of Vision

Giorgio Del Noce and Elena Vittoria Longhi

The male sexual pain in the Diagnostic and Statistical Manual of Mental Disorders Fourth Edition (DSM-IV) has something to do with dyspareunia. However, I can say from experience very few men feel pain during sexual intercourse. The patients that have this kind of pain show organic problems (dermatological, induratio penis, etc.).

In the Diagnostic and Statistical Manual of Mental Disorders Fifth Edition (DSM-5) dyspareunia and vaginismus have been classified as genital/pelvic pain or as a penetration disorder, considering them as disorders only affecting females. This leaves the question that why could not a disorder such as genital pain "sine materia" that is very common among women also affects men. Actually, frequently in medical practice some patients complain of genital pain that cannot be explained by organic causes, while some characteristics could suggest a psychological aetiology [1, 2]. In fact, sexual ailment symptoms are often associated with significant anguish. Frequently, there are alterations in urination, perineum discomfort and sometimes misdiagnosed as chronic prostatitis. Patients with these symptoms often carry out various medical examinations and long and strenuous therapies without seeing significant results. Sometimes, the relationship between the doctor and the patient is affected, which results in the patient referring to other specialists for answers. Male sexual pain usually can begin during adolescence and in some cases can severely affect the quality of life.

The author classifies at least four types of sexual pain disorders.

The first type that occurs quite frequently experiences pain when touched above the testicles and can persist for a lifetime.

Normally, this disorder is discovered during an urological or andrological visit for other motives. The pain is normally described as pain or discomfort by palpation

G. Del Noce (✉)
Promea Institute, Turin, Italy

E. V. Longhi
Department of Sexual Medical Center, San Raffaele Hospital, Milano, Italy

E. V. Longhi (ed.), *Managing Psychosexual Consequences in Chronic Diseases*,
https://doi.org/10.1007/978-3-031-31307-3_38

of the testicles. It rarely occurs spontaneously. Generally, it does not cause serious/ grave suffering for the patient, who normally has a regular life, also sexually and considers this hypersensibility only as a characteristic of their body. It is often correlated with a positive medical history of surgical operations such as hypospadias and cryptorchidism and/or frequent genital medical examinations at paediatric age. It could perhaps be considered a defensive reaction to what we could consider a kind of sexual abuse for the child. The pain sometimes only occurs when the palpation is conducted by foreign hands and not by the subject himself. Normally, treatments are not required as the patient is able to live without problems whilst being affected by this disorder. In some cases, it can be useful to explain to the patient the probable causes of the disorder that increases awareness of possible psychological factors.

The second type may be quite related to penodynia. Also, in this case the pain is discovered occasionally following an andrological visit. The patient normally shows discomfort especially when the glans is uncovered, which is almost never performed. The patient does not always experience pain, but very often feels discomfort or other unpleasant sensations. Often, the patient is informed by the doctor that their poor hygiene has caused these symptoms. This humiliation sometimes does not assist the patient. In not all cases, phimosis is present. Sometimes, there is only a long prepuce. The symptoms could be defined as a true case of allodynia. The affected patients are able to have sexual intercourse and curiously during sexual intercourse very few symptoms occur. During sexological consultations, often the patient presents signs of conflict with their genitalia.

In these patients, premature ejaculation is frequent. These patients usually have an andrological examination with the intention of circumcision, which usually has a long postoperative recovery period.

The third type may be compared to a very true case of vaginismus. The patient cannot even tolerate any contact near the penis and make the same actions and movements as a vaginismus female. Due to this, the patients are unable to have sexual intercourse. The causes of these symptoms are usually associated with significant psychological distress, but fortunately the third type is quite rare.

The fourth and final type may be defined as a real case of male dyspareunia. The patients experience pain in the pelvic–perineum region during sexual intercourse and especially during ejaculation. They are characterised by alterations to penile and perineal sensibility, with the feeling of hypogastric weight. Often, it is found that there is an erectile dysfunction present. Normally, symptoms of overactive bladder are also present, and due to this, it is often diagnosed as prostatitis, even if in reality no organic treatment/therapy is effective. In fact, if we analyse the symptoms of nonbacterial chronic prostatitis we can often find patients that fit into this category. However, some characteristics are identifiable in the patient's medical history. First of all, they often feel a sense of anguish and sometimes panic. In fact, frequently these patients go to the emergency department, even if their symptoms are vague. There is an absolute discordance between the extent of the modest symptoms and the suffering of the patients that often lasts for many years despite the countless amount of medical examinations and attempted treatments. Frequently, the patients suffering from this disorder are comparable to somatisation (gastritis, colitis, intolerances and dermatologic diseases). The physician that sees patients with this type of disorder usually finds that they have a file with an extensive medical history of examinations and previous medical visits. The physician tends to confirm a diagnosis of prostatitis and add other medical visits or examinations to the patient's file. The patient–doctor relationship then becomes conflicting, and assisting the patient to find a permanent medical solution becomes difficult as the patient is satisfied with temporary improvements.

Treatment

Normally, all the patients suffering from genital pain undergo an andrological or urological visit without considering the problem from a psychological aspect. In the first and second types, generally a treatment is not necessary. The patients suffering from penodynia should be carefully considered, since in some cases general counselling allows for a psychological problem to be highlighted, which, however, is not always necessary to cure. When carrying out a circumcision in a case of phimosis, it is necessary to take into account that the post-operative progress is not good. The circumcision that normally would be carried out using local anaesthetic, in some cases requires the use of an additional sedative, due to the fact that the patient transforms tactile sensibility into pain. Circumcision is normally able to vanish the symptoms, but generally does not assist with the patients' psychological problems even if sometimes the patients' need/want for surgery is unconsciously born from the will to overcome their sexual difficulty.

In the third type of counselling, the patient is important, also to clarify that even if a circumcision operation is undertaken, it would not resolve the problem. Generally, circumcision is carried out in a deep state of narcosis. However, postoperative progress is absolutely more complex. Unfortunately, the patient typically has many expectations about the results of the surgery, which usually turn out to be disappointing, since subsequently the emergence that the cause of the sexual disorder is due to psychological reasons can convert and develop into other disorders, which continue to prevent normal sexuality. It is useful for the patient to be accompanied by psychological/psychiatric support, but it is an extremely difficult path and simply sanding the patient to a psychological consultation is generally not effective. It is important that the andrologist offers the first psychological support.

The fourth type of disorder affects a significant number of patients, and the symptoms presented in the clinic are extremely variable. Consequently, treating these patients is difficult, and when treating, it is necessary to use an integrated approach. From an aspect, it is necessary to maintain contact with the body, and medical examinations are useful to exclude the presence of associated diseases. Medical treatment can also be useful to reduce symptoms related to this disorder. A treatment that can be very efficient in reducing symptoms is anti-depressant medication. However, this treatment is often rejected by the patient, and sometimes, unconsciously he shows unbearable side effects. In fact, it is necessary to try to help the patient be aware that the disorder could originate from psychological reasons. However, it should never be said that the patient does not have a medical issue, because the pain felt is real, but doubt could be established. For example, the anguish and anxiety that patients feel are not caused by symptoms, but that they are symptoms and are caused by psychological malaise. The effectiveness of this approach depends on the time that these symptoms began to exist. If the disorder has been present in the patient for a significant period of time, it is quite unlikely that the patient can be easily healed. It is not said that healing means the disappearance of symptoms, but with this type of disorder, often it is enough to inform the patient to be aware of the psychological aetiology of the disorder. We must take into account that the use of some pharmaceutical antidepressants can interfere with sexual activity. On the other hand, the result is excellent in the case of premature ejaculation. From a perspective of multidisciplinary and integrated methodology, the patients were treated with drugs and/or with sexual therapy according to the integrated Kaplan method and/or with techniques for the rehabilitation of the pelvic floor. In particular, the use of TENS (transcutaneous electrical nerve stimulation) is highly effective for its antalgic effects. In fact, it allows a significant relaxation of the pelvic floor and locally stimulates the production of endorphins. The method is very effective in controlling hyper-contraction on the perineal floor, even present among patients affected by the 4th type of disorder. In fact, frequently patients with this disorder suffer also from anal problems that interfere with defecation. The tension of the perineum is often the cause of the pain. The therapy has to be evaluated case by case, and rigid protocols are not so easily applicable.

Clinical Case of the First Type

A 17-year-old patient comes with his mother for an andrological consultation for an issue of bilateral testicular pain. The teenager has suffered from a late drop of the testicles. The patient tenses while being examined and pushes away the hands of the physician, which makes it difficult to palpate the testicles as the patient is defensive as says to be suffering from pain. The physician understands the situation and subtlety addresses the mother to closely observe the next part of the examination. From a distance, the physician asks the teenager to palpate the testicles himself. This is done so without any problems as the patient is able to touch both of his testicles without feeling pain. The mother remained astonished, and the physician began to explain the possible reasons behind the symptoms that it is likely the teenager became hypersensitive resulting from frequent medical visits during infancy and reassured the mother of the low extent of the problem.

Clinical Case of the Second Type

A 28-year-old patient was referred to see an andrologist by a sexual psychologist. The patient was having difficulty in sexual relations resulting from premature ejaculation. The examinations conducted by the physician showed hematochemical examinations to be regular, with no reference to any particular disorder. The examination objectively showed no signs of illness, but as soon as the physician began to examine to penis and the glans, the patient began to suffer and asked the physician to cease the examination. The glans were examined in a regular manner, but the very act of examining the penis provoked significant suffering to the patient, which confirmed high sensitivity. The physician then asked the patient to try and find the glans himself. The man says he is able to do it often without problems. However, it was noticed that he did not seem to understand what to do. When asked if he was able to expose the glans during an erection, the man affirmed not to know it and to have never done it. There was no evidence of pain during masturbation, nor during sexual activity. The patient did not desire a circumcision, and the physician encouraged him to conduct exercises exposing the glans. After talking with the sexual psychologist, it became evident that the patient has a conflicting relationship with sex.

Clinical Case of the Third Type

A 23-year-old patient consulted for a circumcision. Even if the patient did not have a true case of phimosis, it was almost impossible for the physician to touch the glans during the examination. In fact, the patient even before being touched reacted by pushing away the hand of the physician because of the pain felt in view of the physical contact (anticipatory pain); however, the patient did not show emotions (alexithymia) and this characteristic is quite frequent in these cases. The mother of this patient also gave insight that even from an infant age, this man did not like being caressed or touched in an affectionate way. The patient reports to have never had sexual intercourse, nor relations in an affectionate way. In fact, he stated that with this problem it would be unthinkable to have an intimate relationship, and for this reason has submitted to have treatment, and a circumcision with the hope that it would resolve all his problems. The postoperative recovery resulted in being very complex, with countless check-up visits. In the end, the patient declared to be satisfied with the result. A year later after the operation, the patient continued to not have intimate relations and the physician gave its full availability to help him.

Clinical Case of the Fourth Type

A 30-year-old patient came for a urological examination complaining of ejaculation pain for the last 13 years. The man is married with two children and has a good relationship with his wife. The patient presented a file of medical history with numerous ultrasound scans and cultural examinations. The man had been given various antibiotic treatments over the years, for chronic prostatitis. This diagnosis was confirmed with testing that found the presence of prostate calcifications. Throughout the consultation, various behaviours and comments made by the patient ("I feel pain with only the thought of ejaculation") drove the urologist to ask open questions. The physician realised that this patient liked to talk and by the end of the consultation came close to the desk and revealed a fact that he had always hidden from everyone: when he was 17 years old, he was subjected to violent sexual abuse by two people. The patient had let out a wealth of detail about the episode to the physician, and at the end of the consultation, he asked: "Do you think that this could be the cause of my disorder?" Actually, the patient is in psychological therapy and has obtained promising results through the rehabilitation of the pelvic floor.

Second Clinical Case of the Fourth Type

A 31-year-old patient came for an andrological consultation for an arousal and erectile sexual disorder with constant ejaculatory pain. In previous examinations, the patient was diagnosed with chronic prostatitis and had used various medications as treatment, without seeing any significant improvement. He presented many recurring somatic symptoms and others often changing. In the past 3 years, he had carried out almost 20 blood tests for hematochemical examinations, 15 cultural tests of semen, urine and faeces, an electromyography and a gastric biopsy. He was visited by many specialists: an ophthalmologist, a dermatologist, a neurologist, a gastroenterologist, an allergist, an immunologist, a rheumatologist, a stomatologist, a nephrologist, and he had also been to an immunopathological and rare disease centre. The andrologist tried to direct the patient towards a colleague who is both sexologist and psychiatrist, and after a difficult initial approach, it was understood that the patient had not accepted the investigation of his problem despite it being evident that he suffered from severe depression. The patient interrupted and left the consultation to visit a different andrologist/urologist.

Discussion and Conclusion

If we search vulvodynia on the Internet, we can find around 500,000 items, but if we look penodynia up we can find only 519 items, which are above all due to dermatologic causes. If you search penodynia in PubMed you can find only two articles [1, 3] (1200 for vulvodynia). In reality, in surgical andrological activities, male genital sine materia pains are very often referred and emphasised. In the DSM-5, the described patients could be placed in the category of somatic symptom and related disorders, but we do not think it is the link with male genitalia that characterises these patients. Chronic pain is highly linked with anxiety and depression [2, 4–6]. It is often associated with substantial financial, occupational, psychological and social burdens. However, if the chronic pain involves the genitals, it is more likely to be related to relational and/or intrapsychic factors. In publications and literature studies, we can find very few articles that treat male genital pain with symptoms of psychological suffering. Yet, among normal general day-to-day consultations cases similar to those described in this article are frequent [7, 8]. Unfortunately, medical culture lacks a holistic vision of the patient and between psychiatric/psychological and medicine there is not an integrated approach. The patients are usually only referred to a psychiatrist when the illness is at a severe level and sometimes irreversible. This does not happen in other specialties where a consultation is requested, even if it is only precautional. It is now accepted that a psychological disorder such as depression can provoke and cause physical symptoms and annoyance to patients, and surely, a precocious treatment of the disorder can help to achieve the best results [9–13]. Finally, I think that, up to now, male sexual pain has been studied in a superficial way and that there are many aspects that need to be further investigated and reported.

Sexuality and Quality of Life

A study by Emiliano Screponi et al. [14] linked the pathology of chronic prostatitis with ejaculation disorder. Although the aetiology of premature ejaculation is commonly thought to be psychological, organic causes must be ruled out before therapy can begin. Among pathological causes, major neurological disorders (multiple sclerosis, spina bifida and spinal cord tumour) are rare. On the other hand, penile hypersensitivity and reflex hyperexcitability have been investigated in several studies [15] using the penile biothesiometer or genital somatosensory-evoked potentials, which have shown that these conditions could be important factors contributing to premature ejaculation. **Another important organic cause is** prostatitis [16]. E. Screponi's study evaluated segmented urine samples before and after prostate massage and prostate secretion samples in 46 patients reporting premature ejaculation and 30 control patients by bacteriological localisation studies. The incidence of premature ejaculation in subjects with chronic prostatitis was also evaluated. Results. Prostate inflammation was found in 56.5% and chronic bacterial prostatitis in 47.8% of the subjects with premature ejaculation. When compared with controls, these new findings were statistically significant ($P < 0.05$).

A similar investigation was carried out by Rany Shauloul et al. [17]: a total of 153 heterosexual men aged 29–51 years with premature ejaculation and another 100 healthy male subjects were included as a control group. Sequential microbiological samples were obtained according to the standardised protocol of Meares and Stamey. Nonbacterial prostatitis was defined by evidence of prostatic inflammation but negative urine and prostatic fluid cultures in men with various genitourinary symptoms. Results: there was no significant difference between patients and control subjects with regard to age, education or frequency of intercourse. Prostatic inflammation was found in 64% and chronic bacterial prostatitis in 52% of patients with premature ejaculation, respectively, showing statistical significance compared to control subjects ($P < 0.05$).

Again, the survey by Smith KB et al. [18] compared the sexual and relational functioning of 38 male patients with chronic prostatitis/chronic pelvic pain syndrome (CP/CPPS) and their partners with a control group of 37 couples.

Compared to control males, men with CP/CPPS reported significantly greater sexual dysfunction and symptoms of depression. In addition, symptoms of depression mediated the relationship between some aspects of sexual function. However, men with CP/CPPS did not report a significant decrease in sexual satisfaction or relationship functioning compared to the control group. Partners of CP/CPPS patients reported significantly more pain during intercourse, vaginismus and depressive symptoms than partners of control couples. Furthermore, CP/CPPS patients and their partners did not differ significantly in sexual functioning and satisfaction, relationship functioning and symptoms of depression. The sexual functioning of the patient significantly predicted the sexual functioning of the female partner. This study was the first to evaluate partners of men with CP/CPPS. Patients and partners in this study reported lower levels of sexual functioning in some domains, but were comparable to control couples on measures of relationship satisfaction and functioning.

Is it possible to assess the association between sexuality/sexual orientation and chronic bacterial prostatitis?

Konstantinos Stamatiou et al. [19] investigated this with 389 patients (retrospectively 1783 visits from 2009 to 2019) by reviewing clinical notes of visits and routine follow-ups. The mean age was 45.5 years. According to their report, 92.28% were heterosexual, 6.16% homosexual and 1.54% bisexual.

Regarding sexuality, 26.6% reported multiple sexual unions, while 73.4% reported single sexual unions. There was a statistically significant association between chronic bacterial prostatitis as an initial diagnosis and having multiple sexual relationships. In contrast, the association between CBP and sexual orientation was not statistically significant. Similarly, no significant association was established between treatment outcome and having multiple sexual partners. This suggests that the connection between sexual practices and the onset of CBP should be further investigated in order to reach scientific conclusions.

We must not exclude the pathogenic sphere. Dino Papes et al. [20] conducted a prospective observational study at the University Hospital for Infectious Diseases "Dr Fran Mihaljevic", Zagreb, Croatia, from 2012 to 2015. A total of 254 patients who had been diagnosed with CP/CPPS in other institutions were enrolled. The diagnosis was based on history, NIH-CPSI, clinical examination and two- or four-glass testing according to guidelines, with the exclusion of other causes of pelvic pain [21].

All patients had pelvic pain for at least three months and complained of lower urinary tract symptoms. Urethral swabs and standard four-glass Meares–Stamey tests were performed. Patients provided standard first-emptying VB1 and midstream VB2 samples. After 2 min of prostate massage, expressed prostatic secretions (EPS) were collected. Finally, all patients provided a post-massage urine sample (VB3). If EPS could not be obtained, only VB3 was analysed. Patients who were not diagnosed according to current guidelines were taking antibiotics or had positive urethral swab, and VB1 and VB2 cultures were excluded.

Quantitative segmented cultures and bacterial identification and the number of leucocytes were determined in the emptied urine samples and EPS in the microbiology laboratory. The samples were cultured on a solid medium. Microbial growth was assessed after 24 and 48 h. Pathogens were identified by biochemical/serological techniques.

C. trachomatis was detected by PCR (Abbott real-time PCR, Abbott Molecular Diagnostics, USA); Mycoplasma genitalium and Ureaplasma urealyticum by semiquantitative culture and Mycoplasma duo and SIR (Mycoplasma test, Bio-Rad Laboratories) antimicrobial susceptibility testing; and T. vaginalis by additional culture on modified diamond medium. All patients were treated with antibiotics (doxycycline, azithromycin, metronidazole) according to the agent isolated. (Statistical analysis was performed using MedCalc for Windows, version 16.0—MedCalc Software, Belgium).

Results: the median age of patients was 41.4 years (IQR: 33–50, range: 24–62). The median duration of symptoms was six months (IQR: 5–8, range: 3–18). The median NIH-CPSI score was 19 (IQR: 7–22, range: 13–41). The median leucocyte count in EPS/VB3 was 5 (IQR: 3–8, range: 0–35). Of 254 patients, 30 had positive urethral swabs and VB1 or VB2 cultures. EPS or VB3 cultures were contaminated in seven patients. Of the remaining 217 patients, EPS was obtained in 85 (39.2%) and VB3 alone was tested in the remaining 132 (60.8%) patients. There were 35/217 positive cultures (16.1%): 16 EPS+VB3 cultures and 19 VB3 cultures in the group in which no EPS was obtained. A total of 22/217 (10.1%) cultures were positive for sexually transmitted diseases. There was no contamination of those EPS and VB3 cultures. All PCRs for *C. trachomatis* were negative.

There is no doubt that the dual diagnosis of andrology and sexology must contribute to the definition of the diagnosis and the personalised sexological therapeutic and rehabilitation model.

The review of medical records seems to confirm this comparative approach [22].

The study by Magri et al. [22] included 285 patients with chronic prostatitis and erectile dysfunction (ED).

The medical records of patients who were first diagnosed with PC in a specialist first-level urological outpatient clinic were reviewed.

The frequency of ED was higher among subjects who showed higher total scores on the two questionnaires administered, namely the NIH-Chronic Prostatitis Symptoms Index (NIH-CPSI) and the International Prostate Symptoms Score (IPSS). No significant relationship emerged between the frequency of ED and the differential classification of prostatitis into Cat. II chronic bacterial prostatitis or Cat. III CP/chronic pelvic pain syndrome. The presence of haemospermia and premature ejaculation was associated with an approximately fourfold increased risk of erectile dysfunction.

In contrast: the study conducted by Chung et al. [23] reported a high prevalence of erectile dysfunction (ED) among patients with chronic prostatitis/chronic pelvic pain syndrome (CP/CPPS). The prevalence of ED ranged from 15.0 to 40.5% in men in China with CP/CPPS; however, previous studies focusing on the prevalence of ED among patients with CP/CPPS have all neglected to explore the extent of this association.

To examine the association between erectile dysfunction (ED) and a previous diagnosis of chronic prostatitis/chronic pelvic pain syndrome (CP/CPPS) using a population-based dataset, a total of 3194 males, aged $\geq$18 years when first diagnosed with ED, were identified, and 15,970 controls were randomly selected. In total, 667 (3.5%) of the 19,164 subjects sampled had been diagnosed with CP/CPPS before the index date; CP/CPPS was found in 276 (8.6%) cases and in 391 (2.5%) controls ($P < 0.001$). Analysis indicated that cases were more likely to have previous CP/CPPS after adjustment for patient's monthly income, geographic location and level of urbanisation and hypertension, diabetes, coronary artery disease, kidney disease, obesity and alcohol abuse/addiction syndrome status, compared to controls.

Conclusion

The National Institutes of Health (NIH) has redefined prostatitis into four distinct entities.

Category I is acute bacterial prostatitis. It is an acute prostatic infection with a uropathogen, often with systemic symptoms of fever, chills and hypotension. Treatment is based on antimicrobials and bladder drainage because the inflamed prostate can block urinary flow.

Category II prostatitis is called chronic bacterial prostatitis. It is characterised by recurrent episodes of documented urinary tract infections with the same uropathogen and causes pelvic pain, urinary symptoms and ejaculatory pain. It is diagnosed by localisation cultures that are 90% accurate in locating the source of recurrent infections within the lower urinary tract. Asymptomatic inflammatory prostatitis comprises NIH category IV. This entity is, by definition, asymptomatic and is often diagnosed incidentally during the evaluation of infertility or prostate cancer.

The clinical significance of category IV prostatitis is not known and it is often left untreated.

Category III prostatitis is called chronic prostatitis/chronic pelvic pain syndrome (CP/CPPS). It is characterised by pelvic pain for more than three of the preceding 6 months, urinary symptoms and painful ejaculation, without documented urinary tract infections by uropathogens. The syndrome can be devastating, affecting 10–15% of the male population and causing nearly 2 million outpatient visits each year [23].

References

1. Dauendorffer JN, Renaud-Vilmer C, Cavelier-Balloy B. Diagnosis and management of penodynia. Ann Dermatol Venereol. 2014;14:383–6.
2. Schover LR. Psychological factors in men with genital pain. Cleve Clin J Med. 1990;57:697–700.

3. Dauendorffer JN, Renaud-Vilmer C, Bagot M, Cavelier-Balloy B. Circumcision-induced penodynia. Ann Dermatol Venereol. 2012;139:566–7.
4. Bair MJ, Robinson RL, Katon W, Kroenke K. Depression and pain comorbidity: a literature review. Arch Intern Med. 2003;163:2433–45.
5. Verdu B, Decosterd I, Buclin T, Stiefel F, Berney A. Antidepressants for the treatment of chronic pain. Drugs. 2008;68:2611–32.
6. Hosthota A, Bondade S, Monnappa D, Basavaraja V. Penodynia and depression. Dermatol Online. 2016;2:240–1.
7. Guy A, Bronselaer JM, Schober HFL, Meyer-Bahlburg GT, Vlietinck R, Hoebeke PB. Male circumcision decreases penile sensitivity as measured in a large cohort. Br J Urol Int. 2013;111:820–7.
8. Morris BJ, Krieger JN. Does male circumcision affect sexual function, sensitivity or satisfaction? A systematic review. J Sex Med. 2012;10:2644–57.
9. Katz J, Rosenbloom BN, Fashler S. Chronic pain, psychopathology, and DSM-5 somatic symptom disorder. Can J Psychiatr. 2015;60(4):160–7.
10. Naim M, Ende D. A new approach to the treatment of non-specific male genital pain. Br J Urol Int. 2011;107(suppl 3):34–7.
11. Nickel JC, Mullins C, Tripp DA. Development of an evidence-based cognitive behavioral treatment program for men with chronic prostatitis/chronic pelvic pain syndrome. World J Urol. 2008;26:167–72.
12. Delavierre D, Rigaud J, Sibert L, Labat J-J. Approche symptomatique des douleurs péniennes chroniques. Prog Urol. 2010;20:958–61.
13. La coppia: Nuove realtà, nuovi valori, nuovi problem, Franco Angeli ed, 1: 255.
14. Screponi E, Carosa E, di Stasi SM, Pepe M, Carruba G, Jannini EA. Prevalence of chronic prostatitis in men with premature ejaculation. Urology. 2001;58(2):198–202.
15. Colpi GM, Fanciullacci F, Beretta S, et al. Sacral potentials evoked in subjects with true premature ejaculation. Andrology. 1986;18:583–6.
16. Stanley E. Eiaculazione precoce. BMJ. 1981;282:1521–2.
17. Shamloul R, Nashaar A. Chronic prostatitis in premature ejaculation: a cohort study of 153 men. J Sex Med. 2006;3:150–4.
18. Smith KB, Pukall CF, Tripp DA, et al. Sexual and relationship functioning in men with chronic prostatitis/chronic pelvic pain syndrome and their partners. Arch Sex Behav. 2007;36:301–11.
19. Stamatiou K, Samara E, Perletti G. Sexuality, sexual orientation and chronic prostatitis. J Sex Marital Ther. 2021;47(3):281–4. https://doi.org/10.1080/0092623X.2020.1871142.
20. Meares EM, Stamey TA. Bacteriological localization models in the bacterial prostate and urethritis. Investig Urol. 1968;5:492–518.
21. Magistro G, Wagenlehner FM, Grabe M. Contemporary management of chronic prostatitis syndrome/chronic pelvic pain. Eur Urol. 2016;69:286–97.
22. Magri V, Perletti G, Montanari E, et al. Chronic prostatitis and erectile dysfunction: results of a cross-sectional study. Ital Arch Urol Androl. 2008;80(4):172–5. PMID: 19235435.
23. Murphy AB, Macejko A, Taylor A, et al. Prostatite cronica. Droghe. 2009;69:71–84. https://doi.org/10.2165/00003495-200969010-00005.

Benign Prostatic Hypertrophy

Marco Giandotti and Elena Vittoria Longhi

Introduction

Benign prostatic hypertrophy is a very common anatomic–pathological condition of men after 45 years of age. It is estimated that around 50% of men who have reached the age of 50 are affected, while in the over-seventies, according to different studies, it reaches over 75–80%. Histologically, it is a fibroadenoma that originates, for reasons not yet clarified, from the peri-urethral transitional component of the prostate gland. This condition is not in itself to be considered a clinically relevant pathology except when, as frequently happens, it becomes a cause of bladder outflow obstruction (BOO). In this case, the diagnostic classification and treatment become extremely important, not only to alleviate any related symptoms, but above all in order to avoid complications still too often recurrent today as we will see later, such as recurrent urinary tract infections, the renal failure and acute urinary retention (AUR).

Main Medical Characteristics

There is no strict correlation between BPH and cervico-urethral obstruction. Not all patients with prostate adenomas have a clinically relevant obstruction, therefore as patients obstructed, even markedly, without a significant BPH being detectable, as, for example, in the case of bladder neck sclerosis. The extent of the BPH is absolutely not correlated with the degree of obstruction, in the sense that the prostate is

M. Giandotti (✉)
Urology and Oncology Unit, Pio XI Institute, Rome, Italy

E. V. Longhi
Department of Sexual Medical Center, San Raffaele Hospital, Milano, Italy

© Springer Nature Switzerland AG 2023

491

E. V. Longhi (ed.), *Managing Psychosexual Consequences in Chronic Diseases*,
https://doi.org/10.1007/978-3-031-31307-3_39

particularly voluminous, and it can be much less obstructive than the prostate with adenomas of a few grams. This depends on several factors, first of all the pathological conformation that the hypertrophic prostate takes; in particular, the development of a median lobe according to a real cork wedged in the urethra, as well as a predominantly sub-cervical development, limits the 'drawing' of the bladder neck during the voiding phase. Another factor that probably plays an essential role in the interpretation of dynamic voiding correction is the prevalence of fibrotic or calcific tissue in the glandular context, which, leading to greater rigidity, hinders the opening of the prostatic urethra.

The symptomatology of BOO is scholastically divided into two types: filling phase disorders and emptying phase disorders. The former include frequency, nocturia, urgency and urge incontinence; the second part of the inheritance, the weak and discontinuous, the delayed drops and the feeling of incomplete bladder emptying sometimes involves the use of the abdominal press to facilitate urination. In reality, this classification does not have a pure schematic value, since the symptoms of the first group are always associated with a difficult voiding bladder, while the other symptoms can also imply different pathologies, such as inflammatory states, neoplastic pathologies of the bladder and neurophysiological vescical sphincter alterations. In these cases, a careful differential diagnosis is of fundamental importance, as we will see later.

It is important to underline that there are patients in obstructive conditions that are also very marked, but paucisymptomatic. They are very insidious forms, and they are those that often lead to acute urinary retention whose temporary resolution requires the urgent insertion of a bladder catheter. We rarely encounter patients, strongly obstructed, who do not have any of the irritative symptoms, but simply a hypovalid stream, sometimes discontinuous, which moreover is often not spontaneously reported by the patient, as it is considered 'normal for age', that is not important and certainly less troublesome than the nocturia, the urgency, etc.; although the reason for these different clinical presentations of the BOO is still unclear, the fact remains that these patients, in particular, are more likely to experience detrimental detrusor underactivity and dangerous bladder overdistension or the AUR.

The complications of the BOO obstruction include urinary tract infections, often linked to the accumulation of urine in the bladder, and urinary insufficiency linked to high pressures that occur in the lower urinary tract in patients with important post-voiding residue and which constitute an impediment to the outflow of urine from the kidneys. The formation of bladder diverticula and bladder stones is also worth mentioning.

Main Tools for the Diagnosis

The diagnosis of benign prostatic hypertrophy is very easy. Often, a simple digitorectal exploration is sufficient to detect a homogeneous enlargement of the gland, which stands for the presence of a prostate adenoma; an ultrasound examination confirms the diagnosis, but as previously explained, the most important thing to define is the degree of any BOO that is determined. The treatment is in fact aimed primarily at solving the present obstructive condition and contextually the related symptomatology. Thus, in support of the anamnesis and digitorectal exploration, we can use simple investigations, such as IPSS or other questionnaires that assign a score to the symptoms, the voiding diary, laboratory tests (urine test, PSA and creatininemia) and uroflowmetry, which allows to directly appreciate the stream, supra-pubic vesico-prostatic ultrasonography that indicates the thickness of the bladder wall, the coexistence of any complications such as the presence of diverticula or bladder stones, the amount of the post-voiding residual urine, approximately calculating the prostate volume and evaluating the presence of median lobe or other anatomical conditions that may represent an obstacle to bladder emptying; in addition, in the context of differential diagnosis, it allows us to exclude bladder formation, inflammatory conditions of the prostate and prostatic neoplasms.

Second-level diagnostic investigations are trans-rectal ultrasound, dynamic examination, cystoscopy or imaging techniques, especially in the case of differential diagnosis. While the first is aimed at anatomically defining the diagnosis, the others are mainly aimed at the differential diagnosis and urodynamic examination against the overactive bladder, a symptomatic picture that is confused or often integrated with BOO and the other towards other obstructive conditions or neoplastic pathologies.

Main Non-Surgical Treatments

We have different categories of drugs for the treatment of BPH, such as follows:

- Phytotherapeutics
- Alfa-blockers
- 5-alpha-reductase inhibitors
- Anticholinergics
- Beta-3 agonists

Among the phytotherapics, we mainly remember the Serenoa repens, which is indicated above all as a decongestant of the prostate gland and therefore has a role, often in association with other drugs, especially towards the improvement of symptoms; the alphalithycs have an action aimed at relaxing the muscular component of the bladder neck and the prostate gland in order to allow a greater opening of the cervico-urethral area and reduce resistance to bladder emptying; among these, we mention alfuzosin, doxazosin, terazosin, tamsulosin and the more recent silodosin that distinguish among them for the always increasing selectivity for the alpha-1 receptors mostly represented at the level of the prostatic urethra, thus supporting a greater efficacy and the reduction in side effects, especially with regard to the cardiovascular system. The 5-alpha-reductase inhibitors, finasteride and dutasteride, act instead hindering the enzyme that determines the transformation of testosterone into its active form, dihydrotestosterone, causing a slowing down of prostatic growth and the consequent reduction in the gland volume up to 30%.

Anticholinergics, including oxybutynin, tolterodine and solifenacin, and beta-3-agonists, mirabregon, are used for treatment, alone or in association with alpha-lithic if a picture is present at the same time obstructive, due to voiding disorders, characteristic of detrusor overactivity.

Other drugs may find use in cases of complications related to incomplete bladder emptying, such as antibiotics for the treatment of infectious complications.

Main Surgical Treatment

When medical therapy is ineffective or the degree of cervico-urethral obstruction is very marked, surgical treatment is found. Based on the European guidelines, the indications are as follows:

- Marked reduction in flowmetric indices
- Pathological post-voiding residue
- Refractory obstruction against medical therapy
- Symptomatic obstruction and intolerance to medical therapy
- Obstruction with renal failure
- Acute or chronic urinary retention
- Complicated obstruction

Today, we have a wide variety of surgical techniques available, which are mainly indicated based on the size of the adenoma, but also based on any patient comorbidity, technical availability and costs.

Undoubtedly, the most widely used surgical treatment is definitely TURP, transurethral resection of the prostate, monopolar or bipolar. The use of bipolar electrical energy has made it possible to extend the surgical indications also to the treatment of very large adenomas, both for the greater speed that the technique allows and for the reduced risk of TUR syndromes.

The alternatives for particularly voluminous prostates are trans-bladder adenomectomy, which is progressively losing ground to more innovative and less invasive methods, such as laser enucleation (in Olmio or Tullio) and laparoscopic or robotic adenomectomy.

The interventions that use the laser are multiple and vary between them for the source that is used (NTP, thulium, holmium etc.) and based on the modalities with which the intervention takes place: vaporisation, vaporesection and enucleation. The vaporisation is indicated for the treatment of small prostates in patients with anticoagulant therapy that cannot be suspended. The laser treatment that is becoming more widespread due to its effectiveness, lack of side effects and indication on prostates of almost unlimited size is HOLEP, which is enucleation by holmium laser.

Less invasive techniques, but still not widely used in current surgical practice, are as follows:

- Temporary implantation nitinol device (TIND), which unlike simple urethral stents has the purpose of producing a necrosis of adenomatous tissue.
- UroLift, which is the implantation of small anchors in the adenomatous tissue.
- AquaBeam, which uses the pressure of a jet of water to remove the tissue on the guide of ultrasound images.
- Embolisation of the prostatic artery, which obviously produces prostate tissue necrosis.
- Rezum, which instead uses the thermal energy of steam producing a colliquative necrosis.

In contrast with other minimally invasive procedures that utilise conductive heat transfer, such as transurethral needle ablation or transurethral microwave therapy (TUMT).

Sexuality and Quality of Life

Numerous studies have shown an association between the use of finasteride and the occurrence of sexual dysfunction and depressive syndrome, which may persist after discontinuation of the drug (post-finasteride syndrome). Reduced levels of DHT and neuroactive 5AR metabolites in CNS areas crucial to sexual activity and mood seem to be responsible for the syndrome.

The official website www.pfsfoundation.org/ defines post-finasteride syndrome (PFS) as 'a clinical condition characterised by the persistence of sexual, neurological and physical side effects after drug withdrawal in patients who have taken finasteride, a type II 5-alpha-reductase inhibitor, for alopecia or prostatic hypertrophy'.

The symptoms are as follows:

- Sexual Symptoms: reduction in the size of the penis and testicular volume and reduction in seminal fluid quantity.
- Systemic Physical Symptoms: gynaecomastia, chronic asthenia, muscular hypertrophy, dry skin and increase in body weight and fat mass; on a biochemical level, reduction in HDL total cholesterol and increase in triglycerides.
- Neurological Symptoms: reduction in memory, slowing of cognitive processes, depression, anxiety and insomnia.

Numerous studies have shown an increase in sexual dysfunction (DS) when taking 5ARI in patients with BPH and lower urinary tract symptoms (LUTS), which are in themselves an important risk factor for DS, and in healthy young men with androgenetic alopecia. In particular, these subjects complain of hypoactive sexual desire at a rate varying between 1.5 and 10%; erectile temperature between 0.75 and 15.8%; and orgasmic difficulties or reduction in seminal volume between 0 and 7.7% [1].

Based on these data, the Medicines and Healthcare Products Regulatory Agency of the UK and the Swedish Medical Products Agency revised the patient information leaflet to include the concept of 'persistence of erectile dysfunction (ED) after discontinuation of treatment'. [2]

To confirm this, a retrospective study conducted by Irwig et al. [3] evaluated 71 patients treated with finasteride for alopecia (age: 21–46 years; mean duration of treatment: 28 months), with normal pre-therapy sexual function, but with the occurrence of ED during treatment persisting more than 3 months after discontinuation [3]. Follow-up was assessed through telephone interviews and by administering the Arizona Sexual Experience Scale (ASEX) questionnaire, which investigates five domains of sexuality: desire, arousal, erectile function, ability to achieve orgasm and orgasmic satisfaction.

The average duration of sexual side effects after withdrawal was 40 months. In 20% of cases, symptoms were still present after 6 years. 94% of the patients complained of ED, 92% of hypoactive sexual desire and 69% of ejaculatory disturbances.

Among the non-sexual symptoms, asthenia was reported in 27%, cognitive difficulties in 26%, depression in 20% and anxiety in 20% [4].

In addition to DS, other symptoms such as altered seminal parameters and volume (11%), shaft deformities (19%), reduced spontaneous erections (9%), reduced testicular volume and soreness (15%) and impaired cognitive ability and depression (17%) were persistent.

Another study by Irwig et al. [5, 6] investigated depressive symptoms and suicidal thoughts in former finasteride users who developed persistent sexual side effects despite discontinuation of finasteride.

Between 2010 and 2011, standardised interviews were administered to former finasteride users ($n = 61$) with persistent sexual side effects. Demographic information, medical and psychiatric histories and information on drug use, sexual function and alcohol consumption were collected. All former users were healthy men without underlying sexual dysfunction, chronic medical conditions, current or past psychiatric conditions or use of oral prescription drugs before or during finasteride use [7].

A control group of men ($n = 29$), recruited from the community, had male pattern hair loss but had never used finasteride and denied any history of psychiatric conditions or psychiatric drug use. The primary outcomes were the prevalence of depressive symptoms and the prevalence of suicidal thoughts as determined by the Beck Depression Inventory II (BDI-II); all subjects self-administered this questionnaire at the time of the interview and up to 10 months later.

Results: Rates of depressive symptoms (BDI-II score $\geq$ 14) were significantly higher in former finasteride users (75%; 46/61) compared with the control group (10%; 3/29) ($P < 0.0001$). Moderate or severe depressive symptoms (BDI-II score $\geq$20) were present in 64% (39/61) of patients taking finasteride and 0% in the control group. Suicidal thoughts were present in 44% (27/61) of former finasteride users and in 3% (1/29) of the control group ($P < 0.0001$).

Conclusion

Scientific literature has shown that metabolic syndrome (MS) plays an important role in the development and progression of benign prostatic hypertrophy (BPH). Among the factors of metabolic syndrome, dyslipidaemia (i.e. low HDL levels and hypertriglyceridemia) is the major risk factor. In particular, dyslipidaemia induces severe prostatic inflammation, which is considered to be the main pathogenetic mechanism for the development and progression of BPH. Therefore, in this perspective both the use of MS drugs and the improvement of lifestyle could play an important role in preventing and/or slowing down the development of the disease. Additionally, the clinical diagnostic procedure could benefit from sexological counselling to make the patient and partner co-responsible for the pharmacological consequences of the therapy by highlighting the limitations and redesigning a sexuality that is nonetheless effective for a better quality of life.

References

1. Gur S, Kadowitz PJ, Hellstrom WJ. Effects of 5-alpha reductase inhibitors on erectile function, sexual desire and ejaculation. Expert Opin Drug Saf. 2013;12:81–90.
2. Traish AM, Hassani J, Guay AT, et al. Negative side effects of 5α-reductase inhibitor therapy: persistent decreased libido and erectile dysfunction and depression in a subset of patients. J Sex Med. 2011;8:872–84.
3. Irwig MS, Kolukula S. Persistent sexual side effects of finasteride for male pattern hair loss. J Sex Med. 2011;8:1747–53.
4. Irwig MS. Persistent sexual side effects of finasteride: could they be permanent? J Sex Med. 2012;9:2927–32.
5. Pinsky MR, Gur S, Tracey AJ, et al. The effects of chronic 5-alpha-reductase inhibitor (dutasteride) treatment on rat erectile function. J Sex Med. 2011;8:3066–74.
6. Irwig MS. Depressive symptoms and suicidal thoughts among former users of finasteride with persistent sexual side effects. J Clin Psychiatry. 2012;73(9):1220–3. https://doi.org/10.4088/JCP.12m07887. Epub 2012 Aug 7. PMID: 22939118.
7. Pizzocaro A, Motta G, Negri L, et al. Post-finasteride syndrome: between myth and reality. Endocrinologist. 2014;15:112–7.

Interstitial Cystitis/Bladder Pain Syndrome

Carmen Maccagnano, Rodolfo Hurle, and Elena Vittoria Longhi

Introduction

Painful bladder syndrome or interstitial cystitis/bladder pain syndrome (IC/BPS) is a chronic debilitating disease, defined by a variable combination of symptoms during micturition and sexual intercourse.

Women are more affected than men by a factor of 5:1 to 10:1 [1, 2].

The most involved ethnicity is Caucasian (superior to 90%), and it manifests itself around an average of 30 years of age [3–6].

The average latency between the manifestation of symptoms to the diagnosis of IC/BPS is about five years (range: 1 month–30 years), and the disease usually progressively gets worse with time [7–11].

The prevalence ranges between 0.5 and 17%, according to both the employed definition and the diagnostic criteria, with a range between 0.5 and 17% [2, 12, 13].

The underlying mechanism of IC/BPS has not been identified yet; the possible causes include chronic systemic inflammation, subclinical infections, urothelial dysfunction, immunological disorders, genetics, and alterations in central pain processing.

Because of the lack of a definite cause, the treatment options are different but no one has a complete efficacy.

C. Maccagnano (✉)
Urotechnology Center, Scientific Institute "Istituto Auxologico Italiano", Milan, Italy

R. Hurle
Department of Urology, Humanitas Research Hospital IRCCS, Rozzano, MI, Italy
e-mail: rodolfo.hurle@humanitas.it

E. V. Longhi
Department of Sexual Medical Center, San Raffaele Hospital, Milano, Italy

© Springer Nature Switzerland AG 2023
E. V. Longhi (ed.), *Managing Psychosexual Consequences in Chronic Diseases*,
https://doi.org/10.1007/978-3-031-31307-3_40

Table 1 Symptoms of IC/BPS

Urinary symptoms	Sexual symptoms	Pain
Urgency	Dyspareunia	Pelvic pain
Frequency		Perineal pain
Nocturia		Irradiation to – Groin – Testicle – Sacrum – Vagina/vulva
Pain relieving after micturition		

Main Medical Characteristics

Patients (pts) usually reported a variable combination of the symptoms reported in Table 1.

Main Tools for the Diagnosis

The definition of the syndrome varies around the world and according to the different Scientific Societies, lacking clear diagnostic criteria and being based primarily on expert opinion. It is important to note that BPS is a diagnosis of exclusion [14–16].

Firstly, the common tools for the entire world are reported below.

History

It should include the following:

1. Pain characteristics:

    (a) Symptom location (suprapubic, perineal, eventual irradiations).
    (b) Symptom descriptors (pain, pressure, or discomfort).
    (c) Exacerbating factors (increases with increasing bladder content, relieved by voiding, and aggravated by food or drink).

    It is important to note that up to 30% may not initially manifest pain [17–20].
2. Any triggers (such as dietary factors) associated with LUTS (see Table 2).

    A variable percentage from 30% to 90% of pts report that certain foods trigger symptoms. This could be due to the passage of irritating solutes across a disrupted urothelium [20, 21]. In this scenario, another important role can be played by neuronal "cross-talk" between the gastrointestinal (GI) and the urinary tract by which inflammation and irritation of the GI tract may lead to urinary

Table 2 Food that gets worse the symptoms in IC/BPS

Acid foods
Citrus fruits and juices
Tomatoes
Vinegar
Pickled foods
Fermented foods
Spicy foods
Vitamin C
Artificial sweeteners
Coffee (also decaffeinated)
Carbonated beverages
Alcohol

tract pain [22, 23]. Finally, some authors have identified a peripheral or central neuronal upregulation that may interact with diet and trigger symptoms [24, 25]. The relationship of pain with menstruation should be analyzed.

3. Any symptoms related to the other pelvic organs. The highest rates of comorbidity are associated with fibromyalgia, chronic fatigue, and irritable bowel syndrome (IBS).

   In addition to those associations, IC/BPS has also been found to be associated with the temporal–mandibular joint disorder, endometriosis, migraines, asthma, inflammatory bowel disease, and systemic lupus erythematosus [26, 27]. There is a high overlap of IC/BPS with IBS and increasing evidence of similar overlapping with upper GI disorders, including functional disorders and gastro-esophageal reflux disease [28–31].

4. A detailed description of urinary symptoms, with particular attention to voiding volumes and frequency; therefore, the use of a frequency volume chart is recommended for the initial evaluation [15].

5. Any previous pelvic operations, previous urinary tract infections (UTIs), previous pelvic radiation treatment, and auto-immune diseases.

6. The use of a validated symptom and quality-of-life scoring instrument is recommended for initial assessment and follow-up, and the O'Leary–Sant Interstitial Cystitis Symptom and Problem Index (ICSI/ICPI) is highlighted by most guidelines [15].

Physical Examination

It should include the following:

1. Physical examination of the abdomen, pelvis, genitalia, and prostate in men, with specific attention paid to areas of tenderness.

2. Neurological and musculoskeletal examination, including pelvic floor muscle examination for tenderness and trigger points.

Laboratory Examination

1. Urine dipstick and urine culture should be performed to exclude UTIs, and culture for tuberculosis, Ureaplasma, and Chlamydia should be included if sterile pyuria is present [15].
2. Urine cytology should be tested, especially in pts who are at high risk of urothelial malignancy.
3. PSA in males >40 years.

Cystoscopy/Hydrodistention /Bladder Biopsy

Cystoscopy has to be performed as part of the initial evaluation so as to exclude other underlying pathologies that may mimic IC/BPS [10, 15]. The association with hydrodistention (HD) has the aim to identify Hunner's lesions, which are localized, reddened mucosal areas with small vessels radiating toward a central scar, with a fibrin deposit or coagulum attached to this area. This site ruptures with increasing bladder distension, with petechial oozing of blood from the lesion and the mucosal margins in a waterfall manner. The presence of Hunner's lesions has been associated with more severe symptoms and smaller bladder capacity, and their identification may help to lead to treatment strategies [32, 33].

Bladder biopsy is not approved by all guidelines, and this examination is usually considered optional and excludes other pathologies.

Pelvic Imaging

The role of pelvic imaging (ultrasound with the evaluation of post- voiding volume, computed tomography, and magnetic resonance) is only to exclude other conditions, if clinically suspected [15].

Urodynamics

Uroflowmetry has to be performed in all pts, because it is a simple examination that can give important information about the urinary flow, in both females and males.

Urodynamics is considered an optional test that should only be performed for pts with a complicated history that suggests the possibility of alternative diagnoses (e.g., voiding dysfunction, bladder obstruction, overactive bladder, and stress urinary incontinence).

The diagnostic criteria have changed over the years, but no consensus has been reached among the most relevant Scientific Societies (Table 3).

We also have reported the differential diagnosis and test to be considered in the diagnostic workup in Table 4.

Table 3 Diagnostic criteria and IC/BPS definition according to Scientific Societies

Organization	Reference	Definition	Duration
ESSIC European Society for the Study of Interstitial Cystitis	van de Merwe [31]	Chronic pelvic pain, pressure, or discomfort perceived to be related to the urinary bladder, accompanied by at least one other urinary symptom like the persistent urge to void or frequency. Confusable diseases as the cause of the symptoms must be excluded	6 months
AUA American Urological Association CUA Canadian Urological Association	Hanno [26] and Cox [28]	An unpleasant sensation (pain, pressure, discomfort) perceived to be related to the urinary bladder, associated with lower urinary tract symptoms, in the absence of infection or other identifiable causes	6 weeks
ICS International Continence Society	Abrams [34]	PBS: pelvic pain related to bladder filling "accompanied by other symptoms such as increased daytime and night-time frequency, in the absence of proven urinary infection or other obvious pathology" IC: if histological findings or cystoscopic features	No duration
NIDDK National Institute of Diabetes and Digestive and Kidney Diseases	Gillenwater [35]	(a) Glomerulations or "Hunner's ulcers" on cystoscopic examination (b) Pain associated with either filling of the urinary bladder or urinary urgency (c) Not meet extensive exclusion criteria from cystometry, treatment response, other diagnoses	9 months

Table 4 Differential diagnosis and test to be considered in the diagnostic workup

Bladder-related	Test to consider
Cancer	Cystoscopy Urinary cytology
Stones	Ultrasound
Urethral diverticula	Urodynamics, Pelvic MR
Iatrogenic	Test to consider
Radiation-induced cystitis	Cystoscopy Urinary cytology
Drug-induced cystitis	Cystoscopy Urinary cytology
Infections	Test to consider
Acute	Urine analysis Urine culture
Recurrent	Urine analysis Urine culture
Gynecological	Test to consider
Endometriosis	Pelvic examination Pelvic MR Laparoscopy
Vulvodynia	Pelvic examination
Cervical, uterine, or ovarian cancer	Pelvic examination Pelvic ultrasound

Table 5 Lines of therapy in IC/BPS

Medical	
First	Diet Behavioral changes Reduction in psychological stress Pelvic floor training
Second	Physical therapy Oral medications
Surgical	
Third	Bladder intravesical therapy Cystoscopy with HD under anesthesia and fulguration of Hunner's lesions
Fourth	BoNT/A Neuromodulation
Fifth	Urinary diversion

Treatment

It is important to explain to pts that, unfortunately, there is no curative treatment, but symptoms can be managed to improve quality of life, also considering a strong placebo effect and encouraging realistic expectations for pts themselves [10, 15, 36]

The principles of the management of these pts are as follows:

1. Target interventions to the patient's specific symptoms
2. Focus on maximizing function, not completely resolving symptoms
3. Considering starting multiple treatments simultaneously in case of severe symptoms
4. Stopping ineffective treatments after a reasonable therapeutic trial [9, 10, 37]

Treatment should start at more conservative levels and then advance as necessary toward more invasive options and often concomitant treatment. The lines of therapy are resumed in Table 5.

Main Nonsurgical Treatment

Behavioral Changes

Behavioral factors that worsen IC/BPS symptoms are extremely personal, but their variability includes stress, constrictive clothes, sexual intercourse, and intake of some particular foods, as indicated before in the text.

Pts can be encouraged to cut out these potential noxious stimuli food one at a time and assess if avoidance of certain food and behaviors improves symptoms [36, 38].

Pelvic Floor Exercises

A pelvic examination can reveal hypertonic pelvic floor muscles; in this context, physical therapy should be recommended for most pts because it is often very effective in terms of improving symptoms, increasing latency between voids, and increasing void volumes [39–45].

Additionally, therapy with an expert in myofascial trigger point release, connective tissue release, and muscle coordination training can lead to symptom improvement in over 50% of pts and has shown significant improvement compared to sham therapy in one randomized controlled trial with the contribution of highly trained therapists [43–45].

Reduction in Psychological Stress

Stress can then have a vicious cycle effect and worsen IC/BPS symptoms and further decrease the quality of life [38].

Self-care and stress reduction can improve symptoms and improve pts' sense of control in their treatment strategy [28, 46, 47].

Acupuncture

Most studies remain poor in quality or power, and more research is needed. However, because acupuncture is safe and relatively inexpensive, it is recommended as an option [9, 10, 37]. One study reported a greater than 50% reduction in pelvic pain in both males and females in 11 of 14 pts treated with up to 8 weeks of acupuncture therapy twice a week [46].

Oral Medications

Oral medications are considered second-line therapies. These are variably recommended by the different guidelines. For details, see Table 6.

Long-term oral antibiotics and systemic steroids are not recommended [9, 10].

Table 6 Standard dosages for commonly used treatments for BPS/IC

Medication	Mechanism of action	Dosage	Side effects
Hydroxyzine	H1-histamine receptor antagonist Block of mast cell activation	10–50 mg at bedtime	• Sedation
Amitriptyline	Tricyclic antidepressant that suppresses the reuptake of serotonin and noradrenalin at presynaptic nerve ends and the anticholinergic reaction of the central nervous system and peripheral nerves, which in turn leads to sedation due to an antihistamine reaction in the central nervous system	25–75 mg at bedtime (initiate at 10 mg and titrate weekly)	• Dry mouths • Constipation • Sedation • Weight gain • Blurred vision • Nausea
Gabapentin	Gabapentin is a structural analog of γ-aminobutyric acid It has been effectively used in various chronic pain treatments and is especially good for treating neuropathic pains	300–2100 mg divided 3 times a day	• Abnormal eye movements • Clumsiness or unsteadiness • Constipation • Diarrhea • Difficulty speaking • Drowsiness or tiredness • Dry mouth • Nausea
Cimetidine	H2-histamine receptor antagonist Block of mast cell activation	400 mg bid	• Drowsiness • Dry mouth
Pentosan polysulfate	Reinforcement of GAG layers and reduction in urothelial permeability		• Nausea • Vomiting • Diarrhea • Headache • Reversible alopecia

Intravesical Therapies

Intravesical therapies, which require referral to a specialist, consist of a direct introduction of pharmacological treatment into the bladder via a catheter with the aim of replenishing the defective GAG layer in BPH and/or relief pain [9, 10, 15]. They have to be considered in those pts with severe symptoms who do not improve with less invasive treatments. The most common intravesical therapies are dimethyl sulfoxide, lidocaine, heparin, and chondroitin sulfate, alone or in combination. Most have limited data on effectiveness and provide relief for only a short period of time [48]. Monthly maintenance therapy for those who respond is recommended [9, 10]. Dimethyl sulfoxide (the only FDA-approved intravesical treatment) is typically instilled weekly for 6 weeks. The most common side effect is pain [48, 49].

Main Surgical Treatment

Cystoscopy with Hydrodistention

Cystoscopy with HD and eventually mucosal fulguration of Hunner's lesions (under anesthetic) have to be considered as a third-line option, with up to 80% cure rate, but with more associated risks including bladder rupture [6, 50–53]. However, relief of symptoms from HD therapy has been shown to decline over the time scale of months, with a wide variation in efficacy thought to be partly due to many different practices for HD itself [3–6]. Almost half of the pts will require retreatment within the timeframe of 2–5 years [7, 8].

Botulinum Toxin A Detrusor Injection

Intradetrusor botulinum toxin A (BoNT/A) is considered as the fourth line of treatment.

BoNT/A is a neuro toxic protein that can be injected intravesically into the detrusor muscles and has been shown to lead to an improvement in IC/BPS symptoms through flaccid paralysis of the detrusor [9, 10]. Observational studies and randomized prospective studies of this off-label use have also supported a high response rate to BoNT/A among IC/BPS pts, but long-term data are lacking, and pts need to be open to performing self-catheterization if they have initial urinary retention [11–13].

Sacral Neuromodulation

This approach showed effectiveness in some refractory cases in multiple prospective, nonrandomized studies [14–16].

Nevertheless, neuromodulation should be limited to pts with significant symptom burden who have failed multiple conservative treatment options, due to the high cost and absence of results from randomized studies.

Radical Surgical Treatments

Radical surgical treatments include diversion with or without cystectomy and substitution cystoplasty. Very few pts will ever progress to this level of treatment, but small studies suggest that this can relieve pts of irritating voiding symptoms and particularly may be useful for those with a fixed small bladder capacity. Unfortunately, some pts will continue to report pain symptoms persisting even after these radical procedures [39, 50].

Appendix

Pain control, both pharmacological and non-pharmacological, should be part of the treatment plan and managed like other chronic pain conditions, including urinary analgesics, nonsteroidal anti-inflammatory drugs, non-opioid medications, and opioid analgesia. A comprehensive program may be needed to adequately manage pain [7, 50].

Patient enrollment in research trials should be considered at any point in the treatment process [7, 8]. The Multidisciplinary Approach to the Study of Chronic Pelvic Pain Research Network is one resource (https://www.niddk.nih.gov/news/archive/2016/multidisciplinary-approach-study-chronic-pelvic-pain).

Sexuality and Quality of Life

IC/BPS is a bladder disorder, which remains largely unrecognized. It affects more women than men, and its etiology remains unclear. No pathognomonic test for IC/BPS is available. It is common for treatment to become less and less effective over time and for symptoms to reappear after a few months. Furthermore, it is difficult to determine whether an improvement is caused by medication or simply by spontaneous remission. A number of aggravating factors have been described that are likely to precipitate pain due to IC. They include stress, sexual intercourse, tight clothing, exercise, and certain foods such as acidic beverages, coffee, spices, alcohol, soda, tea, and chocolate. At the sensory level, investigating the pain aspect, in addition to the five senses (sight, hearing, touch, taste, and smell) clinical studies have tracked: the exteroceptive function (cutaneous, musculoskeletal, visceral), which includes sensitivity to touch, pressure, and vibration (mechanoreception), thermal sensitivity (thermoception), and sensitivity to noxious stimuli [54, 55].

The presence of urinary burning sensations is most often the result of a local inflammation caused by microbial or other factors. Due to their frequency, isolated UTIs are largely the predominant cause, but rarer causes should not, however, be excluded [56, 57].

From these early references, it is widely recognized in the literature that IC/BPS is a debilitating disease characterized by urgency, frequency, and pelvic pain [58, 59]. Sexual dysfunction in female pts with IC/BPS consists of dyspareunia, altered sexual desire, disturbance of arousal and orgasm, and insufficient lubrication that adversely affects pts' quality of life.

IC/BPS often manifests as "classic" cystitis: burning sensation, pain in the lower abdomen, need to urinate frequently and urgently (up to 60 times throughout the day and night), and vaginal pain, which precludes the sexual act. The entire urogenital area is involved. Pelvic floor and acute pain cannot be treated well with common analgesics. IC/BPS is a multifactorial syndrome that combines stressful events, psychological symptoms, and urinary system disorders. Be that as it may, the literature agrees on a multidisciplinary approach: urological, gynecological, physical rehabilitative, and psychotherapeutic [60].

However, this pathology often coexists with other clinical conditions, such as follows:

Chronic fatigue syndrome
Fibromyalgia
Irritable bowel syndrome
Sjögren's syndrome
Chronic headache
Depression and anxiety, vulvodynia [61]

Related symptoms correspond to different phenotypes of IC/BPS, as demonstrated by the National Research Network MAPP phenotyping initiative, supported by the National Institute of Diabetes and Digestive and Kidney Disease (NIDDK), one of the National Institutes of Health [62].

The literature indicates that approximately 5% of pts diagnosed with IC/BPS present with symptoms persisting for more than 2 years, characterized by a poorly elastic bladder with poor continence and the presence of severe pain.

It appears that the mean age of onset of the condition is older in Europe than in the United States, due to the different diagnostic criteria used. Pts initially report a single symptom, such as dysuria, frequent micturition, and pain, with a possible subsequent multi-symptomatic picture. The onset with a well- defined symptomatology is not infrequent and symptoms tend to progressively intensify for several hours, days, or weeks [63]. The scientific literature has often described the painful symptomatic course of these pts as "silent suffering," because they suffer relentless pain associated with frequent micturition and nocturia [64]. This is followed by sleep disturbances (due to persistent pain and nocturia), chronic fatigue, and depression.

Perceived pain is highly variable; it may be suprapubic and similar to a sense of heaviness or discomfort related to bladder filling, which improves with emptying; other pts experience **urinary painful dysesthesia** that radiates from the pelvis to the urethra, vulva, vagina, and rectum, or may affect the extra-genital area such as the lower abdomen or back.

It also seems that the perception of pain is more intense in female pts than in men.

It is therefore understandable that the quality of life and sexuality of pts are greatly compromised by the impact of this pathology [65]. Moreover, **the impact on QoL is severe**, and comparable to that of other pathologies such as rheumatoid arthritis or end-stage renal insufficiency, and is worse than that of endometriosis.

Regarding the **impact on sexuality** and interpersonal relationships, a study conducted by the Interstitial Cystitis Association (ICA) found that at least **90% of affected pts are unable to have complete sexual intercourse** with their partners [62]. Also, from the female point of view, the percentage affects 85% of pts with IC (due to pelvic, vestibular, vaginal pain, and **vulvodynia**).

Besides increased conflict, the partners of the pts report difficulties in the couple's relationship due to impatience, aggressiveness, and emotional distance caused by the symptoms of the disease.

The situation is no different for men. Pts complain of erectile dysfunction, hypoactive desire, anhedonia, and fatigue during attempts at sexual performance, which they describe as "impossible" and useless. A sort of reluctance is caused by the destructive aspect of the symptoms and the intolerant fatigue of the caregivers.

Anticipatory anxieties about possible further pain during penetration make pts freeze from the stage of foreplay, conditioning arousal, and the already poor vaginal lubrication. The therapies for depression and generalized anxiety disorder contribute to lower the threshold level of passion in the couple and increasing the level of individual isolation [66].

Conclusion

The management of IC/BPS could evolve with an improved understanding of this condition, which involves both central and peripheral contributors. It is fundamental to employ multimodal therapies early on, following a thorough evaluation of all potential contributing factors, especially given the nature of pelvic cross-organ sensitization. The consideration remains that the relational and sexual symptomatic consequences imply a severe limitation of the pts' QoL in every context: social, personal, professional, sexual, affective, and interpersonal. Communication in a team with several multidisciplinary specialists can have, even from this point of view, a role of welcome, encouragement, and empathy, stimulating pts not to make the pathology the only project of life. The psychosexologist in this case could also contribute to the maintenance of compliance with the multi-therapeutic plan of the patient and caregiver.

References

1. Jhang J-F, Kuo H-C. Patho-mechanism of interstitial cystitis/bladder pain syndrome and mapping the heterogeneity of disease. Int Neurourol J. 2016;20(Suppl 2):S95–104.
2. Huffmann M, Slak A, Hoke M. Bladder pain syndrome. Prim Care. 2019;46(2):213–21.
3. Koziol JA. Epidemiology of interstitial cystitis. Urol Clin North Am. 1994;21(1):7–20.
4. Huffman MM, Slack A, Hoke M. Bladder pain syndrome. Prim Care. 2019;46(2):213–21.
5. Chaiken DC, Blaivas JG, Blaivas ST. Behavioral therapy for the treatment of refractory interstitial cystitis. J Urol. 1993;149(06):1445–8.

6. Christofi N, Hextall A. An evidence-based approach to lifestyle interventions in urogynaecology. Menopause Int. 2007;13(04):154–8.
7. Parsons CL, Koprowski PF. Interstitial cystitis: successful management by increasing urinary voiding intervals. Urology. 1991;37(03):207–12.
8. FitzGerald MP, Payne CK, Lukacz ES, et al. Randomized multicenter clinical trial of myofascial physical therapy in women with interstitial cystitis/painful bladder syndrome and pelvic floor tenderness. J Urol. 2012;187(6):2113–8.
9. Moldwin RM, Fariello JY. Myofascial trigger points of the pelvic floor: associations with urological pain syndromes and treatment strategies including injection therapy. Curr Urol Rep. 2013;14(5):409–17.
10. Weiss JM. Pelvic floor myofascial trigger points: manual therapy for interstitial cystitis and the urgency-frequency syndrome. J Urol. 2001;166(06):2226–31.
11. Whitmore KE. Self-care regimens for patients with interstitial cystitis. Urol Clin North Am. 1994;21(01):121–30.
12. Webster DC, Brennan T. Use and effectiveness of physical self- care strategies for interstitial cystitis. Nurse Pract. 1994;19(10):55–61.
13. Lee S-H, Lee B-C. Use of acupuncture as a treatment method for chronic prostatitis/chronic pelvic pain syndromes. Curr Urol Rep. 2011;12(4):288–96.
14. Colaco MA, Evans RJ. Current recommendations for bladder instillation therapy in the treatment of interstitial cystitis/bladder pain syndrome. Curr Urol Rep. 2013;14(5):442–7.
15. Dyer AJ, Twiss CO. Painful bladder syndrome: an update and review of current management strategies. Curr Urol Rep. 2014;15(2):384.
16. Marcu I, Campian EC, Tu FF. Interstitial cystitis/bladder pain syndrome. Semin Reprod Med. 2018;36:123–35.
17. Ahmad I, Sarath KN, Meddings RN. Sequential hydrodistention and intravesical instillation of hyaluronic acid under general anaesthesia for treatment of refractory interstitial cystitis: a pilot study. Int Urogynecol J Pelvic Floor Dysfunct. 2008;19(4):543–6.
18. Platte RO, Parekh M, Minassian VA, Poplawsky D. Spontaneous bladder rupture following cystoscopy with hydrodistention and biopsy in a female patient with interstitial cystitis. Female Pelvic Med Reconstr Surg. 2011;17(3):149–52.
19. Jhang J-F, Kuo H-C. Patho-mechanism of interstitial cystitis/bladder pain syndrome and mapping the heterogeneity of disease. Int Neurourol J. 2016;20(2):95–104.
20. Cervigni M, Nasta L, Schievano C, Lampropoulou N, Ostardo E. Micronized palmitoylethanolamide-polydatin reduces the painful symptomatology in patients with interstitial cystitis/bladder pain syndrome. Biomed Res Int. 2019;2019:9828397.
21. Sant GR. Etiology, pathogenesis, and diagnosis of interstitial cystitis. Rev Urol. 2002;4(1):9–15.
22. Grover S, Srivastava A, Lee R, et al. Role of inflammation in bladder function and interstitial cystitis. Ther Adv Urol. 2011;3(1):19–33.
23. Davis NF, Brady CM, Creagh T. Interstitial cystitis/painful bladder syndrome: epidemiology, pathophysiology and evidence-based treatment options. Eur J Obstet Gynecol Reprod Biol. 2014;175:30–7.
24. McLennan MT. Interstitial cystitis: epidemiology, pathophysiology, and clinical presentation. Obstet Gynecol Clin N Am. 2014;41(3):385–95.
25. Davis NF, Gnanappiragasam S, Thornhill JA. Interstitial cystitis/painful bladder syndrome: the influence of modern diagnostic criteria on epidemiology and on Internet search activity by the public. Transl Androl Urol. 2015;4(5):506–51.
26. Hanno PM, Burks DA, Clemens JQ, et al. AUA guideline for the diagnosis and treatment of interstitial cystitis/bladder pain syndrome. J Urol. 2014;185(6):2162–70.
27. Cox A, Golda N, Nadeau G, et al. CUA guideline: diagnosis and treatment of interstitial cystitis/bladder pain syndrome. Can Urol Assoc J. 2016;10(5–6):E136.
28. Berry SH, Elliott MN, Suttorp M, et al. Prevalence of symptoms of bladder pain syndrome/interstitial cystitis among adult females in the United States. J Urol. 2011;186(2):540–4.
29. Jones CA, Nyberg L. Epidemiology of interstitial cystitis. Urology. 1997;49(5):2–9.

30. Clemens JQ, Link CL, Eggers PW, Kusek JW, Nyberg LM Jr, McKinlay JB, BACH Survey Investigators. Prevalence of painful bladder symptoms and effect on quality of life in black, hispanic and white men and women. J Urol. 2007;177(4):1390–4.
31. van de Merwe JP, Nordling J, Bouchelouche P, et al. Diagnostic criteria, classification, and nomenclature for painful bladder syndrome/interstitial cystitis: an ESSIC proposal. Eur Urol. 2008;53(1):60–7.
32. Malde S, Palmisani S, Al-Kaisy A, Sahai A. Guideline of guidelines: bladder pain syndrome. BJU Int. 2018;122(5):729–43.
33. Warren JW, Brown J, Tracy JK, Langenberg P, Wesselmann U, Greenberg P. Evidence-based criteria for pain of interstitial cystitis/painful bladder syndrome in women. Urology. 2008;71:444–8.
34. Abrams P, Baranowski A, Berger RE, Fall M, Hanno P, Wesselmann U. A new classification is needed for pelvic pain syndromes–are existing terminologies of spurious diagnostic authority bad for patients? J Urol. 2006;175(6):1989–90.
35. Gillenwater JY, Wein AJ. Summary of the National Institute of Arthritis, Diabetes, Digestive and Kidney Diseases Workshop on Interstitial Cystitis, National Institute of Health, Bethesda, Maryland, August 28-29, 1987. Urology. 1988;140(1):203–6.
36. Driscoll A, Teichman JM. How do patients with interstitial cystitis present? J Urol. 2001;166:2118–20.
37. Ito T, Ueda T, Homma Y, Takei M. Recent trends in patient characteristics and therapeutic choices for interstitial cystitis: analysis of 282 Japanese patients. Int J Urol. 2007;14:1068–70.
38. Parsons CL. Interstitial cystitis: epidemiology and clinical presentation. Clin Obstet Gynecol. 2002;45(1):242–9.
39. Parsons CL, Bullen M, Kahn BS, Stanford EJ, Willems JJ. Gynecologic presentation of interstitial cystitis as detected by intravesical potassium sensitivity. Obstet Gynecol. 2001;98(1):127–32.
40. Shorter B, Lesser M, Moldwin RM, Kushner L. Effect of comestibles on symptoms of interstitial cystitis. J Urol. 2007;178(1):145–52.
41. Rudick CN, Chen MC, Mongiu AK, Klumpp DJ. Organ cross talk modulates pelvic pain. Am J Physiol Regul Integr Comp Physiol. 2007;293(3):R1191–8.
42. Christianson JA, Liang R, Ustinova EE, Davis BM, Fraser MO, Pezzone MA. Convergence of bladder and colon sensory innervation occurs at the primary afferent level. Pain. 2007;128(3):235–43.
43. Friedlander JI, Shorter B, Moldwin RM. Diet and its role in interstitial cystitis/bladder pain syndrome (IC/BPS) and comorbid conditions. BJU Int. 2012;109(11):1584–91.
44. Herati AS, Shorter B, Srinivasan AK, et al. Effects of foods and beverages on the symptoms of chronic prostatitis/chronic pelvic pain syndrome. Urology. 2013;82(6):1376–80.
45. Alagiri M, Chottiner S, Ratner V, Slade D, Hanno PM. Interstitial cystitis: unexplained associations with other chronic disease and pain syndromes. Urology. 1997;49(5):52–7.
46. Rodríguez MAB, Afari N, Buchwald DS, National Institute of Diabetes and Digestive and Kidney Diseases Working Group on Urological Chronic Pelvic Pain. Evidence for overlap between urological and nonurological unexplained clinical conditions. J Urol. 2009;182(5):2123–31.
47. Nickel JC, Tripp DA, Pontari M, et al. Psychosocial phenotyping in women with interstitial cystitis/painful bladder syndrome: a case control study. J Urol. 2010;183(1):167–72.
48. Birder LA, Hanna-Mitchell AT, Mayer E, Buffington CA. Cystitis, co-morbid disorders and associated epithelial dysfunction. Neurourol Urodyn. 2011;30(5):668–72.
49. Nastaskin I, Mehdikhani E, Conklin J, Park S, Pimentel M. Studying the overlap between IBS and GERD: a systematic review of the literature. Dig Dis Sci. 2006;51(12):2113–20.
50. Messing E, Pauk D, Shaeffer A, et al. Associations among cystoscopic findings and symptoms and physical examination findings in women enrolled in the Interstitial Cystitis Data Base (ICDB) Study. Urology. 1997;49(5):81–5.

51. Lamale LM, Lutgendorf SK, Hoffman AN, Kreder KJ. Symptoms and cystoscopic findings in patients with untreated interstitial cystitis. Urology. 2006;67:242–5.
52. Bosch PC. Examination of the significant placebo effect in the treatment of interstitial cystitis/bladder pain syndrome. Urology. 2014;84(2):321–6.
53. Rapkin AJ, Kames LD. The pain management approach to chronic pelvic pain. J Reprod Med. 1987;32(5):323–7.
54. Kosek E, Hansonn P. Modulatory influence on the perception of vibration and thus heterosensory conditioning (HNCS) in patients with fibromyalgia and health subjects. Ache. 1997;70(1):41–51.
55. Julien N, Goffaux P, Arsenault P, Marchand S. Diffuse pain in fibromyalgia is related to a deficiency in endogenous pain inhibition. Ache. 2005;114(1-2):295–302.
56. Freemason P. Medullary circuits for nociceptive modulation. Curr Opin Neurobiol. 2012;22(4):640–5.
57. Plaghki L, Mouraux A, Le Bars D. Pain physiology. EMC Rehabil Med. 2018;25(1):1–22.
58. Chiu B, Tai HC, Chung SD, Birder LA. Botulinum toxin A for bladder pain syndrome/interstitial cystitis. Toxins. 2016;8:201.
59. Bogart LM, Suttorp MJ, Elliott MN, Clemens JQ, Berry SH. Prevalence and correlations of sexual dysfunction among women with bladder pain syndrome/interstitial cystitis. Urology. 2011;77:576–80.
60. Puliatti M, Fiacchi S, Silipigni F. Psychological aspects and psychotherapy of women with interstitial cystitis. Cognitive-behavioral therapy and EMDR: an integrated approach [Psychological aspects and psychotherapy of women with interstitial cystitis]. Cognitive-behavioral therapy and EMDR: an integrated approach. Psychosom Med. 2007;52(3):101–3.
61. Clauw DJ, Schmidt M, Radulovic D, et al. The relationship between fibromyalgia and interstitial cystitis. J Psychiatr Res. 1997;31:125–31.
62. Sutcliffe S, Colditz GA, Pakpahan R, et al. Changes in symptoms during urologic chronic pelvic pain syndrome symptom flares: findings from one site of the MAPP Research Network. Neurourol Urodyn. 2013;34(2):188–95.
63. Davisa NF, Bradyb CM, Creagha T. Interstitial cystitis/painful bladder syndrome: epidemiology, pathophysiology and evidence based treatment options. Eur J Obstet Gynecol Reprod Biol. 2014;175C:30–7.
64. Persu C, Cauni V, Gutue S, et al. From interstitial cystitis to chronic pelvic pain. J Med Life. 2010;3:167–74.
65. Berry SH, Hayes RD, Suttorp M, et al. Health-related quality of life impact of interstitial cystitis/painful bladder syndrome and other symptomatic disorders. Qual Life Res. 2013;22:1537–41.
66. Vesela R, Aronsson P, Andersson M, et al. The potential of non-adrenergic, non-cholinergic targets in the treatment of interstitial cystitis/painful bladder syndrome. J Physiol Pharmacol. 2012;63:209–16.

Chronic Prostatitis

Omidreza Sedigh and Elena Vittoria Longhi

Introduction to Chronic Disease

The term "chronic prostatitis" in everyday practice defines a symptomatic prostatic disease that continues for a long time (at least 3–6 months). A wide spectrum of signs and symptoms due to the inflammation of the gland can be observed.

Over the last few years, many classifications and definitions have been proposed.

The last classification of prostatitis and chronic pelvic pain syndrome distinguished five different types of prostatitis according to symptoms, laboratory, and histological findings (Table 1) [1].

Table 1 classification of prostatitis and chronic pelvic pain syndrome

NIH classification	Definition
Category I Acute bacterial prostatitis	Acute infection of the prostate gland
Category II Chronic bacterial prostatitis	Recurrent infection of the prostate gland
Category IIIA Inflammatory CPPS	White blood cells in semen/EPS/voided bladder urine 3 (VB3 or post-prostatic drainage)
Category IIIB Non-inflammatory CPPS	No white blood cells in semen/EPS/VB3
Category IV Asymptomatic inflammatory prostatitis	• Abnormal semen analysis • Elevated PSA values • Incidental findings in prostate biopsy

NIDDK NIH classification of prostatitis, *CPPS* chronic pelvic pain syndrome

O. Sedigh (✉)
Reconstructive Urology and Andrology of Humanitas, Gradenigo, Turin, Italy

E. V. Longhi
Department of Sexual Medical Center, San Raffaele Hospital, Milano, Italy

© Springer Nature Switzerland AG 2023
E. V. Longhi (ed.), *Managing Psychosexual Consequences in Chronic Diseases*,
https://doi.org/10.1007/978-3-031-31307-3_41

According to this classification, categories II and III (IIIA-B) can be included in the heterogeneous group of "chronic prostatitis."

Main Medical Characteristics

The main difference between the two categories is the isolation of bacteria in the microbiological tests only in type II prostatitis, whereas pathogens are never found in type III [2].

Clinical manifestations are due to a persistent infection in type II prostatitis, while persisting inflammation without infection is the basis of the other type.

Type III is split into two subcategories according to the presence of white blood cells (WBCs) in the semen; in type IIIB, WBC is not found but inflammation is carried out by other paths.

Symptoms usually last more the three months and can be similar between the two groups [1]. Patients complain a classical manifestation of "urinary tract infection symptoms like": frequent micturition, burning and feeling of incomplete voiding. Besides these, a wide broad of atypical symptoms can be reported. Pain in the perineal area, in the rectum, in the low back, in the gonads, and during ejaculation is usually the most annoying presentation. Pelvic floor muscles and sexual dysfunction, anxiety, depression, and other psychological disorders usually appear progressively with a deep impact on the quality of life [3, 4].

Validated questionnaires are available (e.g., NIH-CPSI) to assess all these symptoms and to check the response to therapies [5].

The cause of bacterial prostatitis is identified in a persisting infection, whereas a clear cause lacks in CPPS [1]. The etiological mechanisms of CPPS are complex and still not clear. Many pathological paths have been described and probably different factors are always involved. Initial triggers (one or more) lead to the activation of self-maintaining inflammation and pain, which finally involves many organs and systems spreading in the multiform manifestations. Central and peripheral nervous systems are certainly involved in the abnormal response of the nociception system [6]. Local tissue modifications of histology, immunological milieu, and neurotransmitter receptors result in the amplification of the peripheral stimulus and central pain perception [7].

Main Tools for the Diagnosis

A history of symptoms, with a special focus on onset evolution, is crucial to get the diagnosis. Organic disorders like cancer and anatomical or neurological syndrome that may mimic chronic prostatitis need to be ruled.

The presence of bacteria differentiates type II and type III prostatitis, and its investigation is the most important diagnostic step. Pathogens are usually not found in a simple mid-stream urine sample. Analysis of segmented urine and prostatic secretion by the Meares–Stamey test is really effective to distinguish type II and type III. Semen analysis can be considered as well [8].

The physical examination can confirm the clinical suspect and rule out other diseases. There are no specific prostatic findings. Pain may be evoked in various trigger points (prostate, rectum, pudendal nerve, etc.).

To define which symptoms are prevalent is crucial to tailor the proper therapy or consultations. Various questionnaires (IPSS, NIH-CPSI, etc.) are available to quantify the amount of symptoms and to follow patients and their response to therapies [5]. Imaging has a minimal role in the diagnostic workout, and it is useful to rule out other organic problems.

Main Nonsurgical Treatments

Considering how heterogeneous the causes are, a wide spectrum of therapies is possible. Monotherapies are usually not indicated, and patients require a multimodal and multidisciplinary approach to manage causes and symptoms. Pharmacological and physical therapies are available. Treatments are partially different for types II and III [1].

Pharmacological Therapies

Since infection is the background of chronic bacterial prostatitis, antibiotics are the first- line therapy. Long- term targeted therapies are always recommended when an antibiogram is available. Fluoroquinolones penetrate relatively well the prostate and are the empiric therapy of choice. Standard administration should last for about 4 weeks. Quinolone resistance is progressively increasing, and other antibiotics (e.g., cotrimoxazole) have to be considered in many cases. In case of recurrent CBP, each episode can be treated with antibiotics or long-term antibiotic prophylaxis can be administrated for a duration of at least 6 months [9]. Due to the wide multifactorial genesis of CPPS, mono-therapy is usually not enough to achieve symptom relief. The therapeutic approach should focus on the different symptomatic patterns in a multimodal setting, tailoring the therapy to every specific case.

Initial infection is probably the "primum movens" of chronic inflammation. Long- term antibiotics are usually given also in this group, with heterogeneous results.

Since the early 2000s, immunological mechanisms responsible for chronic inflammation in chronic prostatitis have been clearly shown. Thus, medications able to interrupt this molecular mechanism can have a primary therapeutic role. Nonsteroidal anti-inflammatory drugs (NSAIDs) induce a favorable effect on prostatic inflammation by reducing prostaglandin synthesis. For this reason, patients with dominantly pain-related symptoms may be given NSAIDs with a great improvement of symptoms improving total symptoms, pain, and QoL. Some herbal medicines act in a similar manner with negligible side effects also for long- term use [10].

Neuromodulating medications have a widespread indication in the treatment of neuropathic pain, which is probably due to a persisting activation of sensitive terminations. The proposal of analgesic neuromodulation comes from some studies concerning the effects of a neuromodulatory drug, pregabalin, in increasing dosages over 6 weeks of treatment, reducing pain- related symptoms. However, patients did not report symptom resolution but mostly a modest improvement in pain symptoms. These medications should only be prescribed as a second-line treatment [11].

Alpha-adrenergic blockers have been widely tested and used, showing moderate beneficial effects, especially in patients with obstructive symptoms. Many other medications were and are under investigation (5 alpha-reductase inhibitors, muscle relaxants, anticholinergic drugs, intra-prostatic injection of botulinum toxin A, etc.); they can be used with heterogeneous results but cannot be recommended as standard therapies so far.

Psychological symptoms may benefit from specific drugs and non- pharmacological therapies. Tricyclic antidepressants (e.g., amitriptyline) and selective serotonin reuptake inhibitors are largely used with good efficacy [12].

Non-Pharmacological Therapies

Prostatic, perineal, or pelvic floor massage and myofascial trigger point release have been proposed with good results as a beneficial treatment modality for patients complaining of perineal soreness and difficulty in bladder/rectal evacuation. Referring patients to a specific physiotherapist is strongly recommended.

Other physical interventions include electromagnetic therapy, microwave thermo-therapy, extracorporeal shockwave therapy, acupuncture, and posterior tibial nerve stimulation/transcutaneous electrical nerve stimulation (TENS). All these treatments proved to be effective in some patients with specific symptoms. They cannot be proposed for all cases but they should be included in single specific tailored settings [12].

Main Surgical Treatments

Surgical treatment is not considered a standard in the treatment of chronic prostatitis. EAU guidelines do not suggest surgery (e.g., TURP, simple prostatectomy, and radical prostatectomy) as a viable option. Small sample studies exploring the role of TURP and radical prostatectomy in this specific setting were analyzed by a systematic review in 2017. The curative rate ranged from 70 to 95%, but reliable conclusions cannot be carried out due to the very low level of evidence and the lack of randomized trials [13]. In conclusion, surgery should not be considered a standard option in the armamentarium for the treatment of chronic prostatitis. Patients may be informed about this option underlining its "experimental setting" as a last resort [1].

Sexuality and Quality of Life

The focus of a study conducted by Dominique Delavierre et al. [14] was to learn about the habits of French urologists in the diagnostic and therapeutic management of chronic prostatitis. In June 2003, 810 urologists, members of the French Association of Urology and practicing in France, received by mail a questionnaire on the diagnosis and therapy of chronic prostatitis.

One hundred and twenty-four (15%) responded, and 61% diagnosed less than 11 new cases of chronic prostatitis per year. Sixty-five percent were not aware of the then- new classification proposed in the USA in 1995 by the NIH (National Institutes of Health), aimed at removing this pathology from the rigid picture of prostate, refocusing on the notion of pain, and introducing the notion of chronic pelvic pain syndrome in men. While 83% had often or always performed microbiological testing, only 10% had often or always performed a Meares and Stamey test involving the analysis of prostate secretions after massage. Some 68% had never done so. On the other hand, 76% had performed an ECB of the 1st urinary stream, 61% of the 2nd stream, and 76% a semen culture. Antibiotics were prescribed often or always by 73% (82% using fluoroquinolones and 43% using the trimethoprim-sulfamethoxazole combination). Even in the absence of microbiological evidence of infection, 41% often or always prescribed antibiotics, 89% sometimes or often prescribed alpha-blockers, 89% sometimes, often, or always prescribed nonsteroidal anti-inflammatory drugs, 81% sometimes, often, or always prescribed analgesics, and 52% sometimes or often prescribed anxiolytics. Sixty-six percent sometimes or often sought advice from other specialists.

Chronic pelvic-perineal pain appears to be disabling and unacknowledged. It reflects injuries that are sometimes obvious and often unrecognized. Understanding it, and therefore treating it, requires knowledge of its pathophysiology. Its particular location and unique innervation often lead to different and often puzzling presentations. The specialties involved should be numerous (urology, gastroenterology, psychology, algology, gynecology, and rheumatology) in order to improve understanding of the pathology and patient motivation during treatment [15].

The main problems of chronic prostatitis regarding male sexuality include the following:

1. Premature ejaculation.
2. Painful and difficult ejaculation.
3. Erectile dysfunction due to the patient's anxious-depressive state.

4. Low sexual frequency, relationship difficulties in the couple, intolerance of the partner, obsessiveness in the mechanical verification of erection by the patient with autoeroticism.
5. Possible decline in fertility.
6. Chemico-physical modifications of the prostatic secretion with alterations in the coagulation and subsequent liquefaction of sperm and modifications in both the number and mobility of spermatozoa.
7. Obstruction of the various ejaculatory ducts due to the succession of various histological changes caused by the inflammatory process.
8. The production of auto-antibodies with the immune release of sperm antigens.
9. The occurrence of an inflammatory and infectious process with a consequent inhibiting action on the mobility of spermatozoa caused by the germs themselves and by the infectious process.
10. Possible inflammatory involvement of the epididymis (scrotal pain).

Regarding Difficulties with Ejaculation

The inflammatory process of the prostate gland occurs in both acute and chronic prostatitis, but also in urethritis (inflammation of the urethra) or vesiculitis (inflammation of the seminal vesicles).

The pain appears at the time of or immediately after ejaculation and may last for hours or even a few days; hemospermia (blood in the seminal fluid) may also be associated.

The discomfort and pain are localized to the perineum—inguinal region—testicles—suprapubic region.

Retrograde ejaculation may occur: caused by the closure of the bladder neck with rhythmic contractions of the pelvic floor muscles and consequent release of the external striated sphincter.

Partner discomfort often appears to be the male motivation (in addition to pain) for a uro-andrological consultation. Stress about partner demotivation is often one of the reasons for failure to perform even after symptoms have remitted.

In particular, painful ejaculation [16] is a pelvic–perineal pain triggered by ejaculation or orgasm. Its prevalence is between 1 and 4% of the general population. Particularly localized to the penis, the pain most often lasts less than 5 minutes. Benign prostatic hypertrophy, chronic pelvic pain syndrome, radical prostatectomy, prostate brachytherapy, and some antidepressant treatments are the best -documented etiologies of painful ejaculation to be found in the literature. The link between painful ejaculation and urogenital infections is likely but has not been clearly established and evaluated.

A very detailed study [17] explored the hypothesis of a link between chronic inflammation of the prostate and the development of prostate cancer among black men by examining sexual activity, sexually transmitted diseases, and prostatitis in a population-based study of 129 patients and a control group of 703 aged 40–79 years. After examining the group of patients (black and white) with chronic prostatitis and following adjustment for age, income, cigarette smoking, and history of digital rectal examination and prostate-specific antigen testing in the previous 5 years, it was observed that a history of gonorrhea infection and prostatitis increased the odds of prostate cancer 1.78- fold (95 % CI: 1.13, 2.79) and 4.93- fold (95 % CI: 2.79, 8.74), respectively. Men who reported 25 or more sexual partners were 2.80 (95 % CI: 1.29, 6.09) times more likely to be diagnosed with cancer than men with five or fewer partners. The highest proportion of neoplastic risk was found among black men.

Chronic prostatitis is also a common condition in Africa.

The descriptive cross-sectional study by Banza et al. [18] evaluated 25 patients with documented acute prostatitis treated at Lubumbashi University Clinics over a four-year period from 2015 to 2018. Data were collected through a survey form based on different study parameters divided into three categories, namely epidemiological data including age, study period and residence, clinical data with subjective signs, objective signs, general status, and rectal examination findings and paramedical data divided into laboratory and imaging tests.

Results: Acute prostatitis associated with non-cancerous prostate accounted for 1.27% of all surgical diseases and 7.66% in urology. The most affected age group was 19–37 years (64% of cases), and the mean age was 33.16 ± 2.4 years. Seventeen patients (68%) were followed up in the outpatient clinic and eight (32%) in the hospital. Clinically, fever above 38.5 °C was found in 15 patients (60%), dysuria in 11 patients (44%), acute urinary retention in three patients (12%), burning during urination in eight patients (32%), pain syndrome in 21 patients (84%), and painful prostate on rectal examination in 18 patients (72%).

In the final analysis, chronic prostatitis is caused by an infection in 5–10% of cases, and other entities are called "chronic pelvic pain syndrome." Current classifications are based on the presence or absence of inflammation or infection in prostatic secretions. The new clinical phenotype concept "UPOINT" offers seven domains:

1. Urinary
2. Psychosocial
3. Organ-specific
4. Infectious
5. Neurological
6. Systemic
7. Related to muscle tension

The therapeutic approach is based on the first use of antibiotics with or without alpha-blockers. The role of psychological and sexological support remains essential.

The patient in these cases discusses virility, sexual role, the guilt of not gratifying the partner, physical and sexual inadequacy, and reluctance to experience drug therapy as a source of well-being.

Finally, an Italian study by Bartoletti et al. [19] assessed the risk factors of chronic prostatitis, enrolling 5540 patients from 28 Italian urological centers, with subjects being between 25 and 50 years of age with symptoms of chronic prostatitis/ chronic pelvic pain syndrome. Results: Of 5540 male urological outpatients, 764 with chronic prostatitis/chronic pelvic pain syndrome were enrolled, of whom 225

(29.4%) presented for the first time and 539 (70.6%) had received prior treatment. The prevalence of the syndrome was thus 13.8%, while the estimated incidence was 4.5%.

Cigarette smoking, a high-calorie diet with low fruit and vegetable intake, constipation, meteorism, slow digestion, a sexual relationship with more than one partner, and coitus interruptus were more likely in patients with chronic prostatitis/chronic pelvic pain syndrome than in controls (each $p < 0.001$). The syndrome had a negative influence with regard to sexual desire, erectile dysfunction, and premature ejaculation ($p < 0.001$). The Meares and Stamey test was positive in 13.3% of patients and 2.9% of controls.

Other evidence comes from the Finnish study by Mehik et al. [20], which conducted a population-based cross-sectional survey in the two northernmost provinces of Finland (Oulu and Lapland). A total of 2500 male residents aged 20–59 years were randomly selected to complete a questionnaire on prostatitis. Responses were received from 1832 men, with a response rate of 75%.

The overall lifetime prevalence of prostatitis was 14.2%. The risk of having or having had prostatitis increased with age, being 1.7 times greater in men aged 40–49 than in those aged 20–39 and 3.1 times greater in those aged 50–59. The overall incidence was 37.8/10,000 person-years.

More than a quarter of the 261 men who had or had had symptoms of prostatitis (27%) suffered from it at least once a year, while 16% suffered from persistent symptoms; 63% of men with prostatitis had the worst symptoms during the winter (November–March). Neither education nor profession had much influence on the occurrence of prostatitis, but divorced and single men had a lower risk than married men. Most patients felt that they had not received enough information about the disease on their first visit to a general practitioner.

Conclusion

There is no doubt that chronic prostatitis appears to be a very recurrent pathology and a painful one. Each patient experiences a state of exasperation with regard to the symptomatology and hypersensitive sensations in the urogenital area, even in the remission or latency phase. Sexual dysfunctions and mood disorders, although less severe, continue to affect intimacy and couple relationships while also limiting single patients in social relationships and in spontaneously experiencing intimate encounters for fear of failure. The psychosexologist, in addition to medication, could give these patients a new way of approaching sexuality, soothe pain or discomfort during intimate relations, and lower the level of anxiety and frustration due to a compromised and often painful body. Sexual exercises are in fact an excellent tool, in addition to counseling, to relearn the timing and mode of the response of physicality. Regaining confidence in their body and self-learning the responses of the body map would allow patients to educate their partners to a more spontaneous and satisfying intimacy.

References

1. EAU guidelines on Urological infections 2019.
2. Zhang J, Liang C, Shang X, Li H. Chronic prostatitis/chronic pelvic pain syndrome: a disease or symptom? Current perspectives on diagnosis, treatment, and prognosis. Am J Mens Health. 2020;14(1):1557988320903200.
3. North CS, Hong BA, Lai HH, Alpers DH. Assessing somatization in urologic chronic pelvic pain syndrome. BMC Urol. 2019;19(1):130.
4. Fitzgerald MP, Link CL, Litman HJ, Travison TG, McKinlay JB. Beyond the lower urinary tract: the association of urologic and sexual symptoms with common illnesses. Eur Urol. 2007;52:407.
5. Litwin MS, McNaughton-Collins M, Fowler FJ, Nickel JC, Calhpun EA, Pontari MA, Alexander RB, Farrar JT, O'Leary MP. The National Institutes of Health chronic prostatitis symptom index: development and validation of a new outcome measure. Chronic Prostatitis Collaborative Research Network. J Urol. 1999;162:369.
6. McMahon SB, Dmitrieva N, Koltzenburg M. Visceral pain. Br J Anaesth. 1995;75:132.
7. Kutcha J, Yania MS, Asavasoponb S, Kiragesa DJ, et al. Altered resting state neuromotor connectivity in men with chronic prostatitis/chronic pelvic pain syndrome: a MAPP: Research Network Neuroimaging Study. Neuroimage Clin. 2015;8:493.
8. Meares EM, Stamey TA. Bacteriologic localization patterns in bacterial prostatitis and urethritis. Investig Urol. 1968;5:492.
9. Magri V, Montanari E, Marras E, Perletti G. Aminoglycoside antibiotics for NIH category II chronic bacterial prostatitis: a single-cohort study with one-year follow-up. Exp Ther Med. 2016;12(4):2585–93. https://doi.org/10.3892/etm.2016.3631.
10. Franco JV, Turk T, Jung JH, et al. Non-pharmacological interventions for treating chronic prostatitis/chronic pelvic pain syndrome. Cochrane Database Syst Rev. 2018;5(5):CD012551. https://doi.org/10.1002/14651858.CD012551.pub3.
11. Yang CC. Neuromodulation in male chronic pelvic pain syndrome: rationale and practice. World J Urol. 2013;31(4):767–72. https://doi.org/10.1007/s00345-013-1066-7. Epub 2013 Apr 26.
12. Pirola GM, Verdacchi T, Rosadi S, Annino F, De Angelis M. Chronic prostatitis: current treatment options. Res Rep Urol. 2019;11:165–74. https://doi.org/10.2147/RRU.S194679.
13. Sjhoeb DS, Schlager D, Booker M, Watterauer U, et al. Surgical therapy of prostatitis: a systematic review. World J Urol. 2017;35:1659–68.
14. Delavierre D. Prostatite chronique et syndrome douloureux pelvien chronique de l'homme. Enquête auprès des urologues français. Prog Urol. 2007;17(1):69–76.
15. Riant T. Comprendre les douleurs pelvi-périnéales chroniques en 2021. Douleurs. 2021;22(2):75–93.
16. Delavierre D, Sibert L, Rigaud J, Labat J-J. L'éjaculation douloureuse. Prog Urol. 2014;24(7):414–20.
17. Sarma AV, McLaughlin JC, Wallner LP, Dunn RL, Cooney KA, Schottenfeld D, Montie JE, Wei JT. Sexual behavior, sexually transmitted diseases and prostatitis: the risk of prostate cancer in black men. J Urol. 2006;176(3):1108–13.
18. Banza MI, Kasanga TK, Mukakala AK, et al. Acute prostatitis associated with non-cancerous prostate at the Lubumbashi University Clinics: epidemiological and therapeutic characteristics. Pan-Afr Med J. 2020;37:290.
19. Bartoletti R, Cai T, Mondaini N, et al. Prevalence, incidence estimation, risk factors and characterization of chronic prostatitis/chronic pelvic pain syndrome in urological hospital outpatient clinics in Italy: results of a multicenter case-control observational study. Diary Urol. 2007;178(6):2411–5.
20. Mehik A, Hellström P, Lukkarinen O, Sarpola A, Järvelin M. Epidemiology of prostatitis in Finnish men: a population-based cross-sectional study. Int BJU. 2000;86(4):443–8.

Appendix

Those interested in clinical research can access these questionnaires, broken down by topic and found in the relevant chapters.

1. Psychological impact of chronic coronary artery disease—**Revised Dyadic Adjustment Scale**
2. Psychological impact of chronic valvular heart disease—*STAI X-1 di Spielberger STAI X-1 di Spielberger*
3. Alzheimer's disease: diagnosis and therapy—*Caregiver Burden Inventory (CBI) (Novak M. e Guest C., Gerontologist, 29, 798–803, 1989)*
4. Rheumatoid arthritis, osteoarthritis: diagnosis and treatment—**Health Assessment Questionnaire (HAQ)** (Salaffi F, Carotti M, Cervini C. Health Assessment Questionnaire: the Italian version of a tool for assessing the quality of life in patient with rheumatoid arthritis. Adria Med 1997;19:5–11)
5. Coeliac disease in children and young adult
   Questionnaire for assessing adherence to the gluten-free diet (The questionnaire "Assessment of dietary compliance in celiac children using a standardized dietary interview" Wessels et al.—DOI: 10.1016/j.clnu.2017.04.010)
6. Periodontal disease—*Review of the Main Sexual Tests Used National and Worldwide:*

   - **ANDROTEST** Corona G., Mannucci E., Petrone L., Balercia G., Fisher dC., Chiarini V., Forti G., Maggi M., 2006. Breve intervista strutt
   - **ASEX** (Arizona Sexual Experience Scale) McGahuey C.A., Gelenberg A.J., Laukes C.A., Moreno F.A., Delgado P.L., McKnight K.M., Manber R., 2000
   - **ASKAS** (Aging Sexuality Knowledge and Attitudes Scale) White, 1982. Il questionario per la conos
   - **BISF-W** (Brief Index of Sexual Functioning for Women) Taylor, Rosen & Leiblum, 1994
   - **BSFI-W** (Brief Sexual Function Inventory) JE Taylor; Rosen RC; Leiblum SR., 2004

© Springer Nature Switzerland AG 2023
E. V. Longhi (ed.), *Managing Psychosexual Consequences in Chronic Diseases*,
https://doi.org/10.1007/978-3-031-31307-3

- **EDITS** (Erectile Dysfunction Inventory of Treatment Satisfaction) Althof SE et Corty EW, 1998
- **FSFI** (Female Sexual Function Index) Rosen R et al., 2000
- **HSAS** (Hendrick Sexual Attitude Scale) Hendrick S. et Hendrick C., 1987
- **IIEF** (International Index of Erectile Function) Rosen RC, Riley A., G. Wagner, Osterhol IH, J. Kirkpatrick, Mishra A., 1997
- **IPE** (Index of Premature Ejaculation) Althof S. et al., 2006
- **ISS** (Index of Sexual Satisfaction) Hudson W.W., Corcoran K., Fischer J., 2000
- **MFSQ** (McCoy Questionnaire of Female Sexuality) McCoy N., Matyas J., 1996
- **MSI-R** (Marital Satisfaction Inventory) Douglas K. Snyder, Ph.D., 1997
- **SAI-2** (Sexual Addiction Inventory) Avenia F., 2004
- **SBI** (Sexual Behavior Inventory) Bentler P.M., 1968
- **SESII-W** (Sexual Excitation/Sexual Inhibition Inventory for Women) Cynthia A. Graham, Stephanie A. Sanders, Robin R. Milhausen, 2005
- **SSS-W** (Sexual satisfaction scale and discomfort in women) Meston CM, Trapnell P., 2005
- **TSS** (patient and partner Treatment Satisfaction Score) M. Kubin, E. Trudeau, K. Gondek, E. Seignobos, AR Fugl-Meyer, 2004

7. **HIV**—*The WHOQOL-HIV has been developed from an extensive test of 115 questions, plus the WHOQOL-100 in 10 centres around the world. These questions represent the finalised version of the WHOQOL-HIV to be used for field trials.*
8. **Osteoarthritis**—*HAQ II (Health Assessment Questionnaire II) and HAQ-Questionnaire*
9. **Premature ovarian failure**—*SF-36*
10. **Chronic Migraine**—*MIDAS Questionnaire*
11. Type 1 and type 2 diabetes mellitus: differences, diagnosis, and treatments—*Parent Report for Children (ages 8–12 Years) and Hypoglycemia Fear Survey II Questionnaire*
12. **Eating disorders**—*EPSI*
13. **Cancers of the female genital tract**   *FACT—version 4*
14. **Male Sexual Pain and Chronic Prostatitis**—*NIH-Chronic Prostatitis Symptom Index (NIH-CPSI)*
15. **Down Syndrome**—*The Adaptive Behaviour Dementia Questionnaire (ABDQ)*
16. **Endometriosis and Fertility**—*CDC HRQOL -14*
17. **Benign Prostatic Hypertrophy** *BECK II and BDI-II*
18. **Interstitial Cystitis/Bladder Pain Syndrome**—*Pelvic Pain and Urgency/ Frequency Patient Symptom Scale (PUF Scale)*
19. Hashimoto Thyroiditis—*european health questionnaire (EQ-5D)*
20. **The Chronic Thyroid Diseases**—*Ryff's Psychological Well-Being Scales (PWB); ThyDQoL Questionnaire*
21. *HYPOGONADISM—Medical Outcomes Study Questionnaire Short Form 36 Health Survey (SF-36)*

22. **Psoriasis in adolescents and adults**—*Psoriasis Area and Severity Index (PASI) Worksheet*
23. **Main Medical Characteristics of Osteoporosis**—*Quality of Life Questionnaire* **(Qualeffo-41)**
24. **Parkinson**—*Montgomery Depression Rating Scale (MADRS)*
25. **Persistent Depressive Disorder (Dysthymia) and Recurrent Unipolar Major Depressive Disorder**—*SSS "Sexual Satisfaction Scale" (1975) M.P. Whitley, S.B. Poulsen—University of Washington School of Nursing*
26. **Vascular and Degenerative Retinal Disease**—*National Eye Institute Visual Functioning Questionnaire 25 (VFQ-25 version 2000)*
27. **Crohn's Disease**—*Crohn's disease activity index (CDAI)—State-Trait Anxiety for Adults STAI form Y-1 and Y-2*
28. **Osteoarthritis**—*The Western Ontario and Mcmaster Universities Osteoarthritis Index (WOMAC)*
29. **Multiple Sclerosis**—*SF 36 Questionnaire*
30. **Prostate cancer and radiotherapy**—*EPIC Questionnaire (The Saskatchewan Prostate Assessment Pathway has been developed to support patients and their families in the diagnosis and treatment of prostate cancer.)*
31. **Male Infertility**—*DASS 21*
32. **Klinefelter**—*Self-Assessment Manikin (SAM) (Margaret M. Bradley, Peter J. Lang, Measuring emotion: The self-assessment manikin and the semantic differential, Journal of Behavior Therapy and Experimental Psychiatry, 25, Issue 1,1994, 49–59)*

MIX
Papier aus verantwortungsvollen Quellen
Paper from responsible sources
FSC® C105338

If you have any concerns about our products,
you can contact us on
ProductSafety@springernature.com

In case Publisher is established outside the EU,
the EU authorized representative is:
Springer Nature Customer Service Center GmbH
Europaplatz 3, 69115 Heidelberg, Germany

Printed by Libri Plureos GmbH
in Hamburg, Germany